Comprehensive
POSTANESTHESIA CARE

Comprehensive
POSTANESTHESIA CARE

Edited by

Morris Brown, M.D.
Professor of Anesthesiology
Wayne State University School of Medicine
Chairman, Department of Anesthesiology
Sinai Hospital of Detroit
Detroit, Michigan

Eli M. Brown, M.D.
Professor and Chairman
Department of Anesthesiology
Wayne State University School of Medicine
Detroit, Michigan

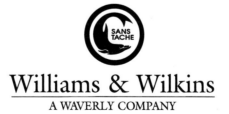

Williams & Wilkins
A WAVERLY COMPANY

BALTIMORE • PHILADELPHIA • LONDON • PARIS • BANGKOK
BUENOS AIRES • HONG KONG • MUNICH • SYDNEY • TOKYO • WROCLAW

Editor: Carroll C. Cann
Managing Editor: Tanya Lazar
Production Coordinator: Peter J. Carley
Book Project Editor: Robert D. Magee
Illustration Planner: Peter J. Carley
Cover Designer: Karen Klinedinst
Typesetter: Port City Press, Inc.
Printer: Port City Press, Inc.
Digitized Illustrations: Port City Press, Inc.
Binder: Port City Press, Inc.

351 West Camden Street
Baltimore, Maryland 21201-2436 USA

Rose Tree Corporate Center
1400 North Providence Road
Building II, Suite 5025
Media, Pennsylvania 19063-2043 USA

Accurate indications, adverse reactions and dosage schedules for drugs are provided in this book, but it is possible that they may change. The reader is urged to review the package information data of the manufacturers of the medications mentioned.

Printed in the United States of America.

First Edition.

Library of Congress Cataloging-in-Publication Data

Comprehensive postanesthesia care / edited by Morris Brown, Eli M.
    Brown.
        p.   cm.
    Includes bibliographical references and index.
    ISBN 0-683-01116-2
    1. Postoperative care.   2. Post anesthesia nursing.   3. Recovery rooms.
  I. Brown, Morris.   II. Brown, Eli M.
    [DNLM: 1. Postanesthesia Nursing—methods.   2. Anesthesia
  Recovery Period.   3. Postoperative Care.   4. Anesthesia Department, Hospi-
  tal—organization & administration.   WY 154 C737 1997]
  RD51.C56   1997
  617'.919—dc20
  DNLM/DLC
  for Library of Congress   96-14627
                                                                   CIP

The publishers have made every effort to trace the copyright holders for borrowed material. If they have inadvertently overlooked any, they will be pleased to make the necessary arrangements at the first opportunity.

To purchase additional copies of this book, call our customer service department at **(800) 638-0672** or fax orders to **(800) 447-8438**. For other book services, including chapter reprints and large quantity sales, ask for the Special Sales department.

Canadian customers should call **(800) 268-4178**, or fax **(905) 470-6780**. For all other calls originating outside of the United States, please call **(410) 528-4223** or fax us at **(410) 528-8550**.

Visit Williams & Wilkins on the Internet: **http://www.wwilkins.com** or contact our customer service department at **custserv@wwilkins.com**. Williams & Wilkins customer service representatives are available from 8:30 am to 6:00 pm. EST. Monday through Friday, for telephone access.

96 97 98 99
1 2 3 4 5 6 7 8 9 10

Dedication

To Estelle, wife and mother, for her constant encouragement and to Rhonda, Erica, and Jeremy for being who they are.

Preface

The care of patients after anesthesia and surgery can be the most challenging time of the perioperative period. Recent advances in technique, the advent of new pharmacologic agents, and a greater understanding of physiologic mechanisms have dramatically changed postoperative care. Indeed, with advances in anesthetic and surgical techniques, more acutely and chronically ill patients, once considered too sick for surgical intervention, are encountered daily in the operating suite. It is, therefore, incumbent on all personnel who care for patients postoperatively to be knowledgeable about anticipated normal postoperative changes and the complications that may develop during recovery from anesthesia and surgery. Certainly, as the patient population has become more complex and the clinical problems more diverse, practitioners and trainees require a better understanding of problems which can occur in the postoperative period and how to manage them. This text is intended to serve as a reference for all who care for patients in the postoperative period. We have selected authors from a wide variety of practice backgrounds to provide a comprehensive approach to the care of postoperative patients. Because the 35 authors represent 20 institutions, the text is intended to provide the scientific information to form the basis of practice rather than description of local practice pattern.

This book is divided into 3 sections. The first section provides a general overview of the development of postanesthesia care units, equipment, and monitoring requirements in the PACU, and general clinical considerations. The second section provides a description of the physiology, pathophysiology, and management of the patient in the postoperative period by organ system. We have chosen this approach rather than surgery-specific considerations because technology and advances in medical management have resulted in elimination of some surgical procedures and development of new ones. It is our belief that an understanding of underlying physiology by organ system will be more valuable than description of current practice by procedure. The final section, provides a review of the administrative structure, physical design, and continuing quality improvement program for postanesthesia care units. Hopefully, this format will provide ready reference material for all who care for patients in the postoperative period.

We wish to express our deepest appreciation for the efforts of Marilyn Robinson, for her time, energy, and effort in the preparation of the manuscript without, which this book would not be possible.

Contributors

Arnold J. Berry, M.D.

Professor of Anesthesiology
Emory University School of Medicine
Atlanta, Georgia

Eli M. Brown, M.D.

Professor and Chairman, Department of
   Anesthesiology
Wayne State University School of Medicine,
Detroit, Michigan

Morris Brown, M.D.

Professor of Anesthesiology, Wayne State University
   School of Medicine
Chairman, Department of Anesthesiology, Sinai
   Hospital of Detroit
Detroit, Michigan

O.W. Brown, M.D., J.D.

Clinical Assistant Professor, Wayne State University
   School of Medicine
Chief, Section of Vascular Surgery, Sinai Hospital
Detroit, Michigan

Gregory Crosby, M.D.

Evan P. and Marion Helfaer Professor Chairman
Department of Anesthesiology
University of Wisconsin
Madison, Wisconsin

Krishnaprasad Deepika, M.D.

Associate Professor of Clinical Anesthesiology,
Department of Anesthesiology, University of Miami
   School of Medicine
Miami, Florida

Stephen F. Dierdorf, M.D.

Professor of Anesthesia, Indiana University School
   of Medicine
Indianapolis, Indiana

John H. Eichhorn, M.D.

Professor and Chairman, Department of
   Anesthesiology
University of Mississippi School of Medicine and
   Medical Center
Jackson, Mississippi

Thomas W. Feeley, M.D.

Professor of Anesthesia, Stanford University School
   of Medicine
Associate Director of Intensive Care Units, Stanford
   University Medical Center
Stanford, California

Andrew Gettinger, M.D.

Associate Professor of Anesthesiology, Dartmouth
   Medical School Director, Critical Care Medicine
   Dartmouth-Hitchcock Medical Center
Lebanon, New Hampshire

Steven C. Hall, M.D.

Arthur C. King Professor of Pediatric Anesthesia
Anesthesiologist-in-Chief, Children's Memorial
   Hospital
Professor of Anesthesia, Northwestern University
   Medical Center
Chicago, Illinois

Charles B. Hickok, M.D.

Assistant Professor of Anesthesiology
Co-Director Ambulatory Anesthesia
The George Washington University Medical Center
District of Columbia

Susan W. Krechel, M.D.

Associate Professor of Anesthesiology
University of Missouri—Columbia
Columbia, Missouri

Mali Mathru, M.D.

Professor of Anesthesiology
University of Texas Medical Branch
Galveston, Texas

Roger S. Mecca, M.D.

Clinical Assistant Professor, Department of
   Anesthesiology
Yale University School of Medicine
New Haven, Connecticut
Chairman, Department of Anesthesiology
Danbury Hospital
Danbury, Connecticut

Geraldine Mitchell, R.N., B.S.N., M.S.

Director of the Operating Room
Henry Ford Health System
Detroit, Michigan

John R. Moyers, M.D.

Professor
Department of Anesthesia
University of Iowa College of Medicine
Iowa City, Iowa

Michael F. Mulroy, M.D.

Staff Anesthesiologist
Department of Anesthesiology
Virginia Mason Clinic
Seattle, Washington

Gary Okum, M.D.

Assistant Professor of Anesthesiology
MCP/Hahnemann University
Philadelphia, Pennsylvania

Brian D. Owens, M.D.

Staff Anesthesiologist,
Department of Anesthesiology
Virginia Mason Medical Center
Seattle, Washington

Tanya Oyos, M.D.

Assistant Professor
Department of Anesthesia
The University of Iowa
Iowa City, Iowa

Charise T. Petrovitch, M.D.

Chairperson and Director
Department of Anesthesia
Providence Hospital
District of Columbia

Donald S. Prough, M.D.

Professor and Chair,
Department of Anesthesiology
The University of Texas Medical Branch
Galveston, Texas

Athos J. Rassias, M.D.

Assistant Professor of Anesthesiology, Dartmouth
Medical School
Anesthesiologist/Intensivist, Dartmouth-Hitchcock
Medical Center
Lebanon, New Hampshire

Henry Rosenberg, M.D.

Professor and Chairman,
Department of Anesthesiology
MCP/Hahnemann University,
Philadelphia, Pennsylvania

Martin J. Serrins, M.D.

Assistant Clinical Professor
Yale University School of Medicine,
New Haven, Connecticut
Medical Director, Inpatient Operating Room
Danbury Hospital,
Danbury, Connecticut

Stephen V. Sharnick, M.D.

Medical Director, Ambulatory Surgical Unit
Danbury Hospital
Danbury, Connecticut

Karen S. Sibert, M.D.

Assistant Professor of Anesthesiology
Chief, General Services Division, Department of
Anesthesiology
Duke University Medical Center
Durham, North Carolina

Robert N. Sladen, M.B., MRCP(UK), FRCP(C)

Associate Professor of Anesthesiology and Surgery
Vice-Chairman, Department of Anesthesiology
Co-Director, Surgical Intensive Care Unit
Duke University Medical Center
Durham, North Carolina

Stephen A. Vitkun, M.D.

Associate Professor of Clinical Anesthesiology and
Medicine
(Pulmonary/Critical Care)
University at Stony Brook
Stony Brook, New York

Herbert D. Weintraub, M.D.

Professor of Anesthesiology
Interim Chairman, Department of Anesthesiology
George Washington University Hospital
District of Columbia

Contents

III. ADMINISTRATIVE CONSIDERATIONS

I
General Considerations

1

DEVELOPMENT OF POSTANESTHESIA CARE UNITS

Morris Brown

HISTORICAL PERSPECTIVE

The immediate postoperative care of patients after anesthesia and surgery is an essential part of the perioperative period. It has long been recognized that a specialized area is necessary in proximity to operating theaters to observe patients after surgical interventions (1). However, it was not until the 1920s that a formal postanesthesia care unit (PACU) was established in the United States (2). Shortly thereafter, it became apparent to the medical community that the establishment of a PACU was necessary to provide the level of care required for patients during the immediate postoperative period. By the 1940s, PACUs were opened in several states in this country and in Europe. By World War II, PACUs became common in the United States (3).

The critical importance of the PACU was established in 1947, when the Anesthesia Study Commission of the Philadelphia County Medical Society reported a highly significant outcome study in which there was a reduction in postoperative morbidity and mortality in patients who had been provided with specialized postanesthesia care within an established PACU (4). By 1949, the Operating Room Committee for New York Hospital categorically stated, "An adequate recovery room service is a necessity to any hospital undertaking modern surgical therapy" (5). As more complex surgical procedures were performed on more severely ill patients, the

PACU served as the site not only for the routine recovery of commonly performed surgical procedures but also as the facility for the postoperative care of critically ill patients. Indeed, the PACU was the forerunner of the present day intensive care unit (2). Even today, many of the same principles in caring for critically ill patients are applicable in the PACU. Clearly, the PACU must provide a setting for patients to be closely monitored after the physiologic trespass caused by anesthesia and surgery to allow prompt recognition and early intervention of any problems. Nonetheless, the primary goal of the PACU remains to monitor and treat the postoperative patient while recovery from anesthesia and surgery is safely accomplished. After recovery, the patient should be transferred from the PACU for further recuperation in the most appropriate environment, be it at home, on a hospital ward, or in the intensive care unit.

ORGANIZATIONAL STRUCTURE

Medical Director

The care of patients in the PACU is multidisciplinary by necessity. It requires input from physicians, nurses, and respiratory care personnel, as well as several ancillary services. The leadership responsibilities of the PACU, however, most commonly fall to a physician from the Department of Anesthesiology in conjunction with a nurse manager. Indeed, it is in the standards for postanesthesia care promulgated by the American Society of Anesthesiologists that "the general medical supervision and coordination of patient care in the PACU should be the responsibility of an anesthesiologist" (6). These individuals provide the leadership for patient care, staff education, and research activities within the PACU. The policies and procedures that govern the PACU should incorporate standards set by the American Society of Anesthesiologists (ASA), the American Society of Post-Anesthesia Nurses (ASPAN), and the Joint Commission on Accreditation of Health Care Organization (JCAHO) (6, 7). It should be noted that standards for postanesthesia care apply to postanesthesia care in all locations. In addition to setting policies and procedures, the medical director of the PACU assumes responsibility for the coordination of medical care as well as establishing admission and discharge criteria and other protocols for patient care. In addition, the director must set standards for record keeping. The director must ensure that "there is a physician available at all times capable of managing complications and providing cardiopulmonary resuscitation for patients in the PACU" (6). Further, the medical director should be an active participant in the Quality Improvement Program for the PACU. Other responsibilities for the medical director should include an active teaching role for the staff of the PACU, as well as initiating and coordinating research activities. Finally, the medical director must ensure that proper funding is available to the PACU for appropriate equipment, patient care programs, research, and staff education.

Nurse Manager

The nurse manager works in conjunction with the medical director of the PACU. The nurse manager must possess the clinical skills and teaching and managerial abilities necessary for the successful functioning of the PACU. Responsibilities of the manager include the development and implementation of the policies and procedures of the PACU. The manager must also play an integral role in the quality improvement program of the PACU and must validate that approved policies and procedures are followed and appropriate documentation is carried out.

Staffing Consideration

Staffing required for a PACU is dependent on the type of surgical cases, the volume of patients seen, and the hours of operation of the PACU. Both ASA and ASPAN acknowledge professional nursing care in the immediate and second-phase postanesthesia settings is essential for the delivery of quality care to patients. Because of the vulnerability of patients in a perioperative setting, profession nurses with specific education, experience, and knowledge about the immediate postoperative period are required to recognize and help manage anesthesia- and surgery-related complications. Specific competencies must be defined and periodically assessed. Many institutions require PACU staff members to have previous critical care nursing experience, although this is by no means universal. Clearly, nurses in a PACU must have the ability to recognize problems quickly, to react appropriately, and to render skilled care in a timely fashion.

An anesthesiologist must be readily available to manage, assist, and advise the nursing staff in the management of patients in the postanesthesia phase. Other personnel, including a ward clerk, operating room (OR) assistants, respiratory care practitioners, and radiology technicians, assist in ensuring that the PACU functions smoothly. In addition, there may be several physicians involved in the care of the postoperative patient. To ensure that there are no breakdowns in patient care, it is essential that patient care responsibilities are clearly delineated and that good communication exists among all caregivers in the PACU. For example, wound care and postoperative bleeding clearly fall within the purview of the surgeon, whereas airway management and pain control are the responsibility of the anesthesiologist. However, there may be several areas of overlap so that good communication between services providing care for patients in the PACU is essential to avoid conflict or duplication and provide optimal patient care.

Educational Opportunities

The PACU provides an outstanding educational opportunity for healthcare professionals. Indeed, it is a requirement of the Residency Review Committee for Anesthesiology and the Accreditation Council for Graduate Medical Education that residents gain experience in the care of postoperative patients. Because subspecialty anesthesia training experience emphasizes the theoretical background, subject material, and practice of the subspecialty of anesthesiology, it is a requirement that residents in anesthesiology have a rotation in recovery room care (8). This rotation provides residents a unique opportunity to observe patients after anesthesia and to provide treatment for a variety of clinical scenarios in the immediate postoperative period after anesthesia and surgery. In addition, the PACU provides an excellent learning opportunity for both nurses and ancillary personnel. Finally, because of the large number of patients seen in a busy PACU, there is also ample opportunity for clinical research. The PACU provides an excellent opportunity for collaborative interdepartmental projects.

REFERENCES

1. Nightingale F. Notes on hospitals. 3rd ed. London: Longman, 1863;89.
2. Hilberman M. The evolution of intensive care units. Crit Care Med 1975;3:159.
3. Dunn FE, Shipp MG. The recovery room: a war time economy. Am J Nurs 1943;43:279.
4. Ruth HS, Hangen FP, Grave DD. Anesthesia study commission: findings of eleven years of activity. JAMA 1947;135:881.
5. Charbon GA, Livingston HM. Planning recovery room for adequate care. Hospitals 1949;23:35.
6. Americans Society of Anesthesiologists. Standards for postanesthesia care. Park Ridge, IL: American Society of Anesthesiologists, 1994.
7. Joint Commission on Accreditation Healthcare Organization. 1994 Accreditation manual for hospitals. Volume II. Scoring guidelines. Oakbrook Terrace, JCAHO, 1993.
8. American Medical Association. Program requirements for residency education in anesthesiology. Graduate Medical Education Directory 1994–1995. Chicago: American Medical Association, 1994.

2

EQUIPMENT AND MONITORING REQUIREMENTS

John H. Eichhorn

Immediate postanesthesia care in the postanesthesia care unit (PACU) is a topic of increasing interest and attention for health care professionals and others. One major reason for this emphasis is the significant reduction in intraoperative anesthetic catastrophes that has occurred in recent years (1, 2). Because the intraoperative phase of the perioperative experience currently receives much less negative attention, events (including catastrophes) and questionable outcomes in the PACU loom larger by comparison and become the focus of new attention. PACU care is not therapeutic but is, instead, facilitative to the healing interventions associated with surgery and other procedures requiring anesthesia. Therefore, there is essentially a zero tolerance for error. Justifiably, maximum effort should be directed at making the PACU as safe, effective, and efficient as possible. Although beyond the scope of this chapter, awareness of common complications occurring in the PACU (3, 4) is important. One key component of preventing and mitigating complications associated with PACU care is the availability of appropriate equipment for the caregivers. Application of the appropriate monitoring practices will aid in identifying untoward patient developments as early as possible in their evolution and will give the responsible personnel the maximum possible time to react and prevent patient damage. Only relatively recently in the evolution of PACU care has there been organized examination of and emphasis on both equipment and monitoring. The American Society of Postanesthesia Nurses (ASPAN) includes sections on both equipment and monitoring in its thoughtful and well-crafted standards (5), which are mandatory reading for existing and prospective PACU managers and staff. In addition to this current text, older textbooks on recovery rooms and their function may provide additional viewpoints (6–8).

PACU EQUIPMENT

The staff of a PACU must have the necessary equipment to provide all routine care to regular patients and to handle any possible postanesthetic problem or complication that conceivably could be expected in the patient population served by that PACU. Specific requirements and recommendations will vary considerably among various units, depending on the nature of the involved health care facility, patient population, surgical case load, and types of surgical procedures performed in the associated operating suite. These factors must be analyzed carefully by the responsible physicians, nurses, and facility administrators to create a projected list of likely and unlikely events in regard to demands for equipment in the PACU. Once accomplished, decisions must be made regarding what equipment will be secured, maintained, and kept at all times in the PACU itself and what additional equipment will be kept in the operating room (OR) suite (including the anesthesia work and storage rooms) but "immediately available" at all times to the PACU in the event of an emergency. These decisions will vary widely depending on the mix of surgical patients admitted to the PACU. A PACU in a large university medical center surgical suite that performs a high volume of thoracic surgery must keep a chest tube tray and probably also a thoracotomy tray or pack in the center of the PACU, whereas a thoracotomy tray may not be indicated for a PACU in a freestanding day surgery clinic that is mainly used for cosmetic plastic surgery and eye cases. Beyond the basic equipment necessary for each PACU bedspace in all facilities, each category or type of equipment will require careful evaluation of the appropriate level of equipment involvement. Securing and maintaining complex equipment that is never used is an unjustified expense. Discussion of the factors that will help make those determinations is included in the various categories outlined below.

Stretchers

All PACU stretchers must have movable side rails, which when in the raised position, can safely hold a sleeping or even thrashing patient on the bed. Stretchers must have reliable brakes that lock the wheels so that any routine or emergency intervention can be performed safely. Because it is likely patients will be transported on these stretchers, a bag of fluid for an intravenous infusion must be able to be hung from a pole, preferably at the foot of the stretcher. All stretchers used in a PACU must be able to be changed quickly into the Trendelenburg position. So-called "shock blocks" of wood, which go under the wheels at the foot of the stretcher and require a number of people with sufficient strength to lift the foot end of the stretcher, afford no flexibility regarding degree of tilt and sometimes create a dangerous situation in which the stretcher may roll off the blocks, endangering the patient. Therefore, because patients are often hypotensive enough to require the head-down position, stretchers in which the head can be mechanically lowered are necessary.

Associated with the choice of stretcher is the sensitive topic of patient restraints. At some time in every PACU, disoriented and thrashing patients will need to be restrained to prevent self-injury. It is beyond the scope of this chapter to discuss the philosophical and nursing care issues involved. However, if buckled leather restraints are needed, they must be included in the equipment list for the PACU and the compatibility of the restraints with the stretchers must be verified.

Monitors

The number of electronic monitors needed in a PACU is much more controversial than the type of monitors required. For purposes of this discussion, reference is to "phase I recovery," or initial recovery directly after being admitted to the PACU from the OR. This is distinct from "phase II recovery," which is the subsequent step, intermediate stage, or "step down" for same-day-surgery patients who will eventually be discharged. It is clear that phase II patients need less intense care; the equipment necessary for this type of care will be discussed in the chapter on ambulatory care (Chapter 20) and is also discussed in textbooks on ambulatory anesthesia (9, 10).

Although the applicable standards for phase I recovery do not necessarily specify the quantities of the various types of monitors that must be available, routine interpretation of the published material and current practice mandates that there should be an electrocardiogram (ECG) monitor and a pulse oximeter for each bedspace. Monitoring equipment manufacturers now make and sell a wide variety of "combination boxes," in which a single case and electronic chassis contain combinations of monitors in a compact arrangement. An ECG and a pulse oximeter combined in a single case is a prime example. It is clear that there must be a means to measure blood pressure continuously at each PACU bedspace. In all cases, a traditional manual sphygmomanometer should be available, usually with a mounted manometer gauge on the headwall of the bedspace connected by a coiled stretchable rubber tubing to the cuff, which should be kept in a small wire basket mounted adjacent to the manometer. Even if an electronic noninvasive blood pressure monitor (NIBP) is located at each bedspace, the manual sphygmomanometer may *not* be omitted, because it provides the necessary backup device that ensures uninterruptible capability of measuring blood pressure (and also of confirming the accuracy of the NIBP). As suggested, by the late 1990s, it is likely that many, if not most, PACUs will have an NIBP monitor for each bedspace. This feature can be included in the single electronic monitoring case mounted on the headwall (with the ECG and pulse oximeter) for simplicity and economy of space.

Likewise, the PACU staff must be able to measure temperature quickly and accurately at all times for all patients. There are many ways to accomplish this. One way, of course, is an electronic thermometer built in to the single electronic monitoring case mounted on the wall. Many manufacturers will configure any combination of features the customer desires, particularly if the order for monitors is large enough. A second option is a hand-held electronic thermometer at each bedspace, but this would entail unnecessary expense. The logical alternative is a small rolling equipment pole with an electronic thermometer mounted on it for transport when needed. Of course, a traditional manual glass thermometer should be available as backup at each location or for cases with special needs.

A similar approach can be taken regarding a Doppler ultrasound instrument. Certainly, in a PACU that receives a considerable number of patients who have had major vascular surgery, Doppler equipment is often needed. If this is not available, arrangements must be made to borrow a Doppler instrument when needed. Often, both the OR and the anesthesia service have Doppler equipment and can commit in advance to lending it when needed. Such commitments must be secured, however, and written into the PACU policy and

procedure manual; it cannot be assumed that the necessary equipment will be made available when the need arises. Relying on borrowing important but rarely used equipment requires planning and discussion so that no delays or glitches occur when the instruments are needed as key components of safe, effective patient care.

Whether the PACU electronic monitors should have the capacity to measure pressures depends on the patient population, as noted above. If patients in the PACU routinely have arterial and venous catheters that were used for pressure monitoring during anesthesia, then the PACU staff must continue monitoring these patients in the same manner. If there are only a few such patients, then an appropriate limited number of monitors on roll-around carts with the capacity to measure two (or three) pressures would be reasonable. If pressure monitoring is required for many patients, then it is logical to install two or three pressure channels in the electronic monitors mounted on the headwalls of most or all bedspaces.

All PACUs in which pressures are measured must deal with the sometimes difficult problem of compatible transducers. Coordination of equipment purchases and choice of supplies with the other parts of the facility is important. In most modern settings, the monitors in the OR and PACU are compatible with regard to the transducers employed. Any invasive monitoring catheters from the OR are simply left attached to the disposable transducers used during the procedure, and then the PACU staff plugs these transducers into the PACU pressure monitors. If the patient is transferred to another care setting with an invasive catheter still in place, the transducer can go along if it is compatible with the pressure monitor at the destination. In the past, particularly before disposable transducers were common, individual ideas and desires in different units of a large facility sometimes led to purchases of incompatible monitors that failed to allow movement of common transducers from unit to unit along with a patient. Current demands for efficiency and cost consciousness are eliminating such incompatibilities.

If there is an appreciable number of patients with pulmonary artery catheters, then the PACU should have its own cardiac output computer(s). If, however, there is only an occasional pulmonary artery catheter to manage, then the PACU staff must arrange for ready access to a cardiac output computer when needed.

The question of whether capnographs should be included in the multifunction electronic monitor on the wall of each bedspace is resolved somewhat similarly. Occasionally, an intensive care unit (ICU) patient will have to be held in the PACU because of lack of beds in the ICU. If such a circumstance is rare, a freestanding rolling monitor with capnography would be appropriate. If, however, this situation occurs frequently, capnographs should be included in most or all of the wall-mounted monitors in the bedspaces. A same-day-surgery center dealing almost exclusively with healthy elective patients will not need electronic capnographs but must have some way to verify correct endotracheal tube placement (see the "Crash Carts" section below).

Disposables and Small Items

Although disposables and small items sometimes are not considered "equipment," the PACU must have, in abundance, all of the small equipment and supplies associated with acute hospital care on a general floor and in an ICU, particularly items such as emesis basins and dressing material to reinforce wound dressings. Sample lists of appropriate items to include in the PACU bedspace have been published (5, 8). These items include the equipment for all possible types of oxygen administration, all sizes and types of suction and other catheters, and all relevant sizes of oral and nasal airways. One key point is that there should be a *self-inflating* resuscitator (positive-pressure valved breathing bag with a removable mask) with its oxygen tubing attached permanently in each bedspace, often in a plastic bag hanging from a hook on the headwall. In the past, such devices usually were reusable and often the exclusive property of respiratory therapists. Most institutions currently use disposable sets to avoid the expense of cleaning and resterilization and the risk of cross-contamination among patients. Consequently, these potentially lifesaving pieces of equipment have become more readily available. Many physicians consider it the standard of care to have a resuscitator in every PACU bedspace at all times. A flashlight, scissors, a clamp set, and a suture set should also be located in every bedspace.

The availability of equipment to facilitate and encourage the use of universal precautions is very important. Gloves, gowns, eye protection, and full-face shields should be available. It is reasonable to have a stock of all necessary protective supplies in every PACU bedspace.

Crash Carts

The immediate availability of a fully equipped emergency or "crash" cart is a PACU standard of care. The ASPAN standards list the contents of a prototypical emergency cart (5). The quantities needed depend on the volume and nature of the patient population. In a large hospital with a large volume of complex surgical patients, a common standard is one crash cart for each 15 to 20 PACU bedspaces. Although few PACUs require more than one crash cart, for those that do, patient and staff location and traffic flow must be studied to determine optimum placement of the emergency equipment.

Certain specialty resuscitation equipment is very important. It is sometimes difficult to justify to very budget-conscious administrators that specific items are needed in a critical situation even though they are rarely used. For PACUs that have pediatric patients, pediatric defibrillator paddles are just as important as the regular adult-sized ones. An external pacemaker is considered virtually a routine resuscitation resource and should be present in every PACU (including pediatric pads, if appropriate). A regular pacemaker with pacing wire insertion kits should also be a routine item. In the rare circumstance when it is needed, it is needed immediately; there is no time for it to be retrieved from another location. Furthermore, because many PACU nurses may not have had prior experience with pacemakers, thorough inservice training and refresher courses on the use of these devices are mandatory.

In a cardiac arrest situation, a patient who had not been intubated previously will require immediate intubation. Therefore, it is reasonable to suggest that there be a way to verify correct intubation by identification of exhaled carbon dioxide. There has been controversy regarding the applicability of this modality during cardiopulmonary arrest because of the possibility that cardiopulmonary resuscitation (CPR) may provide insufficient circulation of the blood to return significant amounts of carbon dioxide to the lungs for exhalation. In such circumstances, a correctly placed endotracheal tube may not reveal any carbon dioxide, leading to the false impression that the tube is not in the trachea. Nevertheless, it is appropriate that there be either an electronic capnograph in the PACU to connect to the endotracheal tube or, in the crash cart, a stock of the filter-paper, color-change indicators. The physician directing the resuscitation must interpret the indication of either device in the context of the clinical situation.

All patient care units must be prepared for a total power failure. Often, the bottom of the crash cart is a good place to keep extra lanterns and flashlights, as well as at least one extra resuscitator bag to allow manual ventilation of an intubated patient who may be on a ventilator. The crash cart should be sealed between checks to help decrease the "disappearance" of these very useful items.

Difficult Intubation and Airway Management Equipment

In addition to the crash cart, a cart that is specifically dedicated to intubation and airway equipment is required. This type of cart is not commercially available; therefore, the responsible anesthesiologists and PACU staff must collaborate and create a set of equipment appropriate to the surgical population served. As noted above, there are certain items that are so important that they must be immediately available in the PACU to treat a life-threatening crisis. The items that fall into this category will vary among PACUs. Whether the OR should be counted as a "distant location" depends on the physical layout of the facility. Certainly, if the OR is on a different floor or is farther than a 1-minute brisk walk, then more equipment must be kept in the PACU.

The same-day-surgery PACU must have basic airway equipment, including an appropriate assortment of laryngoscope handles and blades and endotracheal tubes, along with a retrograde intubation wire kit and a kit for emergency cricothyrotomy and subsequent ventilation. The latter is very important. In all situations, if a catheter such as a 14-gauge intravenous catheter is placed percutaneously through the cricothyroid membrane into the trachea, a resuscitator bag (or even a breathing bag on an anesthesia machine) is not sufficient to get oxygen into the lungs through the comparatively small orifice available. A direct source of wall-pressure oxygen (up to 55 psi) is required to insufflate sufficient oxygen through the catheter to maintain oxygenation while alternative solutions are sought. In an OR, the oxygen flush valve of the anesthesia machine can function as this source. In the PACU, if no anesthesia machine is immediately available, it is necessary to have a "jet ventilator" device (often known as a "Saunders injector") that attaches directly to the oxygen wall outlet and can be configured to attach to all of the devices that can be used for emergency cricothyrotomy. Such an oxygen insufflating device, either left in the intubation/airway cart in the PACU or *immediately* available very nearby, is mandatory for difficult intubation/airway situations. Copies of the American Society of Anesthesiologists (ASA) practice parameter for management of the difficult airway (11) should be included with this equipment and reviewed by all staff periodically (such as at the time of mock code drills organized by the nursing service). There are many other devices intended to help manage the difficult intubation/airway. The devices chosen for inclusion in the intubation/airway cart of a PACU will depend on the problems of the surgical patient population. It should be noted, however, that even a routine outpatient peripheral procedure can turn into an airway emergency. As noted, all PACUs should have the capability of verifying correct placement of an endotracheal tube in the trachea by identification of exhaled carbon dioxide. If a capnograph is not available in the unit, then the difficult intubation/airway cart include filter-paper, color-change indicators to demonstrate the presence of exhaled carbon dioxide when the airway is secured.

Any PACU that handles intubated patients must have its own set of respiratory measurement devices. Although respiratory therapists usually carry their own equipment, frequently PACU nurses or involved physicians will seek information about a patient's ventilatory status without involving a respiratory therapist. Therefore, a box (often on top of the difficult intubation/airway cart) should contain a spirometer and an inspiratory force meter ("NIF gauge") and the appropriate disposable adapters to allow connection of these devices to an endotracheal tube.

Whether anesthesiologists choose to secure extra items for the PACU difficult intubation/airway cart will depend on their experience and available budgets. Light wands are relatively inexpensive. There are a variety of laryngoscopes with unusual configurations, mirrors, or other designs, all of which are intended to facilitate successful intubation after failure with traditional approaches. The use of fiberoptic bronchoscopes in management of the difficult airway has become so ubiquitous that at least having access to this type of equipment, if not actually having it permanently on the cart, has become a standard of care. The fiberoptic bronchoscope has

so many other uses for intubated and ventilated patients (verification of placement, plug suction, segmental atelectasis inflation, lavage, etc.) that there is good reason for a PACU to have its own. Occasionally, the use of a rigid ventilating bronchoscope is necessary in certain critical life-threatening scenarios. These situations include tracheal collapse, other external compression on the trachea, masses within the trachea or mainstem bronchus, or foreign bodies. A ventilating rigid bronchoscope passed beyond the obstruction and functioning as a stent will restore ventilation dramatically. Immediate availability of a selection of such bronchoscopes (from the OR or actually on the PACU intubation/airway cart is mandatory because of specific situations in which they may be lifesaving.

The need for a separate tray of surgical instruments to perform a more formal tracheostomy in a PACU emergency will vary among facilities. The patient population and physical relationship with the OR will help make this determination. Input should be sought from the involved surgical services. Many larger PACUs have such a tray because in an acute emergency, the delay in retrieving it from the OR could result in mortality or severe morbidity.

The desirability of keeping an ICU ventilator on standby for emergencies in a PACU is debatable. The ASPAN standards (5) refer to this as a suggestion. In emergency situations in which an airway has been secured and requires mechanical ventilation in an unstable patient, it seems reasonable and appropriate to hand ventilate with the resuscitator bag mentioned above until the respiratory therapists deliver and set up a ventilator. PACUs that regularly receive patients who need mechanical ventilation must develop a suitable system to handle this situation, because usually there is sufficient time to plan and organize before the patient arrives in the PACU.

Fluid Therapy

All types and sizes of bags of intravenous fluid that are likely to be administered to postoperative patients should be stored in the PACU in quantities that relate to projected use. Plasma expanders must also be stored in the PACU for immediate use. At least one manual mechanism for rapid pressurized infusion of fluid (inflatable bags with mesh netting to hold the intravenous bag, plastic boxes with enclosed inflatable bladders, mechanical crank-driven compression plate) must be kept in the PACU in sufficient numbers so that more than one patient at a time can receive high-volume fluid resuscitation. Whether there is a role for an electric-pump power infuser in the PACU will depend on the nature of the patients admitted. A PACU that routinely receives patients who have had liver transplants, for example, will have many opportunities to use a power fluid/blood infuser. Most PACUs, however, will be adequately equipped with the manual devices with the caveat that, if necessary, a power infuser can be obtained from the OR.

The necessary kits and catheters for all manners of intravenous monitoring and infusions and intra-arterial monitoring (including long catheters for femoral arterial lines) should be kept in the PACU. The exact mix and numbers will depend on the nature of the surgical case load of the associated OR. If pulmonary artery catheters are not unusual in the patient mix normally moving through a PACU, then it is likely that there will be occasions when pulmonary artery lines will need to be inserted in the PACU. Therefore, all of the necessary associated materials must be immediately available on site.

Temperature Management Equipment

The need for electronic thermometers is noted above under "Monitors." Unintentional hypothermia seen in patients upon admission to a PACU, although perhaps less frequent than only a few years ago, remains a definite problem. Equipment to warm these patients has become very common in PACU's and likely will achieve the status of a standard of care soon. All PACU's that admit patients who have had body cavity surgery or any surgery that continues for an extended time need to have the equipment necessary to treat hypothermia. Blankets heated in a warming cabinet in the PACU are a traditional and useful therapy. Fluid warmers certainly are useful and indicated for inclusion as routine PACU equipment. However, unless there is massive infusion of fluid, these items are more useful to prevent a further drop in temperature rather than as the primary method to warm a cold patient. Hot-air blankets, properly applied for a sufficient period, seem to effectively warm hypothermic patients. These units are functionally large hair dryers connected by a hose to a plastic and paper "blanket" of connected air chambers that inflates to about 2 inches thick. Placed close enough to the patient's skin, heat transfer into the patient can take place, reversing the hypothermia. In institutions that have extensively equipped their PACUs with these devices, the costs are justified by virtue of fewer complications of hypothermia and earlier discharge from the PACU.

Even though malignant hyperthermia (MH) should be diagnosed, in most cases before the temperature actually rises significantly, the name of the syndrome leads to its association with temperature management. Every PACU must have immediate access to a comprehensive MH treatment cart or kit. The contents of such a kit are described in all major anesthesiology textbooks. The kit includes in one container all of the supplies, equipment, and medications needed. Whereas almost all of the items would be found in a PACU, there is insufficient time to search for and retrieve them in a genuine MH crisis. One item that is unique is the medication dantrolene sodium. Dantrolene is usually kept in an MH kit in the anesthesia work room in the OR. As long as the responsible anesthesia personnel are in agreement and there are no impediments to the equipment (excessive distance, locked doors at night, etc.), it is reasonable for the OR's MH kit to be the designated resource for the PACU. All PACU personnel must know exactly where the kit and the associated refrigerated intravenous fluids are located. It is reasonable to include PACU staff in the mechanism of periodically verifying that the dantrolene vials are not outdated.

Procedure Kits

A cutdown for emergency vascular access is a minor but important procedure that should be possible literally at a moment's notice in a PACU. Therefore, a cutdown tray or kit should be kept in a central location in every PACU at all times. If it is an OR pack, even double-wrapped in plastic, it will expire every several months and must be exchanged for a new kit.

As noted above, all PACUs must have the capability of supporting an emergency chest tube placement. The causes of tension pneumothorax associated with surgery and anesthesia are numerous and certain types of surgical interventions may also have a significant risk of postoperative hemothorax. Although life-threatening emergencies can be treated with a temporizing decompressing intravenous catheter in many cases, chest tube placement in the PACU should be readily possible in a very short time. As with other related circumstances, if the need for this intervention is truly rare and if trays and kits from the OR are genuinely immediately available, then the PACU can rely on securing the needed equipment from the OR.

Transport Equipment

Some patients discharged from the PACU will need various types of support during transport. Occasionally, a patient may need to go to another unit for a procedure, such as imaging, and return to the PACU. To facilitate such transport circumstances, the PACU must be equipped at all times with the necessary supporting equipment. Portable oxygen is obvious. Portable suction is less obvious but no less important in situations in which the patient's airway tends to become rapidly ob-

structed with secretions, blood, pulmonary edema fluid, etc. Immediate access to some type of portable suction device that can be used on transport from the PACU is necessary. A transport monitor (with a battery pack kept fully charged and functional) that can display ECG, a pulse oximeter reading, and an arterial pressure tracing/readout is indicated. If such monitors are used frequently throughout an average day, several should be available. Ventilation of intubated patients requiring ventilatory support who are to be transported is usually provided with a manual self-inflating breathing bag connected to the oxygen tank regulator. Small transport ventilators are available in both electric and pneumatically powered models. The advisability of considering such a piece of equipment for inclusion in a PACU will depend on its potential use.

MONITORING IN THE PACU

As has been clearly demonstrated for intraoperative patient monitoring, the presence of qualified professional personnel is the single most important component of patient monitoring. Guidelines exist for the ratio of PACU nursing and support staff to PACU patients, depending on the complexity and conditions of the patients involved (5) (nurse:patient ratio classes of 1:3, 1:2, and 1:1). Likewise, whereas a full set of vital signs must be taken immediately upon admission and immediately before discharge, patient-dependent guidelines exist regarding the frequency and complexity of monitoring during a patient's stay. Each PACU staff must develop its own protocols based on the type of patients, the surgical procedures, and input of the responsible anesthesiologists and surgeons. The judgment of the PACU nurses is also essential to this process.

The ASA's "Standards for Post Anesthesia Care" are presented in Figure 2–1. Parallel to the "Standards for Basic Anesthetic Monitoring," there is emphasis on monitoring oxygenation, ventilation, circulation, and temperature for each patient. The only specific

These Standards apply to postanesthesia care in all locations. These Standards may be exceeded based on the judgment of the responsible anesthesiologist. They are intended to encourage quality patient care, but cannot guarantee any specific patient outcome. They are subject to revision from time to time as warranted by the evolution of technology and practice. Under extenuating circumstances, the responsible anesthesiologist may waive the requirements marked with an asterisk (*); it is recommended that when this is done, it should be so stated (including the reasons) in a note in the patients's medical record.

STANDARD I

ALL PATIENTS WHO HAVE RECEIVED GENERAL ANESTHESIA, REGIONAL ANESTHESIA OR MONITORED ANES-THESIA CARE SHALL RECEIVE APPROPRIATE POSTANESTHESIA MANAGEMENT.[‡]

1. A Postanesthesia Care Unit (PACU) or an area which provides equivalent postanesthesia care shall be available to receive patients after anesthesia care. All patients who receive anesthesia care shall be admitted to the PACU or is equivalent **except** by specific order of the anesthesiologist responsible for the patient's care.
2. The medical aspects of care in the PACU shall be governed by policies and procedures which have been reviewed and approved by the Department of Anesthesiology.
3. The design, equipment and staffing of the PACU shall meet requirements of the facility's accrediting and licensing bodies.

STANDARD II

A PATIENT TRANSPORTED TO THE PACU SHALL BE ACCOMPANIED BY A MEMBER OF THE ANESTHESIA CARE TEAM WHO IS KNOWLEDGEABLE ABOUT THE PATIENT'S CONDITION. THE PATIENT SHALL BE CONTINUALLY EVALUATED AND TREATED DURING TRANSPORT WITH MONITORING AND SUPPORT APPROPRIATE TO THE PATIENT'S CONDITION.

STANDARD III

UPON ARRIVAL IN THE PACU, THE PATIENT SHALL BE RE-EVALUATED AND A VERBAL REPORT PROVIDIED TO THE RESPONSIBLE PACU NURSE BY THE MEMBER OF THE ANESTHESIA CARE TEAM WHO ACCOMPANIES THE PATIENT.

1. The patient's status on arrival in the PACU shall be documented.
2. Information concerning the preoperative condition and the surgical/anesthetic course shall be transmitted to the PACU nurse.
3. The member of the Anesthesia Care Team shall remain in the PACU until the PACU nurse accepts responsibility for the nursing care of the patient.

STANDARD IV

THE PATIENT'S CONDITION SHALL BE EVALUATED CONTINUALLY IN THE PACU.

1. The patient shall be observed and monitored by methods appropriate to the patient's medical condition. Particular attention should be given to monitoring oxygenation, ventilation, circulation and temperature. During recovery from all anesthetics, a quantitative method of assessing oxygenation such as pulse oximetry shall be employed in the initial phase of recovery.* This is not intended for application during the recovery of the obstetrical patient in whom regional anesthesia was used for labor and vaginal delivery.
2. An accurate written report of the PACU period shall be maintained. Use of an appropriate PACU scoring system is encouraged for each patient on admission at appropriate intervals prior to discharge and at the time of discharge.
3. General medical supervision and coordination of patient care in the PACU should be the responsibility of an anesthesiologist.
4. There shall be a policy to assure the availability in the facility of a physician capable of managing complications and providing cardiopulmonary resuscitation for patients in the PACU.

continues

---

† Reproduced with permission from the American Society of Anesthesiologists Directory of Members, 1996:395–396.
‡ Refer to *Standards of Post Anesthesia Nursing Practice 1992* published by ASPAN, for issues of nursing care.

STANDARD V

A PHYSICIAN IS RESPONSIBLE FOR THE DISCHARGE OF THE PATIENT FROM THE POSTANESTHESIA CARE UNIT.

1. When discharge criteria are used, they must be approved by the Department of Anesthesiology and the medical staff. They may vary depending upon whether the patient is discharged to a hospital room, to the Intensive Care Unit, to a short stay unit or home.
2. In the absence of the physician reponsible for the discharge, the PACU nurse shall determine that the patient meets the discharge criteria. The name of the physician accepting responsibility for discharge shall be noted on the record.

Fig. 2–1. American Society of Anesthesiologists (ASA) Standards for Postanesthesia Care.

mandate in the ASA standards is for the use of a pulse oximeter (or the functional equivalent) to monitor and assess patient oxygenation "during the initial phase of recovery," which does not necessarily mean throughout the phase I recovery period. The standard was written to indicate that for a patient arriving in the PACU from the OR, a pulse oximeter should be applied immediately and then used to monitor oxygenation thereafter for a period of time specified by the responsible caregivers as appropriate to the patient, the procedure performed, and the patient's condition. The variability in these parameters is so great as to make definite time interval specifications impossible.

A key component of monitoring is the patient record. In the PACU, the surgeon and assistants, the anesthesiologist(s) and associated anesthetists, and the PACU nurses will independently examine the PACU record, especially the vital signs, and make therapeutic judgments based on the data in that record. Accordingly, basic guidelines are as follows: (*a*) there should be *continuous* monitoring of the patient, and (*b*) vital signs, numerical scores, and notes should be recorded on the printed chart as frequently as necessary ("at appropriate intervals") to capture the pattern of the development and evolution of the PACU admission.

CONCLUSION

The main goals of equipping a PACU are, first, to provide the materials necessary for proficient execution of the routine care that most patients will receive and, second, to facil-

itate preparedness for the unusual or even strikingly rare emergency situations that occur in the immediate postoperative period. In accomplishing the latter, as outlined above, familiarity with the patient population using the PACU is important. The judgment of all involved must be applied and a cooperative effort among all the caregivers is required.

Patient monitoring in the PACU is subject to standards and guidelines but, importantly, is also greatly influenced by the nature of the patients and surgical procedures with the concomitant application of the professional judgment of the staff involved.

REFERENCES

1. Eichhorn JH. Prevention of intraoperative anesthesia accidents and related severe injury through safety monitoring. Anesthesiology 1989;70:572–577.
2. Eichhorn JH. Risk reduction. In: Duncan P, ed. Anesthetic risk and complications. Problems in anesthesia. Philadelphia: JB Lippincott, 1992;6(2):278–294.
3. Rosenfeld BA. Postanesthesia care unit. In: Rogers MC, Tinker JH, Covino BG, Longnecker DE, eds. Principles and practice of anesthesiology. St. Louis: Mosby Year Book, 1993;2359–2386.
4. Hines R, Barash PG, Watrous G, et al. Complications occurring in the postanesthesia care unit: a survey. Anesth Analg 1992;74:503–509.
5. Standards of post anesthesia nursing practice. Richmond: American Society of Postanesthesia Nurses, 1992.
6. Israel JS, DeKornfeld TJ, eds. Recovery room care. Chicago: Year Book Medical Publishers, 1987.
7. Frost EAM, ed. Post anesthesia care unit. St. Louis: CV Mosby, 1990.
8. Hatfield A, Tronson M. The complete recovery room book. Oxford: Oxford University Press, 1992.
9. McGoldrick KE, ed. Ambulatory anesthesiology. Baltimore: Williams & Wilkins, 1995.
10. Wetchler BV, ed. Anesthesia for ambulatory surgery. 2nd ed. Philadelphia: JB Lippincott, 1991.
11. Practice guidelines for management of the difficult airway. Anesthesiology 1993;78:597–602.

3

POSTANESTHESIA RECOVERY

Roger S. Mecca, Martin J. Serrins

Postanesthesia care rendered to patients in a postanesthesia care unit (PACU) has significant impact both on actual clinical outcomes and on the perceived quality of a surgical procedure. In the PACU, patient assessment must be efficient and thorough. Therapeutic interventions must be aggressively implemented for specific clinical problems with a defined endpoint. This approach optimizes postoperative outcomes while minimizing risk, inconvenience, and expense for the patient, the professional staff, and the facility.

Facility design, staffing, and equipment requirements for a contemporary PACU are reviewed in Chapters 1 and 2 (1–5).

VALUE OF PACU CARE

Since the advent of PACUs, "quality" always has been measured with indices related to clinical care. Evolution of admission and discharge criteria, monitoring policies, ratios and mixes of professional staff, and diagnostic or therapeutic care protocols has been oriented solely toward improving clinical outcomes. As the emphasis on cost containment grows (6), the element of "value" is being added to the quality analysis. The value of PACU care might be defined as the actual improvement in clinical outcome per dollar spent on the PACU admission. Analysis of the value of a PACU admission to a patient, a facility, or a health care system will be difficult, because both the impact on clinical outcome and the cost are difficult to measure and control.

The actual impact of PACU care on clinical outcomes is affected by a large number of variables. The mix of patients admitted to a PACU affects the frequency and complexity of postoperative problems that require resolution. Patient mix reflects the incidence and severity of underlying illness, the blend of surgical and anesthetic techniques employed, and the frequency, intensity, and urgency of surgical procedures. Beyond patient mix, the individual training, skill, and bias of surgeons, anesthesiologists, anesthetists, and PACU nurses caring for a given patient also affect how important that patient's PACU admission might be. The staff's effectiveness at recognizing complications and notifying physicians, the quality and availability of diagnostic or consultative services, and the efficiency of instituting therapy are also important. All of these factors are facility specific and vary over time. In addition, regulatory requirements, standards of care, and medicolegal climates vary among different regions or between facilities in the same locale. Given these factors, decisions about "cost effectiveness" of PACU care in a specific facility will be fraught with inaccuracy and controversy if they are based on national averages or broad standards. This difficulty is compounded by the lack of controlled scientific analysis that substantiates the actual clinical importance of many policies, procedures, and interventions commonly employed in PACU care.

With respect to cost, PACU care requires relatively expensive space, staff, and hardware.

The actual cost of PACU care in a facility is affected by many different factors. Admission and discharge policies determine which patients and for how long each patient will "consume" PACU resources. The mix of professional staff (e.g., amount of training and experience; salaries and benefit levels) and staffing ratios (e.g., number of patients per care giver; number of clerical, transport, and support staff) determine the hourly personnel cost to provide PACU care. The type of physician support (e.g., dedicated versus on-demand medical coverage, response times) affects efficiency of care. The level of routine monitoring provided affects capital expenditure for equipment and operating expenditure for disposable components (e.g., electrocardiogram [ECG] pads, disposable oximetry probes). Of course, the patient mix affects expenditures for staffing and for equipment such as monitors, intravenous pumps, and ventilators. Routine diagnostic testing increases the cost for securing and processing tests and sometimes adds an additional cost for professional interpretation. Administration of standard therapy (e.g., oxygen, antiemetics, respiratory therapy) increases the expenditure per patient for drugs and disposables and can add to the staffing resources required per patient.

Despite this complexity, increasing emphasis on containment of health care expenditures will force each surgical facility to evaluate the value of PACU care. PACU directors face the challenge of balancing the potentially conflicting goals of optimizing clinical outcome while minimizing expenditure per patient. When making changes to decrease cost, it is important to distinguish between perceived and actual cost savings. For example, decreasing the number of postoperative surgical patients admitted to PACU by 5% would seem to generate savings for an institution. However, if this reduction in admissions does not lead to a reduction in an actual expenditure for staffing, hours of PACU operation, or supplies, then the "cost reduction" is illusory. Similarly, use of inexpensive medications that are equally effective as more expensive agents makes good

economic sense, especially when the difference in cost is very large. However, if using a more expensive medication yields a greater savings by reducing the length of PACU stay or avoiding unnecessary overnight admission, then the investment in the more expensive medication may be warranted.

Medical and administrative leaders in each PACU must collaboratively examine practices and determine which are truly important and which are "wasteful." Innovative policies and practices must be created that guarantee safe care, fulfill regulatory requirements, and minimize cost. Obviously, superfluous expenditures such as inappropriate PACU admissions, useless testing, unnecessary therapy, and delayed discharge should be eliminated. Beyond this, establishing a dividing line between cost-effective postanesthesia care and unsafe, negligent clinical practice is a matter of individual professional judgment and personal conscience. The author recommends always erring on the side of patient safety regardless of cost.

LEVELS OF POSTOPERATIVE CARE

Every patient benefits from some degree of observation and support while the physiologic impact of anesthesia and surgery wanes. Whether surgery is performed on an ambulatory or an inpatient basis, the level of postoperative care that a patient actually requires is determined by severity of underlying illness, duration and complexity of anesthesia and surgery, and the potential for postoperative complications. Evolution of surgical and anesthetic care has broadened the spectrum of physiologic disruption that patients exhibit after surgery. Some patients still arrive in the PACU requiring a level of monitoring and intervention equal to that required in a critical care unit. However, an ever-increasing percentage of patients exhibit minimal depression on admission. For these patients, use of less invasive surgical techniques, short-acting anesthetic medications with fewer side effects, and regional or continuous infusion anesthesia can generate less somatic and autonomic disturbance after surgery. The frequency and severity of untoward cardiovascular, respiratory, or central nervous system (CNS) events has certainly decreased. This overall improvement in postoperative condition is evidenced by the increasing complexity of procedures currently being performed on an ambulatory basis. Given this broadening spectrum of postoperative conditions and the emphasis on cost containment, providing varying levels of postanesthesia care might provide patients with exactly the level of care needed.

Matching the level of care to actual patient requirements has many advantages. Patient satisfaction is a key indicator of success for practices and surgical facilities. Patients recovering from relatively minor procedures are often more satisfied with their postoperative experiences if they are separated from patients recovering from major procedures. Not only are they spared upsetting sights and sounds, but they are not inconvenienced by policies that mandate extensive assessment, low-yield interventions, and a long duration of PACU stay, which are more appropriate for higher intensity patients. Providing "nonhospital" amenities such as recliners, reading material, television, music, and food can greatly improve perceptions about surgical care without affecting actual clinical quality or safety. Earlier inclusion of family members in lower-intensity settings is a positive feature for many patients, especially when procedures are performed on children. In addition, diverting lower-intensity patients to a less intensive postanesthesia setting fosters a reduction in unit cost of a surgical procedure while allowing the facility to divert scarce staffing resources to patients with greater needs. This, of course, assumes that care is safe and appropriate for the patient's condition.

There are several ways in which a facility might safely provide different levels of postanesthesia care. Creation of separate PACUs for inpatients and ambulatory patients can foster a streamlining of PACU care for more straightforward cases. If separation is not feasible, then creating policies and procedures that more closely link the level of monitoring and coverage to the degree of postoperative impairment can achieve similar results within one PACU. If ambulatory patients are transferred from a PACU to a discharge area after surgery, practitioners might consider allowing selected patients to bypass the "phase I" PACU altogether and to be admitted directly to the discharge area. If recovery and discharge are both accomplished within the PACU, revision of the stage at which a patient "enters" the continuum can achieve similar results.

If a choice is made to provide different levels of postoperative care, the quality and intensity of care available in the "full service" PACU cannot be diminished in the process of establishing lower intensity settings. Existing protocols governing clinical care should be periodically reviewed for appropriateness, but they should not be categorically changed or discarded solely in the name of progress.

Regulatory requirements imposed on facilities by local, state, and national agencies can impede implementation of innovative, progressive care policies. Regulations and codes are sometimes out of date, poorly substantiated by valid scientific analysis, and interpreted by regulators whose clinical experience was derived in a different era. This problem can be especially pronounced in high-intensity areas such as the PACU. If the public demands that surgical facilities reduce the cost of care, then a degree of flexibility and logic must be incorporated into the regulatory bureaucracy so that appropriate changes can be made to meet this demand.

POSTOPERATIVE TRIAGE

If a facility provides several levels of postanesthesia care, then patients must be carefully evaluated to determine which level of care is most appropriate. Individualized decisions about level of care should be based on a patient's clinical condition and on the potential that a complication will occur that will require intervention. Triage decisions about using alternatives to PACU care must fully satisfy the requirement that patients be treated in a non-discriminatory fashion. Artificial cutoffs based on age, American Society of Anesthesiologists (ASA) classification, ambulatory versus inpatient status, or type of insurance should not be used to determine the type of care a patient receives. Equally obvious are the needs to preserve a wide margin of safety and to provide care that acknowledges established PACU standards (see Fig. 2–1.) (5). The level of postoperative observation that a patient requires should be assessed before a patient is transferred from the operating room after surgery. Whenever a doubt exists concerning a patient's ability to recover safely in a lower-intensity setting, the patient should be admitted to a "full service" PACU for comprehensive postanesthesia care.

Patients undergoing superficial procedures under local infiltration or peripheral regional anesthetics such as digital or field blocks can usually bypass PACU admission and recover safely in areas with less intensive monitoring and coverage, even when mild sedation is employed. In some instances, healthy patients undergoing more extensive procedures (e.g., hernia repairs, arthroscopic procedures, minor joint procedures) under local or plexus blockade might also be admitted to a less intensive setting. This decision should be made after considering the alternative unit's capacity to deal with the patient's needs for analgesia and the likelihood that a surgical or anesthetic complication might occur.

As anesthetic techniques improve, practitioners will frequently encounter patients who actually meet the facility's PACU discharge criteria at the end of the anesthesia in the operating room. This raises an interesting question: if assessment before PACU admission indicates that a patient is ready for PACU discharge, what is the purpose of admitting the patient to the PACU rather than to the next step in the postoperative continuum? Obvious concerns arise about the accuracy and reliability of PACU discharge criteria and about the possibility of acute, unexpected complications. The concept of bypassing the PACU after general or major regional anesthetics requires further exploration before it is widely implemented.

SAFETY IN THE PACU

The PACU medical director, the PACU staff, and the facility's risk manager are responsible for ensuring that the PACU environment is as safe as possible under all potential conditions. Beyond obvious provisions for physiologic monitoring, therapeutic equipment, and policies governing clinical care, other important elements should be considered when evaluating patient safety in the PACU. Staffing levels and staff training must be closely managed to ensure that appropriate coverage and skill mix are available to deal with unforeseen clinical crises. The PACU staff must remain current with evolving trends in anesthesiology, surgery, and PACU care as well as with important ancillary training such as advanced cardiac life support. Under ideal circumstances, all nurses caring for patients in a PACU setting should have full PACU certification and staffing ratios should never fall below accepted standards (5). However, evolving constraints on expenditures may force a relaxation of stringent staffing criteria in many healthcare facilities. If this occurs, each medical director must guarantee that less skilled staff are appropriately supervised and that sufficient skilled personnel are always available to deal with worst-case scenarios.

Minimizing risk of injury to patients during the PACU course is an underemphasized role of the PACU medical director. It is essential to ensure proper maintenance of equipment and appropriate use of bed rails and restraints. Each PACU should have an aggressive program to minimize risk of incidental injury to patients, especially early in the PACU course, when patients are emerging from general anesthesia or are still impaired by a regional anesthetic. For example, risk of ocular injury is high during emergence from general anesthesia. Corneal abrasion can be caused by contact of oxygen apparatus with the unguarded eye during emergence or by a digital pulse oximeter probe when a patient rubs his/her eyes. Entrapment of sensitive body parts or small pieces of apparatus beneath a patient can cause soft tissue injury. Risk of incidental injury is particularly high for patients who suffer emergence reactions characterized by disorientation, thrashing, and physical combativeness. Violent movements may disrupt suture lines and dislodge tracheal tubes, invasive monitors, or drains. Contusion can occur during contact with bed rails or equipment.

In addition to protecting against accidental injury, the PACU staff is responsible for acting as the patient's agent during periods of impaired consciousness. The patient's right to informed consent must be strictly safeguarded if additional procedures are required during the PACU course. Every attempt must be made to preserve each patient's personal privacy and dignity and to minimize the psychological impact of unpleasant or frightening events that unavoidably occur in a busy PACU. The environment must also preclude any possibility of personal insult or assault during the recovery period. Access to the PACU should be strictly regulated and security services should be readily available at all times. A prudent director should try to avoid unmonitored PACU coverage by one staff member for prolonged periods and should avoid having personnel care for members of the opposite sex whenever practical. Certainly, any hint of impropriety on the part of a staff member should be dealt with immediately.

It is equally important for the medical director to ensure that the PACU environment is safe for professionals. All staff and admitting practitioners must strictly adhere to established policies for infection control, including universal precautions for blood-borne pathogens when caring for patients and handling specimens or waste. Suitable masks, gloves, eye protection, and other safety devices must always be readily available. Safe practices for disposal of needles and other "sharps" are essential. PACU staff should be strongly en-

couraged to receive appropriate vaccinations, including hepatitis B vaccinations. Procedures that protect staff from exposure to respiratory pathogens such as tuberculosis and other pathogens such as methicillin-resistant staphylococcus must also be observed. Adequate personnel should be available so that individuals do not risk personal injury while lifting and positioning patients or while dealing with patients suffering physical emergence reactions. Policies governing documentation and limits of clinical responsibility should be reviewed by the facility's risk management process to protect staff against unnecessary medicolegal exposure. Obviously, personnel policies protecting staff against discrimination, harassment, and unfair labor practices must be observed.

ADMISSION PROCEDURES

Although a facility might make its PACU policies more flexible, there are absolute minimum levels of observation and care that should be provided whenever a patient is admitted to a PACU.

Vital Signs

Every patient admitted to a PACU should have ventilatory rate and character, heart rate, and systemic blood pressure recorded on admission. Assessment every 5 minutes for the first 15 minutes and every 15 minutes thereafter is a reasonable minimum. Axillary or oral temperature should be documented at least on admission and discharge and more frequently if appropriate. Rectal or esophageal temperature determinations can be employed if estimation of core temperature is important, although for most postoperative patients, this yields little additional benefit and some incremental risk. Qualitative assessment of level of consciousness, skin color, and airway patency are essential. Clear, contemporaneous documentation of all vital signs on the PACU record is important for medical decision-making and for reconstruction of PACU events if a peer review or medicolegal analysis is required in the future. It is equally important to carefully specify the time that each reading was recorded.

Physiologic Monitoring

Every patient admitted to the PACU should be monitored continuously with at least a pulse oximeter and a single-lead ECG (7). Cost-containment efforts should not erode this basic monitoring standard. These modalities can alert staff to imminent cardiovascular or pulmonary dysfunction, with a minimal cost for capital equipment, supplies, and labor. Employment of automated noninvasive blood pressure devices is recommended when feasible. Routine, continuous capnographic monitoring during the postoperative period is probably not warranted in view of cost, yield, and patient inconvenience (8). However, patients requiring mechanical ventilation or those at risk of compromised ventilatory function should be monitored with capnography or arterial blood gas (ABG) determinations as appropriate. Invasive monitoring initiated in the operating room should be continued throughout the PACU course or until discontinued in the PACU. Equipment necessary for transducer measurement of central venous, systemic arterial, pulmonary arterial, and intracranial pressures must be available if the unit receives patients requiring these modalities. It is vital that readings from all of the patient's physiologic monitors be legibly and contemporaneously recorded with a clear time delineation on the PACU record.

Postoperative Testing

Considering the acuity and severity of the clinical problems encountered in the PACU, a full spectrum of diagnostic capabilities must be provided. Straightforward laboratory testing, electrocardiography, and portable radiography must be available in the PACU at a moment's notice. In addition, a facility should provide priority access to more eso-

teric diagnostic modalities such as ultrasonography, computerized axial or magnetic resonance imaging, electromyography, and evoked potentials. Availability of skilled consultants to assist anesthesiologists and surgeons with interpretation of results is essential.

It is increasingly clear that every attempt should be made to avoid routine postoperative testing. Numerous studies have indicated the low yield of routine testing for preoperative evaluation (9–12). In the PACU, diagnostic tests should be individually ordered to address specific clinical concerns based on preoperative history, intraoperative events, or postoperative presentation (13). PACU medical directors should closely evaluate standard testing protocols in terms of benefit versus risk. Benefit of a routine postoperative test might be defined as the likelihood that the test will yield a result that will improve the patient's clinical outcome. Risk can be viewed as the likelihood that the patient will suffer a negative outcome from the test, either from a direct injury during the test procedure or because the test result prompts an inappropriate alteration in treatment that generates morbidity. Objective evaluation reveals that statistical risk of routine testing is real and often greater than the statistical benefit of the test.

For narrow categories of patients, some rationale might exist for ordering specific tests by protocol. For example, automatically securing a postoperative serum glucose determination for every insulin-dependent diabetic or a postoperative ECG for every patient with symptomatic coronary artery disease may improve overall efficiency of care with a defensible risk/benefit ratio. In the author's opinion, routine postoperative testing should never be performed solely to provide ammunition for defense against potential malpractice litigation. Documentation of a thorough postoperative assessment and an intelligently selected battery of tests is much more helpful to demonstrate that sound and appropriate judgment were used during PACU care.

Transfer of Responsibility

Every patient should be delivered to the PACU by a licensed member of the anesthesia care team. On admission, anesthesiology personnel should manage the patient at least until PACU staff have secured admission heart rate and rhythm, blood pressure, and ventilatory rate. A succinct clinical report should be delivered and documented by PACU staff in a readily accessible location. This report should incorporate sufficient information to allow a physician who is unfamiliar with the patient to rapidly evaluate and intervene if a postoperative complication arises (14). The report should include physician's orders for diagnostic tests and a brief description of why those tests are important. Therapeutic regimens unique to the patient should be clearly outlined, including specific endpoints to be reached. Finally, the responsible anesthesiologist should be clearly identified, along with a means of rapidly contacting him or her. A standardized format printed on the PACU record is useful to ensure documentation of pertinent data, especially when anesthesiology personnel deliver a report that conforms with the format. An example of a PACU report format is outlined in Table 3–1.

Before responsibility for the patient's care is turned over to PACU personnel, a final evaluation should be performed. Airway patency, vital signs, and ECG rhythm must be confirmed. The level of analgesia should be adjusted if necessary. Degree of arousal should be assessed, and evolving emergence reactions should be appropriately handled before leaving the patient. An evaluation for minor complications such as lacerated lips, injured teeth, or corneal abrasion is important. Ensuring the function of therapeutic equipment, intravenous catheters, and monitoring devices is prudent. Responsibility must not be turned over to PACU personnel until airway, ventilatory, and hemodynamic status is satisfactory and the PACU personnel are capable of safely providing all aspects of the care required by the patient.

Table 3–1.   Components of a PACU Admission Report

1. *Preoperative History*
   Medication allergies or reactions
   Underlying medical illness
   Chronic medications
   Previous surgical procedures
   Premedications
   Acute problems (ischemia, trauma, acid-base, dehydration)
   NPO status

2. *Intraoperative Information*
   Surgical procedure and surgeon
   Type of anesthetic and agents used
   Intraoperative vital sign ranges
   Relaxant/reversal status
   Time/amount of narcotic administration
   Type/amount of intravenous fluids
   Drugs given (steroids, diuretics, antibiotics, vasoactive medicines)
   Estimated blood loss and urine output
   Intraoperative laboratory findings
   Unexpected surgical or anesthetic events

3. *Current Status*
   Airway patency
   Ventilatory adequacy
   Heart rate and heart rhythm
   Systemic pressure
   Level of consciousness
   Intravascular volume status
   Size and location of intravenous catheters
   Function of invasive monitors
   Endotracheal tube position
   Presence of anesthetic devices (e.g., epidural catheters)
   Overall impression

4. *Postoperative Instructions*
   Acceptable ranges for vital signs, urine output, and blood loss
   Anticipated cardiovascular, airway, or ventilatory problems
   Orders for therapeutic interventions with clear goals before discharge
   Surgical instructions (positioning, wound care)
   Diagnostic tests to be secured
   Location of responsible physician

ROUTINE THERAPY

Therapeutic interventions should always be tailored to the individual patient's specific needs. However, a few inexpensive interventions are so commonly beneficial to postoperative patients that they can be routinely employed. For example, almost every patient who has undergone a procedure significant enough to require PACU care will exhibit some reduction in body temperature on admission. Routine application of low-intensity interventions for "warming" are justified, both for patient comfort and in some instances to actually facilitate restoration of normal body temperature. Perception of hypothermia is strongly affected by peripheral thermal receptors that monitor surface temperature in the hands and other exposed surfaces. "Satisfying" these receptors with a comfortable ambient temperature, warm blankets, or radiant warmers will often attenuate postoperative shivering and lessen the patient's perception of being cold. Actual impact of these interventions on body temperature is relatively minor. For true hypothermia, more aggressive rewarming with heating blankets, warming of intravenous fluids, reflective thermal coverings, and heated nebulizers (for intubated patients) should be instituted by individual order.

Administration of supplemental oxygen is another therapeutic intervention that is often routinely used at PACU admission. Supplemental oxygen increases alveolar partial pressure of oxygen (PaO_2). In areas of the lung where ventilation is limited when compared with perfusion (low V/Q units), increasing PaO_2 can improve partial pressure of arterial oxygen (PaO_2) and arterial hemoglobin saturation. In addition, increasing PaO_2 in the functional residual capacity prolongs the time interval between interruption of effective ventilation and appearance of serious hypoxemia. Clinically, this provides staff with more time to identify and rectify an upper airway obstruction or an acute reduction in minute ventilation before hypoxemia reaches a level that causes end-organ damage. The medical risk of administering supplemental oxygen to a patient is almost negligible, although risk of eye injury from oxygen apparatus in somnolent patients is real. One could question whether the cost of disposable oxygen apparatus balances the benefits gained by administering oxygen to healthy, awake patients in the PACU, especially when a regional technique has been employed. In the author's opinion, every patient who is admitted to a PACU after general anesthesia or deep sedation should be administered supplemental oxygen, regardless of the level of arterial oxygen saturation on admission. Problems with upper airway patency and ventilation are the second most frequently encountered postoperative complications after nausea and vomiting (15). Numerous studies have shown that hypoxemic episodes occur with alarming frequency, even in healthy adults and children who have met PACU discharge criteria (16–20). It is difficult to predict which patients are at risk for hypoxemia, when in the PACU course hypoxemia will occur, and what the actual impact of a hypoxemic episode will be (21). Whenever a concern exists about the safety of allowing a PACU patient to ventilate with room air, supplemental oxygen should be administered. For healthy young patients admitted after regional anesthetics and/or light sedation, a physician might choose to waive supplemental oxygen. However, if that patient's risk for respiratory compromise is judged to be so low that supplemental oxygen is not cost effective, it may be that the patient's condition does not warrant PACU admission at all. In contrast to supplemental oxygen, there is little rationale for routine administration of medications in a PACU. Analgesics and antiemetics are two classes of medications that might be employed in a "routine" regimen, either prophylactically or in response to pain or nausea, respectively. In the author's opinion, medications should always be selected and dosed based on an individual patient's history, actual clinical presentation, and the specific therapeutic endpoint desired. Routine administration of analgesics, antiemetics, or other medications should be avoided. This is not to imply that standardized medication administration is necessarily bad care. Use of well conceived, standardized protocols to treat routine problems is efficient, offers the opportunity for scientific comparison of approaches, and forms the cornerstone for the "practice guideline" approach to clinical care. However, protocols must be initiated after consideration of each individual patient's history, current status, and the desired therapeutic endpoints. This evaluation should be carried out by a physician or by a designee who uses established criteria under a physician's authority. Automatically implementing a medication regimen that blankets all patients eliminates the value of an individual evaluation in the PACU and adds an unnecessary element of medical and legal risk to the treatment. The same principle holds true for protocols aimed at artificially selected patient groupings based on age, type of surgical procedure, or ambulatory status.

PAIN MANAGEMENT

Relieving surgical pain with minimal analgesic side effects is a primary goal in PACU care. Beyond achieving patient comfort, relief of pain reduces sympathetic nervous system (SNS) response and helps control postoperative hypertension, tachycardia, and agitation.

To avoid masking symptoms from another condition or a complication, it is important to check that the nature and degree of pain is appropriate for the operative procedure before administering analgesics or sedatives (22). For a given surgical procedure, the degree of postoperative pain will vary with the anesthetic technique (23), perhaps related to the manner in which intraoperative pain is processed by the CNS. Cognitive appreciation of postoperative pain sometimes correlates poorly with SNS responses. Some patients exhibit severe hypertension, tachycardia, and even cardiac dysrhythmias with minimal complaint of discomfort, whereas others perceive severe pain without signs of increased SNS activity. This divergence may be related to psychological, cultural, and cardiovascular variations among individuals.

Whenever possible, one should use innocuous interventions such as reassurance and re-positioning to reduce discomfort. Incisional pain can be treated effectively with intermittent administration of long-acting intravenous opiates such as morphine or meperidine. Shorter-acting agents such as fentanyl are useful in ambulatory settings. The desired clinical endpoint is relief of pain without undue depression, even if large doses of narcotics are necessary. Intravenous titration allows incremental assessment of both analgesia and respiratory or cardiovascular depression, because peak effects evolve rapidly. Intramuscular administration is less desirable, given the requirement for larger doses, delayed onset, unpredictable uptake, and unnecessary tissue trauma. Rectal administration of analgesics is appropriate for selected pediatric patients. Oral and transdermal analgesics have little role in immediate postoperative recovery but may be useful for ambulatory patients for post-PACU analgesia. Non-narcotic analgesics such as ketorolac or ibuprofen offer little advantage over narcotics in the PACU. Supplementation with these agents seems to reduce the total dosages of narcotics required to achieve postoperative analgesia, but the validity of this impression is unclear (24–26). Clonidine's role as a postoperative analgesic is still being explored (27–30).

Fear, anxiety, and disorientation often accompany pain after surgery, especially during emergence from general anesthesia. When treating postoperative discomfort, it is important to differentiate between requirements for analgesia and sedation and to choose an appropriate medication regimen. Opioids exhibit sedative properties that are relatively weak compared to their analgesic and depressant effects, and inferior to those of sedative medications. Similarly, analgesic properties of most sedatives are very weak. When a patient exhibits a strong psychogenic component of postoperative discomfort, incremental titration of an intravenous sedative such as diazepam or midazolam can attenuate anxiety and fear and improve the effectiveness of analgesic interventions.

When assessing postoperative pain, recall that hypovolemic patients are at risk for hypotension after elimination of painful stimuli. Analgesia reduces SNS outflow, which can in turn cause both venous and arterial vasodilation. In hypovolemic patients relying on SNS activity to support cardiovascular dynamics, this can generate precipitous hypotension. Vasodilation and hypotension can be worsened by histamine release secondary to opioid administration. A normotensive or hypotensive patient complaining of severe postoperative pain must be carefully assessed before administration of analgesics, especially if tachycardia is evident. Pain is also a potent stimulus for arousal and ventilation. Reduction of postoperative pain in combination with depressant effects of analgesics can precipitate hypoventilation with consequent respiratory acidemia and hypoxemia.

It is vital to remember that hypoxemia, respiratory acidemia, or cerebral hypoperfusion will generate symptoms and signs of SNS activity that mimic those of postoperative pain. If parenteral analgesics or sedatives are administered in such an instance, underlying hypoventilation, airway obstruction, or hypotension may become worse, causing sudden deterioration and cardiopulmonary arrest. Because patients suffering from these life-threatening conditions are often agitated and confused, evaluating levels of arousal and orientation, along with cardiovascular and pulmonary status, usually separates them from patients with true pain. However, differentiation can be difficult in patients who are confused and combative during emergence from general anesthesia.

Other analgesic modalities are available that provide postoperative pain relief through and beyond the PACU stay. Intravenous narcotic loading in the PACU is important for smooth transition to postoperative patient-controlled analgesia (PCA). Patients can assume control of PCA in the PACU or after transfer, depending on program design and individual preference. Nausea and pruritus limit the effectiveness of PCA for some patients. These side effects are sometimes eliminated by switching the opioid used for PCA or by treating with antihistamines or narcotic antagonists.

Injection of narcotics into the epidural or subarachnoid space during anesthesia can yield prolonged postoperative analgesia for selected patients (31–35). Both immediate and delayed ventilatory depression can occur. Immediate respiratory depression is probably related to vascular uptake, whereas delayed respiratory depression probably is caused by a spread in cerebral spinal fluid. Use of epidural or intrathecal narcotics mandates careful postoperative monitoring of ventilation. Nausea and pruritus are also bothersome side effects of spinal narcotics. Addition of clonidine may enhance analgesia and decrease the risk of side effects from epidural opiates (27, 36–38). The efficacy and safety of adding local anesthetics or vasoconstrictors to subarachnoid or epidural narcotics for extended postoperative management varies with individual patients, physician philosophy, and program design.

Placement of long-acting regional analgesic blocks for selected patients can effectively reduce postoperative pain, improve ventilatory function, and control SNS activity. Intraoperative local anesthetic infiltration in joints, soft tissues, or incisions decreases intensity of postoperative pain (39). Administration of caudal analgesia is very effective for pediatric patients after inguinal or genital procedures. After painful shoulder and upper extremity procedures, an analgesic interscalene block can yield almost complete relief with only moderate motor impairment. Percutaneous intercostal blocks can reduce analgesic requirements after thoracic or high abdominal incision (thoracotomy, cholecystectomy, chest tube placement, gastrostomy, multiple rib fractures), although beneficial effects on postoperative pulmonary function are questionable (40–43). Provision of continuous infusions of local anesthetics through an indwelling epidural catheter for postoperative analgesia can be effective for patients with severe thoracic or abdominal pain and may assist in weaning from mechanical ventilation after major abdominal surgery (44, 45). Input of positive suggestion during surgery might have some influence on analgesic requirement and recovery course (46, 47). Other modalities for pain relief, such as acupuncture, transcutaneous nerve stimulation, "white noise," and hypnosis have relatively limited use in the immediate postoperative period (48).

Analgesic modalities that extend beyond the PACU require careful planning and anticipation of potential risks. One should plan extended postoperative pain therapy before induction of surgical anesthesia and orient the anesthetic and PACU care with that course of therapy in mind. If an extended therapy later proves inadequate, caution should be used before adding a second innovative modality. Experience of floor personnel and degree of monitoring available must be carefully considered.

PERSISTENT SEDATION

Occasionally, a practitioner encounters a patient whose return to consciousness in the PACU seems delayed. When evaluating prolonged unconsciousness after general anesthesia, the level of preoperative responsiveness should be checked to rule out preexisting cerebral dysfunction. The possibility of unrecognized drug or alcohol intoxication should be assessed. The time and amount of medications with sedative properties that were administered preoperatively and intraoperatively should be noted. Any unusual intraoperative events should be thoroughly reviewed. The rate and character of spontaneous ventilation should be assessed, because the degree of ventilatory depression can help gauge residual anesthetic depth. Evaluation of heart rate, rhythm, and systemic blood pressure can indicate the prevailing level of autonomic tone and adequacy of cerebral perfusion. Pupillary size and response should be evaluated, although the real diagnostic value of this observation is questionable. A firm tactile stimulus is often more effective than a verbal stimulus to elicit arousal.

Residual sedation from anesthetic medications is the most frequent cause of postoperative somnolence (49). After a reasonably conducted anesthetic, arousal will usually occur within 60 to 90 minutes of admission to the PACU, even in patients who are susceptible to sedation. Long-acting sedatives used for premedication or in the anesthetic technique can contribute to postoperative somnolence. Prolonged unconsciousness from volatile anesthetics is more likely when high inspired concentrations are continued through the end of surgery or after long surgical procedures in obese patients. Sedation caused by intraoperative narcotic or sedative administration is generally dose related.

To evaluate residual sedation, low-dose intravenous naloxone can be administered (0.04-mg increments every 2 minutes up to 0.2 mg) to reverse sedative effects of intraoperative narcotics. Titration of naloxone allows reversal of respiratory depression and sedation without precipitating dangerous reversal of analgesia (50). In the absence of massive overdose, it is unlikely that unconsciousness is related to residual narcotic sedation if spontaneous ventilation and arousal do not improve after 0.2 mg of intravenous naloxone. Flumazenil, a new benzodiazepine antagonist, will reverse the central sedative effects of midazolam and diazepam (51–53). Intravenous physostigmine (1.25 mg) will sometimes counteract sedation caused by inhalation anesthetics and other sedative medications (54, 55). If these interventions fail to generate arousal after a reasonably conducted anesthetic, it is unlikely that prolonged unconsciousness is related to residual anesthetic sedation. However, it is possible that an unrecognized preoperative overdose with depressant oral medication might be causing prolonged sedation in an emergency patient. CNS depression secondary to intravenous local anesthetic toxicity or inadvertent subarachnoid injections can also mimic postoperative coma, although this diagnosis is usually obvious in view of intraoperative events.

Rarely, profound residual neuromuscular paralysis might prevent a noticeable response to stimuli and mimic unconsciousness in the PACU. This conceivably could occur after gross relaxant overdosage or inadvertent omission of reversal agent or in patients with unrecognized neuromuscular disease or phase II blockade caused by pseudocholinesterase deficiency or excessive succinylcholine administration. However, any observation of spontaneous ventilation, motion, or motor reflex activity eliminates residual paralysis as the cause of unresponsiveness.

After residual effects of anesthetic agents and relaxants have been ruled out, other causes of unresponsiveness should be evaluated. A suspicion that a patient is feigning unresponsiveness can be easily evaluated by checking for an eyelid reflex or a startle response to an unexpected sound. If suspicion persists, an ECG machine can be used to document a psychogalvanometric response to upsetting verbal input or a startle. Similar to a lie detector, it is almost impossible for a patient to control the results of this test. Patients who were exhausted preoperatively will often be difficult to rouse after a general anesthetic. This is especially true for children when emergency surgery at night disrupts the normal sleep pattern. Evaluation of serum glucose will rule out severe hypoglycemia or hyperosmolar coma from hyperglycemia. Suspicion that unresponsiveness may be caused by hypoglycemia is an indication for an immediate empiric trial of intravenous 50% dextrose. Evaluation of serum electrolyte concentrations and osmolarity will check for iatrogenic hyposmolar states such as acute hyponatremia. Oximetry should eliminate unrecognized hypoxemia as a cause, whereas arterial blood gas analysis or capnometry is useful to check for severe hypercarbia, which might be causing CO_2 narcosis. Body temperature should be assessed, because hypothermia below 33°C can impair consciousness and increase the potency and duration of depressant medications. Core temperatures below 30°C can cause fixed dilation of pupils, absence of reflexes, and coma.

If the foregoing analysis does not reveal a diagnosis, a thorough neurologic evaluation in consultation with a neurologist is appropriate. Subclinical grand mal seizures from an underlying seizure disorder or delirium tremens can present with unresponsiveness in the PACU. Severe intraoperative hypotension, dysrhythmias, hypoxemia, or hypercarbia must be considered as potential causes of cerebral anoxia. The possibility of unrecognized head trauma and increasing intracranial pressure must be considered for injured patients. Intraoperative cerebral thromboembolism is another possibility, especially for patients recovering from cardiac, proximal major vascular, or invasive neck surgery (56, 57) or for those who have undergone internal jugular, subclavian, or intra-arterial cannulation. Patients with atrial fibrillation, symptomatic carotid bruits, or hypercoagulable states are also at increased risk for cerebral embolism. Paradoxical air embolism through a right-to-left intracardiac shunt or intracerebral hemorrhage secondary to intraoperative hypertension can also cause postoperative cerebrovascular accidents (58). Of course, for patients recovering from intracranial surgery, increased intracranial pressure from bleeding, edema, or pneumocephalus must also be considered (59). Postoperative cerebrovascular accidents for other patients are rare and usually occur later in the postoperative course (60).

ALTERED MENTAL STATUS

Sometimes a patient will manifest abnormal mental reactions in the PACU, ranging from confusion and lethargy through physical combativeness and extreme disorientation. Delirium and confusion during emergence entails real medical risks to the patient and disturbs other patients and staff in the PACU. Agitated patients can exhibit high levels of SNS activity with tachycardia and hypertension, which can cause serious medical complications. Forceful, thrashing movements can jeopardize suture lines, orthopedic fixations, vascular grafts, drains, tracheal tubes, and indwelling catheters. Risk of incidental trauma such as corneal abrasions, contusions, and sprains also increases. Least appreciated is the risk of injury to PACU staff struggling to contain a combative patient.

A psychological response to emergence from general anesthesia is undoubtedly the most frequent cause of emergence reactions. Lack of integration of higher cerebral functions can interfere with the patient's ability to process and appropriately react to sensory input. Many emerging patients are somnolent and slightly disoriented, with sluggish mental reactions that clear gradually. Wide emotional swings can occur, causing uncontrollable weeping or laughter. Sometimes a patient will exhibit significant combativeness with escalating physical resistance to positioning and restraint. Predicting which patients will have unusual reactions is difficult. Children and younger adults are more prone to extreme emergence reactions than elderly patients, although delirium is a frequent problem for elderly patients (61, 62). Separation from the parents increases anxiety in young children. Women seem more prone to weeping, whereas men more frequently manifest combative responses. Incidence of stormy emergence is probably higher after surgical procedures such as breast or testicular biopsies, which have a high level of anxiety or emotional significance. Patients with significant preoperative personality aberrations will exhibit those aberrations during emergence. A higher frequency of emergence problems occurs in patients with mental retardation, clinically evident psychiatric disorders, organic brain dysfunction, or hostile preoperative interactions. A language barrier that precludes reassuring input from PACU staff can accentuate an emergence reaction. Modes of expressing pain and fear rooted in ethnic, cultural, or individual personality differences can play a role (63). When oral fixation or endotracheal intubation impedes a patient's ability to communicate, resulting fear or frustration can exaggerate an emergence reaction.

Patients taking psychogenic medications or those premedicated with long-acting sedatives can exhibit clouded sensorium and disorientation in the PACU. Patients who abuse alcohol, narcotics, barbiturates, cocaine, or other illicit drugs might exhibit bizarre emergence behavior caused by acute intoxication or unrecognized withdrawal. Disorientation and combativeness occur after use of parenteral scopolamine as premedication or antiemetic and can be treated with intravenous physostigmine (64). Droperidol, metoclopramide, and ranitidine rarely can also cause dysphoria or confusion (65). Long-term preoperative meperidine therapy or atropine premedication can also cause postoperative delirium (66, 67). Ketamine has been implicated in causing postoperative dysphoria and hallucination, although adverse reactions in the PACU are rare. Use of etomidate for induction can contribute to postoperative restlessness (68).

Noxious stimuli during emergence certainly amplify confusion, agitation, and aggressive behavior. Every effort should be made to ensure adequate analgesia early in the PACU course. Painful gastric distention with entrapped gas or urinary bladder distention will generate marked agitation in an emerging patient, as will tight dressings, painful phlebotomy, or discomfort from endotracheal tubes, nasogastric tubes, urinary catheters, or infiltrated vascular catheters. Corneal abrasions, small pieces of equipment left beneath the patient, or entrapment of sensitive body parts can cause discomfort that is difficult to pinpoint. Nausea and dizziness are distressing, as is severe pruritus from medications. Some patients are far more comfortable in a semisitting position during emergence and will struggle vigorously to sit up when supine. This occurs frequently in patients with obesity, symptomatic gastroesophageal reflux, or pulmonary congestion. Patients will often fight vigorously against physical restraint from personnel or binders and then quiet when the restraint is relaxed. Weakness from partial neuromuscular relaxation is terrifying to a patient and will elicit severe anxiety and agitation during emergence, even when ventilation is adequate. Violent, uncoordinated motion characteristic of partial paralysis can make a patient appear disoriented and combative. Lack of strength, peculiar flapping motions, and quantitative electrical nerve stimulation are helpful in making the differential diagnosis.

Confusion, delirium, or combativeness can also indicate serious dysfunction of major organ systems. Moderate hypoxemia in an emerging patient often causes clouded mentation, disorientation, and agitation resembling that caused by pain. Postoperative delirium may be related to less serious degrees of hypoxemia (69). Hypercarbia without acidemia is generally asymptomatic unless $PaCO_2$ is so high that CO_2 narcosis causes somnolence and disorientation. Respiratory acidemia elicits profound agitation, especially when hypercarbia is caused by poor ventilatory mechanics or airway obstruction. Hypercarbia caused by respiratory center depression generates less agitation because higher CNS functions are also depressed. Limitation of lung inflation by tight chest dressings, gastric distention, decreased pulmonary compliance, or delivery of low tidal volumes during mechanical ventilation will gradually cause a dissatisfaction with ventilation similar to air hunger. This phenomenon is probably mediated by stretch receptors in pulmonary parenchyma that respond to changes in lung volume. Resulting agitation can be profound, even with adequate oxygenation and ventilation. Inability to generate a forceful cough or clear secretions is distressing, as is increased work of breathing from increased small airway resistance or partial upper airway obstruction.

Cardiovascular problems can accentuate anxiety during emergence. Early interstitial pulmonary edema causes symptoms of chest fullness and air hunger before airway flooding occurs. Perception of frequent ventricular ectopy is also distressing, especially if undue concern is expressed by the staff. Inadequate peripheral perfusion and lactic acidemia can cause anxiousness and mild disorientation. If systemic blood pressure falls so low that cerebral perfusion is not maintained, a patient can exhibit lethargy, severe disorientation, agitation, or combativeness. Administration of sedative or analgesic medications to such a patient for a mistaken diagnosis of anxiety or pain can generate a catastrophic cerebral event.

Several metabolic abnormalities affect lucidity. Acute hyponatremia after transurethral prostatic resection causes a hyposmolar state that markedly clouds the sensorium. Also, cerebral fluid shifts should be considered after dialysis, massive fluid infusion, or repletion of severe dehydration. Hyperglycemia from excessive glucose infusion or insufficient insulin can cloud consciousness during recovery if hyperosmolarity is severe. Severe hypoglycemia will cause significant agitation or markedly diminished responsiveness during recovery.

After common causes of delirium have been ruled out, the possibility of a primary neurologic problem must be considered. Seizure activity can mimic agitation and combativeness or can make the patient appear disoriented, somnolent, and confused during the postictal phase. One should suspect seizures in patients with head trauma, chronic alcohol intoxication, cocaine abuse, or epilepsy. Acute cerebral embolism, hemorrhage, or infarct sometimes presents with changes in level of consciousness, orientation, or ability to vocalize clearly (70).

The therapy for altered mental status varies with etiology. Waiting for residual anesthetic effects to resolve is usually sufficient. Most emergence reactions improve within 10 minutes. Verbal reassurance that surgery is completed and status is acceptable can be invaluable. Using the patient's and surgeon's name frequently and stressing time and location help reestablish orientation. When possible, patients should be allowed to select their own position. Offending stimuli should be removed or minimized. Adequate analgesia is essential. Small doses of a parenteral sedative can help relieve fear or anxiety and smooth emergence. Identifying whether a patient is reacting to pain or anxiety is important, because narcotics are relatively poor sedatives whereas benzodiazepines or barbiturates are ineffective analgesics. In the author's opinion, physical restraint by staff or through the use of binding should be used only as a last resort to protect a patient from injury.

If aggressive evaluation reveals that altered mental status is a symptom of a physiologic abnormality (e.g., hypoxemia, acidemia, hypoglycemia, hypotension), sedative or analgesic medications should not be administered. Instead, the underlying problem causing the physiologic abnormality should be treated.

DISCHARGE CRITERIA

When discharging a patient from a PACU, a practitioner certifies that in his or her judgment, the patient's level of postoperative impairment has resolved to a point that a much lower intensity of care is appropriate. This usually implies that the patient no longer needs close observation, frequent evaluation of vital signs, comprehensive physiologic monitoring, or the immediate availability of specialized staff. Obviously, the consequences of poor judgment can be catastrophic for both the patient and the practitioner.

Ideally, each patient should be evaluated individually for discharge by an anesthesiologist using a consistent set of general criteria (Table 3–2). Discharge criteria can be modified or waived in view of an individual patient's unique condition or the characteristics of the patient's destination. However, in most instances, discharge criteria should be strictly observed. If a specific criterion requires frequent waiver, then it should be revalidated to ensure that it is not outdated or overly strict. Discharge criteria must be used with caution and perspective in a PACU. Patients exhibit a wide spectrum of problems with varying presentations. Scoring systems that attempt to quantify physical status and readiness for discharge can be useful to facilitate a thorough assessment but should not replace individual patient assessment (71, 72). The type and severity of underlying disease, anesthetic and recovery course, and postoperative destination

should be carefully considered. Numerical thresholds for vital signs, physiologic monitoring indices, or test results must never replace assessment with respect to a given patient's condition. Assessment of ambulatory patients must be particularly meticulous, given the low level of care and observation available outside the medical facility.

As cost containment in surgical care accelerates, practitioners may be pressured either to bypass the PACU or to shorten the PACU interval when admission is deemed appropriate. Few data are available to elucidate whether a minimum length of stay is required for appropriate PACU care. It is prudent to assume that if a patient requires PACU admission, he or she should remain for a period sufficient to allow a full evaluation of physical and mental condition and the initiation and assessment of appropriate therapy. Sufficient time must also be available to permit emergence of reasonably anticipated postoperative problems or complications. In the author's experience, at least 30 minutes is required for straightforward cases. If selected patients are objectively ready for discharge in less than 30 minutes, then the appropriateness of those admissions might be examined.

Several general criteria should be applied when assessing a patient for discharge from a PACU. A postoperative patient should be sufficiently oriented to assess his own physical condition and to summon assistance if necessary. Protective airway reflexes and neuromuscular function must be sufficiently recovered to preclude airway obstruction or aspiration of secretions or vomitus. Ventilation and oxygenation should be acceptable based on physical examination, oximetry, capnometry, or other appropriate quantitative indices. Sufficient ventilatory reserve should be evident to cover minor deterioration in an unmonitored setting. Systemic blood pressure, heart rate, and indices of intravascular volume and peripheral perfusion should be within acceptable ranges for that patient and relatively constant for at least 20 minutes. Shivering should be resolved before discharge, although warming

Table 3–2. Guidelines for Discharge Evaluation from a PACU[a]

General Conditions:	Responds to verbal input and follows simple instructions
	Oriented to time, place, and surgical procedure
	Adequate strength and mobility for appropriate self-care
	Absence or control of specific, acute surgical complications
	Suitable control of nausea and emesis
	Destination appropriate for patients's status
Control of Pain:	Ability to localize and estimate surgical pain
	Adequate analgesia achieved
	At least 15 minutes since last parenteral narcotic
	Appropriate postdischarge analgesic orders
Airway Maintenance:	Protective reflexes (swallow, gag, expulsion) intact
	Absence of obstruction, stridor, retraction
	Need for artificial airway support resolved
Ventilation and oxygenation:	Ventilatory rate greater than 10, less than 30
	Forced vital capacity more than twice tidal volume
	Adequate ability to cough and clear secretions
	Qualitatively acceptable work of breathing
Systemic Blood Pressure:	Within ±20% resting preoperative value
	"Acceptable" color without splotches, paleness, cyanosis
	Appropriate orders for persistent hypertension
Heart Rate and Rhythm:	Relatively constant for at least 15 minutes
	Resolution or evaluation of new dysrhythmias
	Acceptable intravascular volume status
	Any suspicion of myocardial ischemia rectified
Renal Function:	Urine output greater than 30 ml · hr^{-1} (catheterized patients)
	Appropriate color and appearance of urine, evaluation of hematuria
	Follow-up orders regarding output if voiding has not occurred
Metabolic/Laboratory:	Acceptable hematocrit level considering hydration and blood loss
	Suitable blood glucose and electrolyte balance
	Results of chest x-ray, electrocardiogram, and other tests reviewed as appropriate
Ambulatory Patients:	Suitable control of nausea after ambulation
	Able to ambulate without dizziness, undue weakness, hypotension

[a] Every patient need may not meet all criteria. Clinical judgment must always supersede established guidelines for the condition. However, if doubt exists about clinical condition or patient safety, discharge should be delayed.

to normal body temperature is not absolutely required. An acceptable level of analgesia must be achieved before transfer. To reliably assess peak effects of analgesics, patients should be observed for a minimum of 15 minutes after the last dose of intravenous narcotic or sedative. Longer periods of observation may be prudent after reinforcement of regional anesthetic techniques. Patients should be observed for 15 minutes after discontinuation of supplemental oxygen to detect unexpected hypoxemia. Likely adverse surgical sequelae and acute exacerbations of underlying conditions such as coronary artery disease, hypertension, or asthma should be assessed before discharge. Results of postoperative diagnostic tests should be reviewed. If these generic criteria cannot be met, postponement of discharge or transfer to a specialized unit for appropriate care and monitoring is advisable.

After a decision is made to discharge a patient from the PACU, several key elements should be reviewed to ensure safe transfer to the next area or to home. Personnel responsible for physically transporting the patient should have acumen and skills commensurate with the individual patient's potential needs during transport. For example, an aide might be sufficient to transport a healthy patient to an ambulatory discharge area, but a PACU nurse or a physician should accompany a critically ill patient to an intensive care unit. Sufficient help should be available to move additional equipment such as infusion pumps, drainage devices, and oxygen apparatus, especially if they are still in use during transfer. When monitoring or resuscitative equipment is required, it should be available and carefully checked before departure, especially when the destination is far from the PACU. It is often prudent to assign two individuals to transport a tenuous patient, especially if an elevator ride is required to reach the receiving unit. On arrival, a clear report must be delivered to the practitioners assuming responsibility for the patient's care, including a brief history, a summary of events in the operating room and PACU, and a projection of likely needs or anticipated problems. The comprehensiveness of this report will vary with the individual circumstance. When patients are discharged directly from the PACU to home, clear written instructions must be provided about wound care, resumption of previous medication regimens, use of analgesics, and other procedure-specific information. Each patient must be provided with a means to rapidly contact a skilled practitioner if unexpected problems arise after discharge.

REFERENCES

1. Willock MM, Willock GM. Design of the recovery room. In: Israel JS, Dekornfeld TJ, eds. Recovery room care. Chicago: Yearbook Medical Publishers, 1987;6.
2. Finch JS. Equipment and monitoring. In: Israel JS, Dekornfeld TJ, eds. Recovery room care. Chicago: Yearbook Medical Publishers, 1987;25.
3. Willock MM. Management and staffing. In: Israel JS, Dekornfeld TJ, eds. Recovery room care. Chicago: Yearbook Medical Publishers, 1987;84.
4. DeFranco M. Planning the physical structure of the PACU. In: Frost EAM, ed. Post anesthesia care unit. St Louis: CV Mosby Co., 1990;187.
5. Standards of post anesthesia nursing care. Richmond: American Society of Post Anesthesia Nurses, 1992.
6. Johnstone RE, Martinec CL. Costs of anesthesia. Anesth Analg 1993;76(4):840–849.
7. Yelderman MH, New W. Evaluation of pulse oximetry. Anesthesiology 1983;59:349.
8. Kavanagh BP, Sandler AN, Turner KE, et al. Use of end tidal PCO_2 and Tc PCO_2 as noninvasive measurement of arterial PCO_2 in extubated patients recovering from general anesthesia. J Clin Monit 1992;8(3):226–230.
9. Roizen MF, Kaplan EB, Schreider BD, et al. The relative roles of the history and physical examination, and laboratory testing in the preoperative evaluation for outpatient surgery: the "Starling" curve in preoperative laboratory testing. Anesthesiol Clin North Am 1987;5:15–26.
10. Marr BJ, Hansen TR, Warner MA. Preoperative laboratory screening in healthy Mayo patients: cost effective elimination of test and unchanged outcomes. Mayo Clin Proc 1991;66:155–159.
11. Tape TG, Mushlin AI. How useful are routine chest X-rays of preoperative patients at risk for postoperative chest disease? J Gen Intern Med 1988;3:15–19.
12. Turnbull JM, Buck C. The value of preoperative screening investigations in otherwise healthy individuals. Arch Intern Med 1987;147:1101–1108.
13. Cooper MH, Primrose JN. The value of postoperative chest radiology after major abdominal surgery. Anaesthesia 1989;44:306–309.
14. Orkin LR, Shapiro G. Admission, assessment and general monitoring. In: Frost EAM, Andrews IC, eds. Recovery room care. International anesthesiology clinics. Boston: Little, Brown & Co., 1983;1.
15. Hines HR, Barash PG, Watrous G, et al. Complications occurring in the postanesthesia care unit: a survey. Anesth Analg 1992;74:503–509.
16. Zvara MJ, Labaille T, Benlabed M, et al. Does significant postoperative arterial desaturation occur with regional anesthesia? Anesthesiology 1989;71(3A):A898.
17. Moller JT, Wittrup M, Johansen SH. Hypoxemia in the postanesthesia care unit: an observer study. Anesthesiology 1900;73:890.
18. Russell GB, Graybeal JM. Persistent occurrence of postoperative arterial oxygen desaturations despite oxygen therapy. Anesthesiology 1990;73(3):A540.
19. Kimovec MA, Grutsch JF, Napcil JA. Incidence of postoperative hypoxemia prior to recovery room discharge. Anesthesiology 1989;71(3A):A373.
20. Tomkins DP, Gaukroger PB, Bentley MW. Hypoxia in children following general anaesthesia. Anaesth Intensive Car 1988;16:177.
21. Rose DK, Cohen MM, Wigglesworth DF, et al. Critical respiratory events in the postanesthesia care unit: patient, surgical, and anesthetic factors. Anesthesiology 1994;81(2):410–418.
22. Henderson JJ, Parbrook GD. Influence of anesthetic technique on postoperative pain. Br J Anaesth 1976;48:587.
23. Tverskoy M, Coxacov C, Ayache M, et al. Postoperative pain after inguinal herniorrhaphy with different types of anesthesia. Anesth Analg 1990;70:29–36.
24. Wong HY, Carpenter RL, Kopacz, et al. A randomized, double-blind evaluation of ketorolac tromethamine for postoperative analgesia in ambulatory surgery patients. Anesthesiology 1993;78(1):6–14.

25. Higgins MS, Givogre JL, Marco AP, et al. Recovery from outpatient laparoscopic tubal ligation is not improved by preoperative administration of ketorolac or ibuprofen. Anesth Analg 1994;79(2):274–280.

26. Ready LB, Brown CR, Stahlgren LH, et al. Evaluation of intravenous ketorolac administered by bolus or infusion for treatment of postoperative pain: a double-blind, placebo-controlled, multicenter study. Anesthesiology 1994;80(6):1277–1286.

27. Bonnet F, Boico O, Rostaing S, et al. Clonidine induced analgesia in postoperative patients: epidural versus intramuscular administration. Anesthesiology 1990;72:423–427.

28. Segal IS, Jarvis DA, Duncan SR, et al. Perioperative use of transdermal clonidine as an adjunctive agent. Anesth Analg 1989;68:S79.

29. Bernard JM, Lechevalier T, Pinaud M, et al. Postoperative analgesia by IV clonidine. Anesthesiology 1989;71(3A):A154.

30. De Kock M, Crochet B, Morimont C, et al. Intravenous or epidural clonidine for intra- and postoperative analgesia. Anesthesiology 1993;79(3):525–531.

31. Chrubasik J, Wiemers K. Continuous-plus-on-demand epidural infusion of morphine for postoperative pain relief by means of a small, externally worn infusion device. Anesthesiology 1985;62:263.

32. Lanz E, Kehrberger E, Theiss D. Epidural morphine: a clinical double blind study of dosage. Anesth Analg 1985;64:786.

33. Cuschieri, RJ, Morran CG, Howie JC, et al. Postoperative pain and pulmonary complications: comparison of three analgesic regimens. Br J Surg 1985; 72:495.

34. Kavanagh BP, Katz J, Sandler AN. Pain control after thoracic surgery: a review of current techniques. Anesthesiology 1994;81(3):737–759.

35. Cousins MJ, Mather LE. Intrathecal and epidural administration of opioids. Anesthesiology 1984; 61:276.

36. Bonnet F, Boico O, Rostaing S, et al. Extradural clonidine analgesia in postoperative patients. Br J Anaesth 1989;63:465–469.

37. Motsch J, Graber E, Ludwig K. Addition of clonidine enhances postoperative analgesia from epidural morphine: a double blind study. Anesthesiology 1990; 73:1067–1073.

38. Mendez R, Eisenbach JC, Kashtan K. Epidural clonidine analgesia after cesarean section. Anesthesiology 1990;73:848–853.

39. Allen GC, St. Amand MA, Lui ACP, et al. Postarthroscopy analgesia with intraarticular bupivacaine/morphine: a randomized clinical trial. Anesthesiology 1993;79(3):475–480.

40. Bridenbaugh PO, Du Pen SL, Moore DC. Postoperative intercostal nerve block analgesia versus narcotic analgesia. Anesth Analg 1973;52:81.

41. Toledo-Pereyra LH, DeMeester TR. Prospective randomized evaluation of intrathoracic intercostal nerve block with Dupicaine on postoperative ventilatory function. Ann Thorac Surg 1979;27(3):203.

42. Ross WB, Tweedle JH, Leong YP, et al. Intercostal blockade and pulmonary function after cholecystectomy. Surgery 1989;105:166–169.

43. Miguel R, Hubbell D. Postoperative pain management and pulmonary function after thoracotomy: a prospective randomized study. Anesthesiology 1990;73(3):A777.

44. Shuman RL, Peters RG. Epidural anesthesia following thoracotomy in patients with chronic obstructive airway disease. J Thorac Cardiovasc Surg 1976; 71:82.

45. Pflug AE, Murphy TM, Butler SH. The effects of postoperative peridural analgesia in pulmonary therapy and pulmonary complication. Anesthesiology 1974;41:8.

46. Evans C, Richardson PH. Improved recovery and reduced postoperative stay after therapeutic suggestions during general anaesthesia. Lancet 1988; 4:491–493.

47. Boeke S, Bonke B, Bouwhuis-Hoogerwerf ML, et al. Effects of sounds presented during general anaesthesia on postoperative course. Br J Anaesth 1988; 60:697–702.

48. McCallum MID, Glynn CJ, Moore RA, et al. Transcutaneous electrical nerve stimulation in the management of acute postoperative pain. Br J Anaesth 1988;61:308–312.

49. Denlinger JK. Prolonged emergence and failure to regain consciousness. In: Orkin FK, Cooperman LH, eds. Complications in anesthesiology. Philadelphia: JB Lippincott, 1983;368–379.

50. Longnecker DE, Grazis PA, Eggers GWN. Naloxone for antagonism of morphine induced respiratory depression. Anesth Analg 1973;52:447–453.

51. Jensen S, Knudsen L, Kirkegaard L, et al. Flumazenil used for antagonizing the central effects of midazolam and diazepam in outpatients. Acta Anaesthesiol Scand 1989;33:26–28.

52. Ghoneim MM, Dembo JB, Block RI. Time course of antagonism of sedative and amnesic effects of diazepam by flumazenil. Anesthesiology 1989;70:899–904.

53. Ghouri AF, Ramirez Ruiz MA, White PF. Effect of flumazenil on recovery after midazolam and propofol sedation. Anesthesiology 1994;81(2):333–339.

54. Bourke DL, Rosenberg M, Allen PD. Physostigmine: effectiveness as an antagonist of respiratory depression and psychomotor effects caused by morphine or diazepam. Anesthesiology 1984;61:523–528.

55. Hill GE, Stanley TH, Seutker CR. Physostigmine reversal of postoperative somnolence. Can J Anaesth 1977;24(6):707–711.

56. Skillman JJ. Neurologic complications of cardiovascular surgery: I. procedures involving the carotid arteries and abdominal aorta. In: Hindman BJ, ed. Neurological and psychological complications of surgery and anesthesia. Boston: Little, Brown & Co., 1986;135–158.

57. Shaw PJ. Neurologic complications of cardiovascular surgery: II. procedures involving the heart and thoracic aorta. In: Hindman BJ, ed. Neurological and psychological complications of surgery and anesthesia. Boston: Little, Brown & Co., 1986;159–174.

58. Hindman BJ. Perioperative stroke: the non-cardiac surgical patient. In: Hindman BJ, ed. Neurological and psychological complications of surgery and anesthesia. Boston: Little, Brown & Co., 1986;101–110.

59. Toung TJ, McPherson RW, Ahn H, et al. Pneumo-cephalus: effects of patient position on the incidence and location of aerocele after posterior fossa and upper cervical cord surgery. Anesth Analg 1986;65(1):65–70.

60. Larsen SF, Zaric D, Boysen G. Postoperative cerebrovascular accidents in general surgery. Acta Anaesthesiol Scand 1988;32:698–701.

61. Williams-Russo P, Urquhart BL, Sharrock NE, et al. Post operative delirium: predictors and prognosis in elderly orthopedic patients. J Am Geriat Soc 1992; 40:759–767.

62. O'Keefe ST, Ni Chonchubhair A. Postoperative delirium in the elderly. Br J Anaesth 1994;73(5): 673–687.

63. Taenzer P, Melzack R, Jeans ME. Influence of psychological factors in postoperative pain, mood, and analgesic requirements. Pain 1986;24:331–342.

64. Smiler BG, Bartholomew EG, Sivak BJ. Physostigmine reversal of scopolamine delirium in obstetric patients. Am J Obstet Gynecol 1973;116:326–329.

65. Schroeder JA, Wolfe WM, Thomas MH, et al. The effect of intravenous ranitidine and metoclopramide on behavior, cognitive function, and affect. Anesth Analg 1994;78(2):359–364.

66. Eisendrath SJ, Goldman B, Douglas J, et al. Meperidine induced delirium. Am J Psychiatry 1987; 144:1062–1065.

67. Hammon K, Demartino BK. Postoperative delirium secondary to atropine premedication. Prog Anesthesiol 1985;32:107–108.

68. Heath PJ, Kennedy DJ, Ogg TW, et al. Which intravenous induction agent for day surgery? A comparison of propofol, thiopentone, methohexitone, and etomidate. Anaesthesia 1988;43:365–368.

69. Aakerlund LP, Rosenberg F. Postoperative delirium: treatment with supplementary oxygen. Br J Anaesth 1994;72(3):286–290.

70. Oliver SB, Cucchiara RF, Warner MA, et al. Unexpected focal neurologic deficit on emergence from anesthesia: a report of three cases. Anesthesiology 1987;67:823–826.

71. Aldrete JA, Kroulik D. A postanesthetic recovery score. Anesth Analg 1970;49:924.

72. Steward DJ. A simplified scoring system for the postoperative recovery room. Can J Anaesth 1975; 22:111.

II

Clinical Aspects of Postanesthesia Care: Physiology, Pathophysiology, and Management

4

FLUID AND ELECTROLYTE MANAGEMENT

Mali Mathru, Donald S. Prough

Trauma and surgery acutely alter the volumes and composition of the intracellular and extracellular spaces. Subsequent therapeutic infusion of fluids, primarily intended to replenish blood volume and maintain cardiac output, further alters compartmental volumes and composition. Both hypovolemia, which increases the risk of organ hypoperfusion and injury, and hypervolemia, which increases the risk of pulmonary edema, are potential hazards of perioperative fluid therapy. In addition to acute changes in intravascular, interstitial, and intracellular volume, surgical patients may develop potentially harmful disorders of the concentrations and total body content of important electrolytes. Precise perioperative management of fluids and electrolytes may minimize surgical morbidity and mortality.

PHYSIOLOGY

Body Fluid Compartments

Accurate replacement of fluid deficits necessitates an understanding of the distribution spaces of water, sodium, and colloid (Fig. 4–1). Total body water (TBW), the distribution volume of sodium-free water, approximates 60% of total body weight, or 42 L in a 70-kg person. TBW consists of intracellular volume (ICV), which constitutes 40% of total body weight (28 L in a 70-kg person), and extracellular volume (ECV), which constitutes 20% of body weight (14 L). Plasma volume (PV),

approximately 3 L, equals about one-fifth of ECV, the remainder of which is interstitial fluid (IF). Red cell volume, approximately 2 L, is part of ICV.

The ECV contains most of the sodium in the body, with equal sodium concentrations ([Na^+]) in the PV and IF, i.e., plasma [Na^+] is approximately 140 mEq·L^{-1}; intracellular [Na^+] is approximately 10 mEq·L^{-1}. The predominant intracellular cation is potassium; the intracellular concentration ([K^+]) is approximately 150 mEq·L^{-1}, in contrast to a [K^+] in ECV of approximately 4.0 mEq·L^{-1}. Albumin, the most important oncotically active constituent of ECV, is unequally distributed in PV (~4 g·dL^{-1}) and IF (~1 g·dL^{-1}) and is virtually excluded from ICV. The IF concentration of albumin varies greatly among tissues. TBW is the distribution volume for sodium-free water; ECV is the distribution volume both for crystalloid solutions in which [Na^+] is approximately 140 mEq·L^{-1} and for colloid, although colloid usually is distributed primarily within the PV.

Distribution of Infused Fluids

Assume that a 70-kg patient has suffered an acute blood loss of 2000 mL, approximately 40% of the predicted 5-L blood volume. Also assume that shed blood is to be replaced with 5% dextrose in water (D5W), lactated Ringer's solution, or 5% or 25% human serum albumin. The formula describing the effects of fluid infusion on PV is as follows:

Fig. 4–1. The distribution volume of water, approximately 60% of total body weight, includes both the extracellular (ECV) and intracellular volume (ICV). Sodium is distributed primarily in the ECV. If capillary integrity is preserved, the concentration of colloid is higher in the plasma volume (PV) than in interstitial fluid (IF). RBC = red blood cells. $[Na_i^+]$ and $[Na_e^+]$ = intracellular and extracellular concentrations of sodium, respectively; $[K_i^+]$ and $[K_e^+]$ represent intracellular and extracellular concentrations of potassium.

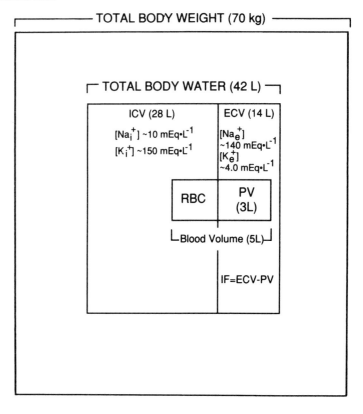

Expected PV increment = volume infused × normal PV/distribution volume

Rearranging the equation yields the following:

Volume infused = expected PV increment × distribution volume/normal PV

To restore blood volume using D5W (which distributes throughout TBW) would require 28 L:

$$28\ L = 2\ L \times 42\ L/3\ L$$

where 2 L is the desired PV increment, 42 L = TBW in a 70-kg person, and 3 L is the normal estimated PV.

To restore blood volume using lactated Ringer's solution (which distributes through-out ECV) would require infusion of approximately 9.3 L:

$$9.3\ L = 2\ L \times 14\ L/3\ L$$

where 14 L = ECV in a 70-kg person.

If 5% albumin or 6% hetastarch, both of which exert oncotic pressure similar to or slightly greater than that of plasma, were infused, most of the volume initially would remain in the PV (the approximate distribution volume), perhaps attracting additional interstitial fluid intravascularly. Twenty-five percent human serum albumin, a hyperoncotic fluid, expands PV by approximately 400 mL for each 100 mL infused, because of translocation of interstitial fluid.

Regulation of Extracellular Fluid Volume

Both low-pressure and high-pressure receptors detect changes in blood volume and blood pressure. Low-pressure intrathoracic volume receptors, located within the great veins, cardiac atria, and pulmonary capillaries, readily detect decreases in blood volume. High-pressure arterial receptors, found within the carotid sinuses, aortic arch, and intrarenal arterioles, are sensitive to decreased perfusion pressure.

To preserve circulating blood volume and organ perfusion, afferent signals from volume and pressure receptors must be converted to efferent signals. In response to decreased renal perfusion pressure, intrarenal barore-ceptors initiate renin release, which increases the production of angiotensin II and aldosterone, which in turn increase blood pressure, increase afferent glomerular arteriolar resistance, and enhance sodium reabsorption. Activation of the sympathetic nervous system, secretion of antidiuretic hormone (ADH), and suppression of atrial natriuretic peptide (ANP) release also serve to increase systemic vascular resistance and conserve sodium and water during volume depletion. Thirst and salt craving stimulate increased intake of water and sodium. Insufficiency or pharmacologic antagonism of these systems may aggravate hypovolemia.

Renal adaptation to hypovolemia (and decreased cardiac output) occurs through three primary mechanisms: a reduction in renal blood flow (RBF), a reduction in glomerular filtration, and increased tubular reabsorption of sodium and water (1). Initially, RBF is maintained (i.e., RBF is autoregulated) as perfusion pressure decreases by reductions in renal afferent arteriolar resistance. Further decreases in cardiac output may decrease the fraction of cardiac output delivered to the kidneys. Increases in renal vascular resistance redistribute blood flow from the kidneys in an attempt to preserve perfusion of other tissues.

As RBF decreases, the efferent arterioles constrict, primarily in response to angiotensin II and norepinephrine, thereby increasing the filtration fraction (FF), according to the equation:

$$FF = \text{(afferent arteriolar plasma flow-efferent arteriolar plasma flow)/afferent arteriolar lasma flow} \times 100$$

Renal perfusion during acute hypovolemia is determined by the balance between renal vasoconstrictive factors (the renal sympathetic nerves, angiotensin II, and catecholamines) and vasodilatory mechanisms (intrinsic renal autoregulation and the renal vasodilatory effects of prostaglandins) (2). Although RBF autoregulates (remains constant over a wide range of perfusion pressures), autoregulation may be impaired or lost during severe, acute hypovolemia (3, 4). Renal sympathetic stimulation with secretion of α-adrenergic catecholamines (2) and angiotensin II increases renal vascular resistance. Hypovolemia also redistributes renal perfusion from outer cortical nephrons to inner cortical nephrons (5), in which longer loops of Henle, which penetrate more deeply into the hypertonic renal medulla, are capable of greater sodium conservation.

To preserve PV, reabsorption of filtered water and sodium is enhanced by changes mediated by the hormonal factors ADH, ANP, and aldosterone. Although a change in serum osmolality of only 1 to 2% significantly alters ADH secretion from the posterior pituitary, a 10 to 20% decrease in blood volume is necessary before ADH secretion increases (Fig. 4–2) (6). ADH acts primarily on the medullary collecting ducts and to a lesser extent on the cortical collecting tubules to increase water permeability, resulting in greater water reabsorption and the excretion of smaller volumes of more highly concentrated urine. Water excretion is further reduced in volume-depleted patients by impaired delivery of tubular fluid to distal nephron sites and by ADH-independent water reabsorption by the collecting ducts.

In contrast to increased secretion of ADH, ANP secretion is decreased during hypovolemia. ANP, released from the cardiac atria in response to increased atrial stretch, exerts vasodilatory effects and increases the renal ex-

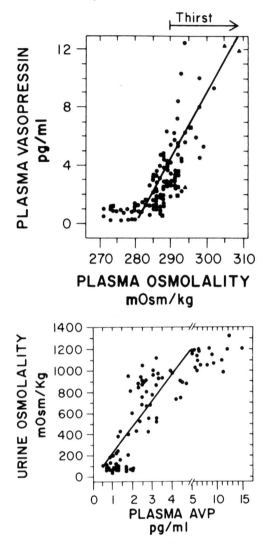

Fig. 4–2. *Top,* As plasma osmolality increases beyond a threshold of approximately 280 mOsm·kg⁻¹, plasma arginine vasopressin (antidiuretic hormone) progressively increases. *Bottom,* As plasma concentrations of arginine vasopressin (AVP) increase, urinary osmolality progressively increases to reach a plateau of approximately 1200 mOsm·kg⁻¹. (Reproduced with permission from Hall J, Robertson G. Diabetes insipidus. Prob Crit Care 1990;4:342–354.)

cretion of sodium and water (7–11). Many of the physiologic effects of ANP seem to be hemodynamically mediated, increasing the glomerular filtration rate (GFR) and resulting in diuresis.

In volume-depleted states, sodium conservation results both from decreased filtration of sodium (decreased GFR) and from increased tubular reabsorption of sodium. Aldosterone, the most important humoral regulator of sodium reabsorption, is produced by the adrenal cortex as the final product of a series of endocrine events. Hypoperfusion stimulates the release of renin from the granular cells of the juxtaglomerular apparatus. Renin catalyzes the conversion of angiotensinogen to angiotensin I. Angiotensin-converting enzyme converts angiotensin I to angiotensin II, and finally, angiotensin II stimulates the adrenal cortex to synthesize and release aldosterone (12–14). Acting primarily in the distal tubules, high concentrations of aldosterone may reduce urinary excretion of sodium nearly to zero.

The kidney also contains large quantities of prostaglandin metabolites that appear to modulate changes in renal vascular tone and glomerular filtration produced by other hormones (15). Vasodilator prostaglandins may play a crucial role in protecting the kidney from the effects of systemic vasoconstrictor hormones and for maintaining RBF during hypovolemia. The protective effect of endogenous renal prostaglandins may be lost if renal circulatory compromise develops in patients receiving nonsteroidal anti-inflammatory drugs (16).

FLUID REPLACEMENT THERAPY

Maintenance Requirements for Water, Sodium, and Potassium

In healthy adults, sufficient water is required to balance gastrointestinal losses of 100 to 200 mL·day⁻¹, insensible losses of 500 to 1000 mL·day⁻¹ (half of which is respiratory and half cutaneous), and urinary losses of 1000 mL·day⁻¹. When deciding whether to replace urinary losses exceeding 1000 mL·day⁻¹, it is prudent to consider whether increased urinary output represents an appropriate physiologic response to ECV expansion

Table 4–1. Maintenance Water Requirements

Weight (kg)	$ml \cdot kg^{-1} \cdot h^{-1}$	$ml \cdot kg^{-1} \cdot day^{-1}$
1–10	4	100
11–20	2	50
21–n	1	20

or an inability to conserve salt or water. Two simple formulas are used interchangeably to estimate maintenance water requirements (Table 4–1).

Renal sodium conservation is highly efficient. Although the average adult requires 75 mEq daily, sodium excretion can decrease to less than 10 mEq per day during chronic sodium depletion. Because the kidneys also efficiently excrete excess sodium, patients with normal cardiac and renal reserve tolerate sodium intake far in excess of normal daily requirements. Renal conservation and excretion of potassium are less efficient. Daily potassium requirements slightly exceed 40 mEq. Physiologic diuresis typically induces an obligate potassium loss of at least $10~mEq \cdot L^{-1}$ of urine. Other electrolytes such as chloride, calcium, and magnesium require no short-term replacement, although they must be supplied during chronic intravenous fluid maintenance.

Combining the above, the predicted daily maintenance fluid requirements for healthy, 70-kg adults is $2500~mL \cdot day^{-1}$ of a solution with a $[Na^+]$ of $30~mEq \cdot L^{-1}$ and a $[K^+]$ of 15 to $20~mEq \cdot L^{-1}$. However, in practice, the $[Na^+]$ in postoperatively administered fluids is typically $77~mEq \cdot L^{-1}$. Approximately one half of the volume of this fluid, colloquially termed "half-normal" saline, is sodium-free water. Intraoperatively, fluids containing free water are rarely employed in adults, largely because of the necessity for replacing losses of PV and IF, both of which are sodium rich.

Dextrose

Traditionally, glucose-containing intravenous fluids have been given in an effort to prevent hypoglycemia and limit protein catab-

olism. However, because of the hyperglycemic response associated with surgical stress, only infants and patients receiving insulin or drugs that interfere with glucose synthesis are at risk for hypoglycemia. Iatrogenic hyperglycemia can limit the effectiveness of fluid resuscitation by inducing an osmotic diuresis and, in animals, may aggravate global and focal neurologic ischemic injury (17, 18). The clinical influence of hyperglycemia on neurologic injury in humans is less well defined. Although hyperglycemia is associated with worse outcome in both ischemic (19) and traumatic (20) brain injury, it is likely that the increase in blood glucose in patients is, in fact, a hormonally mediated accompaniment of more severe injury (19). Sieber et al. have concisely summarized the issue of intraoperative glucose administration by stating, "glucose administration is indicated during clinical situations where hypoglycemia is likely to occur" (21).

SURGICAL FLUID REQUIREMENTS

Water and Electrolyte Composition of Fluid Losses

Surgical patients require replacement of PV and ECV losses secondary to wound or burn edema, ascites, and gastrointestinal secretions. Wound and burn edema and ascitic fluid are protein-rich and contain electrolytes in concentrations similar to plasma. If ECV is adequate and renal and cardiovascular function are normal, all gastrointestinal secretions (Table 4–2) can be replaced using lactated Ringer's solution or 0.9% ("normal") saline. Substantial loss of gastrointestinal fluids requires replacement of other electrolytes (i.e., potassium, magnesium, phosphate). However, if cardiovascular or renal function is impaired, more precise replacement may require frequent assessment of serum electrolytes. Chronic gastric losses may produce hypochloremic metabolic alkalosis that can be corrected with 0.9% saline; chronic diarrhea may produce hyperchloremic metabolic acidosis

Table 4–2.   Average Volumes and Electrolyte Composition of Gastrointestinal Secretions

Source	Volume (ml · day^{-1})	[Na$^+$] (mEq · L^{-1})	[K$^+$] (mEq · L^{-1})	Cl$^-$ (mEq · L^{-1})	HCO$_3^-$ (mEq · L^{-1})
Gastric	1500	60	10	130	—
Ileal	3000	140	5	104	30
Pancreatic	400	140	5	75	115
Biliary	400	140	5	100	35

that may be prevented or corrected by infusion of fluid containing bicarbonate or bicarbonate substrate (i.e., lactate).

Fluid Shifts During Surgery

Replacement of intraoperative fluid losses must compensate for the acute reduction of functional IF that accompanies trauma, hemorrhage, and tissue manipulation. This reduction, often called "third-space" loss (22, 23), is surprisingly extensive. Upper abdominal surgery not involving major hemorrhage is associated with a 15% decline in functional ECV, the reservoir available for physiologic repletion of PV in response to hypovolemia (22). Otherwise healthy subjects undergoing gastric or gallbladder surgery demonstrate a decline in ECV of nearly 2 L and an acute 13% decline in GFR when they receive no intraoperative sodium (22). In contrast, patients who receive lactated Ringer's solution maintain ECV and increase GFR by 10%. In more extensive surgical procedures, the decrease in ECV is presumably much greater.

No data describe acute changes in PV, IF, and ICV during acute, unresuscitated shock in humans. In response to mild hemorrhage in humans, the net transfer of IF to PV is as rapid as 500 mL every 10 minutes (24). In contrast, during prolonged experimental hemorrhagic shock, both sodium and water accumulate intracellularly (25). Shock depletes energy stores and impairs cellular membrane function (26). Shock-induced alterations in cellular membrane function and intracellular concentrations of sodium seem to return to normal after systemic hemodynamic

stability is restored. Patients studied during the first 10 days after resuscitation from massive trauma in fact demonstrated a slight percentage decrease in ICV (27); however, total body weight was increased as a consequence of a 55% increase in IF volume (Fig. 4–3) (27). As would be expected, because of the reduction of colloid osmotic pressure in traumatized patients, the ratio of IF to blood volume is increased, exceeding 5:1 in some patients (27).

Based on the above considerations, guidelines have been developed for replacement of fluid losses during surgical procedures. The simplest formula provides, in addition to maintenance fluids and replacement of estimated blood loss, 2 to 4 mL·kg^{-1}·h^{-1} for procedures involving minimal trauma, 6 to 8 mL·kg^{-1}·h^{-1} for those involving moderate trauma, and 8 to 10 mL·kg^{-1}·h^{-1} for those involving extreme trauma.

Mobilization of Expanded Interstitial Fluid

An important corollary of IF expansion is the mobilization and return of accumulated fluid to the ECV and the PV, colloquially termed "deresuscitation." For most patients, mobilization occurs on approximately the third postoperative day, although it may occur sooner or later, depending on patient characteristics, the severity and duration of the initial insult, and the development of postoperative complications such as acute renal failure or sepsis. If the cardiovascular system and kidneys can effectively transport and excrete mobilized fluid, no important physiologic consequences

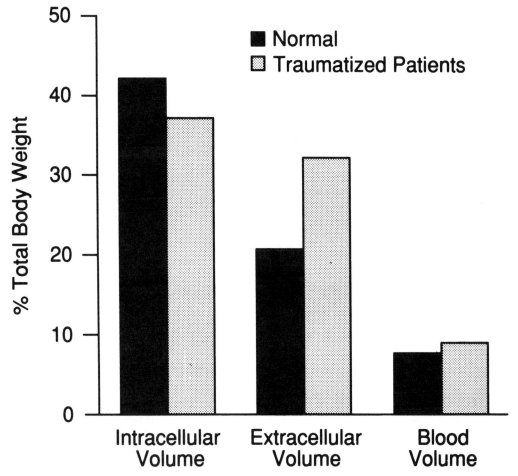

Fig. 4–3. In comparison with normal individuals, patients recently subjected to severe trauma (fluid and blood requirements exceeding an average of 21 L on the day of admission) have a slight decrease in intracellular volume (as percentage of body weight) and an increase in extracellular volume and blood volume. (Data redrawn with permission from Böck JC, Barker BC, Clinton AG, et al. Post-traumatic changes in, and effect of colloid osmotic pressure on the distribution of body water. Ann Surg 1989;210:395–405.)

follow. However, if the cardiovascular system is unable to accommodate the increase in intravascular volume or the kidneys are unable to increase urinary volume (i.e., because of renal insufficiency or stress-induced secretion of ADH), hypervolemia and pulmonary edema may occur.

COLLOIDS, CRYSTALLOIDS, AND HYPERTONIC SOLUTIONS

Physiology and Pharmacology

Intravenous fluids vary in oncotic pressure, osmolarity, and tonicity. Osmotically active particles attract water across semipermeable membranes until equilibrium is attained. The osmolarity of a solution refers to the number of osmotically active particles per liter of solution. In contrast, osmolality is a measurement of the number of osmotically active particles per kilogram of solvent. Serum osmolality (in $mmol \cdot kg^{-1}$) can be estimated as follows:

$$Osmolality = ([Na^+] \times 2) + (Glucose/18) + (BUN/2.3)$$

where $[Na^+]$ is expressed in $mEq \cdot L^{-1}$, serum glucose is expressed in $mg \cdot dL^{-1}$, and BUN is blood urea nitrogen expressed in mg·dL^{-1}. Sugars, alcohols, and radiographic dyes that increase osmolality may further increase the measured value, generating an increased "osmolal gap" between the calculated and measured values.

A hyperosmolar state occurs whenever the concentration of osmotically active particles is high. A hypertonic state occurs when an osmotically active solute is concentrated in the ECV. Thus, both uremia (increased BUN) and hypernatremia (increased serum sodium) increase serum osmolality. However, because urea distributes throughout TBW, an increase in BUN, unlike an increase in [Na$^+$], does not cause hypertonicity. Sodium, largely restricted to the ECV, causes osmotically mediated redistribution of water from ICV to ECV. The term "tonicity" is also used colloquially to compare the osmotic pressure of a solution to that of plasma. A fluid in which the osmotic pressure is similar to that of plasma is termed isotonic. Hypotonic solutions exert lower osmotic pressures than plasma; hypertonic solutions exert higher osmotic pressures.

Although only a small proportion of the osmotically active particles in blood consist of plasma proteins, those particles are essential in determining the equilibrium of fluid between the interstitial and plasma compartments of ECV. Because systemic capillary beds are only semipermeable to plasma proteins, interstitial protein concentrations remain lower than plasma. The reflection coefficient (σ) describes the permeability of capillary membranes to individual solutes, with 0 representing free permeability and 1.0 representing complete impermeability. For example, σ for albumin ranges from 0.6 to 0.9 in various capillary beds. Because capillary protein concentrations exceed interstitial concentrations, the osmotic pressure exerted by plasma proteins (termed "colloid osmotic pressure" or "oncotic pressure") is higher than interstitial oncotic pressure and tends to preserve PV. The filtration rate of fluid from the capillaries into the interstitial space is the net result of a combination of forces, including the gradient from intravascular to interstitial colloid osmotic pressures and the hydrostatic gradient between intravascular and interstitial pressures. The net fluid filtration at any point within a systemic or pulmonary capillary is represented by Starling's law of capillary filtration (Fig. 4–4), as expressed in the equation:

$$Q = kA \left[(P_c - P_i) + \sigma(\pi_i - \pi_c) \right]$$

where Q = fluid filtration, k = capillary filtration coefficient (conductivity of water), A = the area of the capillary membrane, P_c = capillary hydrostatic pressure, P_i = interstitial hydrostatic pressure, π_i = interstitial colloid osmotic pressure, and π_c = capillary colloid osmotic pressure.

The IF volume is determined by the relative rates of capillary filtration and lymphatic drainage; homeostatic mechanisms acutely accommodate limited amounts of excess fluid. P_c, the most powerful factor favoring fluid filtration, is determined by capillary flow, arterial resistance, venous resistance, and venous pressure (28). Increased capillary filtration alters the balance of forces in the Starling equilibrium. Usually, the rate of water and sodium filtration exceeds protein filtration, resulting in preservation of π_c, dilution of π_i, and preservation of the oncotic pressure gradient, the most powerful factor opposing fluid filtration. When coupled with increased lymphatic drainage, preservation of the oncotic pressure gradient limits the accumulation of IF. Although IF contains less protein than plasma, the interstitium contains glycosaminoglycans and proteoglycans that absorb fluid. As increased IF decreases the concentrations of glycosaminoglycans and proteoglycans, fluid and protein drain more freely into the lymphatics (29). If P_c is increased at a time when lymphatic drainage is maximal, then IF accumulates, forming edema. In chronic edematous states, IF pressure is reduced by enhanced lymphatic drainage through dilated lymphatic vessels (30). The proteoglycans in the vascular basement membrane also help to maintain normal vascular permeability. Dilution of this

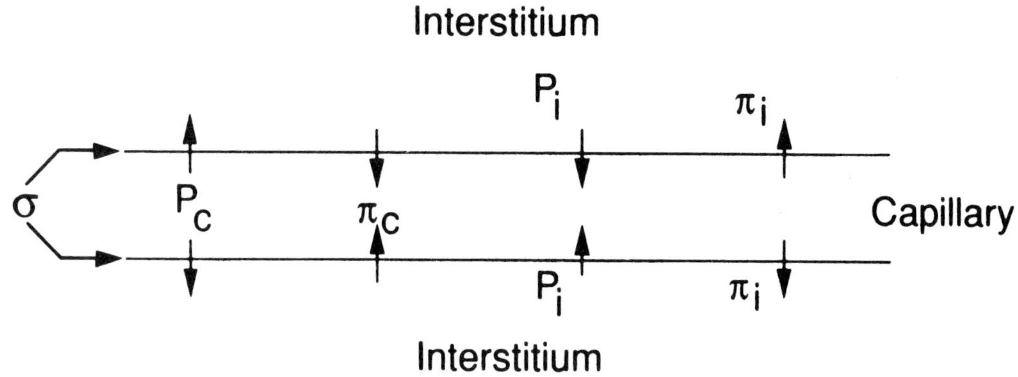

Interstitium

Fig. 4–4. Movement of fluid between the capillaries and the interstitium is a function of hydrostatic pressure in the capillaries (P_c) and in the interstitium (P_i) and oncotic pressure in the capillaries (π_c) and in the interstitium (π_i). The permeability of the capillary membrane to albumin is described by the reflection coefficient, σ.

proteoglycan matrix increases while dehydration of the interstitium reduces vascular permeability (28).

Clinical Implications of Choices Between Alternative Fluids

If membrane permeability is intact, fluids containing colloids such as albumin or hydroxyethyl starch preferentially expand PV rather than IF volume. Concentrated colloid-containing solutions (i.e., 25% albumin) may exert sufficient oncotic pressure to translocate substantial volumes of IF into the PV. PV expansion unaccompanied by IF expansion offers apparent advantages: lower fluid requirements, less peripheral and pulmonary edema accumulation, and reduced concern about the cardiopulmonary consequences of later fluid mobilization.

However, exhaustive research has failed to establish the superiority of either colloid-containing or crystalloid-containing fluids. Colloid solutions require a smaller initial infused volume, generate a more prolonged increase in PV, and are associated with less peripheral edema but are not less likely to increase intracranial pressure (Table 4–3). Crystalloid is less expensive, tends to increase glomerular filtration, and more effectively replaces depleted IF. However, crystalloid fluids exert short-lived hemodynamic effects in comparison to colloid and, when used for massive resuscitation, invariably produce peripheral edema. Crystalloid solutions are also associated with pulmonary edema, usually as a result of increased left atrial pressure, perhaps in combination with a reduction of the gradient between π_c and pulmonary P_c. The disadvantages of colloid-containing fluids include greater expense, coagulopathy (especially with dextran), a reduction in ionized calcium (with albumin), impaired cross-matching (with dextran), a reduction in GFR, and osmotic diuresis (with low molecular weight dextran). Finally, in disease states associated with increased alveolar capillary permeability (i.e., sepsis or the adult respiratory distress syndrome), infusion of colloid may aggravate pulmonary edema. If microvascular permeability increases (i.e., σ decreases), as commonly occurs in response to injury, infection, or prolonged tissue hypoperfusion, the gradient between π_c and π_i diminishes. In the absence of an oncotic pressure gradient, the hydraulic gradient is unopposed and minimal increases in P_c can result in clinically important edema accumulation.

Although hydroxyethyl starch, the most commonly used synthetic colloid, is less expensive than albumin, large doses produce laboratory evidence of coagulopathy (31).

Table 4–3.   Advantages and Disadvantages of Colloid Versus Crystalloid Intravenous Fluids

Solution	Advantages	Disadvantages
Colloid	Smaller infused volume Prolonged increase in plasma volume Greater peripheral edema	Greater cost Coagulopathy (dextran > HES) Pulmonary edema (capillary leak states) Decreased GFR Osmotic diuresis (low-molecular-weight dextran)
Crystalloid	Lower cost Greater urinary flow Replaces interstitial fluid	Transient hemodynamic improvement Peripheral edema Pulmonary edema (protein dilution plus high PAOP)

HES, hydroxyethyl starch; GFR, glomerular filtration rate; PAOP, pulmonary artery occlusion pressure.

However, 6.0% hydroxyethyl starch, used in recommended volumes, is not apparently associated with clinically important coagulopathy (32–35). Gold et al. randomly assigned 40 patients undergoing repair of abdominal aortic aneurysms to receive either 5.0% albumin or 6.0% hydroxyethyl starch in a dose of 1 g·kg⁻¹ (approximately 1200 mL of the albumin solution or 1100 mL of the hydroxyethyl starch solution in a 70-kg adult) (32). All objective measurements of coagulation status at all intervals were comparable and within normal limits. Blood loss, total fluid required, and subjective assessment of surgical bleeding were similar. The use of hydroxyethyl starch also produced no clinical coagulopathy in patients undergoing major abdominal surgery (33) or cardiac surgery (34, 35).

Part of the difficulty in defining the superiority of crystalloid or colloid fluids is directly attributable to the difficulty of defining comparable experimental endpoints (Table 4–4) (36, 37). Because PV expansion persists longer after colloid administration, substantially greater quantities of crystalloid must be given to maintain comparable systemic hemodynamics. In general, to achieve comparable PV expansion, isotonic crystalloids must be infused in volumes at least four to five times greater than volumes of iso-oncotic colloid solutions. Infusion of iso-oncotic colloid solutions significantly increases PV for at least 2 hours after infusion (38). The necessity for infusion of four to five times as much crystalloid as colloid, reflecting the fact that PV

is only one-fifth of ECV, may be exaggerated in hypoproteinemic traumatized patients, in whom the ratio may be much higher (27).

More recently developed experimental models compare crystalloid and colloid solutions in specific, clinically modeled situations. Baum et al., comparing lactated Ringer's solution to 6.0% hydroxyethyl starch dissolved in 0.9% saline in animals infused with *Escherichia coli* lipopolysaccharide, evaluated mesenteric blood flow, mesenteric oxygen delivery, ileal hydrogen ion concentration, and ileal and pulmonary extravascular water (39). In that model, which mimics some aspects of clinical sepsis, clinically relevant doses of lactated Ringer's solution or 6.0% hydroxyethyl starch produced comparable effects on the critical endpoint of oxygen delivery while producing the expected differences in extravascular fluid accumulation. The efficacy with which various colloids restore oxygen transport after surgical hemorrhagic shock has been investigated in a more complex porcine model, consisting of temporary exteriorization of the small intestine accompanied by incremental hemorrhage and replacement (40). Colloid solutions, in contrast to Ringer's acetate solution, produced superior restoration of cardiac output, oxygen delivery, and oxygen consumption. Although the results are intriguing, one possible interpretation is that an insufficient volume of Ringer's acetate was infused.

One of the most intriguing developments in colloid research is the possibility that pentafraction, the generic name attached to hydro-

Table 4–4. Possible Endpoints for Comparison of Resuscitation Fluids

Endpoint	Advantages	Disadvantages
Equal volume	Simple calculation	Different acute effects and time course
Equal sodium load	Simple calculation	Different acute effects and time course
Equal preload (i.e., CVP, PAOP)	Simple, continuous measurement	Determined by multiple, simultaneously changing variables
Equal cardiac output	Simple measurement, easily repeated	Misleading if fluids differently affect hemoglobin concentration
Equal DO_2	Logical, physiologically appealing endpoint	Difficult calculation to perform frequently; calculated from two simultaneously changing variables
Equal VO_2	Physiologically important variable	Difficult calculation to perform frequently; calculated from simultaneously changing variables

CVP, central venous pressure; PAOP, pulmonary artery occlusion pressure; DO_2, systemic oxygen delivery; VO_2, systemic oxygen consumption.
Reproduced with permission from Prough DS, Johnston WE. Fluid resuscitation in septic shock: no solution yet. Anesth Analg 1989;69:699–704.

xyethyl starch molecules of a specific size range (100,000 to 1,000,000 daltons), may actually counteract increases in capillary permeability associated with a variety of lesions, including myocardial ischemia (41), scalded rat jejunum (42), ischemic muscle (43), and endotoxin-damaged lung (44). In such models, fluid accumulation in injured tissue and permeability to protein are substantially reduced. If these data can be confirmed in clinical states associated with increased permeability, pentafraction may offer major therapeutic advantages in hypovolemic patients with sepsis or adult respiratory distress syndrome.

Pulmonary Implications of Colloid Osmotic Pressure

Much of the acrimonious controversy regarding the merits of perioperative fluid therapy with either colloids or crystalloids stems from the theoretical effects of the two types of fluids on the risk of pulmonary edema in patients who have diseases that increase pulmonary P_c, decrease π_c, or decrease σ. Some clinicians preferentially administer colloid solutions, hoping to reduce the risk of pulmonary edema by increasing π_c. Hypoproteine-mia in critically ill patients has been associated with the development of pulmonary edema (45, 46) and with increased mortality (47). However, either crystalloid or colloid administration may precipitate pulmonary edema in patients who have valvular heart disease, decreased left ventricular compliance, or decreased left ventricular contractility (i.e., heart failure). Increased left atrial pressure increases filtration from PV into IF and, if fluid accumulates, into the alveoli. Expansion of PV with colloid, unlike expansion with crystalloid, resolves slowly; if pulmonary edema develops, diuretic therapy is often required.

The administration of large volumes of crystalloid solutions dilutes serum protein concentrations, reducing π_c and enhancing interstitial accumulation of fluid. However, increasing filtration of protein-poor fluid dilutes pulmonary π_i, increases P_i, and enhances lymphatic flow. These physiologic defenses must be overwhelmed before the accumulation of interstitial fluid results in clinically apparent pulmonary edema.

There seems to be no clinically important differences in pulmonary function after administration of crystalloid or colloid solutions in the absence of hypervolemia (48–51). After

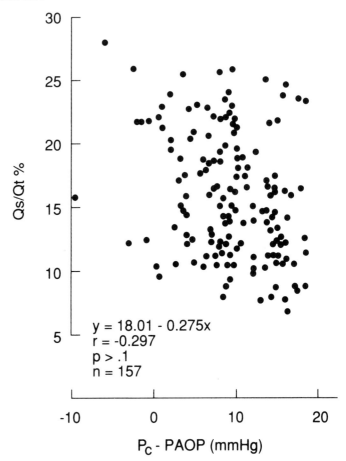

Fig. 4–5. There is poor correlation between intrapulmonary shunt fraction (Qs/Qt%) and the difference between colloid oncotic pressure (COP) and pulmonary capillary wedge pressure (PCWP) in patients undergoing major surgical procedures. (Reproduced with permission from Virgilio RW, Smith DE, Zarins CK. Balanced electrolyte solutions: experimental and clinical studies. Crit Care Med 1979;7: 98–106.)

$$y = 18.01 - 0.275x$$
$$r = -0.297$$
$$p > .1$$
$$n = 157$$

experimentally increasing microvascular permeability, Pearl et al. found no differences between increases in extravascular lung water induced by colloid or crystalloid (52).

In surgical patients at risk for the development of pulmonary edema, pulmonary artery catheterization may facilitate management. If the σ for albumin is likely to be decreased, pulmonary fluid accumulation becomes highly dependent on pulmonary P_c; therefore, pulmonary artery occlusion pressure (PAOP) should be maintained at the lowest practical level. However, if increased microvascular permeability occurs in conjunction with hypovolemia, administration of fluid to improve organ perfusion directly conflicts with the goal of minimizing pulmonary P_c. Theoretically, hemodynamic monitoring coupled with volume expansion with colloid should minimize edema formation. However, Virgilio et al. found no correlation in surgical patients between intrapulmonary shunt fraction (Q_s/Q_t) and the π_c-PAOP gradient (Fig. 4–5) (53).

Implications of Crystalloid and Colloid Infusions for Intracranial Pressure

Because the cerebral capillary membrane, the blood-brain barrier, is highly impermeable to protein, clinicians have assumed that administration of colloid-containing solutions should increase intracranial pressure (ICP) less than crystalloid solutions. In fact, in rabbits subjected to isovolemic hemodilution with 6.0% hetastarch or lactated Ringer's solution, the latter fluid was associated with a significant increase in ICP and brain water; no significant changes occurred in animals that had received 6.0% hetastarch (54). In dogs subjected to hemorrhagic shock in the presence of an intracranial mass lesion, resuscitation with 6.0% hetastarch resulted in a significantly lower ICP than did resuscitation with lactated Ringer's solution (55). However, in both studies, the difference probably occurred because 6.0% hetastarch is dissolved in 0.9% saline ($[Na^+]$ = 154 $mEq \cdot L^{-1}$). In contrast to 0.9% saline, lactated Ringer's solution ($[Na^+]$ = 130 $mEq \cdot L^{-1}$) is slightly hyposmotic relative to serum. In anesthetized rabbits subjected to plasmapheresis, a reduction in plasma osmolality of 13 $mOsm \cdot kg^{-1}$ (baseline value = 295 $mOsm \cdot kg^{-1}$) increased cortical water content and ICP; a reduction in oncotic pressure from 20 to 7 mm Hg produced no significant change in either variable (56). Subsequent studies in animals after forebrain ischemia (57) and cryogenic brain injury (58, 59) also clearly indicate that oncotic pressure exerts little if any effect on brain water accumulation. A prolonged reduction in colloid osmotic pressure generates peripheral edema but not cerebral edema (59).

Clinical Implications of Hypertonic Fluid Administration

An ideal alternative to conventional crystalloid and colloid fluids would be inexpensive, would produce minimal peripheral or pulmonary edema, and would generate sustained hemodynamic effects. In addition, the value for resuscitation of civilian or military trauma victims would be enhanced if the solution were effective, even if administered in smaller volumes than conventional fluids. Based on data gathered during the past decade, hypertonic, hypernatremic solutions seem to fulfill some of these criteria (Table 4–5).

Although investigators have studied various hypertonic resuscitation solutions for much of this century (60–64), current enthusiasm results from the work of Velasco et al. (65). They employed small volumes (6.0 $mL \cdot kg^{-1}$) of 7.5% hypertonic saline (HS) as the sole resuscitative measure in lightly anesthetized dogs that had been subjected to sufficient hemorrhage (averaging 23 ± 2.1 $mL \cdot kg^{-1}$) to reduce mean arterial pressure (MAP) to 45 to 50 mm Hg for 30 minutes. Hypertonic saline restored systolic blood pressure and cardiac output and increased mesen-

Table 4–5. Hypertonic Resuscitation Fluids: Advantages and Disadvantages

Solution	Advantages	Disadvantages
Hypertonic crystalloid	Inexpensive Promotion of urinary flow Small initial volume Improved myocardial contractility(?) Arteriolar dilation Reduced peripheral edema Lower intracranial pressure	Hypertonicity Precipitation of subdural hematoma Transient effect
Hypertonic crystalloid plus colloid (in comparison to hypertonic crystalloid alone)	Sustained hemodynamic response Reduced subsequent volume requirements	Added expense Coagulopathy (dextran > HES) Osmotic diuresis Impaired cross-match (dextran) Hypertonicity

HES, hydroxyethyl starch.
Reproduced with permission from Prough DS, Johnston WE. Fluid resuscitation in septic shock: no solution yet. Anesth Analg 1989;69:699–704.

teric blood flow to greater than control values for 6 hours after resuscitation. All animals in a group that had undergone slightly greater hemorrhage survived after infusion of 4.0 mL·kg^{-1} of 7.5% saline (65). Although post-treatment serum osmolality exceeded 330 mOsm·kg^{-1}, no animal showed adverse effects attributable to acute hypertonicity. Mattox et al. reported improved survival in traumatized patients initially resuscitated with 7.5% saline and requiring surgery (66).

Traditional goals of resuscitation have focused on restoring systemic hemodynamics but have paid less attention to reversing microvascular dysfunction induced by ischemia and reperfusion. Persistent reduction in regional perfusion despite successful restoration of systemic hemodynamics is one proposed mechanism of multisystem organ failure. Recent in vivo experimental evidence suggests that 7.2% NaCl + 10% HES attenuates leukocyte-endothelial interactions induced by shock and reperfusion. This improvement in microvascular perfusion is attributed to shrinkage of endothelial cells, thereby improving perfusion and facilitating the passage of leukocytes through the microvascular network (67).

The primary mechanism by which HS solutions improve systemic hemodynamics is through PV expansion (68). The beneficial effects of HS solutions also have been attributed to decreases in afterload, activation of pulmonary vagal reflexes, or increased cardiac contractility. However, in a recent canine study, Constable et al. demonstrated that infusion of 7.2% HS (4.0mL·kg) produced a negative inotropic effect (69). It remains to be determined whether HS elicits a similar negative inotropic effect in hypovolemic humans (69).

Although hyperosmotic saline solutions (usually 250 to 300 mEq·L^{-1} sodium) have been used for many years for burn resuscitation (62), recent studies in animals and humans suggest that highly hyperosmotic (7.5% sodium chloride in 6.0% dextran 70) (70) or less hyperosmotic saline (250 mEq·L^{-1} so-

dium) (71) are of limited value. In sheep subjected to a scald burn of 40% of body surface area, resuscitation with hyperosmotic saline-dextran (4 mL·kg^{-1}) only transiently improved hemodynamics (70) and, in comparison to conventional isosmotic (0.9% saline) resuscitation, was associated with a slightly longer interval before additional fluid therapy was required (70). In burned adults randomly assigned to receive lactated Ringer's solution or hyperosmotic saline to achieve comparable hemodynamic endpoints, the hyperosmotic solution did not decrease total fluid requirements, improve tolerance to feedings, or decrease edema accumulation (71).

Hypertonic solutions exert favorable effects on cerebral hemodynamics, in part because of the reciprocal relationship between plasma osmolality and brain water (56). ICP increases during resuscitation from hemorrhagic shock with lactated Ringer's solution but remains unchanged if 7.5% saline is infused in a sufficient volume to comparably improve systemic hemodynamics (72). In anesthetized rabbits, hypertonic lactated Ringer's solution (252 mEq·L^{-1} [Na$^+$]) maintains a lower ICP than 0.9% saline after isovolemic hemodilution (73). In hemorrhaged rats subjected to mechanical brain injury, brain water content in the injured hemisphere increases regardless of the resuscitation solution, but water content is lower in uninjured brain after resuscitation with a hyperosmotic solution (74). In dogs with intracranial mass lesions, hypertonic solutions may also restore regional cerebral blood flow better than slightly hypotonic solutions (75). However, recent data also suggest that differences between fluids of varying tonicity may become negligible if fluid resuscitation continues after immediate stabilization (76). In a randomized clinical study, Vassar et al. evaluated the effects of 250 mL of sodium chloride with and without 6% or 12% dextran 70 for the prehospital resuscitation of hypotensive trauma patients. The authors found that the addition of dextran to HS solution did not improve the blood pressure changes associated with administration of hypertonic saline alone. A small subgroup of patients with Glasgow Coma Scale scores lower than 8, but without severe anatomic injury, seemed to benefit most from the 7.5% sodium chloride (77).

Resuscitation with hyperosmotic solutions requires ongoing attention to maintenance of intravascular volume, because systemic hemodynamic improvements are short-lived. After initial improvement, both cerebral blood flow and cardiac output rapidly decline after single-dose resuscitation of hypovolemic (72) or oleic acid-injured (78) animals with either lactated Ringer's solution or hypertonic saline. In experimental endotoxic shock, acute improvements in MAP, cardiac output, and left ventricular stroke work associated with a combination hypertonic/hyperoncotic solution had greatly diminished by 60 minutes after infusion, despite continued maintenance of PAOP with additional fluid (79).

The transient effects of hypertonic saline administration represent a major obstacle to wider clinical application. Possible strategies that might prolong the therapeutic effects include continued infusion of hypertonic saline, subsequent infusion of blood or conventional fluids, or addition of colloid to hypertonic resuscitation. In hemorrhaged animals, adding 6.0% dextran 70 to 7.5% saline increased the duration of hemodynamic improvement when compared with equal volumes of hypertonic saline, sodium bicarbonate, or sodium chloride/sodium acetate (80). In traumatized patients, the combination of 6.0% dextran 70 in 7.5% saline for initial resuscitation increases blood pressure without adverse effects (81).

Initial concerns regarding the adverse neurologic sequelae of hypertonic resuscitation seem to have been premature. First, the increment in serum sodium in response to addition of concentrated sodium is less than would be expected (82). Second, patients tolerate acute increases in serum sodium to 155 to 160 $mEq \cdot L^{-1}$ without apparent harm (81, 83). Third, central pontine myelinolysis, which follows rapid correction of severe hyponatremia (84, 85), seems to be most likely after correc-

tion of chronic hyponatremia (86) and has not been observed in clinical trials of hypertonic resuscitation (81). Fourth, Wisner et al. used nuclear magnetic resonance spectroscopy to examine, in a rodent model of hemorrhagic shock, the effects of resuscitation on cerebral metabolism (87). They demonstrated that intracellular pH was lower after resuscitation with HS compared with lactated Ringer's solution. However, this decrease was not accompanied by changes in high-energy metabolites, suggesting that there was no anaerobic glycolysis. The reduction in intracellular pH was attributed to cellular dehydration and the resulting concentration of intracellular hydrogen ions (87).

The least encouraging observations regarding hyperosmotic resuscitation involve models of uncontrolled hemorrhage (88, 89), in which restoration of blood pressure increases bleeding and may adversely affect mortality (89). Although hyperosmotic solutions may offer superior prehospital restoration of blood pressure (66, 77), Bickell et al. reported that prehospital resuscitation was associated with increased mortality in comparison to resuscitation only after arrival in the operating room (90).

The clinical efficacy of hypertonic resuscitation in comparison to conventional fluids remains unclear, because most preclinical studies have compared the effects of single boluses of experimental and control fluids. Although such a design may duplicate acute field resuscitation after military or civilian trauma, routine fluid resuscitation rarely consists of a single bolus; instead, fluid administration continues until clinical signs indicate that no additional fluid is required. If single boluses of equal volumes of fluids of markedly differing tonicity are compared, the results of the comparison are predictable. Therefore, 6.0 $mL \cdot kg^{-1}$ of 0.9% saline should not be expected to produce hemodynamic effects equivalent to 6.0 $mL \cdot kg^{-1}$ of 7.5% saline. An attempt to simulate the clinical situation necessitates a choice among a variety of possible goals of resuscitation (Table 4–4). PAOP reflects the interaction of multiple variables, including blood volume, venous capacitance, and left ventricular afterload, diastolic compliance, and contractility. Consequently, comparison of two or more resuscitation regimens that alter more than one variable may generate misleading conclusions. For example, because hypertonic fluids reduce systemic vascular resistance, systolic ventricular ejection may improve, leading to decreased PAOP; theoretically, therefore, more fluid would be necessary to increase PAOP to the level produced by a colloid solution. Conversely, if hypertonicity-induced venoconstriction reduces the size of the capacitance bed, as suggested by Velasco et al. (65), a given blood volume should produce a greater PAOP. Therefore, the observation that hypertonic solutions do not reduce the volume of fluid required after the initial bolus may apply only if PAOP is used as the goal of resuscitation.

More physiologically sophisticated goals, also based on invasive monitoring, have been proposed. A predetermined level of systemic oxygen delivery (DO_2) is a theoretically attractive endpoint for resuscitation. It combines in a single term cardiac output (Q) and arterial oxygen content (CaO_2) according to the equation:

$$DO_2 = Q \cdot CaO_2 \cdot 10$$

where the factor 10 corrects CaO_2, usually measured in mL $O_2 \cdot dL^{-1}$, to mL$\cdot L^{-1}$.

However, because non-blood–containing fluid resuscitation both increases cardiac output and decreases hemoglobin concentration, the application of DO_2 as a goal poses practical difficulties. For example, in animals with oleic acid-induced pulmonary edema, cardiac output acutely increased 70% in response to infusion of HS whereas hemoglobin concentration decreased 12%; therefore, DO_2 increased. However, as the effects of fluid infusion on cardiac output dissipated, the hemoglobin remained lower than preinfusion values, resulting in a small decline in DO_2 from preinfusion levels. Despite the straightforward

arithmetic implications of simultaneous increases in cardiac output and decreases in CaO_2, many clinicians attempt to increase cardiac output (whether or not it is directly measured) as a goal during rapid volume expansion.

Will clinicians routinely use hypertonic or combination hypertonic/hyperoncotic fluids for resuscitation in the future? At present, there is no clear answer. Burn resuscitation is the only clinical situation in which hypertonic resuscitation solutions are commonly employed. Pending further preclinical work, the theoretical advantages of such fluids seem most attractive in the acute resuscitation of hypovolemic patients who have decreased intracranial compliance.

FLUID STATUS: ASSESSMENT AND MONITORING

Assessment of Hypovolemia and Tissue Hypoperfusion

Two contrasting methods are used to assess the adequacy of intravascular volume. The first method, conventional clinical assessment, is appropriate for most patients; the second method, goal-directed hemodynamic management, may be superior for high-risk surgical patients.

Conventional Clinical Assessment

Clinical quantification of blood volume and ECV is difficult. The clinician must first recognize settings in which deficits are likely, such as protracted gastrointestinal losses, bowel obstruction, bowel perforation, preoperative bowel preparation, chronic hypertension, chronic diuretic use, sepsis, burns, pancreatitis, and trauma. The physical signs of hypovolemia are insensitive and nonspecific. Suggestive evidence includes oliguria, supine hypotension, and a positive tilt test. Oliguria implies hypovolemia, although hypovolemic patients may be nonoliguric and normovolemic patients may be oliguric because of renal failure or stress-induced endocrine responses. Supine hypotension implies a blood volume deficit exceeding 30%. However, arterial blood pressure within the normal range could represent relative hypotension in an elderly or chronically hypertensive patient. Substantial depletion of blood volume and organ hypoperfusion may occur despite an apparently normal blood pressure and heart rate.

In the tilt test, one of the traditional methods of assessing intravascular volume depletion, a positive response is defined as an increase in heart rate ≥ 20 beats·min^{-1} and a decrease in systolic blood pressure ≥ 20 mm Hg when the subject assumes the upright position. However, a high incidence of false positive and false negative findings limits the value of the test. Classic studies (91) demonstrate that young, healthy subjects can withstand acute loss of 20% of blood volume while exhibiting only postural tachycardia and variable postural hypotension. Similar studies have not been performed in elderly patients, patients with autonomic dysfunction, patients on chronic hypertensive therapy, and patients who have reduced cardiovascular reserve. Twenty to thirty percent of elderly patients may demonstrate orthostatic changes in blood pressure despite normal blood volume (92).

In normal subjects, heart rate and blood pressure did not change when abruptly moved to the 45° head-up position, but noninvasively measured cardiac index significantly decreased and systemic vascular resistance significantly increased (93). Surprisingly, a heterogeneous group of critically ill patients exhibited no significant alterations in any variable when tilted to 45° (93). In volunteers, withdrawal of 500 mL of blood (94) was associated with a greater increase in heart rate on standing than before blood withdrawal but no significant difference in the response of blood pressure or cardiac index.

Orthostatic changes in filling pressure, coupled with assessment of the response to fluid infusion, may represent a more sensitive test of the adequacy of circulating blood volume. In patients with chronic renal failure (95),

baseline central venous pressure (CVP), which averaged 0.1 cm H_2O, declined precipitously to a mean value of –9.7 cm H_2O when the patients assumed a 45° sitting posture. Infusion of fluid slightly increased the mean supine CVP to 2.3 cm H_2O but eliminated the marked postural decline in CVP.

Laboratory evidence that suggests hypovolemia or ECV depletion includes hemoconcentration, azotemia, low urinary sodium, metabolic alkalosis, and metabolic acidosis. Hematocrit, a poor indicator of intravascular volume, changes in relationship to the magnitude of hemorrhage, the time elapsed since hemorrhage, and the volume of asanguineous replacement fluid. Hematocrit is virtually unchanged by acute hemorrhage; later, hemodilution occurs as fluids are administered or as fluid shifts from the interstitial to the intravascular space. If intravascular volume has been restored, hematocrit measurement will reflect red cell mass more accurately and can be used to guide transfusion.

Both BUN and serum creatinine (SCr) may be increased if hypovolemia has been sufficiently prolonged. However, BUN, normally 8.0 to 20 mg·dL^{-1}, is increased not only by hypovolemia but also by high protein intake, gastrointestinal bleeding, or accelerated catabolism. Hepatic dysfunction decreases urea synthesis. Serum creatinine, a product of muscle catabolism, may be misleadingly low in elderly adults, females, and debilitated or malnourished patients. In contrast, in muscular or acutely catabolic patients, serum creatinine may exceed the normal range (0.5 to 1.5 mg·dL^{-1}) because of more rapid muscle breakdown. If the ratio of BUN:SCr exceeds the normal range (10 to 20), one should suspect dehydration or one of the individual factors that alter the serum concentration of the two metabolites. In prerenal oliguria, enhanced sodium reabsorption should reduce urinary sodium to ≤ 20 mEq·L^{-1} and enhanced water reabsorption should increase urinary concentration (i.e., urinary osmolality > 400; urine/plasma creatinine ratio > 40:1). However, the sensitivity and specificity of measurements of urinary sodium, osmolality, and creatinine ratios may be misleading in acute situations. Although hypovolemia does not generate metabolic alkalosis, ECV depletion is a potent stimulus for the maintenance of metabolic alkalosis. Severe hypovolemia may result in systemic hypoperfusion and lactic acidosis.

Intraoperative Clinical Assessment

Visual estimation, the simplest technique for quantifying intraoperative blood loss, adds the amount of blood in suction canisters to that absorbed by gauze squares and laparotomy pads and modifies the estimate depending on whether the sponges have been prerinsed in saline. An estimate of blood accumulation on the floor and surgical drapes is then added. Both surgeons and anesthesia providers tend to underestimate losses; the magnitude of the error is directly proportional to the actual blood loss. Weighing blood-soaked gauze squares and laparotomy pads improves accuracy, but this tedious process is confounded by evaporation from the wet materials.

The adequacy of intraoperative fluid resuscitation during hemorrhagic shock cannot be ascertained by any single modality. Commonly measured clinical variables include heart rate, arterial blood pressure, urinary output, arterial oxygenation, and pH. Tachycardia is an insensitive, nonspecific indicator of hypovolemia. In patients receiving potent inhalational agents, maintenance of a satisfactory blood pressure implies adequate intravascular volume. Preservation of blood pressure, accompanied by a CVP of 6 to 12 mm Hg, more strongly suggests adequate replacement. During profound hypovolemia, indirect measurements of blood pressure may significantly underestimate true blood pressure. In patients undergoing extensive procedures, direct arterial pressure measurements are more accurate than indirect techniques; in addition, arterial catheters provide convenient access for obtaining arterial blood samples.

Urinary output usually declines precipitously during moderate to severe hypovolemia. Renal perfusion decreases after moderate hemorrhage in anesthetized mammals (96). Therefore, in the absence of glycosuria or diuretic administration, a urinary output of 0.5 to 1.0 mL·kg^{-1}·h^{-1} during anesthesia suggests adequate renal perfusion. Pulse oximetry is an unreliable indicator of decreased flow (97). Arterial pH is an insensitive reflection of tissue perfusion because pH may decrease only in severe tissue hypoxia. Invasive measurement of cardiac output and PAOP may be more useful for patients with known cardiac disease or those who have recently sustained cardiac trauma (e.g., contusion) (98, 99). However, cardiac output can be normal despite severely reduced regional blood flow. Mixed venous oxygenation, a sensitive indicator of poor systemic perfusion (100), reflects average perfusion in multiple organs and cannot supplant regional monitors such as urinary output.

Oxygen Delivery as a Goal of Management

No intraoperative monitor is sufficiently sensitive or specific to detect hypoperfusion in all patients. Moreover, certain postoperative surgical complications, such as acute renal failure, hepatic failure, and sepsis, may result from unrecognized, subclinical tissue hypoperfusion during the perioperative period. Average cardiac output and DO$_2$ are greater in high-risk surgical patients who survive than in those who succumb to critical illness (101, 102). One key variable that seems to be highly associated with survival is a DO$_2 \geq 600$ mL O$_2$·m^{-2}·min^{-1} (equivalent to a cardiac index of 3.0 L·m^{-2}·min^{-1}, a hemoglobin concentration of 14 g·dL^{-1}, and 98% oxyhemoglobin saturation). Therefore, Shoemaker et al. adjusted hemodynamic therapy in high-risk surgical patients to achieve those hemodynamic values (including a DO$_2$ of 600 mL O$_2$·m^{-2}·min^{-1}) (101). In comparison to a control group that received conventional monitoring, including central venous catheterization, the group treated by goal-directed management had greater survival and decreased complications (101). A subsequent protocol added a second control group that underwent pulmonary artery catheterization without specific management guidelines. As in the first series, the protocol group that received goal-directed therapy had greater survival and fewer complications than either control group. These data suggest that aggressive, goal-directed hemodynamic support in high-risk surgical patients reverses clinically inapparent hypoperfusion and, as a consequence, limits the mortality and morbidity secondary to that process. Similar management also seems to improve outcome in septic patients (102).

However, recent data continue to generate controversy regarding the value of aggressive maintenance of DO_2. Boyd et al. randomized 107 patients to DO_2 greater than or less than 600 mL $O_2 \cdot m^{-2} \cdot min^{-1}$ and demonstrated a decrease in mortality and in the number of complications in the patients managed at the higher level of DO_2 (103). In contrast, Hayes et al. randomized 109 patients to DO_2 greater than or less than 600 mL $O_2 \cdot m^{-2} \cdot min^{-1}$, using a combination of volume and dobutamine. They demonstrated an increase in mortality in the patients maintained at the higher levels of DO_2 and speculated that aggressive elevations in DO_2 may actually have been harmful (104).

ELECTROLYTES

Sodium

PHYSIOLOGIC ROLE

Increases or decreases in total body sodium, the principal extracellular cation and solute, tend to increase or decrease ECV and PV. Because sodium is largely confined to ECV, disorders of sodium concentration (i.e., hyponatremia and hypernatremia) usually result from relative excesses or deficits, respectively, of water. As one of the ions involved in the action potential, sodium also is essential for proper function of both neurologic and cardiac tissue.

Table 4–6. Regulation of Electrolytes

Electrolyte	Regulated by
Sodium	Aldosterone
	ANP
	[NA$^+$] altered by ADH
Potassium	Aldosterone
	Epinephrine
	Insulin
	Intrinsic renal mechanisms
Calcium	PTH
	Vitamin D
Phosphorus	Primarily renal mechanism
	Minor: PTH
Magnesium	Primarily renal mechanisms
	Minor: PTH, vitamin D

ANP, atrial natriuretic peptide; [Na$^+$], sodium concentration; ADH, antidiuretic hormone; PTH, parathyroid hormone.
Reproduced with permission from Zaloga GP, Prough DS. Fluids and electrolytes. In: Barash PG, Bullen BF, Stoelting RK, eds. Clinical anesthesia. Philadelphia: JB Lippincott, 1992;203–236.

Regulation of the quantity and concentration of sodium is accomplished primarily by the endocrine and renal systems (Table 4–6). Total body sodium is primarily regulated by aldosterone, which is responsible for renal sodium reabsorption in exchange for potassium and hydrogen (12). In addition, when the cardiac atria are stretched, secretion of ANP increases renal sodium excretion and decreases PV (8). Sodium concentration is primarily regulated by ADH, although ADH does not regulate sodium balance. Increased secretion of ADH, in response to either osmotic or hemodynamic stimuli, results in reabsorption of water by the kidneys and subsequent dilution of the plasma [Na$^+$]; inadequate ADH secretion results in renal free water excretion, which in the absence of adequate water intake, results in hypernatremia. In response to changes in plasma [Na$^+$], changes in secretion of ADH can vary urinary osmolality from 50 to 1400 mOsm·kg^{-1} and urinary volume from 0.4 to 20 L·day^{-1} (see Fig. 4–2).

HYPONATREMIA

The signs and symptoms of hyponatremia depend on both the rate at which plasma [Na$^+$]

decreases and the severity of the decrease. Symptoms that usually accompany $[Na^+] \leq 120$ mEq·L^{-1}, include central nervous system (CNS) manifestations, gastrointestinal complaints (anorexia, nausea, vomiting), and muscular cramps and weakness. Acute CNS manifestations relate to brain overhydration. Although the blood-brain barrier (which separates blood from interstitial fluid) is poorly permeable to sodium, water equilibrates rapidly. Therefore, a decrease in plasma $[Na^+]$ promptly leads to an increase in both extracellular and intracellular brain water. The magnitude of brain swelling is limited by bulk movement of interstitial fluid into the cerebrospinal fluid and the loss of intracellular solutes (105, 106), including potassium and organic osmolytes (previously termed "idiogenic osmoles") such as taurine, phosphocreatine, myoinositol, glutamine, and glutamate (107–109). Because the brain rapidly compensates for changes in osmolality, the symptoms of acute hyponatremia are considerably more severe than those of chronic hyponatremia at similar levels of plasma $[Na^+]$ (Fig. 4–6). The symptoms of chronic hyponatremia probably relate to depletion of brain electrolytes. Cerebral edema is minimal if hyponatremia is chronic (107, 110). After the brain has adapted by decreasing the intracellular concentrations of potassium and organic osmolytes, rapid correction of hyponatremia may lead to abrupt brain dehydration (Fig. 4–7).

The occasional postoperative occurrence of hyponatremia, mental status changes, and seizures has been attributed historically to intravenous administration of hypotonic fluids and inappropriate secretion of ADH (111). Prospective studies suggest that at least 4.0% of postoperative patients develop plasma $[Na^+] < 130$ mEq·L^{-1} (112). Smaller females are most susceptible to rapid changes in sodium concentration in response to administration of hypotonic intravenous fluids. Administration of 200 mL·h^{-1} of sodium-free water to a 50-kg woman (in whom TBW would be estimated as 50% of body weight, or 25 liters) would reduce plasma $[Na^+]$ by 1.0 mEq·L^{-1}·h^{-1} (113).

An 80-kg, muscular male, in whom TBW would be equal to 60% of body weight (48 L), would require twice as large an infusion of sodium-free water to achieve similar dilution. In extreme cases, administration of hypotonic fluids to healthy, young women after surgery has resulted in severe neurologic symptoms and death secondary to transtentorial herniation (114, 115).

A substantial proportion of postoperative patients, including pediatric patients, develop laboratory evidence of the syndrome of inappropriate ADH secretion (SIADH) (116). These patients develop impaired water excretion and are susceptible to hyponatremia. Although neurologic manifestations are relatively uncommon in postoperative hyponatremia, signs of hypervolemia are occasionally present (112). Careful attention to fluid and electrolyte balance in the postoperative period may minimize the occurrence of symptomatic hyponatremia. However, the actual relationship of hyponatremia and urinary volume to ADH secretion is unclear (117). Many other factors, such as drugs, water intake, and renal function, influence perioperative water balance (118).

Hyponatremia is classified as factitious or true. Factitious hyponatremia occurs when hyperproteinemia or hyperlipidemia displaces water from plasma, thereby producing an apparently low plasma $[Na^+]$. Factitious hyponatremia occurs if protein concentrations are nearly twice normal or if hyperlipidemia is sufficiently severe to produce plasma lactescence. In such patients, serum osmolality is normal (Fig. 4–8). Although $[Na^+]$ is conveniently reported in terms of mEq·L^{-1}, true $[Na^+]$ is expressed per unit volume of plasma divided by the percentage of plasma that is comprised of water. Factitious hyponatremia requires no treatment.

True hyponatremia may be associated with normal, high, or low serum osmolality. In turn, hyponatremia with hypo-osmolality is associated with a high, low, or normal total body sodium and PV. Hyponatremia ($[Na^+] < 135$ mEq·L^{-1}) with a normal or high serum

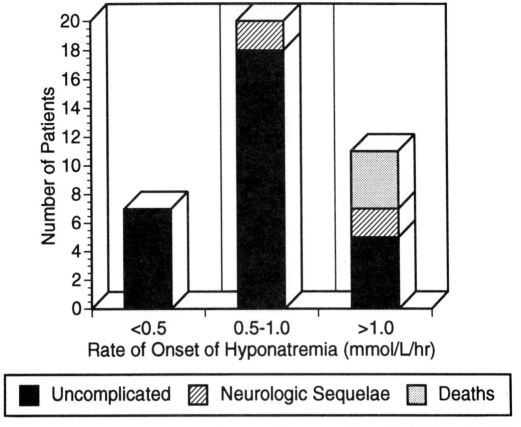

Fig. 4–6. Rate of decrease (in mmol·L·hr) in the serum sodium concentration and the incidence of neurologic sequelae in patients developing acute hyponatremia. (Reproduced with permission from Cluitmans FHM, Meinders AE. Management of severe hyponatremia: rapid or slow correction? Am J Med 1990;88:161–166.)

osmolality results from the presence of a non-sodium solute, such as glucose or mannitol, which does not diffuse freely across cell membranes (see Fig. 4–8). The resulting osmotic gradient causes water to move from the ICV to the ECV, resulting in dilutional hyponatremia. In anesthesia practice, a common cause of hyponatremia associated with a normal osmolality is the absorption of large volumes of sodium-free irrigating solutions during transurethral resection of the prostate (119, 120).

Although plasma [Na⁺] is markedly reduced, plasma osmolality remains nearly normal because of the absorbed irrigant solute, whether that is mannitol, glycine, or sorbitol. Neurologic symptoms are minimal if mannitol is employed because the agent does not cross the blood-brain barrier and is excreted with water in the urine. In contrast, as glycine or sorbitol is metabolized, hyposmolality will gradually develop and cerebral edema may appear as a late complication (120). Metabolism of glycine may also cause neurologic symptoms secondary to ammonia intoxication (120).

A discrepancy exceeding $10 \, mOsm \cdot kg^{-1}$ between the measured and calculated osmolality suggests either factitious hyponatremia or the presence of a nonsodium solute. Hyponatremia with a normal or elevated serum osmolality may also occur in renal insufficiency if excessive free water has been ingested or infused. Although an elevated BUN increases

Fig. 4–7. Brain water and solute in hyponatremia. If normal plasma sodium [Na] (A) suddenly were to decrease, the increase in brain water theoretically would be proportional to the decrease in plasma [Na] (B). However, because of adaptive loss of cerebral intracellular solute, cerebral edema is minimized in chronic hyponatremia (C). Once adaptation has occurred, a rapid return of plasma [Na] concentration toward a normal level results in brain dehydration (D). (Reprinted with permission from Cluitmans FHM, Meinders AE. Management of severe hyponatremia: rapid or slow correction? Am J Med 1990;88:161–166.)

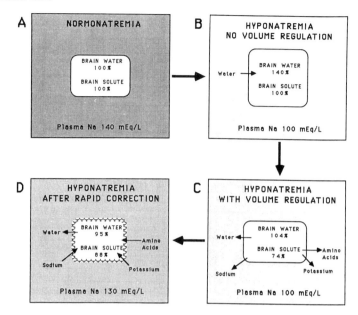

both measured and calculated osmolality, calculation of effective osmolality (2 [Na$^+$] + glucose/18) demonstrates true hypotonicity. BUN, included in the calculation of total osmolality, is excluded from the calculation of effective osmolality because it distributes throughout both ECV and ICV.

Hyponatremia with hyposmolality (see Fig. 4–8) is evaluated by assessing BUN, serum creatinine, total body sodium content, urinary osmolality, and urinary [Na$^+$]. Hyponatremia with increased total body sodium is characteristic of edematous states, i.e., congestive heart failure, cirrhosis, nephrosis, and renal failure. The common denominator among these conditions is decreased effective circulating volume, usually accompanied by edema. Reduced urinary diluting capacity in patients with renal insufficiency can lead to hyponatremia when excess free water is given. Hyponatremia with low total body sodium content (hypovolemia) may occur in association with nonrenal or renal losses of sodium, in response to which volume-responsive ADH secretion sacrifices tonicity to preserve intravascular volume.

A third group of patients develop euvolemic hyponatremia associated with a relatively normal total body sodium and ECV. Although in such patients TBW is usually expanded by 2 to 3 L, edema is rarely evident. Almost invariably because of SIADH, euvolemic hyponatremia is usually associated with excessive ectopic ADH secretion (as occurs with certain neoplasms), excessive hypothalamic-pituitary release of ADH (secondary to stress, pulmonary disease, CNS pathology, or endocrine abnormalities), exogenous ADH administration, pharmacologic potentiation of ADH action, or drugs that mimic the action of ADH in the renal tubules.

Treatment of hyponatremia associated with a normal or high serum osmolality requires reduction of the elevated concentrations of the responsible solute. Uremic, hyponatremic patients are treated by free water restriction or dialysis. Treatment of edematous (hypervolemic), hyponatremic patients necessitates restriction of both sodium and water (Fig. 4–9). Therapy is directed toward improving cardiac output and renal perfusion and using diuretics to inhibit sodium reabsorption. For patients with congestive heart failure, furosemide and an inhibitor of angiotensin-converting enzyme (ACE) may be particularly effective (121), probably because the ACE inhibitor

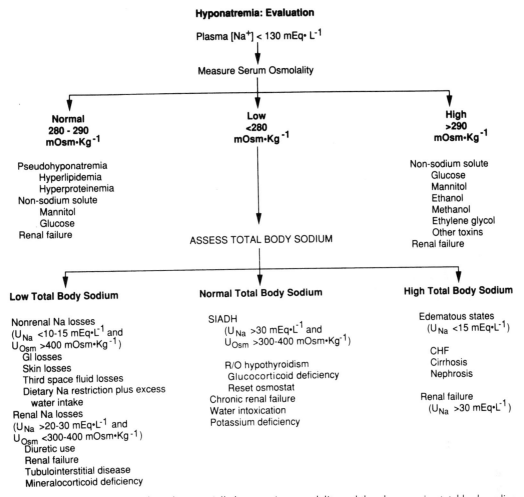

Fig. 4–8. Hyponatremia is evaluated sequentially by assessing osmolality and then by assessing total body sodium.

limits both the thirst and ADH release associated with angiotensin II (113). In hypovolemic, hyponatremic patients, blood volume must be restored, usually by infusion of 0.9% saline, and excessive sodium losses must be curtailed. Correction of hypovolemia usually results in removal of the stimulus for ADH release, accompanied by a rapid water diuresis. If plasma [Na$^+$] increases too rapidly (a urinary output of 500 mL·h^{-1} will increase plasma [Na$^+$] by approximately 2 mEq·L^{-1}·h^{-1} in a 50-kg woman) (113), it may be necessary to administer sodium-free water to avoid excessively rapid correction (122).

The cornerstone of SIADH management is free water restriction and elimination of pre-cipitating causes. Water restriction, sufficient to decrease TBW by 0.5 to 1.0 L·day^{-1}, decreases ECV even if excessive ADH secretion continues. The resultant reduction in GFR enhances proximal tubular reabsorption of salt and water, thereby decreasing free water generation, and stimulates aldosterone secretion. As long as free water losses (i.e., renal, skin, gastrointestinal) exceed free water intake, serum [Na$^+$] will increase. Free water excretion can be increased by administering furosemide.

Neurologic symptoms or profound hyponatremia ([Na$^+$] < 115 to 120 mEq·L^{-1}) require more aggressive therapy. Hypertonic (3%) saline is most clearly indicated for patients who have seizures or patients who

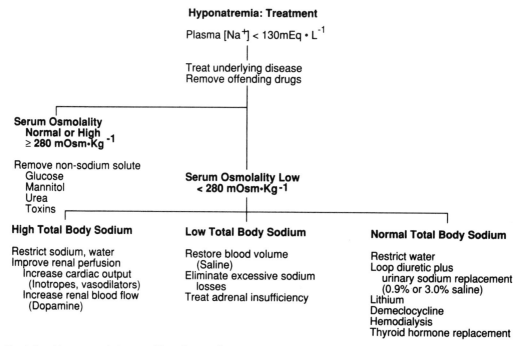

Fig. 4–9. Hyponatremia is treated based on etiology, serum osmolality, and clinical estimation of total body sodium.

acutely develop symptoms of water intoxication secondary to intravenous fluid administration. In such cases, 3% saline could be administered at a rate of 1 to 2 mL·kg^{-1}·h^{-1}, to increase plasma [Na$^+$] by 1 to 2 mEq·L^{-1}·h^{-1}; however, this treatment should not continue for more than a few hours to avoid excessively rapid correction (105, 123). In 25 children treated in this manner, seizures were promptly terminated and there were no delayed neurologic sequelae (124). Three percent saline alone will increase total body sodium as well as TBW; nevertheless, plasma [Na$^+$] may only transiently increase, because ECV expansion results in rapid sodium excretion in the urine. Intravenous furosemide, combined with quantitative replacement of urinary sodium losses with 0.9% or 3.0% saline, can rapidly increase plasma [Na$^+$], in part by increasing free water clearance.

Treatment of hyponatremia in the clinical setting continues to generate controversy. Al-though delayed correction may result in neurologic injury, inappropriately rapid correction also may result in permanent neurologic sequelae (i.e., central pontine myelinolysis or the osmotic demyelination syndrome) (84–86, 125), cerebral hemorrhage, or congestive heart failure. The symptoms of the osmotic demyelination syndrome vary from mild (transient behavioral disturbances or seizures) to severe (including pseudobulbar palsy and quadriparesis) (105, 106, 123, 125, 126). Within 3 to 4 weeks of the clinical onset of the syndrome, areas of demyelination are apparent on magnetic resonance imaging (126, 127). In rats, rapid correction of severe hyponatremia to normonatremic or hypernatremic levels results in severe demyelinating brain lesions; in contrast, rapid correction to mildly hyponatremic levels is associated with less severe pathology (128). The rapidity of correction seems to be a critical factor in both clinical and experimental osmotic demyelination (85,

125). Greater chronicity of hyponatremia predisposes experimental animals to more severe demyelination (86).

Clinical evidence supports the view that rapid correction of hyponatremia to normal levels plays a central role in the development of central demyelinating lesions and the accompanying clinical picture. Based on a retrospective survey, Stern and associates emphasized that neurological complications occurred more frequently if the rate of correction exceeded 0.6 mEq·L^{-1}·h^{-1} (113) (Fig 4–10). Others have argued that the magnitude rather than the rate of correction is responsible for demyelinating lesions (105). Experimental evidence indicates that demyelinating lesions are not observed if the rate of correction is less than 2.5 mEq·L·h or if the magnitude of correction is limited to less than 25 mEq in 24 hours (129). Demyelinating lesions tend to occur if either of these levels are exceeded. Most patients in whom the osmotic demyelination syndrome is fatal have undergone correction of plasma [Na$^+$] of more than 20 mEq·L^{-1}·day^{-1} (125, 130). In addition, it is important to remember that certain groups of patients, i.e., those with chronic alcoholism, malnutrition, and potassium depletion, have

a greater propensity to develop hyponatremia. The clinician is faced with enormous difficulties in calculating the rate at which serum sodium concentration is increased. Karmel and Bear (131), basing their conclusion on a quantitative analysis, pointed out that increases in serum sodium concentrations during treatment of hyponatremia are determined not only by the nature of the infused fluid, but also, to a major degree, by the rate of free water excretion by the kidney.

In treating hyponatremia, plasma [Na$^+$] may be increased by 1 to 2 mEq·L^{-1}·h^{-1}; however, plasma [Na$^+$] should not be increased more than 12 mEq·L^{-1} in 24 hours or 25 mEq·L^{-1} in 48 hours (106, 130, 132–135). Hypernatremia should be avoided. When the plasma [Na$^+$] exceeds 120 to 125 mEq·L^{-1}, water restriction alone is usually sufficient to normalize [Na$^+$]. As acute hyponatremia is corrected, CNS signs and symptoms usually improve within 24 hours, although 96 hours may be necessary for maximal recovery.

Demeclocycline and lithium, although potentially toxic, have been used effectively to reverse SIADH in patients in whom the primary disease process is irreversible. Although better tolerated than lithium, demeclocycline

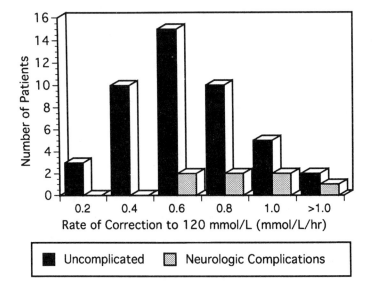

Fig. 4–10. Relationship between the incidence of neurological complications and the rate of correction (in mmol·L·hr) of chronic hyponatremia. In a series of patients with severe chronic hyponatremia (serum sodium ≤ 110 mmol·L), delayed neurological deterioration was observed with increasing frequency when the rate of correction to 120 mmol·L exceeded 0.55 mmol·L. Four of these patients had transient neurological events; three had permanent sequelae, with features suggesting a diagnosis of central potitine myelinolysis. (Reprinted with permission from Sterns RH. Severe symptomatic hyponatremia: treatment and outcome. A study of 64 cases. Ann Intern Med 1987;107:656–664.)

may induce nephrotoxicity, which is a particular concern for patients with hepatic dysfunction. Hemodialysis is occasionally necessary for severely hyponatremic patients who cannot be adequately managed with drugs or hypertonic saline. When hyponatremia has improved, careful fluid restriction is necessary to avoid recurrence of hyponatremia.

HYPERNATREMIA

Because neurons are extremely vulnerable to dehydration, hypernatremia also produces neurologic symptoms, including alterations in the level of consciousness and seizures (6, 136). Most hospitalized patients who have hypernatremia also have severe associated illness (137). Because hypernatremia frequently results from diabetes insipidus or osmotically induced losses of sodium and water, many patients are hypovolemic or bear the stigmata of renal disease. Postoperative neurosurgical patients who have undergone pituitary surgery are at particular risk of developing transient or prolonged diabetes insipidus (138, 139). Polyuria may be present for only a few days within the first week of surgery, may be permanent, or may demonstrate a triphasic sequence: early diabetes insipidus, return of urinary concentrating ability, and then recurrent diabetes insipidus (140). The clinical consequences of hypernatremia are most serious at the extremes of age (137) and when hypernatremia develops abruptly. Brain shrinkage may damage delicate cerebral vessels, leading to subdural hematoma, subcortical parenchymal hemorrhage, subarachnoid hemorrhage, and venous thrombosis. Polyuria may cause bladder distention, hydronephrosis, and permanent renal damage.

By definition, hypernatremia ($[Na^+] > 150$ $mEq \cdot L^{-1}$) indicates an absolute or relative water deficit and is always associated with hypertonicity. The TBW deficit can be estimated from the plasma $[Na^+]$ using the equation:

$$TBW\ deficit = (0.6)\ (weight\ in\ kg)$$
$$- (140/actual\ [Na^+])\ (0.6)\ (weight\ in\ kg)$$

Because hypovolemia accompanies most pathologic water loss, signs of hypoperfusion also may be present. In many patients, before the development of hypernatremia, an increased volume of hypotonic urine suggests an abnormality in water balance (140, 141).

Patients with hypernatremia can be separated into three groups, based on clinical assessment of ECV (Fig. 4–11). The plasma $[Na^+]$ does not reflect total body sodium, which must be estimated based on signs of the adequacy of ECV. The next differential diagnostic decision to be made in polyuric patients, after assessing ECV, is between solute diuresis and diabetes insipidus. As extracellular $[Na^+]$ increases, intracellular water is shifted out of cells and ICV is depleted.

Treatment of hypernatremia produced by water loss consists of water replacement as well as repletion of associated deficits in total body sodium and other electrolytes (Table 4–7). Hypernatremia must be corrected slowly because of the risk of neurologic sequelae such as seizures or cerebral edema (Fig. 4–12) (137, 142). The water deficit should be replaced over 24 to 48 hours, and the plasma $[Na^+]$ should not be reduced by more than 1 to 2 $mEq \cdot L^{-1} \cdot h^{-1}$. Reversible underlying causes should be treated. Hypovolemia should be corrected promptly with 0.9% saline. Once hypovolemia is corrected, water can be replaced orally or with intravenous hypotonic fluids, depending on the ability of the patient to tolerate oral hydration. In the occasional sodium-overloaded patient, sodium excretion can be accelerated using loop diuretics or dialysis, and diuresed or dialyzed volume can be replaced with hypotonic fluids.

Hypernatremia secondary to diabetes insipidus is managed according to whether the etiology is central or nephrogenic (see Table 4–7). Central diabetes insipidus requires replacement of ADH, with care taken to avoid water intoxication. The two most suitable agents for correcting central diabetes insipidus are desmopressin (DDAVP) and aque-

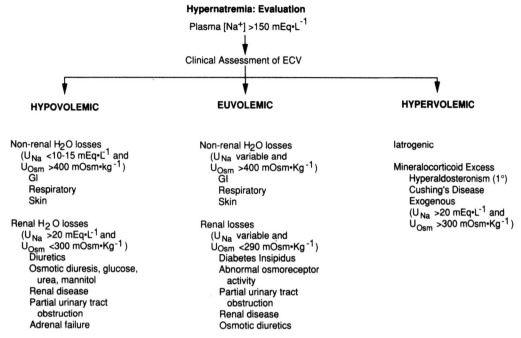

Fig. 4–11. Severe hypernatremia is evaluated by first assessing extracellular volume (ECV). After patients are divided into hypovolemic, euvolemic, and hypervolemic groups, potential etiologic factors are diagnostically assessed.

ous vasopressin. DDAVP, given subcutaneously in a dose of 1 to 4 μg every 12 to 24 hours, is effective for most patients. The medication can also be administered intranasally in a dose of 5 to 20 μg at 12- to 24-hour intervals. DDAVP lacks the vasoconstrictor effects of vasopressin and is less likely to produce abdominal cramping (143–146). Incomplete ADH deficits (partial diabetes insipidus) often are effectively managed with pharmacologic agents that stimulate ADH release or enhance the renal response to ADH. The combination of chlorpropamide (100 to 250 mg·day^{-1}) and clofibrate or a thiazide diuretic has proven effective in patients who respond inadequately to either drug alone. Because the dose of chlorpropamide may be reduced if a thiazide is added, the combination reduces the risk of chlorpropamide-induced hypoglycemia. Chlorpropamide and thiazides may also be effective in treating disorders of the osmoreceptors. In nephrogenic diabetes insipidus, the renal collecting ducts are resistant to the action of ADH. Urinary water losses can be decreased by using salt and water restriction or thiazide diuretics to induce ECV contraction and enhance fluid reabsorption in the proximal tubules.

Table 4–7. Hypernatremia: Acute Treatment

Sodium Depletion (hypovolemia)
  Hypovolemia correction (.9% saline)
  Hypernatremia correction (hypotonic fluids)

Sodium Overload (hypervolemia)
  Enhance sodium removal (loop diuretics, dialysis)
  Replace water deficit (hypotonic fluids)

Normal Total Body Sodium (euvolemia)
  Replace water deficit (hypotonic fluids)
  Control diabetes insipidus
    Central diabetes insipidus:
      DDAVP, 10–20 μg intranasally; 2–4 μg s.c.
      Aqueous vasopressin, 5 U q 2–4 hours i.m. or
        s.c.
    Nephrogenic diabetes insipidus:
      Restrict sodium, water intake
      Thiazide diuretics

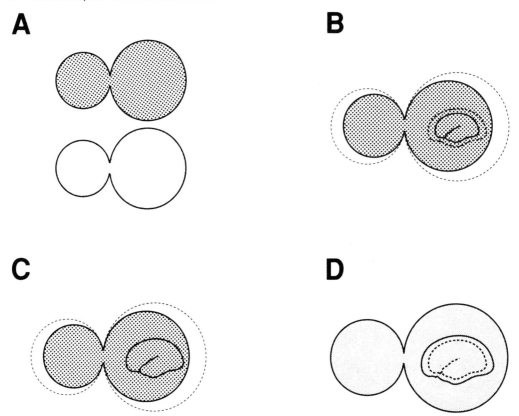

Fig. 4–12.   *A,* The concentration of sodium is reflected in the intensity of the stippling: the upper figure, representing extracellular volume (smaller circle) and intracellular volume (larger circle), is more heavily stippled, i.e., serum sodium is higher. *B,* In response to an acute increase in serum sodium resulting from water loss, both intracellular and extracellular volume substantially decrease. The brain (schematically illustrated) shrinks in proportion to the reduction in intracellular volume in other tissues. *C,* However, owing to the production of idiogenic osmoles, the brain rapidly restores its intracellular volume, despite the persistent reduction in intracellular volume in other tissues and in extracellular volume. *D,* With excessively rapid correction of hypernatremia (the reduction in serum sodium is reflected in the decrease in the intensity of stippling), the brain expands to greater than its original size. The resulting increase in cerebral edema and intracranial pressure can cause severe neurologic damage. (Modified with permission from Feig PU. Hypernatremia and hypertonic syndromes. Med Clin North Am 1981;65:271–290.)

Potassium

PHYSIOLOGIC ROLE

Potassium, the predominant intracellular cation, normally has an intracellular concentration of 150 mEq·L^{-1}, whereas the extracellular concentration is only 3.5 to 5.0 mEq·L^{-1}. Serum potassium concentration ([K$^+$]) is about 0.5 mEq·L^{-1} higher than plasma [K$^+$] because of cell lysis during clotting. Total body potassium in a 70-kg adult is approximately 4256 mEq, of which 4200 mEq is intracellular, 56 mEq is extracellular, and only 12 mEq is located in the plasma volume. Potassium plays an important role in cell membrane physiology, especially that of excitable membranes in the CNS and heart. Potassium is essential in maintaining resting membrane potentials and in generating action potentials. Thus, changes in extracellular potassium strongly influence excitation of cardiac tissue.

Total body potassium and potassium concentration are primarily regulated by three hormones: aldosterone, epinephrine, and insulin (see Table 4–6). Aldosterone increases renal reabsorption of sodium and renal excretion of potassium. Both epinephrine and insulin shift potassium intracellularly and provide important mechanisms for short-term amelioration of hyperkalemia.

Potassium is also influenced independently by intrinsic renal mechanisms that regulate renal potassium excretion and are especially important in preventing chronic potassium overload. Assuming a plasma [K+] of 4.0 mEq·L⁻¹ and a normal GFR of 180 L·day⁻¹, 720 mEq of potassium is filtered daily. Most is reabsorbed; usually, only the amount ingested (normally 40 to 120 mEq·day⁻¹) is lost. Dietary potassium intake, unless greater than normal, can be excreted as long as GFR exceeds 8.0 mL·min⁻¹. In the proximal renal tubule, 50 to 70% of filtered potassium is passively reabsorbed. After secretion into the descending limb of the loop of Henle, potassium is subsequently reabsorbed from the medullary collecting ducts as part of a recycling loop (147). Potassium excretion is primarily dependent on potassium secretion into the distal convoluted tubules and cortical collecting ducts and is increased by aldosterone, hyperkalemia, high urinary flow rates, and the presence in luminal fluid of nonreabsorbable anions such as carbenicillin, phosphates, and sulfates (148). Within the distal nephron, a magnesium-dependent sodium/potassium ATPase enzyme plays a critical role in potassium reabsorption (149). Magnesium depletion impairs the activity of the enzyme, leading to renal potassium wasting.

HYPOKALEMIA

The signs and symptoms of hypokalemia ([K+] < 3.0 mEq·L⁻¹) reflect the diffuse effects of hypokalemia on cell membranes and excitable tissue. Hypokalemia causes muscle weakness and, when severe, may even cause paralysis (Table 4–8). The ratio of intracellular to extracellular potassium contributes to the resting potential difference across cell membranes and therefore to the integrity of cardiac and neuromuscular transmission. The resting

Table 4–8. Hypokalemia: Clinical Manifestations

Cardiovascular
Dysrhythmias
Electrocardiogram changes
Digitalis toxicity potentiation
Postural hypotension
Impaired pressor responses
Neuromuscular
Weakness
Rhabdomyolysis
Respiratory failure
Hyporeflexia
Confusion
Depression
Renal
Polyuria
Concentrating defect
Metabolic
Glucose intolerance
Potentiation of hypercalcemia, hypomagnesemia

membrane potential (E_m) is calculated from the Nernst equation:

$$E_m = -61 \log r [K_i] + 0.01 [Na_i]/r[K_e] + 0.01 [Na_e]$$

where r = 1.5 (the ratio of sodium to potassium actively transported by the ATPase pump), the subscripts i and e refer to intracellular and extracellular concentrations of sodium or potassium, respectively, and 0.01 is the relative membrane permeability of sodium and potassium. With chronic potassium loss, the ratio of intracellular to extracellular [K+] remains relatively stable; in contrast, acute redistribution of potassium from extracellular to intracellular spaces substantially changes E_m.

Cardiac rhythm disturbances are among the most dangerous complications of potassium deficiency. Acute hypokalemia causes hyperpolarization of the cardiac cell and may lead to ventricular escape activity, re-entrant phenomena, ectopic tachycardias, and delayed conduction. Despite the longstanding concern of anesthesia personnel that preoperative chronic hypokalemia increases the incidence of intraoperative dysrhythmias, a prospective study failed to confirm increased risk (150).

Potassium depletion also induces defects in renal concentrating ability, resulting in polyuria and a reduction in GFR (151–153). Potassium replacement improves GFR; however, the concentrating deficit may not improve for several months after treatment of hypokalemia. If hypokalemia is sufficiently prolonged, chronic renal interstitial damage may occur.

The plasma potassium concentration ($[K^+]$) poorly reflects total body potassium; hypokalemia may occur with normal, low, or high total body potassium stores. As a rule, a chronic decrement of 1.0 $mEq·L^{-1}$ in the plasma $[K^+]$ corresponds to a total body deficit of approximately 200 to 300 mEq. In uncomplicated hypokalemia, the potassium deficit exceeds 300 mEq if plasma $[K^+]$ is <3.0 $mEq·L^{-1}$ and 700 mEq if plasma $[K^+]$ is <2.0 $mEq·L^{-1}$ (154).

Hypokalemia may result from acute redistribution of potassium from the extracellular to intracellular space, in which case total body potassium will be normal or from chronic depletion of total body potassium. Redistribution of potassium into cells occurs when the activity of the sodium-potassium ATPase pump is acutely increased by extracellular hyperkalemia or increased intracellular concentrations of sodium, as well as by insulin, carbohydrate loading (which stimulates release of endogenous insulin), β_2 agonists, and aldosterone. Both metabolic acidosis and respiratory alkalosis lead to decreases in plasma $[K^+]$ (155). Metabolic acidosis and respiratory acidosis tend to cause an increase in plasma $[K^+]$. However, organic acidoses (i.e., lactic acidosis, ketoacidosis) have little effect on $[K^+]$, whereas mineral acids cause significant cellular shifts. Acute hypokalemia is also associated with hypothermia; overzealous replacement of potassium during hypothermia has been associated with hyperkalemia after rewarming (156).

Causes of chronic hypokalemia include those etiologies associated with renal potassium conservation (extrarenal potassium losses; low urinary $[K^+]$) and those with renal potassium wasting. A low urinary $[K^+]$ suggests inadequate dietary intake or extrarenal depletion (in the absence of recent diuretic use). Diuretic-induced urinary potassium losses are frequently associated with hypokalemia, secondary to increased aldosterone secretion, alkalemia, and increased renal tubular flow. Aldosterone does not cause renal potassium wasting unless sodium ions are present; i.e., aldosterone primarily controls sodium reabsorption, not potassium excretion. Renal tubular damage caused by nephrotoxins such as aminoglycosides or amphotericin B may also cause renal potassium wasting.

Initial evaluation of hypokalemia includes a medical history (e.g., diarrhea, vomiting, diuretic or laxative use), physical examination (e.g., hypertension, cushingoid features, edema), measurement of serum electrolytes (e.g., magnesium), and arterial pH assessment. Measurement of 24-hour urinary excretion of sodium and potassium may distinguish extrarenal from renal causes. Plasma renin and aldosterone levels may be helpful in the differential diagnosis.

The treatment of hypokalemia consists of potassium repletion, correction of alkalemia, and removal of offending drugs (Table 4–9). Hypokalemia secondary only to acute redistribution may not require treatment. The need for potassium replacement therapy in mild to moderate hypokalemia ($[K^+]$ 3 to 3.5 $mEq·L^{-1}$) without clear symptoms has been questioned (157). If total body potassium is decreased, oral potassium supplementation is

---

Table 4–9. Hypokalemia: Treatment

Correct Precipitating Factors
  Increased pH
  Decreased $[Mg^{2+}]$
  Drugs

Mild Hypokalemia ($[K^+]$ > 2.0 mEq · L^{-1})
  Intravenous KCl infusion ≤ 10 mEq · h^{-1}

Severe Hypokalemia ($[K^+]$ ≤ 2.0 mEq · L^{-1}, paralysis or electrocardiogram changes)
  Intravenous KCl infusion ≤ 40 mEq · h^{-1}
  Continuous electrocardiogram monitoring

preferable to intravenous replacement. Potassium is usually replaced as the chloride salt because coexisting chloride deficiency may limit renal conservation of potassium.

Potassium repletion must be performed cautiously (i.e., usually at a rate no greater than 10 to 20 mEq·h^{-1}) because the absolute deficit is unpredictable. The plasma [K$^+$] and the electrocardiogram (ECG) must be monitored during rapid repletion (>20 mEq·h^{-1}) to avoid hyperkalemic complications. Particular care should be taken for patients who have concurrent acidemia, type IV renal tubular acidosis, diabetes mellitus, or patients receiving nonsteroidal anti-inflammatory agents, ACE inhibitors, or β blockers, all of which delay movement of extracellular potassium into cells.

Hypokalemia associated with hyperaldosteronemia (e.g., primary aldosteronism, Cushing's syndrome) usually responds favorably to reduced sodium intake and increased potassium intake.

Spironolactone, an aldosterone antagonist, reduces urinary potassium losses in patients who have adrenal hyperplasia. Hypomagnesemia, if present, aggravates the effects of hypokalemia, impairs potassium conservation, and should be treated. Cyclo-oxygenase inhibitors such as aspirin can improve hypokalemia in patients with Bartter's syndrome. Potassium supplements or potassium-sparing diuretics should be given cautiously to patients who have diabetes mellitus or renal insufficiency, which limit compensation for acute hyperkalemia. For patients such as those who have diabetic ketoacidosis, who are both acidemic and hypokalemic, potassium administration should precede correction of acidosis to avoid a precipitous decrease in plasma [K$^+$] as pH increases.

For patients with normal serum potassium accompanied by symptoms of potassium depletion (e.g., muscle fatigue), history of potassium loss or insufficient intake, or patients in whom potassium depletion may be a special threat (e.g., patients on diuretics, digitalis, or β$_2$ agonists), muscle biopsy with measurement of muscle potassium concentration may be a useful procedure to detect and quantify potassium depletion. Quantification of muscle potassium concentration can be used to monitor therapy. Skeletal muscle biopsies may be underused in the evaluation of potassium homeostasis (158).

HYPERKALEMIA

The clinical manifestations of hyperkalemia ([K$^+$] > 5.0 mEq·L^{-1}) primarily involve the neuromuscular and cardiovascular systems. The most lethal manifestations involve the cardiac conducting system and include dysrhythmias, conduction abnormalities, and cardiac arrest (Table 4–10). In anesthesia practice, the classic example of hyperkalemic cardiac toxicity is associated with the administration of succinylcholine to paraplegic or quadriplegic patients (159). If plasma [K$^+$] is <6.0 mEq·L^{-1}, cardiac effects are negligible. As the concentration increases, the ECG shows tall, peaked T waves, especially in the precordial leads. With further increases, the PR interval becomes prolonged, followed by a decrease in the amplitude of the P wave. Finally, the QRS complex widens into a pattern resembling a sine wave, as a prelude to cardiac standstill. Hyperkalemic cardiotoxicity is enhanced by hyponatremia, hypocalcemia, or acidosis. Because progression to fatal cardiotoxicity is un-

Table 4–10. Hyperkalemia: Clinical Manifestations

Cardiovascular
  Tall, peaked T waves
  Decreased P waves
  P-R prolongation
  Atrial asystole
  QRS widening
  Heart block
  Asystole
Neuromuscular
  Paresthesias
  Weakness
  Paralysis
  Confusion

predictable and often swift, the presence of hyperkalemic ECG changes mandates immediate therapy. The life-threatening cardiac effects usually require more urgent treatment than other manifestations of hyperkalemia. However, ascending muscle weakness appears when plasma [K$^+$] approaches 7.0 mEq·L^{-1} and may progress to flaccid paralysis, inability to phonate, and even respiratory arrest (160).

Hyperkalemia may occur with normal, high, or low total body potassium stores. A deficiency of aldosterone, a major regulator of potassium excretion, leads to hyperkalemia in adrenal insufficiency and hyporeninemic hypoaldosteronism, a state associated with diabetes mellitus, renal insufficiency, and advanced age. Because the kidneys excrete potassium, severe renal insufficiency commonly causes hyperkalemia (Table 4–11). Patients with chronic renal insufficiency can maintain normal plasma [K$^+$] despite markedly decreased GFR because urinary potassium excretion depends on tubular secretion rather than glomerular filtration when GFR falls below 8 mL·min^{-1}.

Drugs are currently the most common cause of hyperkalemia (161). Drugs that may limit potassium excretion include nonsteroidal anti-inflammatory drugs, ACE inhibitors, cyclosporine, and potassium-sparing diuretics such as triamterene. Drug effects most commonly occur in patients with other factors that predispose hyperkalemia, such as diabetes mellitus, renal insufficiency, advanced age, or hyporeninemic hypoaldosteronism. ACE inhibitors are particularly likely to produce hyperkalemia in patients who have renal insufficiency (162) or severe congestive heart failure (163).

Table 4–11. Hyperkalemia: Etiology

Hypoaldosteronism
Acute or chronic renal failure
Renal tubular dysfunction
Drugs (e.g., succinylcholine)
Extracellular translocation (acidemia)
Excess potassium intake

Table 4–12. Severe Hyperkalemia:[a] Treatment

Reverse membrane effects
  Calcium (10 mL of 10% calcium chloride i.v. over 10 min)
Transfer extracellular [K$^+$] into cells
  Glucose and insulin (D10W + 5–10 U regular insulin per 25–50 g glucose)
  Sodium bicarbonate 50–100 mEq over 5–10 min)
  β_2 agonists
Remove potassium from body
  Diuretics, proximal or loop
  Potassium-exchange resins (sodium polystyrene sulfonate)
  Hemodialysis
Monitor ECG and serum [K$^+$] level

[a] [K$^+$] > 7.0 mEq · L^{-1} or electrocardiogram changes.

In patients who have normal total body potassium, hyperkalemia may accompany a sudden shift of potassium from the ICV to the ECV because of acidemia, increased catabolism, or rhabdomyolysis. Pseudohyperkalemia, which occurs when potassium is released from cells in blood collection tubes, can be diagnosed by comparing serum and plasma [K$^+$] levels from the same blood sample.

The treatment of hyperkalemia is aimed at eliminating the cause, reversing membrane hyperexcitability, and removing potassium from the body (Table 4–12). Mineralocorticoid deficiency can be treated with 9-α-fludrocortisone (0.025 to 0.10 mg·day^{-1}). Hyperkalemia secondary to digitalis intoxication may be resistant to therapy because attempts to shift potassium from the ECV to the ICV are often ineffective. In this situation, use of digoxin-specific antibodies has been successful.

Hyperexcitability can be antagonized by translocating potassium from the ECV to the ICV, removing excess potassium, or (transiently) by infusing calcium chloride to depress the membrane threshold potential. Acute alkalinization using sodium bicarbonate (50 to 100 mEq over 5 to 10 minutes in a 70-kg adult) transiently promotes movement of potassium from the ECV to the ICV. Bicarbonate can be administered even if pH exceeds

7.40; however, it should not be administered to patients with congestive cardiac failure or hypernatremia. Insulin, in a dose-dependent fashion, causes cellular uptake of potassium by increasing the activity of the sodium/potassium ATPase pump. Insulin increases cellular uptake of potassium best when high insulin levels are achieved by intravenous injection of insulin (164). Therefore, administration of 5 to 10 U of regular insulin intravenously, accompanied by 50 mL of 50% glucose, is an effective way to transiently reduce serum potassium. β_2-adrenergic drugs also increase potassium uptake by skeletal muscle and reduce plasma [K^+] (165), an action that may explain hypokalemia with severe, acute illness (166). β_2 agonists have been used to treat hyperkalemia in a few specific settings (167).

Rapid infusion of calcium chloride (1 ampule of $CaCl_2$ over 3 minutes, or 2 to 3 ampules of 10% calcium gluconate over 5 minutes) may stabilize cardiac rhythm pending more definitive treatment. Calcium should be given cautiously if digitalis intoxication is likely. Potassium may be removed from the body by renal or gastrointestinal routes. Furosemide promotes kaliuresis in a dose-dependent fashion. Sodium polystyrene sulfonate resin (Kayexalate; Sanofi Winthrop, New York, NY) exchanges sodium for potassium. Kayexalate can be given orally (30 g) or as a retention enema (50 g in 200 mL of 20% sorbitol). However, sodium overload and hypervolemia are potential risks. Because these temporizing measures are usually sufficient, emergency hemodialysis is rarely necessary. When used, hemodialysis may remove 25 to 50 $mEq \cdot h^{-1}$. Peritoneal dialysis is less efficient.

Calcium

PHYSIOLOGIC ROLE

Calcium is a divalent cation found primarily in the extracellular fluid. The concentration of free calcium [Ca^{2+}] in the ICV approximates 100 nM, whereas the free [Ca^{2+}] in ECV is approximately 1 mM. Thus, the gradient between ECV and ICV is approximately 10,000 to 1. Circulating calcium consists of a protein-bound fraction (40%), a chelated fraction (10%), and an ionized fraction (50%), which is the physiologically active and homeostatically regulated component (168). Acute acidemia decreases protein-bound calcium (i.e., increases ionized calcium) whereas acute alkalemia increases protein-bound calcium (i.e., decreases ionized calcium). Because mathematical formulae that "correct" total calcium measurements for albumin concentration are inaccurate for critically ill patients (Fig. 4–13) (169), ionized calcium should be measured directly (170).

Calcium serves vital cellular functions. In general, all movement that occurs in mammalian systems requires calcium. Essential for normal excitation-contraction coupling, calcium is also necessary for proper function of muscle tissue, ciliary movement, and mitosis. Calcium is involved in contractile elements that are responsible for secretion in neural tissue (i.e., neurotransmitter release), enzyme secretion, and hormonal secretion from endocrine tissue. Cyclic AMP (cAMP) and phosphoinositides, which are major second messengers regulating cellular metabolism, function primarily through the regulation of calcium movement. Activation of numerous intracellular enzyme systems requires calcium. Important both for generation of the cardiac pacemaker activity and for generation of the cardiac action potential, calcium is the primary ion responsible for the plateau phase of the action potential. Calcium also plays vital functions in membrane and bone structure.

Calcium is regulated through two primary hormones: parathyroid hormone (PTH) and vitamin D (see Table 4–6). Both of these hormones, which are secreted when circulating ionized [Ca^{2+}] decreases, mobilize calcium from bone, increase reabsorption of calcium from the renal tubule, and enhance intestinal absorption of calcium. Metabolites of vitamin D exert a major role in long-term control of circulating calcium. Vitamin D, after ingestion or manufacture of vitamin D in the skin under

Fig. 4–13. Total serum calcium and calculated ionized calcium concentrations are poor indicators of directly measured serum ionized calcium in critically ill surgical patients. *Top,* Total serum calcium versus measured serum ionized calcium in 156 surgical ICU patients. Despite apparent hypocalcemia, based on measurement of total calcium, many patients have normal ionized calcium. *Bottom,* Calculated ionized calcium (using the McLean-Hastings nomogram) is frequently low in surgical ICU patients in whom measured ionized calcium is within the normal range. (Reproduced with permission from Zaloga GP, Chernow B, Cook D, et al. Assessment of calcium homeostasis in the critically ill surgical patient. The diagnostic pitfalls of the McLean-Hastings nomogram. Ann Surg 1985;202:587–594.)

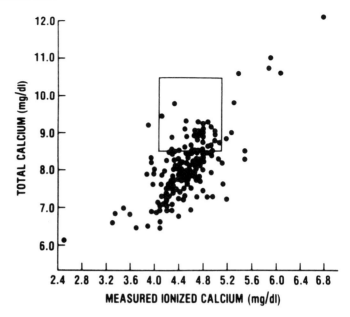

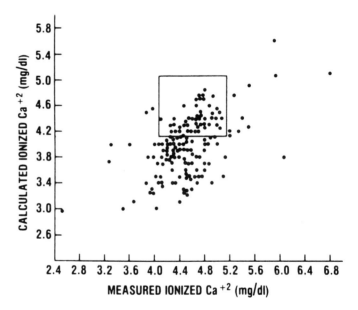

the stimulus of ultraviolet light, is 25-hydroxylated to calcidiol in the liver and then is 1-hydroxylated to calcitriol in the kidney. Calcitriol, the active metabolite, stimulates osseous calcium release, renal calcium reabsorption, and enteric calcium absorption. PTH and vitamin D can maintain a normal circulating $[Ca^{2+}]$, even in the absence of dietary calcium intake, by mobilizing calcium from bone.

HYPOCALCEMIA

The hallmark of hypocalcemia, increased neuronal membrane irritability and tetany (Table 4–13), classically is associated with

Table 4–13. Hypocalcemia: Clinical Manifestations

Cardiovascular	Respiratory
Dysrhythmias	Apnea
Digitalis insensitivity	Laryngeal spasm
Electrocardiogram changes	Bronchospasm
Heart failure	**Psychiatric**
Hypotension	Anxiety
Neuromuscular	Dementia
Tetany	Depression
Muscle spasm	Psychosis
Papilledema	
Seizures	
Weakness	
Fatigue	

Chvostek's or Trousseau's signs. In frank tetany, tonic contraction of respiratory muscles may lead to laryngospasm, bronchospasm, or respiratory arrest. Smooth muscle spasm can result in abdominal cramping and urinary frequency. Mental status alterations include irritability, depression, psychosis, and dementia. Hypocalcemia may impair cardiovascular function and has been associated with heart failure, hypotension, dysrhythmias, insensitivity to digitalis, and impaired β-adrenergic action.

Hypocalcemia (ionized calcium < 4.0 mg·dL^{-1} or 1 mM) occurs as a result of failure of PTH or calcitriol action or because of calcium chelation or precipitation, not because of calcium deficiency alone. PTH deficiency can result from surgical parathyroid gland damage or removal or from parathyroid gland suppression. Parathyroid gland suppression may occur during severe hypomagnesemia or hypermagnesemia. Burns, sepsis, and pancreatitis may suppress parathyroid function and interfere with vitamin D action. Vitamin D deficiency may result from lack of dietary vitamin D or vitamin D malabsorption in patients who lack sunlight exposure. Failure of renal hydroxylation occurs in some patients who have renal failure, sepsis, or rhabdomyolysis. Hyperphosphatemia-induced hypocalcemia may occur as a consequence of overzealous phosphate therapy, from cell lysis secondary

to chemotherapy, or as a result of cellular destruction from rhabdomyolysis.

Hyperphosphatemic hypocalcemia results from calcium precipitation and suppression of calcitriol synthesis. In massive transfusion, citrate may produce hypocalcemia by chelating calcium; however, decreases are usually transient and produce no cardiovascular effects. A healthy, normothermic adult who has intact hepatic and renal function can metabolize the citrate present in 20 units of blood within 1 hour without becoming hypocalcemic (171). However, when citrate clearance is decreased (e.g., by hepatic or renal disease, hypothermia) and when blood transfusion rates are rapid (e.g., >0.5 to 2 mL·kg^{-1}·min^{-1}), hypocalcemia and cardiovascular compromise may occur.

Reduced total serum calcium occurs in as many as 80% of critically ill and postsurgical patients (168). However, fewer patients develop ionized hypocalcemia, including 15 to 20% of critically ill patients (168–170), 20% of patients after cardiopulmonary bypass, and 30 to 40% after multiple trauma. In these situations, ionized hypocalcemia is clinically mild (ionized [Ca^{2+}] > 0.8 mM).

The definitive treatment of hypocalcemia necessitates identification and treatment of the underlying cause (Table 4–14). Symptomatic hypocalcemia usually occurs when serum ionized [Ca^{2+}] is below 0.7 mM. The clinician should determine whether mild ionized hypocalcemia requires therapy, particularly in ischemic and septic states in which experimental evidence suggests that calcium may increase cellular damage (172, 173).

Unnecessary offending drugs should be discontinued. Hypocalcemia resulting from hypomagnesemia or hyperphosphatemia is treated by repletion of magnesium or removal of magnesium or phosphate. Potassium and other electrolytes should be measured and abnormalities should be corrected. Hyperkalemia and hypomagnesemia potentiate hypocalcemia-induced cardiac and neuromuscular irritability. In contrast, hypokalemia protects against hypocalcemic tetany; therefore, cor-

Table 4–14. Hypocalcemia: Acute Treatment

Administer calcium
    i.v.: 10 mL 10% calcium gluconate[a] over 10 min as bolus, followed by 0.3–2 mg elemental calcium $\cdot$ kg^{-1} $\cdot$ h^{-1}
    Oral: 500–100 mg elemental calcium q 6 hours
Administer vitamin D
    Ergocalciferol, 1200 μg $\cdot$ day^{-1} ($T_{1/2}$ = 30 days)
    Dihydrotachysterol, 200–400 μg $\cdot$ day^{-1} ($T_{1/2}$ = 7 days)
    1,25-dihydroxycholecalciferol, 0.25–1.0 μg $\cdot$ day^{-1} ($T_{1/2}$ = 1 day)
Monitor electrocardiogram

[a] Calcium gluconate contains 93 mg elemental calcium per 10-mL vial; $T_{1/2}$ = half-life.
Reproduced with permission from Zaloga GP, Prough DS. Fluids and electrolytes. In: Barash PG, Bullen BF, Stoelting RK, eds. Clinical anesthesia. Philadelphia: JB Lippincott, 1992;203–236.

rection of hypokalemia without correction of hypocalcemia may provoke tetany.

Cardiac surgical patients present special problems in calcium management. Using pressure-volume relationships, Mathru and associates have demonstrated in normocalcemic dogs that the predominant effect of calcium chloride is peripheral vasoconstriction, with transient reduction of myocardial contractility (Table 4–15) (174). However, in hypocalcemic states, calcium infusion significantly improves contractile performance with parallel increases in MAP. Therefore, the inotropic effect of calcium infusions should be of limited value during cardiac surgery (174). Ionized

hypocalcemia should not be overtreated in patients recovering from cardiac surgery. Considerable evidence demonstrates that the administration of calcium after cardiac surgery only increases MAP (175, 176), actually attenuates the β-adrenergic effects of epinephrine (Fig. 4–14) (175), and does not increase vasoconstriction produced by β agonists (176). Calcium salts seem to confer no benefit to patients who otherwise require inotropic or vasoactive agents (177).

The cornerstone of therapy for confirmed, symptomatic, ionized hypocalcemia ([Ca^{2+}] < 0.7 mM) is calcium administration. For patients who have severe or symptomatic hypo-

Table 4–15. Serum Ionized [Ca^{2+}] Concentrations and Hemodynamic Variables 1 Minute After Calcium Administration (5 mg/kg intravenous bolus) in Normocalcemic and Hypocalcemic Dogs[a]

	Normocalcemic		Hypocalcemic		
	Baseline	1 min	Baseline	CPD	1 min
[Ca^{2+}] (mmol/L)	1.24 ± 0.04	1.47 ± 0.06[b]	1.24 ± 0.03	0.76 ± 0.03[b]	1.42 ± 0.22
E$_{lves}$ (mm Hg/mL)	4.06 ± 1.00	2.16 ± 0.90[b]	5.03 ± 0.47	3.76 ± 0.61[b]	4.87 ± 0.64
HR (beats/min)	159 ± 8	260 ± 9	154 ± 6	144 ± 7[b]	148 ± 6[b]
PAOP (mm Hg)	9 ± 2	9 ± 1	7 ± 1	10 ± 2	9 ± 2
MAP (mm Hg)	120 ± 6	137 ± 8[b]	157 ± 6	131 ± 6[b]	154 ± 6
SVR (dyne/s/cm^{-1})	3858 ± 458	4347 ± 596[b]	4067 ± 550	3697 ± 479	4548 ± 904
CO (L/min)	2.7 ± 0.4	2.7 ± 0.4	3.4 ± 0.2	3.0 ± 0.3	3.1 ± 0.4

[a] Dogs were rendered acutely hypocalcemic by CPD administration.
[b] P < .05 vs. baseline.
Values are mean ± SEM (n = 6); E$_{lves}$, slope of the left ventricular end-systolic pressure-volume relationship; CPD, citrate-phosphate-dextrose; HR, heart rate; PAOP, pulmonary artery occlusion pressure; MAP, mean arterial pressure; SVR, systemic vascular resistance; CO, cardiac output.
Reproduced with permission from Mathru M, Rooney MW, Goldberg SA, et al. Separation of myocardial versus peripheral effects of calcium administration in normocalcemic and hypocalcemic states using pressure-volume (conductance) relationships. Anesth Analg 1993;77:250–255.

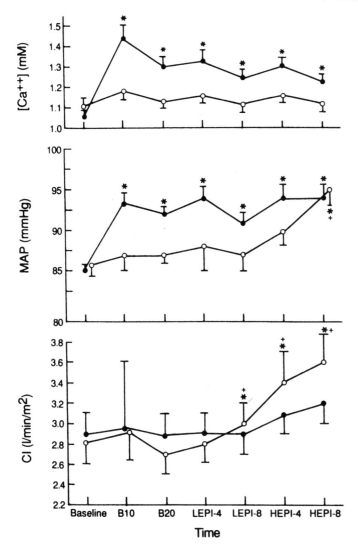

Fig. 4–14. Effects of epinephrine infusion, with (closed circle) and without (open circle) simultaneous infusion of calcium chloride (10 mg·kg^{-1} bolus followed by 2 mg·kg^{-1}·h^{-1} infusion). Baseline, baseline; B10, 10 minutes into calcium and D$_5$W infusion; B20, 20 minutes into calcium and D$_5$W infusion. In 12 adult patients on the first day after aortocoronary bypass surgery, calcium chloride significantly increased ionized calcium levels and mean arterial pressure (* $P <$ .05 in comparison to baseline). Epinephrine was infused in a low dose (LEPI; 10 mg·kg^{-1}·min^{-1}) for 4 minutes and 8 minutes (LEPI-4 and LEPI-8, respectively) and in a high dose (HEPI; 30 mg·kg^{-1}·min^{-1}) for 4 and 8 minutes (HEPI-4 and HEPI-8, respectively). Infused alone, epinephrine significantly increased blood pressure and cardiac output in comparison to predrug (B20) data ($P <$ .05). During the infusion of calcium chloride, epinephrine failed to significantly increase either mean arterial pressure (MAP) or cardiac index (CI). (Reproduced with permission from Zaloga GP, Strickland RA, Butterworth JF IV, et al. Calcium attenuates epinephrine's β-adrenergic effects in postoperative heart surgery patients. Circulation 1990;81:196–200.)

calcemia, calcium should be administered intravenously. In emergency situations in an averaged-sized adult, the "rule of 10s" advises infusion of 10 mL of 10% calcium gluconate (93 mg elemental calcium) over 10 minutes, followed by a continuous infusion of elemental calcium, 0.3 to 2 mg·kg^{-1}·h^{-1} (i.e., 3 to 16 mL·h^{-1} of 10% calcium gluconate for a 70-kg adult). Calcium salts should be diluted in 50 to 100 mL D5W (to limit venous irritation and thrombosis), should not be mixed with bicarbonate (to prevent precipitation), and must be given cautiously to digitalized pa-

tients because calcium increases the toxicity of digoxin. The response to treatment of hypocalcemia can be monitored clinically by using Chvostek's and Trousseau's signs. Continuous ECG monitoring during initial therapy will detect cardiotoxicity (e.g., heart block, ventricular fibrillation). During calcium replacement, the clinician should monitor serum calcium, magnesium, phosphate, potassium, and creatinine. When the ionized [Ca^{2+}] is stable in the range of 4 to 5 mg·dL^{-1} (1.0 to 1.25 mM), oral calcium supplements can substitute for parenteral therapy. Urinary calcium should be monitored in an attempt to avoid hypercalciuria (>5 mg·kg^{-1} per 24 hours) and urinary tract stone formation.

When supplementation fails to maintain serum calcium within the normal range or if hypercalciuria develops, vitamin D may be added. Although the principal effect of vitamin D is to increase enteric calcium absorption, osseous calcium resorption is also enhanced. When rapid changes in dosage are anticipated or an immediate effect is required (e.g., postoperative hypoparathyroidism), shorter-acting calciferols such as dihydrotachysterol may be preferable. The earliest vitamin D metabolite that is deficient should be administered first, to allow the body a chance to regulate activation of the vitamin to calcitriol and replenish other vitamin D metabolites. When the 1-hydroxylase enzyme is deficient, as in renal failure, it is best to administer calcitriol. Because the effect of the vitamin is not regulated, the dosages of calcium and vitamin D should be adjusted to raise the serum calcium into the low normal range.

Physiologic states and concurrently administered drugs may influence therapeutic results. Bone remineralization after initiation of therapy (e.g., after correction of hyperparathyroidism) may increase calcium requirements. When remineralization is complete, a reduction in calcium or vitamin D may be necessary to avoid hypercalcemia. Malabsorption states impair vitamin D absorption more than calcium absorption; major dosage adjustments may be required as malabsorption is corrected. Calciferol requirements are increased in patients receiving bile acid sequestrants (e.g., cholestyramine), barbiturates, phenytoin, corticosteroids, and calciuric diuretics (e.g., furosemide). Requirements are decreased by hypocalciuric diuretics (e.g., thiazides).

Adverse reactions to calcium and vitamin D result in hypercalcemia and hypercalciuria. If hypercalcemia develops, calcium and vitamin D should be discontinued and appropriate therapy should be given. The toxic effects of vitamin D metabolites persist in proportion to their biologic half-lives (ergocalciferol, 20 to 60 days; dihydrotachysterol, 5 to 15 days; calcitriol, 2 to 10 days). Glucocorticoids antagonize the toxic effects of vitamin D metabolites.

HYPERCALCEMIA

Although measurement of ionized [Ca^{2+}] is best for detecting hypercalcemia, most studies of hypercalcemia have defined hypercalcemia using total serum calcium values. Hypercalcemia (total serum calcium > 10.5 mg·dL^{-1} or ionized [Ca^{2+}] > 1.3 mM) causes a variety of pathophysiologic alterations. Patients in whom total serum calcium is less than 11.5 mg·dL^{-1} are usually asymptomatic. Patients with moderate hypercalcemia (total serum calcium 11.5 to 13 mg·dL^{-1}) may show symptoms of lethargy, anorexia, nausea, and polyuria. Severe hypercalcemia (total serum calcium > 13 mg·dL^{-1}) is associated with more severe neuromyopathic symptoms, including muscle weakness, depression, impaired memory, emotional lability, lethargy, stupor, and coma.

Urinary concentrating ability deteriorates early in hypercalcemic patients. Hypercalcemia impairs renal excretory capacity for calcium by irreversibly precipitating calcium salts within the renal parenchyma and by reducing RBF and GFR. In response to hypovolemia, renal tubular reabsorption of sodium results in enhanced renal calcium reabsorption (Fig. 4–15). When hypercalcemia is severe, effective treatment is necessary to prevent progressive dehydration and renal failure leading to further increases in total serum calcium. Skeletal disease may occur secondary to direct osteolysis or humoral bone resorption. The cardiovascular effects of hypercalcemia include hypertension, arrhythmias, heart block, cardiac arrest, and digitalis sensitivity.

Hypercalcemia occurs when calcium enters the ECV more rapidly than the kidneys can excrete the excess. Clinically, hypercalcemia most commonly results from an excess of bone resorption over bone formation, usually secondary to malignant disease, hyperparathy-

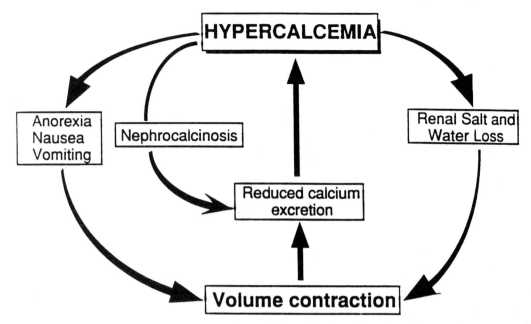

Fig. 4–15. Hypercalcemia initiates a vicious cycle in which renal salt and water loss plus anorexia, nausea, and vomiting result in hypovolemia. The resulting volume contraction further reduces calcium excretion, accentuating hypercalcemia. Nephrocalcinosis further reduces renal function and calcium excretion and results in additional increments in serum calcium. (Reproduced with permission from Davis KD, Attie MF. Management of severe hypercalcemia. Crit Care Clin 1991;7:175.)

roidism, hypocalciuric hypercalcemia, thyrotoxicosis, granulomatous diseases, and immobilization. Hypercalcemia induced by malignant disease results from neoplastic bone destruction or from the secretion of humoral substances that stimulate bone resorption (178–180). Although weakness, weight loss, and anemia associated with primary hyperparathyroidism may suggest malignancy, these may result simply from the primary disease process. Hypercalcemia associated with granulomatous diseases (i.e., sarcoidosis) results from the production of calcitriol by granulomatous tissue (181). To compensate for increased gut absorption or bone resorption of calcium, renal excretion can readily increase from 100 to more than 400 mg·day^{-1}.

The ionized [Ca^{2+}] provides the best diagnostic information. However, a fasting total serum calcium exceeding 10.5 mg·dL^{-1} is a reliable indicator of hypercalcemia. In hypoalbuminemic patients, total serum calcium can be estimated by assuming an increase of 0.8 mg·dL^{-1} for every 1 g·dL^{-1} of albumin concentration below 4.0 g·dL^{-1}. Factors that promote hypercalcemia may be offset by coexisting disorders that cause hypocalcemia, such as pancreatitis, sepsis, or hyperphosphatemia.

Although definitive treatment of hypercalcemia requires correction of underlying causes, temporizing therapy may be necessary to avoid complications and to relieve symptoms. Total serum calcium exceeding 14 mg·dL^{-1} represents a medical emergency associated with frequent complications. General supportive treatment includes hydration, correction of associated electrolyte abnormalities, removal of offending drugs, dietary calcium restriction, and increased physical activity. Because anorexia and antagonism by calcium of ADH action invariably lead to sodium and water depletion, infusion of 0.9% saline will dilute serum calcium, promote renal excretion, and can reduce total serum calcium by

1.5 to 3 mg·dL⁻¹. Urinary output should be maintained at 200 to 300 mL·h⁻¹. As GFR increases, the sodium ion increases calcium excretion by competing with the calcium ion for reabsorption in the proximal renal tubules and loop of Henle. Furosemide further enhances calcium excretion by increasing tubular sodium. Patients who have renal impairment may require higher doses of furosemide. During saline infusion and forced diuresis, careful monitoring of cardiopulmonary status and electrolytes, especially magnesium and potassium, is required. Intensive diuresis and saline administration can achieve net calcium excretion rates of 2000 to 4000 mg per 24 hours, a rate eight times greater than saline alone, but still somewhat less than the rate of removal achieved by hemodialysis (i.e., 6000 mg every 8 hours).

Bone resorption, the primary cause of hypercalcemia, can be minimized by mobilization and drug therapy. Calcitonin, which inhibits osteoclastic bone resorption and increases renal calcium clearance, is most effective in hypercalcemia states resulting from increased bone resorption (e.g., Paget's disease, malignant disease, and immobilization). Calcitonin begins to reduce serum calcium within 1 to 2 hours after drug administration, with the maximal effect evident at 6 to 10 hours. Usually, calcitonin reduces total serum calcium by only 1 to 2 mg·dL⁻¹ (182, 183). After 24 to 48 hours of treatment, resistance to the hypocalcemic effects of calcitonin frequently develops, an effect that may be delayed by coadministration of glucocorticoids. Although calcitonin is relatively nontoxic, more than 25% of patients may not respond. Thus, calcitonin is unsuitable as a first-line drug during life-threatening hypercalcemia.

Mithramycin, a cytotoxic agent, lowers serum calcium primarily by inhibiting bone resorption, probably because of toxicity to osteoclasts (184). Effective for most patients with malignant disease, mithramycin also improves hypercalcemia from other hyper-resorptive causes. The hypocalcemia effect, usually seen within 12 to 24 hours after a single intravenous dose of 25 μg·kg⁻¹, peaks at 48 to 72 hours, and persists for 5 to 7 days. Major toxic effects of mithramycin, more likely to occur in renal insufficiency, include thrombocytopenia, nephrotoxicity, and hepatotoxicity.

Etidronate disodium, a diphosphonate that inhibits both bone resorption and mineralization, lowers serum calcium in many patients with malignant tumors. Daily intravenous administration of etidronate normalizes serum calcium for as long as 2 weeks in many patients with hypercalcemia caused by malignancy (185). Often, however, mithramycin must be added. Pamidronate, an aminobiphosphonate that is 100 times more potent than etidronate as an inhibitor of bone resorption, normalized serum calcium levels in 70% of patients with malignancy-associated hypercalcemia as compared with 41% of patients treated with etidronate (186).

Hydrocortisone is effective in treating hypercalcemic patients with lymphatic malignancies, vitamin D or A intoxication, and diseases associated with production by tumor or granulomas of $1,25(OH)_2D$ or osteoclast-activating factor. Glucocorticoids rarely improve hypercalcemia secondary to malignancy or hyperparathyroidism and may be little better than simple saline infusion (187). Gallium nitrate, an antineoplastic agent recently approved by the U.S. Food and Drug Administration (FDA) to treat malignancy-associated hypercalcemia, reduces bone resorption by reducing the solubility of hydroxyapatite rather than by affecting osteoclasts. Nephrotoxicity is the most common side effect of gallium nitrate; therefore, the agent should not be administered to patients with serum creatinine values greater than 2.5 mg·L⁻¹ or to patients receiving nephrotoxic drugs such as aminoglycosides or amphotericin (188). Infused over a 5-day period, gallium nitrate decreased the total serum calcium concentration in more than 75% of patients with hypercalcemia from malignant disease (188). Indomethacin, a cyclo-oxygenase inhibitor that decreases prostaglandin production, occasionally can be effective in treating rare cases of hypercalcemia that result from excess prostaglandin production. Cyclo-oxygenase inhibitors are ineffective in most patients with hypercalcemia caused by malignancy (189).

Phosphates, which lower serum calcium by causing deposition of calcium in bone and soft tissue, risk extraskeletal calcification of vital organs such as the kidneys and myocardium. Therefore, intravenous phosphates are rarely indicated in hypercalcemia. Because soft-tissue calcification is less likely if phosphates are given orally, the intravenous route should be reserved for patients with life-threatening hypercalcemia or patients in whom other measures have failed. The initial dose of intravenous phosphates should not exceed 50 mM within 8 hours. Patients receiving phosphates should be well hydrated. Slow calcium channel antagonists such as verapamil and nifedipine may also be useful in reversing hypercalcemic cardiotoxicity (190).

Phosphate

PHYSIOLOGIC ROLE

Phosphorus, in the form of phosphate, is distributed in similar concentrations throughout intracellular and extracellular fluid. Eighty-five percent of phosphate is osseous and 15% is nonosseous. Phosphate circulates as the free ion (55%), as the complexed ion (33%), and in a protein-bound form (12%). Blood levels vary widely; the normal total serum phosphate level ranges from 2.7 to 4.5 $mg \cdot dL^{-1}$ in adults. Phosphates play a vital role in energy storage and are responsible for the primary energy bond in ATP and creatine phosphate. Therefore, severe phosphate depletion results in cellular energy depletion. Phosphorus is an essential element of second-messenger systems, including cAMP and phosphoinositides, and a major component of nucleic acids, phospholipids, and cell membranes. As part of 2,3-diphosphoglycerate, phosphate is important for off-loading oxygen from the hemoglobin molecule. Phosphorus also functions in protein-phosphorylation and acts as a urinary buffer.

HYPOPHOSPHATEMIA

Hypophosphatemia is characterized by low levels of phosphate-containing cellular components, including ATP, 2,3-diphosphoglycerate, and membrane phospholipids. Neurologic manifestations of hypophosphatemia include paresthesias, myopathy, encephalopathy, delirium, seizures, and coma (191). Hematologic abnormalities include dysfunction of erythrocytes, platelets, and leukocytes. Muscle weakness and malaise are common. Respiratory muscle failure (192, 193) and myocardial dysfunction (194, 195) are potential problems of particular concern to anesthesiologists. Serious life-threatening organ dysfunction may occur when the serum phosphate (PO_4) concentration falls below 1 $mg \cdot dL^{-1}$.

Common in hospitalized patients (196) and postoperative or traumatized patients (197), hypophosphatemia (PO_4 <2.5 $mg \cdot dL^{-1}$) is caused by three primary abnormalities in PO_4 homeostasis: an intracellular shift of PO_4, an increase in renal PO_4 loss, and a decrease in gastrointestinal PO_4 absorption. High carbohydrate intake, such as occurs with parenteral nutrition, stimulates insulin secretion, which in turn increases cellular PO_4 uptake. Carbohydrate-induced hypophosphatemia is the type most commonly encountered in hospitalized patients. Hypophosphatemia may also occur as catabolic patients become anabolic and during medical management of diabetic ketoacidosis. Acute alkalemia secondary to respiratory or metabolic alkalosis increases intracellular consumption of PO_4 by increasing the rate of glycolysis. Hyperventilation to a $PaCO_2$ of 20 mm Hg may reduce the serum PO_4 level by 2 to 3 $mg \cdot dL^{-1}$ (198). Acute correction of respiratory acidemia may also result in severe hypophosphatemia. In response to acute alkalemia, serum PO_4 frequently falls to 1 to 2 $mg \cdot dL^{-1}$. Respiratory alkalosis probably explains the hypophosphatemia associated with gram-negative bacteremia and salicylate poisoning. Excessive renal loss of PO_4 explains the hypophosphatemia associated with hyperparathyroidism, hypomagnesemia, hypothermia, diuretic therapy, and renal tubular defects in PO_4 absorption. Excess gastrointestinal loss of PO_4 is most commonly secondary to the use of PO_4-binding antacids or to malabsorption syndromes.

Measurement of urinary PO_4 aids in differentiation of hypophosphatemia caused by renal losses from that caused by excessive gastrointestinal losses or redistribution of PO_4 into cells. Extrarenal causes of hypophosphatemia cause avid renal tubular PO_4 reabsorption, reducing urinary PO_4 excretion to less than 100 $mg \cdot day^{-1}$.

Patients who have severe (<1 $mg \cdot dL^{-1}$) or symptomatic hypophosphatemia require intravenous phosphate administration (Table 4–16) (191). In chronically hypophosphatemic patients, 0.2 to 0.68 $mmol \cdot kg^{-1}$ (5 to 16 $mg \cdot kg^{-1}$ elemental phosphorus) should be infused over 12 hours. The dosage is then adjusted as indicated by the serum PO_4 level, because the cumulative deficit in total body phosphate cannot be predicted accurately based on serum levels. Phosphate should be administered cautiously to hypocalcemic patients because of the risk of precipitating more severe hypocalcemia. In hypercalcemic patients, PO_4 may cause soft-tissue calcification. Phosphorus must be given cautiously to patients with renal insufficiency because of impaired excretory ability. During treatment, close monitoring of serum PO_4, calcium, magnesium, and potassium levels is essential to avoid complications including hyperphosphatemia. Oral therapy can be substituted for parenteral PO_4 when the serum PO_4 level exceeds 2.0 $mg \cdot dL^{-1}$. Continued therapy with PO_4 supplements is required for 5 to 10 days to replenish body stores.

Table 4–16. Hypophosphatemia: Acute Treatment

Parenteral phosphate, 0.2 mM–0.68 mM · kg^{-1} (5–16 mg · kg^{-1}) over 12 hours
  Potassium phosphate (contains phosphate, 93 mg · mL^{-1})
  Sodium phosphate (contains phosphate, 93 mg · mL^{-1})

HYPERPHOSPHATEMIA

The clinical features of hyperphosphatemia relate primarily to the development of hypocalcemia and ectopic calcification.

Hyperphosphatemia ($PO_4 > 5.0$ $mg \cdot dL^{-1}$) is caused by three basic mechanisms: inadequate renal excretion, increased movement of PO_4 to the ECV from the ICV, and increased PO_4 or vitamin D intake. Rapid cell lysis from chemotherapy, rhabdomyolysis, and sepsis can cause hyperphosphatemia, especially when renal function is impaired. Frequent iatrogenic causes of hyperphosphatemia include oral PO_4 supplements, PO_4 enemas, and overenthusiastic administration of PO_4 in diabetic ketoacidosis. Renal excretion of PO_4 remains adequate until the GFR falls below 20 to 25 $mL \cdot min^{-1}$. Renal excretion of PO_4 is reduced in hypoparathyroid patients because of the loss of the phosphaturic effects of PTH.

Measurements of BUN, creatinine, GFR, and urinary PO_4 are helpful in the differential diagnosis of hyperphosphatemia. Normal renal function accompanied by high PO_4 excretion (>1500 $mg \cdot day^{-1}$) indicates an endogenous or exogenous oversupply of PO_4. An elevated BUN, elevated creatinine, and low GFR suggest impaired renal excretion of PO_4. Normal renal function and PO_4 excretion less than 1500 $mg \cdot day^{-1}$ suggest increased PO_4 reabsorption (i.e., hypoparathyroidism).

Hyperphosphatemia is corrected by eliminating the cause of the PO_4 elevation and correcting the associated hypocalcemia and hyperphosphatemia. The serum concentration of PO_4 is reduced by restricting intake, increasing urinary excretion with saline and acetazolamide (500 mg every 6 hours), and increasing gastrointestinal losses by enteric administration of aluminum hydroxide (30 to 45 mL every 6 hours). Aluminum hydroxide absorbs PO_4 secreted into the bowel lumen and increases PO_4 loss even if no PO_4 is ingested. Hemodialysis and peritoneal dialysis are effective in removing PO_4 in patients who have renal failure.

Magnesium

PHYSIOLOGIC ROLE

Magnesium is an important, multifunctional, divalent cation located primarily in the intracellular space (intracellular magnesium ~2400 mg; extracellular magnesium ~280 mg). Approximately 50% of magnesium is located in bone, 25% is found in muscle, and less than 1% of total body magnesium circulates in the serum. Of the normal circulating total magnesium concentration (1.6 to 2.4 $mEq \cdot L^{-1}$ or 0.8 to 1.2 $mmol \cdot L^{-1}$ or 1.8 to 3.0 $mg \cdot dL^{-1}$), there are three components: protein-bound (30%), chelated (15%), and ionized (55%), of which only ionized magnesium is active. As a primary regulator or cofactor in many enzyme systems, magnesium is important for the regulation of the sodium-potassium pump, Ca-ATPase enzymes, adenyl cyclase, proton pumps, and slow calcium channels. Magnesium has been called an endogenous calcium antagonist, because regulation of slow calcium channels contributes to maintenance of normal vascular tone, prevention of vasospasm, and perhaps to prevention of calcium overload in many tissues. Because magnesium partially regulates PTH secretion and is important for the maintenance of end-organ sensitivity to both PTH and vitamin D, abnormalities in ionized magnesium concentration ($[Mg^{2+}]$) may result in abnormal calcium metabolism. Magnesium functions in potassium metabolism primarily through regulating sodium-potassium ATPase, an enzyme that controls potassium entry into cells, especially in potassium-depleted states, and controls reabsorption of potassium by the renal tubules. In addition, magnesium functions as a regulator of membrane excitability and serves as a structural component in both cell membranes and the skeleton.

Because magnesium stabilizes axonal membranes, reduction of magnesium concentration decreases the threshold of axonal stimulation and increases nerve conduction velocity. Magnesium also influences the release of neurotransmitters at the neuromuscular junction by competitively inhibiting the entry of calcium into the presynaptic nerve terminals. The concentration of calcium required to trigger calcium release and the rate at which calcium is released from the sarcoplasmic reticulum have been shown to be inversely related to the ambient magnesium concentration. Thus, the net effect of low magnesium concentrations is muscle that contracts more in response to a given stimulus and is tetany-prone.

Serum $[Mg^{2+}]$ is regulated primarily by intrinsic renal mechanisms, although PTH and vitamin D exert minor influences. Whereas both magnesium and PO_4 are primarily regulated by intrinsic renal mechanisms, PTH exerts a greater effect on renal loss of PO_4.

HYPOMAGNESEMIA

The clinical features of hypomagnesemia ($[Mg^{2+}] < 1.7$ $mg \cdot dL^{-1}$), like those of hypocalcemia, are characterized by increased neuronal irritability and tetany (199). Symptoms are rare when the serum $[Mg^{2+}]$ is higher than 1.5 to 1.7 $mg \cdot dL^{-1}$; most symptomatic patients have serum $[Mg^{2+}]$ less than 1.0 $mg \cdot dL^{-1}$. Patients frequently complain of weakness, lethargy, muscle spasms, paresthesias, and depression. When severe, hypomagnesemia may induce seizures, confusion, and coma. Cardiovascular abnormalities include coronary artery spasm, cardiac failure, dysrhythmias, and hypotension. Magnesium is important in the regulation of potassium channels. The interrelationship between magnesium and potassium in cardiac tissue has the greatest clinical relevance in terms of arrhythmias, digoxin toxicity, and myocardial infarction.

Magnesium may influence dysrhythmias by direct effects on myocardial membranes, by altering cellular potassium and sodium concentrations, by inhibiting cellular calcium entry, by improving myocardial oxygen supply and demand, by prolonging the effective refractory period, by depressing conduction, by antagonizing catecholamine action on the conducting system, and by preventing vasospasm (200). Dysrhythmias occurring after myocardial infarction may be related to hypokalemia and hypomagnesemia (201). Consequently, administration of magnesium reduces the incidence of dysrhythmias after myocardial infarction (202). Treatment of hypomagnesemia, which frequently occurs after cardiopulmonary bypass, decreases the incidence of ventricular dysrhythmias after heart surgery from 63% to 22% (203). In addition, magnesium may be useful as treatment for torsades de pointes, even in normomagnesemic patients (204). Because the sodium-potassium pump is magnesium dependent, hypomagnesemia increases myocardial sensitivity to digitalis preparations and may cause hypokalemia as a result of renal potassium wasting. In hypomagnesemic patients, attempts to correct potassium deficits are unsuccessful without simultaneous magnesium therapy. Both severe hypomagnesemia and hypermagnesemia suppress PTH secretion and can cause hypocalcemia. Severe hypomagnesemia may also impair end-organ response to PTH.

Because magnesium is present in many foods, hypomagnesemia rarely results from inadequate dietary intake. The most common causes of hypomagnesemia are inadequate gastrointestinal absorption, excessive magnesium losses, or failure of renal magnesium conservation. Gastrointestinal disease can cause hypomagnesemia by decreasing absorption and increasing magnesium losses in intestinal secretions. Excessive magnesium loss is also associated with prolonged nasogastric suctioning, gastrointestinal or biliary fistulas, and intestinal drains. Renal magnesium wasting complicates a variety of systemic and renal diseases because of the inability of the renal tubule to conserve magnesium. Polyuria, whether secondary to ECV expansion or to pharmacologic (205) or pathologic diuresis, may also result in excessive urinary magnesium excretion. Various drugs and toxins, including aminoglycosides (206), cis-platinum, cardiac glycosides, and diuretics, enhance urinary magnesium excretion and may cause hypomagnesemia. However, patients who have renal disease and reduced GFR frequently develop magnesium retention. Hypoparathyroidism, although frequently associated with hypomagnesemia, seems to be a consequence rather than the cause. Intracellular shifts of magnesium as a result of thyroid hormone or insulin administration may also decrease serum [Mg^{2+}].

Although hypomagnesemia is common in critically ill patients (207), the incidence of serum hypomagnesemia probably underestimates the incidence of total body magnesium depletion (208). Serum values of magnesium may not accurately reflect intracellular magnesium content. Recent studies indicate that peripheral lymphocyte content of magnesium correlates well with skeletal and cardiac magnesium content. Parenteral magnesium tolerance testing is useful in confirming magnesium deficiency in the presence of normal renal function. Measurement of 24-hour urinary magnesium excretion is useful in separating renal from nonrenal causes of hypomagnesemia. Normal kidneys can reduce magnesium excretion to less than 1 to 2 mEq·day^{-1} in response to magnesium depletion. Hypomagnesemia accompanied by high urinary excretion of magnesium (>3 to 4 mEq·day^{-1}) suggests a renal etiology for hypomagnesemia.

Magnesium deficiency is treated by administering magnesium supplements (Table 4–17). One gram of magnesium sulfate provides approximately 4 mmol (8 mEq or 98 mg) of elemental magnesium. Mild deficiencies can be treated with diet alone. Daily magnesium requirements range from 0.3 to 0.4 mEq·kg^{-1}·day^{-1}, in addition to replacement of abnormal losses. Symptomatic or severe hypomagnesemia ([Mg^{2+}] < 1.0 mg·dL^{-1}) should

Table 4–17. Hypomagnesemia: Acute Treatment

Intravenous Mg[a]: 8–16 mEq bolus over 1 hour, followed by 2–4 mEq/h^{-1} as continuous infusion
Intramuscular mg[a]: 10 mEq q 4–6 hours

[a] $MgSO_4$: 1 g = 8 mEq Mg; $MgCl_2$: 1 g = 10 mEq Mg.
Reproduced with permission from Zaloga GP, Prough DS. Fluids and electrolytes. In: Barash PG, Bullen BF, Stoelting RK, eds. Clinical anesthesia. Philadelphia: JB Lippincott, 1992;203–236.

be treated with parenteral magnesium: 1 to 2 g (8 to 16 mEq) of magnesium sulfate as an intravenous bolus over the first hour, followed by a continuous infusion of 2 to 4 mEq·h^{-1}. Therapy should be guided subsequently by the serum magnesium level. The rate of infusion should not exceed 1 mEq·min^{-1}, even in emergency situations, and the patient should receive continuous cardiac monitoring to detect cardiotoxicity. Because magnesium antagonizes calcium, blood pressure and cardiac function should be monitored. In experimental animals, magnesium infusion produces a dose-dependent decrease in systemic vascular resistance, to which hypertensive animals are more susceptible (209). Despite a demonstration of decreased cardiac function in open-chest dogs (210), effects on myocardial contractility and blood pressure seem to be modest under clinical circumstances.

During repletion, the patellar reflexes should be monitored frequently; if they become suppressed, magnesium therapy should be withheld. Repletion of systemic magnesium stores usually requires 5 to 7 days of therapy. When magnesium stores have been replenished, all patients should receive daily maintenance doses of magnesium. Magnesium can be given orally, usually in a dose of 60 to 90 mEq·day^{-1} of magnesium oxide (30% absorbed). Magnesium-containing antacids are poorly absorbed and the dosage is limited by diarrhea. Hypocalcemic, hypomagnesemic patients should receive magnesium as the chloride salt, because the sulfate ion can chelate calcium and further reduce the serum [Ca^{2+}]. Patients who have renal insufficiency have a diminished ability to excrete magnesium and require careful monitoring during therapy.

HYPERMAGNESEMIA

Therapeutic hypermagnesemia is used to treat patients with premature labor, preeclampsia, and eclampsia. Because magnesium blocks the release of catecholamines from adrenergic nerve terminals and the adrenal glands, magnesium has been used to reduce the hypertensive response to tracheal intubation (211) and to reduce the effects of catecholamine excess in patients with tetanus (212) and pheochromocytoma (213). Other rarer causes of mild hypermagnesemia are hypothyroidism, Addison's disease, lithium intoxication, and familial hypocalciuric hypercalcemia.

Most cases of hypermagnesemia ([Mg^{2+}] > 2.5 mg·dL^{-1}) are iatrogenic in origin, resulting from the administration of magnesium-containing preparations, such as antacids, enemas, and parenteral nutrition formulas, especially to patients with impaired renal function. Hypermagnesemia antagonizes the release and effect of acetylcholine at the neuromuscular junction. The result is depressed skeletal muscle function and neuromuscular blockade. Magnesium potentiates the action of nondepolarizing muscle relaxants (214) and decreases potassium release in response to succinylcholine (215). The clinical features of progressive hypermagnesemia are listed in Table 4–18.

The neuromuscular and cardiac toxicity of hypermagnesemia can be acutely, but transiently, antagonized by giving intravenous calcium (5 to 10 mEq) to buy time while more definitive therapy is instituted (216–219). All magnesium-containing preparations must be stopped. Urinary excretion of magnesium can be increased by expanding ECV and inducing

Table 4–18. Hypermagnesemia: Clinical Findings

Clinical findings	Serum [Mg^{2+}] level (mg · dL^{-1})
Normal	1.7–2.4
Therapeutic range (preeclampsia)	5–8
Hypotension	3–5
Deep tendon hyporeflexia	5
Somnolence	8.5
Respiratory insufficiency, deep tendon areflexia	12
Heart block, respiratory paralysis	18
Cardiac arrest	24

Reproduced with permission from Zaloga GP, Prough DS. Fluids and electrolytes. In: Barash PG, Bullen BF, Stoelting RK, eds. Clinical anesthesia. Philadelphia: JB Lippincott, 1992;203–236 diuresis with a combination of saline and furosemide. In emergency situations and for patients with renal failure, magnesium may be removed by dialysis.

REFERENCES

1. Badr KF, Ichikawa I. Prerenal failure: a deleterious shift from renal compensation to decompensation. N Engl J Med 1988;319:623–629.
2. Henrich WL, Anderson RJ, Berns AS, et al. The role of renal nerves and prostaglandins in control of renal hemodynamics and plasma renin activity during hypotensive hemorrhage in the dog. J Clin Invest 1978;61:744.
3. Aukland K, Kirkebo A, Loyning E, et al. Effect of hemorrhagic hypotension on the distribution of renal cortical blood flow in anesthetized dogs. Acta Physiol Scand 1973;87:514.
4. Henrich WL, Pettinger WA, Cronin RE. The influence of circulating catecholamines and prostaglandins on canine renal hemodynamics during hemorrhage. Circ Res 1981;48:424–429.
5. Stone AM, Stahl WM. Renal effect of hemorrhage in normal man. Ann Surg 1970;172:825–836.
6. Hall J, Robertson G. Diabetes insipidus. Prob Crit Care 1990;4:342–354.
7. Salazar FJ, Romero JC, Burnett JC Jr. Atrial natriuretic peptide levels during acute and chronic saline loading in conscious dogs. Am J Physiol 1986;251:R499.
8. Needleman P, Greenwald JE. Atriopeptin: a cardiac hormone intimately involved in fluid, electrolyte, and blood-pressure homeostasis. N Engl J Med 1986;314:828–834.
9. Roy LF, Ogilvie RI, Larochelle P. Cardiac and vascular effects of atrial natriuretic factor and sodium nitroprusside in healthy men. Circulation 1989; 79:383.
10. Cernacek P, Maher E, Crawhall JC, et al. Renal dose response and pharmacokinetics of atrial natriuretic factor in dogs. Am J Physiol 1988;255:R929.
11. Shenker Y. Atrial natriuretic hormone and aldosterone regulation in salt-depleted state. Am J Physiol 1989;257:E583–E587.
12. Laragh JH. The endocrine control of blood volume, blood pressure and sodium balance: atrial hormone and renin system interactions. J Hypertens 1986;4(Suppl 2):S143–S156.
13. Barajas L, Powers K. The structure of juxtaglomerular apparatus (JGA) and the control of renin secretion: an update. J Hypertens 1984;2(Suppl 1):3–12.
14. Briggs JP, Schnermann J. Macula densa control of renin secretion and glomerular vascular tone: evidence for common cellular mechanisms. Renal Physiol 1986;9:193–203.
15. Scharschmidt LA, Lianos E, Dunn MJ. Arachidonate metabolites and the control of glomerular function. Fed Proc 1983;42:3058–3063.
16. Murray MD, Brater DC. Adverse effect of nonsteroidal anti-inflammatory drugs on renal function. Ann Intern Med 1990;112:559–560.
17. Lanier WL, Stangland KJ, Scheithauer BW, et al. The effects of dextrose infusion and head position on neurologic outcome after complete cerebral ischemia in primates: examination of a model. Anesthesiology 1987;66:39–48.
18. Pulsinelli WA, Kraig RP, Plum F. Hyperglycemia, cerebral acidosis, and ischemic brain damage. In: Plum F, Pulsinelli WA, eds. Cerebrovascular diseases. New York: Raven Press, 1985;201–205.
19. Longstreth WT Jr, Diehr P, Cobb LA, et al. Neurologic outcome and blood glucose levels during out-of-hospital cardiopulmonary resuscitation. Neurology 1986;36:1186–1191.
20. Lam AM, Winn HR, Cullen BF, et al. Hyperglycemia and neurological outcome in patients with head injury. J Neurosurg 1991;75:545–551.
21. Sieber FE, Smith DS, Traystman RJ, et al. Glucose: a reevaluation of its intraoperative use. Anesthesiology 1987;67:72–81.
22. Roberts JP, Roberts JD Jr, Skinner C, et al. Extracellular fluid deficit following operation and its correction with Ringer's lactate: a reassessment. Ann Surg 1985;202:1–8.
23. Carrico CJ, Coln CD, Lightfoot SA. Extracellular fluid volume replacement in hemorrhagic shock. Surg Forum 1963;14:10.
24. Lundvall J, Länne T. Large capacity in man for effective plasma volume control in hypovolemia via fluid transfer from tissue to blood. Acta Physiol Scand 1989;137:513–520.
25. Chiao JJC, Minei JP, Shires GT III, et al. In vivo myocyte sodium activity and concentration during hemorrhagic shock. Am J Physiol 1990;258: R684–R689.
26. Shires GT, Cunningham JN, Baker CR, et al. Alterations in cellular membrane function during hemorrhagic shock in primates. Ann Surg 1972; 176:288–295.
27. Böck JC, Barker BC, Clinton AG, et al. Post-traumatic changes in and effect of colloid osmotic pressure on the distribution of body water. Ann Surg 1989;210:395–405.
28. Demling RH. Shock and fluids. In: Chernow B, Shoemaker WC, eds. Critical care: state of the art. Fullerton, CA: Society of Critical Care Medicine, 1986;301–351.
29. Swabb EA, Wei J, Gullino PM. Diffusion and convection in normal and neoplastic tissues. Cancer Res 1974;34:2814.
30. Uhley HN, Leeds SE, Sampson JJ, et al. Role of pulmonary lymphatics in chronic pulmonary edema. Circ Res 1962;11:966–970.
31. Stump DC, Strauss RG, Henriksen RA, et al. Effects of hydroxyethyl starch on blood coagulation, particularly factor VIII. Transfusion 1985;25:349–354.
32. Gold MS, Russo J, Tissot M, et al. Comparison of hetastarch to albumin for perioperative bleeding in patients undergoing abdominal aortic aneurysm surgery: a prospective, randomized study. Ann Surg 1990;211:482–485.
33. Halonen P, Linko K, Myllyla G. A study of haemostasis following the use of high doses of hydroxyethyl starch 120 and dextran in major laparotomies. Acta Anaesthesiol Scand 1987;31:320–324.

34. Palanzo DA, Parr GV, Bull AP, et al. Hetastarch as a prime for cardiopulmonary bypass. Ann Thorac Surg 1982;34:680–683.

35. Sade RM, Crawford FA Jr, Dearing JP, et al. Hydroxyethyl starch in priming fluid for cardiopulmonary bypass. J Thorac Cardiovasc Surg 1982;84:35–38.

36. Prough DS, Johnston WE. Fluid resuscitation in septic shock: no solution yet. Anesth Analg 1989;69:699–704.

37. Davidson I. Fluid resuscitation of shock: current controversies. Crit Care Med 1989;17:1078–1080.

38. Van den Broek WGM, Trouborst A, Bakker WH. The effect of iso-oncotic plasma substitutes: gelatin, dextran 40 (50 g/l) and the effect of Ringer's lactate on the plasma volume in healthy subjects. Acta Anaesthesiol Belg 1989;40:275–280.

39. Baum TD, Wang H, Rothschild HR, et al. Mesenteric oxygen metabolism, ileal mucosal hydrogen ion concentration, and tissue edema after crystalloid of colloid resuscitation in porcine endotoxic shock: comparison of Ringer's lactate and 6% hetastarch. Circ Shock 1990;30:385–397.

40. Linko K, Makelainen A. Cardiorespiratory function after replacement of blood loss with hydroxyethyl starch 120, dextran-70, and Ringer's acetate in pigs. Crit Care Med 1989;17:1031–1035.

41. Zikria BA, Subbarao C, Oz MC, et al. Hydroxyethyl starch macromolecules reduce myocardial reperfusion injury. Arch Surg 1990;125:930–934.

42. Zikria BA, King TC, Stanford J, et al. A biophysical approach to capillary permeability. Surgery 1989;105:625–631.

43. Zikria BA, Subbarao C, Oz MC, et al. Macromolecules reduce abnormal microvascular permeability in rat limb ischemia-reperfusion injury. Crit Care Med 1989;17:1306–1309.

44. Traber LD, Brazeal BA, Schmitz M, et al. Pentafraction reduces the lung lymph response after endotoxin administration in the ovine model. Circ Shock 1992;36:93–103.

45. Rackow EC, Falk JL, Fein IA, et al. Fluid resuscitation in circulatory shock: a comparison of the cardiorespiratory effects of albumin, hetastarch, and saline solutions in patients with hypovolemic and septic shock. Crit Care Med 1983;11:839–850.

46. Rackow EC, Fein IA, Siegel J. The relationship of the colloid osmotic-pulmonary artery wedge pressure gradient to pulmonary edema and mortality in critically ill patients. Chest 1982;82:433–437.

47. Weil MH, Henning RH, Puri VK. Colloid oncotic pressure: clinical significance. Crit Care Med 1979;7:113–116.

48. Hauser CJ, Shoemaker WC, Turpin I, et al. Oxygen transport responses to colloids and crystalloids in critically ill surgical patients. Surg Gynecol Obstet 1980;150:811–816.

49. Lowe RJ, Moss GS, Jilek J, et al. Crystalloid vs. colloid in the etiology of pulmonary failure after trauma: a randomized trial in man. Surgery 1977;81:676.

50. Moss GS, Lowe RJ, Jilek J, et al. Colloid or crystalloid in the resuscitation in hemorrhagic shock: a controlled clinical trial. Surgery 1981;89:434–438.

51. Moss GS, Siegel DC, Cochin A, et al. Effects of saline and colloid solutions on pulmonary function in hemorrhagic shock. Surg Gynecol Obstet 1971;133:53–58.

52. Pearl RG, Halperin BD, Mihm FG, et al. Pulmonary effects of crystalloid and colloid resuscitation from hemorrhagic shock in the presence of oleic acid-induced pulmonary capillary injury in the dog. Anesthesiology 1988;68:12–20.

53. Virgilio RW, Rice CL, Smith DE, et al. Crystalloid vs. colloid resuscitation: is one better? A randomized clinical study. Surgery 1979;85:129–139.

54. Tommasino C, Moore S, Todd MM. Cerebral effects of isovolemic hemodilution with crystalloid or colloid solutions. Crit Care Med 1988;16:862–868.

55. Poole GV Jr, Prough DS, Johnson JC, et al. Effects of resuscitation from hemorrhagic shock on cerebral hemodynamics in the presence of an intracranial mass. J Trauma 1987;27:18–23.

56. Zornow MH, Todd MM, Moore SS. The acute cerebral effects of changes in plasma osmolality and oncotic pressure. Anesthesiology 1987;67:936–941.

57. Warner DS, Boehland LA. Effects of iso-osmolal intravenous fluid therapy on post-ischemic brain water content in the rat. Anesthesiology 1988;68:86–91.

58. Zornow MH, Scheller MS, Todd MM, et al. Acute cerebral effects of isotonic crystalloid and colloid solutions following cryogenic brain injury in the rabbit. Anesthesiology 1988;69:180–184.

59. Kaieda R, Todd MM, Warner DS. Prolonged reduction in colloid oncotic pressure does not increase brain edema following cryogenic injury in rabbits. Anesthesiology 1989;71:554–560.

60. Weed LH, McKibben PS. Experimental alteration of brain bulk. Am J Physiol 1919;48:531–558.

61. Baue AE, Tragus ET, Parkins WM. Effects of sodium chloride and bicarbonate in shock with metabolic acidosis. Am J Physiol 1967;212:54.

62. Monafo WW, Chuntrasakul C, Ayvazian VH. Hypertonic sodium solutions in the treatment of burn shock. Am J Surg 1973;126:778–783.

63. Liang CS, Hood WB. Mechanism of cardiac output response to hypertonic sodium chloride infusion in dogs. Am J Physiol 1978;235:H18–H22.

64. Shackford SR, Sise MJ, Fridlund PH, et al. Hypertonic sodium lactate versus lactated Ringer's solution for intravenous fluid therapy in operations on the abdominal aorta. Surgery 1983;94:41–51.

65. Velasco IT, Pontieri V, Rocha E, et al. Hyperosmotic NaCl and severe hemorrhagic shock. Am J Physiol 1980;239:H664–H673.

66. Mattox KL, Maningas PA, Moore EE, et al. Prehospital hypertonic saline/dextran infusion for posttraumatic hypotension. The U.S.A. Multicenter Trial. Ann Surg 1991;213:482–491.

67. Vollmar B, Lang G, Menger MD, et al. Hypertonic hydroxyethyl starch restores hepatic microvascular perfusion in hemorrhagic shock. Am J Physiol (Heart Circ Physiol) 1994;266:H1927–H1934.

68. Schertel ER, Valentine AK, Rademakers AM, et al. Influence of 7% NaCl on the mechanical properties

of the systemic circulation in the hypovolemic dog. Circ Shock 1990;31:203–214.

69. Constable PD, Muir WW III, Binkley PF. Hypertonic saline is a negative inotropic agent in normovolemic dogs. Am J Physiol 1994;267:H667.

70. Onarheim H, Missavage AE, Kramer GC, et al. Effectiveness of hypertonic saline-dextran 70 for initial fluid resuscitation of major burns. J Trauma 1990;30:597–603.

71. Gunn ML, Hansbrough JF, Davis JW, et al. Prospective, randomized trial of hypertonic sodium lactate versus lactated Ringer's solution for burn shock resuscitation. J Trauma 1989;29:1261–1267.

72. Prough DS, Johnson JC, Stump DA, et al. Effects of hypertonic saline versus lactated Ringer's solution on cerebral oxygen transport during resuscitation from hemorrhagic shock. J Neurosurg 1986;64:627–632.

73. Todd MM, Tommasino C, Moore S. Cerebral effects of isovolemic hemodilution with a hypertonic saline solution. J Neurosurg 1985;63:944–948.

74. Wisner DH, Schuster L, Quinn C. Hypertonic saline resuscitation of head injury: effects on cerebral water content. J Trauma 1990;30:75–78.

75. Prough DS, Whitley JM, Taylor CL, et al. Regional cerebral blood flow following resuscitation from hemorrhagic shock with hypertonic saline: Influence of a subdural mass. Anesthesiology 1991; 75:319–327.

76. Whitley JM, Prough DS, Brockschmidt JK, et al. Cerebral hemodynamic effects of fluid resuscitation in the presence of an experimental intracranial mass. Surgery 1991;110:514–522.

77. Vassar MJ, Fischer RP, O'Brien PE, et al. A multicenter trial for resuscitation of injured patients with 7.5% sodium chloride: the effect of added dextran 70. Arch Surg 1993;128:1003–1013.

78. Johnston WE, Alford PT, Prough DS, et al. Cardiopulmonary effects of hypertonic saline in canine oleic acid-induced pulmonary edema. Crit Care Med 1985;13:814–817.

79. Armistead CW Jr, Vincent J, Preiser J, et al. Hypertonic saline solution-hetastarch for fluid resuscitation in experimental septic shock. Anesth Analg 1989;69:714–720.

80. Smith GJ, Kramer GC, Perron P, et al. A comparison of several hypertonic solutions for resuscitation of bled sheep. J Surg Res 1985;39:517–528.

81. Vassar MJ, Perry CA, Holcroft JW. Analysis of potential risks associated with 7.5% sodium chloride resuscitation of traumatic shock. Arch Surg 1990;125:1309–1315.

82. Spital A, Sterns RD. The paradox of sodium's volume of distribution. Why an extracellular solute appears to distribute over total body water. Arch Intern Med 1989;149:1255–1257.

83. Shackford SR, Fortlage DA, Peters RM, et al. Serum osmolar and electrolyte changes associated with large infusions of hypertonic sodium lactate for intravascular volume expansion of patients undergoing aortic reconstruction. Surg Gynecol Obstet 1987;164:127–136.

84. Norenberg MD, Leslie KO, Robertson AS. Associa-
tion between rise in serum sodium and central pontine myelinolysis. Ann Neurol 1982;11:128–135.

85. Laureno R. Central pontine myelinolysis following rapid correction of hyponatremia. Ann Neurol 1983;13:232–242.

86. Norenberg MD, Papendick RE. Chronicity of hyponatremia as a factor in experimental myelinolysis. Ann Neurol 1984;15:544–547.

87. Wisner DH, Battstelia FD, Freshman SP, et al. Nuclear magnetic resonance as a measure of cerebral metabolism: effects of hypertonic saline. J Trauma 1992;32:351–357.

88. Mazzoni MC, Borgström P, Arfors KE, et al. The efficacy of iso- and hyperosmotic fluids as volume expanders in fixed-volume and uncontrolled hemorrhage. Ann Emerg Med 1990;19:350–358.

89. Gross D, Landau EH, Klin B, et al. Treatment of uncontrolled hemorrhagic shock with hypertonic saline solution. Surg Gynecol Obstet 1990; 170:106–112.

90. Bickell WH, Wall MJ Jr, Pepe PE, et al. Immediate versus delayed fluid resuscitation for hypotensive patients with penetrating torso injuries. N Engl J Med 1994;331:1105–1109.

91. Shenkin HA, Cheney RH, Govons SR, et al. On the diagnosis of hemorrhage in man: a study of volunteers bled large amounts. Am J Med Sci 1944;208:421–436.

92. Lipsitz LA. Orthostatic hypotension in the elderly. N Engl J Med 1989;321:952–957.

93. Gotshall RW, Wood VC, Miles DS. Modified head-up tilt test for orthostatic challenge of critically ill patients. Crit Care Med 1989;17:1156–1158.

94. Wong DH, O'Connor D, Tremper KK, et al. Changes in cardiac output after acute blood loss and position change in man. Crit Care Med 1989;17:979–983.

95. Amoroso P, Greenwood RN. Posture and central venous pressure measurement in circulatory volume depletion. Lancet 1989;2:258–260.

96. Vatner SF, Braunwald E. Cardiovascular control mechanisms in the conscious state. N Engl J Med 1975;293:970–976.

97. Lawson D, Norley I, Korbon G, et al. Blood flow limits and pulse oximeter signal detection. Anesthesiology 1987;67:599–603.

98. Mangano DT. Monitoring pulmonary artery pressure in coronary-artery disease. Anesthesiology 1980;53:364.

99. Shah DM, Browner BD, Dutton RE. Cardiac output and pulmonary wedge pressure: use for evaluation of fluid replacement in trauma patients. Arch Surg 1977;112:1161.

100. Scalea TM, Holman M, Fuortes M, et al. Central venous blood oxygen saturation: an early, accurate measurement of volume during hemorrhage. J Trauma 1988;28:725–732.

101. Shoemaker WC, Appel PL, Kram HB, et al. Prospective trial of supranormal values of survivors as therapeutic goals in high-risk surgical patients. Chest 1988;94:1176–1186.

102. Tuchschmidt J, Fried J, Astiz M, et al. Elevation of cardiac output and oxygen delivery improves outcome in septic shock. Chest 1992;102:216–220.

103. Boyd O, Grounds RM, Bennett ED. A randomized clinical trial of the effect of deliberate perioperative increase of oxygen delivery on mortality in high-risk surgical patients. JAMA 1993;270:2699–2707.

104. Hayes MA, Timmins AC, Yau EHS, et al. Elevation of systemic oxygen delivery in the treatment of critically ill patients. N Engl J Med 1994;330:1717–1722.

105. Berl T. Treating hyponatremia: damned if we do and damned if we don't. Kidney Int 1990;37:1006–1018.

106. Sterns RH. Vignettes in clinical pathophysiology. Neurological deterioration following treatment for hyponatremia. Am J Kidney Dis 1989;XIII:434–437.

107. Lien YH, Shapiro JI, Chan L. Effects of hypernatremia on organic brain osmoles. J Clin Invest 1990;85:1427–1435.

108. Thurston JH, Hauhart RE, Nelson JS. Adaptive decreases in amino acids (taurine in particular), creatine, and electrolytes prevent cerebral edema in chronically hyponatremic mice: rapid correction (experimental model of central pontine myelinolysis) causes dehydration and shrinkage of brain. Metab Brain Dis 1987;2:223–241.

109. Thurston JH, Sherman WR, Hauhart RE, et al. Myo-inositol: a newly identified nonnitrogenous osmoregulatory molecule in mammalian brain. Pediatr Res 1989;26:482–485.

110. Sterns RH, Thomas DJ, Herndon RM. Brain dehydration and neurologic deterioration after rapid correction of hyponatremia. Kidney Int 1989;35:69–75.

111. Deutsch S, Goldberg M, Dripps RD. Postoperative hyponatremia with the inappropriate release of antidiuretic hormone. Anesthesiology 1966;27:250–256.

112. Chung H, Kluge R, Schrier RW, et al. Postoperative hyponatremia. A prospective study. Arch Intern Med 1986;146:333–336.

113. Sterns RH. The management of hyponatremic emergencies. Crit Care Med 1991;7:127.

114. Arieff AI. Hyponatremia, convulsions, respiratory arrest, and permanent brain damage after elective surgery in healthy women. N Engl J Med 1986;314:1529–1535.

115. Fraser CL, Arieff AI. Fatal central diabetes mellitus and insipidus resulting from untreated hyponatremia: a new syndrome. Ann Intern Med 1990;112:113–119.

116. Burrows FA, Shutack JG, Crone RK. Inappropriate secretion of antidiuretic hormone in a postsurgical pediatric population. Crit Care Med 1983;11:527–531.

117. Fieldman NR, Forsling ML, Le Quesne LP. The effect of vasopressin on solute and water excretion during and after surgical operations. Ann Surg 1985;201:383–390.

118. Ayus JC, Arieff AI. Symptomatic hyponatremia: making the diagnosis rapidly. Women of childbearing age are most at risk for encephalopathy. J Crit Ill 1990;5:846–856.

119. Mitnick PD, Bell S. Rhabdomyolysis associated with severe hyponatremia after prostatic surgery. Am J Kidney Dis 1990;XVI:73–75.

120. Rothenberg DM, Berns AS, Ivankovich AD. Isotonic hyponatremia following transurethral prostate resection. J Clin Anesth 1990;2:48–53.

121. Packer M, Medina N, Yushak M. Correction of dilutional hyponatremia in severe chronic heart failure by converting-enzyme inhibition. Ann Intern Med 1984;100:782–789.

122. Oh MS, Uribarri J, Barrido D, et al. Case report: danger of central pontine myelinolysis in hypotonic dehydration and recommendation for treatment. Am J Med Sci 1989;298:41–43.

123. Sterns RH. Severe symptomatic hyponatremia: treatment and outcome. A study of 64 cases. Ann Intern Med 1987;107:656–664.

124. Sarnaik AP, Meert K, Hackbarth R, et al. Management of hyponatremic seizures in children with hypertonic saline: a safe and effective strategy. Crit Care Med 1991;19:758.

125. Sterns RH, Riggs JE, Schochet SS Jr. Osmotic demyelination syndrome following correction of hyponatremia. N Engl J Med 1986;314:1535–1542.

126. Brunner JE, Redmond JM, Haggar AM, et al. Central pontine myelinolysis and pontine lesions after rapid correction of hyponatremia: a prospective magnetic resonance imaging study. Ann Neurol 1990;27:61–66.

127. Miller GM, Baker HL Jr, Okazaki H, et al. Central pontine myelinolysis and its imitators: MR findings. Radiology 1988;168:795–802.

128. Ayus JC, Krothapalli RK, Armstrong DL. Rapid correction of severe hyponatremia in the rat: histopathological changes in the brain. Am J Physiol 1985;248:F711–F719.

129. Verbalis JG, Drutarowsky MD. Adaptation to chronic hyposmolarity in rats. Kidney Int 1988;34:351–360.

130. Cluitmans FHM, Meinders AE. Management of severe hyponatremia: rapid or slow correction? Am J Med 1990;88:161–166.

131. Karmel KS, Bear RA. Treatment of hyponatremia: a quantitative analysis. Am J Kidney Dis 1994;21:439–443.

132. Ayus JC, Arieff AI. Symptomatic hyponatremia: correcting sodium deficits safely. Extent of replacement may be more important than infusion rate. J Crit Ill 1990;5:905–918.

133. Narins RG. Therapy of hyponatremia. Does haste make waste? N Engl J Med 1986;314:1573–1575.

134. Berl T. Treating hyponatremia: What is all the controversy about? Ann Intern Med 1990;113:417–419.

135. Anderson RJ, Chung H, Kluge R, et al. Hyponatremia: a prospective analysis of its epidemiology and the pathogenetic role of vasopressin. Ann Intern Med 1985;102:164–168.

136. Ober KP. Diabetes insipidus. Crit Care Clin 1991;7:109.

137. Snyder NA, Feigal DW, Arieff AI. Hypernatremia in elderly patients. A heterogeneous, morbid, and iatrogenic entity. Ann Intern Med 1987;107:309–319.

138. Black PM, Zervas NT, Candia GL. Incidence and management of complications of transsphenoidal operation for pituitary adenomas. Neurosurgery 1987;20:920–924.
139. Seckl JR, Dunger DB, Lightman SL. Neurohypophyseal peptide function during early postoperative diabetes insipidus. Brain 1987;110:737–746.
140. Verbalis JG, Robinson AG, Moses AM. Postoperative and post-traumatic diabetes-insipidus. Front Horm Res 1985;13:247–265.
141. Robertson GL. Differential diagnosis of polyuria. Annu Rev Med 1988;39:425–442.
142. Griffin KA, Bidani AK. How to manage disorders of sodium and water balance. Five-step approach to evaluating appropriateness of renal response. J Crit Ill 1990;5:1054–1070.
143. Robinson AG. DDAVP in the treatment of central diabetes insipidus. N Engl J Med 1976;294:507–511.
144. Cobb WE, Spare S, Reichlin S. Neurogenic diabetes insipidus: management with dDAVP (1-desamino-8-D arginine vasopressin). Ann Intern Med 1978;88:183–188.
145. Shucart WA, Jackson I. Management of diabetes insipidus in neurosurgical patients. J Neurosurg 1976;44:65–71.
146. Chanson P, Jedynak CP, Dabrowski G, et al. Ultralow doses of vasopressin in the management of diabetes insipidus. Crit Care Med 1987;15:44–46.
147. Jamison RL. Potassium recycling. Kidney Int 1987;31:695.
148. Greger R, Gögelein H. Role of K⁺ conductive pathways in the nephron. Kidney Int 1987;31:1055-1064.
149. Sweadner KJ, Goldin SM. Active transport of sodium and potassium ions. Mechanism, function, and regulation. N Engl J Med 1980;302:777–783.
150. Vitez TS, Soper LE, Wong KC, et al. Chronic hypokalemia and intraoperative dysrhythmias. Anesthesiology 1985;63:130–133.
151. Relman AS, Schwartz WB. The nephropathy of potassium depletion: a clinical and pathological entity. N Engl J Med 1956;255:195.
152. Schwartz WB, Relman AS. Effects of electrolyte disorders on renal structure and function. N Engl J Med 1967;276:383.
153. Torres VE, Young WF Jr, Offord KP, et al. Association of hypokalemia, aldosteronism, and renal cysts. N Engl J Med 1990;322:345.
154. Sterns RH, Cox M, Feig PU, et al. Internal potassium balance and the control of the plasma potassium concentration. Medicine 1981;60:339–351.
155. Adrogué HJ, Madias NE. Changes in plasma potassium concentration during acute acid-base disturbances. Am J Med 1981;71:456–467.
156. Koht A, Cerullo LJ, Land PC, et al. Serum potassium levels during prolonged hypothermia. Anesthesiology 1979;51:S203.
157. Kassirer JP, Harrington JT. Fending off the potassium pushers. N Engl J Med 1985;312:785–787.
158. Norgaard A, Kjeldsen K. Interrelation of hypokalaemia and potassium depletion and its implications: a re-evaluation based on studies of the skeletal muscle sodium, potassium-pump. Clin Sci 1991;81:449–455.
159. Tobey RE. Paraplegia, succinylcholine and cardiac arrest. Anesthesiology 1970;32:359–364.
160. Pollen RH, Williams RH. Hyperkalemic neuromyopathy in Addison's disease. N Engl J Med 1960; 263:273–278.
161. Rimmer JM, Horn JF, Gennari FJ. Hyperkalemia as a complication of drug therapy. Arch Intern Med 1987;147:867–869.
162. Textor SC, Bravo EL, Fouad FM, et al. Hyperkalemia in azotemic patients during angiotensin-converting enzyme inhibition and aldosterone reduction with captopril. Am J Med 1982;73:719–725.
163. Maslowski AH, Nicholls MG, Ikram H, et al. Haemodynamic, hormonal, and electrolyte responses to captopril in resistant heart failure. Lancet 1981;1:71–74.
164. DeFronzo RA, Felig P, Ferrannini E, et al. Effect of graded doses of insulin on splanchnic and peripheral potassium metabolism in man. Am J Physiol 1980;238:E421–E427.
165. Vincent HH, Boomsma F, Man in't Veld AJ, et al. Effects of selective and nonselective β-agonists on plasma potassium and norepinephrine. J Cardiovasc Pharmacol 1984;6:107–114.
166. Brown MJ. Hypokalemia from beta₂-receptor stimulation by circulating epinephrine. Am J Cardiol 1985;56:3D–9D.
167. Allon M, Dunlay R, Copkney C. Nebulized albuterol for acute hyperkalemia in patients on hemodialysis. Ann Intern Med 1989;110:426–429.
168. Zaloga GP, Chernow B. Hypocalcemia in critical illness. JAMA 1986;256:1924–1929.
169. Zaloga GP, Chernow B, Cook D, et al. Assessment of calcium homeostasis in the critically ill surgical patient. The diagnostic pitfalls of the McLean-Hastings nomogram. Ann Surg 1985;202:587–594.
170. Zaloga GP. Evaluation of bedside testing options for the critical care unit. Chest 1990;97:185S–189S.
171. Rutledge R, Sheldon GF, Collins ML. Massive transfusion. Crit Care Clin 1986;2:791.
172. Malcolm DS, Holaday JW, Chernow B, et al. Calcium and calcium antagonists in shock and ischemia. In: Chernow B, ed. The pharmacologic approach to the critically ill patient. Baltimore: Williams & Wilkins, 1988;889.
173. Zaloga GP, Chernow B. The multifactorial basis for hypocalcemia during sepsis. Studies of the parathyroid hormone-vitamin D axis. Ann Intern Med 1987;107:36–41.
174. Mathru M, Rooney MW, Goldberg SA, et al. Separation of myocardial versus peripheral effects of calcium administration in normocalcemic and hypocalcemic states using pressure-volume (conductance) relationships. Anesth Analg 1993;77:250–255.
175. Zaloga GP, Strickland RA, Butterworth JF IV, et al. Calcium attenuates epinephrine's β-adrenergic effects in postoperative heart surgery patients. Circulation 1990;81:196–200.
176. Butterworth JF IV, Strickland RA, Mark LJ, et al.

Calcium does not augment phenylephrine's hypertensive effects. Crit Care Med 1990;18:603–606.

177. Prielipp R, Zaloga GP. Calcium action and general anesthesia. Adv Anesth 1991;8:241–278.

178. Broadus AE, Mangin M, Ikeda K, et al. Humoral hypercalcemia of cancer: identification of a novel parathyroid hormone-like peptide. N Engl J Med 1988;319:556–563.

179. Burtis WJ, Brady TG, Orloff JJ, et al. Immunochemical characterization of circulating parathyroid hormone-related protein in patients with humoral hypercalcemia of cancer. N Engl J Med 1990; 322:1106–1112.

180. Davis KD, Attie MF. Management of severe hypercalcemia. Crit Care Clin 1991;7:175.

181. Adams JS, Singer FR, Gacad MA. Isolations and structural identification of 1,25-dihydroxyvitamin D3 produced by cultured alveolar macrophages in sarcoidosis. J Clin Endocrinol Metab 1985;60:960.

182. Ralston SH, Dryburgh FJ, Cowan RA, et al. Comparison of aminohydroxypropylidene diphosphonate, mithramycin, and corticosteroids/calcitonin in treatment of cancer-associated hypercalcaemia. Lancet 1985;2:907–909.

183. Warrell RP Jr, Israel R, Frisone M, et al. Gallium nitrate for acute treatment of cancer-related hypercalcemia. A randomized, double-blind comparison to calcitonin. Ann Intern Med 1988;108:669–674.

184. Kiang DT, Loken MK, Kennedy BJ. Mechanism of the hypocalcemic effect of mithramycin. J Clin Endocrinol Metab 1979;48:341–344.

185. Hasling C, Charles P, Mosekilde L. Etidronate disodium in the management of malignancy-related hypercalcemia. Am J Med 1987;82:51–54.

186. Gucalp R, Ritch P, Wiernik PH, et al. Comparative study of pamidronate disodium and etidronate disodium in the treatment of cancer-related hypercalcemia. J Clin Oncol 1992;10:134–142.

187. Percival RC, Yates AJP, Gray RES, et al. Role of glucocorticoids in management of malignant hypercalcaemia. Br Med J 1984;289:287.

188. Warrell RP, Murphy WK, Schulman P. A randomized, double-blind study of gallium nitrate compared with etidronate for acute control of cancer-related hypercalcemia. J Clin Oncol 1991;9:1467–1475.

189. Brenner DE, Harvey HA, Lipton A, et al. A study of prostaglandin E_2, parathormone, and response to indomethacin in patients with hypercalcemia of malignancy. Cancer 1982;49:556–561.

190. Zaloga GP, Malcolm D, Holaday J, et al. Verapamil reverses calcium cardiotoxicity. Ann Emerg Med 1987;16:637.

191. Peppers MP, Geheb M, Desai T. Hypophosphatemia and hyperphosphatemia. Crit Care Clin 1991;7:201.

192. Newman JH, Neff TA, Ziporin P. Acute respiratory failure associated with hypophosphatemia. N Engl J Med 1977;296:1101–1103.

193. Aubier M, Murciano D, Lecocguic Y, et al. Effect of hypophosphatemia on diaphragmatic contractility in patients with acute respiratory failure. N Engl J Med 1985;313:420–424.

194. Fuller TJ, Nichols WW, Brenner BJ, et al. Reversible depression in myocardial performance in dogs with experimental phosphorus deficiency. J Clin Invest 1978;62:1194–1200.

195. O'Connor LR, Wheeler WS, Bethune JE. Effect of hypophosphatemia on myocardial performance in man. N Engl J Med 1977;297:901–903.

196. Halevy J, Bulvik S. Severe hypophosphatemia in hospitalized patients. Arch Intern Med 1988; 148:153–155.

197. England PC, Duari M, Tweedle DEF, et al. Postoperative hypophosphatasemia. Br J Surg 1979;66:340–343.

198. Watchko J, Bifano EM, Bergstrom WH. Effect of hyperventilation on total calcium, ionized calcium, and serum phosphorus in neonates. Crit Care Med 1984;12:1055–1056.

199. Salem M, Munoz R, Chernow B. Hypomagnesemia in critical illness: a common and clinically important problem. Crit Care Clin 1991;7:225.

200. Dyckner T, Wester PO. Relation between potassium, magnesium and cardiac arrhythmias. Acta Med Scand Suppl 1981;647:163–169.

201. Kafka H, Langevin L, Armstrong PW. Serum magnesium and potassium in acute myocardial infarction. Arch Intern Med 1987;147:465–469.

202. Rasmussen HS, Suenson M, McNair P, et al. Magnesium infusion reduces the incidence of arrhythmias in acute myocardial infarction. A double-blind placebo-controlled study. Clin Cardiol 1987; 10:351–356.

203. Harris MNE, Crowther A, Jupp RA, et al. Magnesium and coronary revascularization. Br J Anaesth 1988;60:779–783.

204. Tzivoni D, Banai S, Schuger C, et al. Treatment of torsade de pointes with magnesium sulfate. Circulation 1988;77:392–397.

205. Dyckner T, Wester PO. Intracellular magnesium loss after diuretic administration. Drugs 1984; 28:161–166.

206. Zaloga GP, Chernow B, Pock A, et al. Hypomagnesemia is a common complication of aminoglycoside therapy. Surg Gynecol Obstet 1984;158:561–565.

207. Chernow B, Bamberger S, Stoiko M, et al. Hypomagnesemia in patients in postoperative intensive care. Chest 1989;95:391–397.

208. Fiaccadori E, Del Canale S, Coffrini E, et al. Muscle and serum magnesium in pulmonary intensive care unit patients. Crit Care Med 1988;16:751–760.

209. DiPette DJ, Simpson K, Guntupalli J. Systemic and regional hemodynamic effect of acute magnesium administration in the normotensive and hypertensive state. Magnesium 1987;6:136–149.

210. Friedman HS, Nguyen TN, Mokraoui AM, et al. Effects of magnesium chloride on cardiovascular hemodynamics in the neurally intact dog. J Pharmacol Exp Ther 1987;243:126–130.

211. James MFM, Beer RE, Esser JD. Intravenous magnesium sulfate inhibits catecholamine release associated with tracheal intubation. Anesth Analg 1989;68:772–776.

212. James MFM, Manson EDM. The use of magnesium sulphate infusions in the management of very severe tetanus. Intensive Care Med 1985;11:5–12.

213. James MFM. The use of magnesium sulfate in the anesthetic management of pheochromocytoma. Anesthesiology 1985;62:188–190.
214. Ghoneim MM, Long JP. The interaction between magnesium and other neuromuscular blocking agents. Anesthesiology 1970;32:23–27.
215. James MFM, Cork RC, Dennett JE. Succinylcholine pretreatment with magnesium sulfate. Anesth Analg 1986;65:373–376.
216. van Hook JW. Hypermagnesemia. Crit Care Clin 1991;7:215.
217. Virgilio RW, Smith DE, Zarins CK. Balanced electrolyte solutions: experimental and clinical studies. Crit Care Med 1979;7:98–106.
218. Feig PU. Hypernatremia and hypertonic syndromes. Med Clin North Am 1981;65:271–290.
219. Zaloga GP, Prough DS. Fluids and electrolytes. In: Barash PG, Bullen BF, Stoelting RK, eds. Clinical anesthesia. Philadelphia: JB Lippincott, 1992; 203–236.

5

POSTOPERATIVE PAIN MANAGEMENT

Michael F. Mulroy, Brian D. Owens

Pain is the first conscious sensation of many patients in the postanesthesia care unit (PACU). It is a consequence of most surgical procedures and can be the most feared experience for patients undergoing surgery. It is detrimental to their recovery not only because of the negative feelings it engenders but also because of the multiple physiologic reflexes that it initiates. Pain stimulates the catecholamine system to produce increased levels of epinephrine and norepinephrine that cause unwanted tachycardia and hypertension (1). It activates the neuroendocrine system, with further elaboration of glucocorticoids that cause increased fluid retention and further increases in myocardial workload during the perioperative period, as well as multiple other hormonal responses (2, 3). The presence of pain can contribute to reduced coughing, deep breathing, and ambulation, resulting in pulmonary atelectasis and an increased tendency for venous thrombosis. The treatment of pain can involve the use of opioids, which precipitate the development of other postoperative complications, such as nausea and vomiting (4). The combination of pain, nausea, and vomiting may delay PACU discharge, increases the complexity of patient care, and may prevent the discharge of the outpatient (5).

PAIN ASSESSMENT

Unfortunately, there is no simple objective methodology for quantifying pain. Some mechanical devices, such as a pressure algometer, have been developed, but they are basically ineffective in assessing the true severity of pain because each patient's response to a painful stimulus is an individual and variable phenomenon. Age, previous pain experience, educational level, and ethnic background seem to play far more significant roles than the actual physical stimulus in influencing the degree of emotional and physiologic response. In attempting to gauge the severity of a patient's discomfort, crude physical signs may be helpful but frequently result in underestimation of pain intensity by medical providers (6). Facial expression (such as a grimace), sweating, or maintenance of a rigid fixed posture are often indications of severe discomfort. Presence of tachycardia or hypertension may indicate distress but can also be seen with anticipation of discomfort. Unfortunately, in pediatric patients, these signs are often the only indicators of pain available to caregivers (see Chapter 19).

Recently, there has been an increasingly frequent attempt to "quantitate" pain by the use of a subjective, patient-based scoring system. An example of this approach is the "visual analog scale" (VAS); the VAS uses a 10-cm line along which the patient quantifies pain as somewhere between 0 (no pain at all) and 10 (worst pain imaginable). Numerous mechanical devices allow the patient to indicate pain intensity by moving a pointer on a scale. Simply placing a mark on a 10-cm line is equally effective. Most commonly, nurses simply ask the patient to specify a number between 0 and 10. The reliability of the scale as an absolute number to quantify pain in a given patient is poor because of the wide variability of individual responses. The scale is more useful when used as a trend for gauging response to therapeutic interventions. A major problem in the use of the scale arises because the patient is often asked to rate analgesia at rest. Although a VAS of 2 to 3 at rest may correlate well with patient satisfaction and with ability to rest or sleep, the same resting VAS does not guarantee an ability or a willingness to cough well, deep breathe, or ambulate. In fact, an excellent resting VAS may be associated with an inhibition of activity as a result of analgesic side effects, i.e., sedation. Determination of VAS scores both at rest and with activity may be more relevant in assessing adequacy of analgesia and readiness to return to normal function.

SOURCES OF PAIN

The International Association for the Study of Pain defines pain as "an unpleasant sensory and emotional experience associated with actual or potential tissue damage" (7). Unfortunately, it not just a simple one-dimensional electrical impulse from the periphery to the central nervous system. We now know that the nervous system bears little resemblance to a linear-wired electrical circuit. The elaboration of chemical compounds in tissues, the presence of modulating substances at the nerve root and spinal cord level, and the effects of neurotransmitters originating in areas of the brain other than the sensory strip play important roles in the subjective sensation that we call pain. Depending on both physiologic and psychological circumstances, a similar stimulus will elicit markedly different complaints in different individuals. In fact, the difference will be seen in the same individual exposed to similar stimuli at different times. To understand this phenomenon, we need some knowledge of the anatomy and pharmacology of pain transmission.

Sensory stimuli capable of eliciting pain activate free nerve endings known as nociceptors, which respond to pressure-induced deformation, extremes of temperature, or chemical stimuli (8). Chemicals capable of stimulating nociceptors include bradykinin, histamine, serotonin, and potassium. Others that sensitize the nociceptor to stimuli are prostaglandins, leukotrienes, and substance P (9). All of these substances are released in areas of inflammation or tissue damage.

The pain message is transmitted centrally by small, thinly myelinated A-delta or by small, unmyelinated C afferent nerve fibers that terminate at neurons located primarily in laminae I, II (substantia gelatinosa), and V of the dorsal horn of the spinal cord. At this time, the neurotransmitter responsible for pain transmission is not known; however, several excitatory compounds have been localized to the dorsal horn laminae I, II, and V, and they probably play a role. They include substance P and the excitatory amino acids, glutamate, and aspartate (10). Inhibitory substances also modulate pain transmission in the dorsal horn. Islet cells within lamina II contain gamma-aminobutyric acid (GABA) and enkephalin (11). Excitation of the pain receptor fibers in the dorsal root entry zone can cause an activation and tonic firing of the group of wide dynamic range (WDR) neurofibers that are associated with the phenomenon of spinal cord activation or "windup." Presynaptic inhibition of pain transmission from the periphery can occur from neurofibers that release β endorphins and enkephalins and cause hyperpolarization of the A-delta and C fibers. There seem to be multiple opioid receptors at the spinal cord level that affect the response in the modulation of pain perception. Opioids also have an effect at the central cortical level, which accounts for many of their side effects, as well as providing pain relief.

The primary ascending tract for pain transmission within the spinal cord is the spinothalamic tract (STT), which originates in laminae I, V, VII, and VIII. The neurons cross to the contralateral anterior lateral quadrant of the spinal cord within one or two levels of their origin and project rostrally. The tract divides into lateral and medial tracts as it approaches the thalamus. The lateral STT continues to the sensory cortex and provides higher levels of pain perception while the medial branch provides multiple synapses to the brainstem and thalamus and ultimately to diffuse areas of the cortex and limbic systems, which serve the affective aspects of pain (12). Descending pathways originating in the brainstem have significant ability to modulate pain transmission at the level of the dorsal horn. Identified neurotransmitters for this pathway include serotonin and norepinephrine, as well as endogenous opioids. It can be activated by intrathecal or systemic opioid administration, intrathecal administration of $\alpha 2$ agonists, stress, pain, and suggestion (13).

PACU discomfort is related primarily to the surgical incision and is transmitted via the somatic sensory nervous system described above. Simple skin incisions are painful because of the high density of sensory endings in the dermis; however, procedures that include incision of the abdominal muscles, particularly in the midline, are more uncomfortable, whereas lower abdominal transverse incisions seem to produce less discomfort. The pain of periosteal disruption associated with orthopedic surgery is transmitted by the same neurofibers, but the osteotomal distribution is not as precise as the dermatomes of incisional pain.

Surgery can initiate pain by other mechanisms. Distention of smooth muscle in hollow visci or of peritoneal tissue causes a vague discomfort that is often difficult to localize. Unfortunately, this visceral pain is transmitted by less clear pathways than somatic pain. Although some discomfort is mediated through the spinal cord, much of the pain sensation is carried centrally through the vagal afferent fibers, which are less susceptible to blockade by either internal inhibitory pathways or analgesic medications.

THE ANALGESICS

The traditional method of providing analgesia for most pain problems is the use of opioids. Morphine is the archetypal compound and has been the standard of analgesic efficacy for decades. It is highly effective in providing pain relief, acting at the $\mu 1$ and $\mu 2$ receptors in both the spinal cord and the brain. It is a relatively hydrophilic compound and therefore has slow penetration of the lipid membranes of nerve tissue, resulting in a relatively slow onset of action. The same property is responsible for its long duration of action. Morphine is not specific for the $\mu 1$ and $\mu 2$ receptors. Side effects occur because of morphine's activation of other opioid receptors. Although respiratory depression is the most feared complication, it is rare when using modern delivery systems such as patient-controlled analgesia (PCA). Nausea and vomiting are the most common reactions and occur in up to 20% of patients. Other minor side effects, such as pruritis and urinary hesitation, can be troublesome. Itching can occur because morphine is a potent releaser of histamine, but other mechanisms are also involved, especially with spinal applications. Central nervous system effects, such as euphoria or sedation, vary considerably among individuals and can be perceived as either an asset or a liability depending on the clinical circumstances.

Because morphine is associated with frequent and bothersome side effects, and because of the problem of narcotic addiction, several alternatives to morphine have been synthesized and used clinically over the years (Table 5–1). None of the synthetic compounds or chemical derivatives of morphine have succeeded in eliminating either concern. Meperidine is the most popular alternative drug. Although it seems to produce euphoria in many patients, it is significantly less potent and shorter in duration. It is an excellent alternative for a patient who does not tolerate morphine because of side effects. Although meperidine is appropriate for short-term use postoperatively, it produces a toxic metabolite (normeperidine) that can accumulate when doses in the upper range of normal are used or in patients with renal insufficiency. Hydro-

Table 5–1. Oral and Parenteral Analgesic Drugs and Doses

Drug	Intravenous Dose	Intramuscular Dose	Oral Dose	Comment
Potent Opioids				
Fentanyl	25–50 μg			Excellent for immediate pain control in PACU, but short in duration
Meperidine	10–30 mg	50–100 mg		Longer relief
Morphine	2–4 mg	5–10 mg		Longest acting; good drug for transition from acute i.v. use in PACU to i.m. use onward
Hydromorphone	1 mg	1–2 mg		Alternative to others, but high potency may be associated with greater risk of respiratory depression
Intermediate Opioids				
Codeine (Tylenol #3)		130 mg	200 mg	
Oxycodone (Percocet, Percodan, Roxicet, Roxicodone, Tylox)		15 mg	30 mg	
Hydrocodone (Vicodin, Hycodan, Lortab, Tussionex)				
Weak Analgesics				
Aspirin				
Propoxyphene				
Acetaminophen				
Nonsteroidal Analgesics				
Ibuprofen			300–600 mg	
Ketorolac	15–30 mg	15–30 mg		Excellent adjunct to opioids, but cost is high compared to oral NSAIDs

morphone is another alternative that shares many of morphine's characteristics but is more potent. The higher potency (and subsequent lower doses) gives a somewhat narrower range of toxic-to-therapeutic ratio.

The most recent additions to the opioid family have been fentanyl and other synthetic derivatives. As a class, these drugs are more lipophilic than morphine and meperidine, and appear to have a faster speed of onset, which is accompanied by a significantly shorter duration of action. They are effective for intravenous bolus or continuous infusion use. They are not free of the side effects of respiratory depression or addiction potential, although the incidence of nausea may be slightly less. They are useful in the PACU when a rapid onset of analgesia for immediate control of pain and a short duration to facilitate early discharge are prime considerations.

The major attempt to avoid side effects and addiction potential has been the development of the agonist-antagonist class of opioids. These drugs produce limited amounts of analgesia on their own by interaction with the κ receptors in the spinal cord and tend to antagonize the action of morphine at the μ receptors. Although there seems to be less risk of respiratory depression with these drugs, it is not altogether absent. More importantly, they all seem to be have a "ceiling effect" of analgesia, beyond which the addition of further drug does not provide additional pain relief. Although attractive in concept, these drugs seem to have limited clinical utility compared to the traditional opioids.

For mild degrees of pain, codeine and several of its derivatives are available, especially when oral analgesia is appropriate. Codeine, hydrocodone, and oxycodone are all more effective than aspirin but definitely less potent than other opioids. The main advantages are the oral route of administration and a relative lack of significant respiratory depression when compared to morphine. Unfortunately, they are not free of the potential to cause nausea, vomiting, and pruritus. They are frequently combined with aspirin or acetaminophen to enhance analgesic effects (Table 5–1). They are especially effective in providing adequate oral analgesia for patients who are to be discharged to home from the PACU.

Nonsteroidal anti-inflammatory drugs (NSAIDS) are another slightly less potent class of analgesics but with a different mechanism of action. They interfere with the synthesis of the prostaglandin compounds, which serve as augmenters of pain in the periphery and in the spinal cord. The NSAIDS have been effective in producing clinical analgesia, especially in situations involving inflammatory types of pain, such as orthopedic procedures. One of the major advantages of the NSAIDS is the absence of respiratory depression and of nausea. This property makes them an ideal class of drugs for outpatient analgesia. In inpatients, they are effective in reducing narcotic requirements and thereby reducing the severity and frequency of side effects associated with potent opioids. NSAIDs are predominantly oral medications. The one exception is ketorolac, which is available for intramuscular or intravenous injection. This drug (30 to 60 mg) is equivalent to 6 to 8 mg of morphine in clinical trials and is effective in the PACU in supplementing opioid analgesia. It may even be sufficient to provide total analgesia for some outpatients having minor surgical procedures. Although cost-effective as a parenteral medication, the expense of the oral form of ketorolac and a potency similar to other oral NSAIDs make it less attractive than other NSAIDS.

ROUTES OF ADMINISTRATION

With the exception of outpatients having minor surgical procedures, most PACU patients are limited by an inability to use oral forms of analgesics in the immediate recovery period. Opioids are traditionally given by the intramuscular or intravenous route. Although the intramuscular route has been the gold standard for postoperative analgesia and has the appeal of simplicity from the physician's and nurse's point of view, it has several shortcomings. Intramuscular injection is associated with pain from the injection itself, as well as anxiety in the mind of patients concerned about needle sticks. The potential also exists for nerve injury or a hematoma formation with needle injections. Also a major problem with this technique is that the blood levels of opioid are extremely variable. It takes an unpredictable period of time for the blood levels to reach the minimum analgesic concentration. Because of this delay in onset, there is a tendency to inject a larger dose than is needed in order to provide a more rapid rise in blood levels. This leads to an "overshoot" of opioid effect, creating a period of excessive blood levels that may be associated with respiratory depression, nausea, and sedation (Fig. 5–1). When the blood level falls, there is an inevitable drop below the minimum effective analgesic concentration and a period of inadequate analgesia, the stimulus for the patient to request additional medication. The delay in onset of analgesia is compounded by a system that requires a patient request, a caregiver assessment, controlled substance security, and documentation of therapeutic intervention. Multiple clinical studies have documented the inadequacy of this modality of analgesia (14). It is associated with a high frequency of side effects, as well as a high frequency of inadequate analgesia. It is estimated that for most patients there is adequate analgesia for only 35% of the time between injections on an "as needed" intramuscular narcotic dose regimen. Equally important is the adversarial relationship that develops between the patient

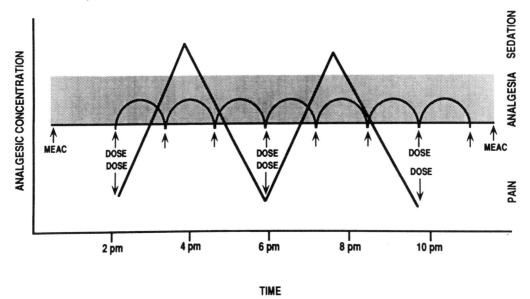

Fig. 5-1. Blood opioid levels with patient-controlled analgesia (PCA). Traditional intramuscular injections create wide fluctuation in blood levels and analgesia, with alternating periods of pain and excessive levels associated with side effects. The use of small incremental injections by the patient in response to varying needs with PCA allows the blood level to be maintained just above the minimum effective analgesic concentration (MEAC) without the potential for side effects. (Reproduced with permission from Ferrante FM, VadeBoncouer TR. Postoperative pain management. New York: Churchill Livingstone, 1993.)

seeking consistent relief of pain and the caregiver focused on life-threatening complications or fear of satisfying drug-seeking behavior.

The concept of the minimum effective analgesic concentration (MEAC) deserves comment. For each of the opioids and for each patient, there is a range of blood level that provides adequate analgesia with minimum side effects. If the blood level falls below the minimum effective concentration, the patient suffers pain. Blood levels above this concentration do not provide additional analgesia but can increase the risk of side effects. The level required obviously varies with each narcotic because of intrinsic variations in potency. More significantly, the MEAC varies considerably among individuals (15). In fact, for meperidine and fentanyl, the MEACs have been found to vary by a factor of 4 among individuals (Fig. 5-2). This wide variation in sensitivity makes a prediction of a single dose for every patient a particularly difficult and frustrating

exercise. Although many opioid regimens recommend doses based on body weight (mg/kg scales), the impressive variability in response suggests that factors other than weight are far more significant in determining individual dose requirements. It is a commonly observed phenomenon that age is one of the primary determinants of narcotic requirement (16). Although it is recognized that elderly patients are more sensitive to analgesics and require lower doses, the opposite phenomenon is often ignored: younger people need higher doses. Age is also a relative term. The physiologic status of the patient is obviously far more important than the chronological assignment of an age category.

Because of unpredictable individual sensitivity and erratic blood levels obtained with traditional intramuscular injection, the use of the intravenous route for narcotic administration is far more appropriate in the PACU. Intravenous injection provides rapid attainment of a therapeutic blood level and an onset

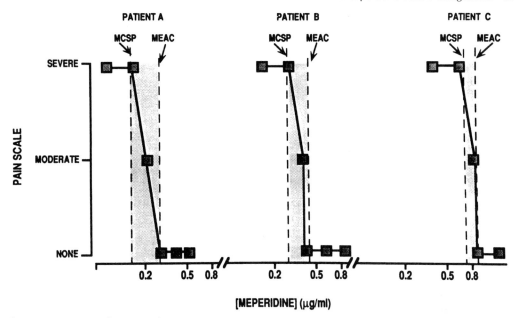

Fig. 5–2. Minimum effective analgesic concentration (MEAC). For each opioid in each patient, there is an MEAC in blood. Above this level, the patient has adequate pain relief. Below this level, analgesia diminishes until the concentration falls below the maximum concentration associated with severe pain (MCSP). The data represent three patients receiving meperidine and demonstrate the wide variation in individual response to opioids, with at least a threefold difference in MEACs in these three patients. (Reprinted from Austin KL, Stapleton JV, Mather LE. Relationship between blood meperidine concentrations and analgesic response: a preliminary report. Anesthesiology 1980;53:460, as modified by Ferrante, with permission.)

of analgesia that allows for early assessment of patient sensitivity and dose requirement. Unfortunately, the rapid onset of action comes with a shorter duration. Nevertheless, it allows more accurate and effective titration and adjustment of patient dosage. It is particularly effective as patients emerge from the residual effects of general anesthetic agents and experience increasing analgesic requirements. The down side of intravenous titration is the amount of nursing time required. Doses must be individually injected, and the patient must be observed closely for respiratory depression associated with the rapid onset of the opioid effect. Nevertheless, this is the most common and effective modality for obtaining acute relief immediately upon arrival in the PACU.

The ideal method of systemic opioid administration would be a continuous infusion that would maintain the patient's blood level at the MEAC. This is not always possible,

because analgesic requirements may vary as the patient emerges from an anesthetic or increases or decreases activity level. The modality that most nearly approaches this ideal is the intravenous titration of small increments of opioid by the patient to meet his or her needs. This concept of intravenous PCA is the most common form of postoperative analgesia currently used in the United States (17). Machines are currently available that allow the patient to inject a small dose of opioid by pushing a button when he or she perceives a need for further analgesia. The machines incorporate a timed interval before the next dose can be administered ("lockout"). This allows the patient to evaluate an analgesic effect from an injected dose before repeating it and thus tends to prevent overdosing. If the patient injects more than is required to maintain their MEAC, the sedation produced will usually prevent them from pushing the button. These machines have proven to be effective in maintaining adequate blood levels of opioids (Fig. 5–1) and can even be employed in the PACU as soon as the patient is awake enough to understand the mechanics of pushing the button. Utility in the PACU can be increased by explaining the system preoperatively.

The important principle in the use of PCA is that the small recommended injections will only maintain a certain blood level of opioid. The effective analgesic concentration must be produced by an injection of a loading dose initially to reach that blood level. This combination of intravenous titration by a PACU nurse followed by the self-administration of small increments to maintain that blood level using intravenous PCA by the patient is an excellent form of analgesia for many surgical patients.

Virtually every opioid has been used in the intravenous PCA mode. The more common drugs are morphine and meperidine, which are available in commercial cartridges for use in the standard commercial machines. Individual pharmacies can prepare specific concentrations of hydromorphone or fentanyl in machine cartridges for patients who are sensitive to the other two drugs. Loading doses and incremental doses must be adjusted for each patient (Table 5–2).

Intravenous PCA is a very simple and effective modality. The machines have been proven to be reliable after initial mechanical problems were solved by the manufacturers (18). A major problem with this methodology occurs when the control of the injection is removed from the hands of the patient, especially by a "caring" family member. When PCA is converted to family-controlled analgesia, the built-in safety mechanism of patient sedation no longer is effective in preventing overdosage. It must be stressed to family members that only the patient should be allowed to push the button. When PCA is used appropriately, it is associated with approximately half the incidence of respiratory depression seen with intramuscular narcotic injection. This is reported as being an approximate 0.5% chance of respiratory depression for PCA, versus 0.9% for intramuscular narcotics (19).

Unfortunately, the small incremental injections provide a relatively short duration of analgesia and the button must be pushed frequently to maintain the blood levels. This means that many postoperative patients do not have uninterrupted sleep on the first postsurgical night. In an attempt to remedy this problem, most infusion pumps are equipped with a "continuous infusion" modality that can be set to administer a small dose on a continuous basis. The assumption is that this background infusion will allow the patient a certain minimal amount of analgesia, to which he or she can add incremental boluses to provide additional analgesia whenever pain intensity or changes in activity produce an increased requirement. Although it was hoped that this would provide better sleep, the usefulness of the continuous infusion modality has been questioned. It does not seem to reduce the narcotic requirement (20), and it has been associated with a few, rare reported cases of respiratory depression attributed to intravenous PCA (19). Continuous infusion plus PCA should be used with caution to avoid the problem of overdosage.

The mechanism of initiating intravenous PCA involves the ordering of a bolus loading dose in addition to the incremental injections and timing of the lockout for each patient. Standard orders for most services include the option for the nursing staff to increase the incremental injection by a 25 or 50% margin if the increments are not providing adequate analgesia for the patient. Similarly, if the duration of the analgesia is insufficient for the pa-

Table 5–2.   PCA Drugs and Doses

	Loading dose (mg)	Increments
Morphine	5–20	0.5–2.5
Meperidine	50–250	10–25
Hydromorphone	1–2	0.05–0.25
Fentanyl	0.075–0.100	0.010–0.050

tient, the lockout interval can be decreased, most typically from 8 to 6 minutes. It is important to include in the orders the option for repeating the bolus dose if, for any reason, the patient's blood levels are falling significantly below the MEAC. This can happen when the IV becomes disconnected or the machine cartridge is exhausted and not replaced for a period of time. Simple use of repeated small increments will take at least four to five half-lives of the drug to reattain the MEAC, and a repeated bolus injection is more appropriate. The choice of drug in intravenous PCA therapy is arbitrary. As with intramuscular injections, all of the opioid analgesics are effective, and the best choice for a given patient is the one that produces the best analgesia with the minimum side effects for that patient. Morphine is often an effective first choice because of its long duration and excellent analgesic potency. Many patients are highly susceptible to the itching, nausea, and sedation produced by this drug. If these side effects are troublesome, simply switching to meperidine is usually an effective solution.

REGIONAL ANESTHESIA TECHNIQUES

The side effects of systemic opioids are troublesome to many patients. Analgesia can be provided by the blockade of the nociceptive stimulus before it arrives at the spinal cord level, reducing the undesirable excitation of pain reception there and preventing perception at the central level. This can be performed by the use of local anesthetics, which are effective in directly blocking pain transmission from the periphery before central perception is attained. A multitude of applications of localized blockade are applicable in the perioperative period.

The simplest of these methods is the performance of a peripheral nerve block, which is especially effective for operations on the extremities. The use of brachial plexus anesthesia has been shown to be effective for hand, arm, and shoulder surgery, especially on an outpatient basis (21–24). Long- or intermediate-acting local anesthetics, such as bupivacaine or mepivacaine, can provide anesthesia not only for the surgery but also for 4 to 12 hours after surgery. In an outpatient setting, this allows the patient to be discharged from the unit before taking any analgesic and avoids the problems of nausea and sedation associated with systemic medication. Similar results have been produced by the use of local anesthesia for ankle blocks or for blockade of the lower leg at the bifurcation of the sciatic nerve in the popliteal fossa (25). The use of femoral nerve block has also been shown to be effective in the relief of pain after knee arthroscopy, especially when extensive painful surgery is performed such as anterior cruciate ligament repair (26).

For simple superficial surgery, wound infiltration with local anesthetics is effective. Here, long-acting drugs such as bupivacaine are the ideal choice. Local infiltration can produce from 6 to 12 hours of anesthesia after superficial operation and can even provide good anesthesia for operations as extensive as hernia repair. Ryan has shown that the use of local infiltration in the wound after a short-acting spinal anesthetic can produce a rapid discharge of patients from the recovery unit with a significantly lower incidence of urinary retention than was found with the use of long-duration anesthetics on an inpatient basis (27). The use of local wound infiltration should be encouraged more frequently for all surgical patients, particularly in the outpatient setting.

For major abdominal procedures, there are other alternatives for regional blockade. For upper abdominal surgery, the use of bilateral intercostal nerve block has been shown to produce excellent analgesia for up to 12 hours postoperatively when bupivacaine is employed. This modality has allowed maintenance of better ventilation in the postoperative period than a control group treated with systemic opioid analgesia. The use of intercostal nerve blockade avoids the central sedation and respiratory depression associated with opioids. A major drawback is that it is a labor-intensive modality and must be repeated every 12 hours to maintain an effective level (28).

Another alternative is the use of a continuous epidural infusion of a dilute local anesthetic solution. A solution such as 0.1 to 0.25% bupivacaine is effective and, in the lower concentration, will reduce the frequency of motor blockade. These concentrations are usually sufficient to provide analgesia and are effective in providing a high level of comfort for postoperative patients for as long as the infusion is continued. Local anesthetic infusions, however, carry significant risks of sensory anesthesia, motor blockade, and sympathetic blockade. These side effects could produce orthostatic hypotension and weakness on ambulation. The presence of full sensory anesthesia can create the potential for nerve injury if a patient is allowed to lie in a position that puts pressure on nerves or other tissues while the perception of pain is ablated by the anesthetic. Although effective, the use of continuous epidural infusions is limited because of these undesirable side effects.

EPIDURAL OPIOIDS

The most exciting development in postoperative analgesia has been the identification of the efficacy of the epidural injection of opioids (29). It has been shown that morphine and other opioids are effective in producing analgesia when injected at the spinal cord level in very small doses. In the case of morphine, the dose of epidural drug required to produce analgesia is one-tenth that of the systemic level, whereas subarachnoid injections will produce analgesia with doses 1/100th of those required systemically. It has been shown that the opioids work at the level of the primary synapses in the dorsal route entry zone to produce effective analgesia, without producing motor, sensory, or sympathetic blockade. Morphine, the original drug tested, is very hydrophilic and spreads extensively through the CSF after injection. With epidural injection, morphine diffuses slowly through the epidural membranes and requires 30 to 60 minutes before onset of analgesia. This slow onset can be overcome at the risk of increased side effects by the use of higher doses. Initial clinical experience with morphine showed that 2 to 5 mg was effective in humans in the epidural space, but doses of 5 to 10 mg were frequently used to provide more rapid onset. The higher doses were frequently associated with undesirable side effects, and the onset of early and prolonged respiratory depression was seen with the 10-mg doses (30). Other side effects such as itching, nausea, and urinary retention were frequent and led to hesitation and concern about the clinical use of epidural narcotics in the early stages.

Fortunately, clinical experience has shown that smaller doses (1 to 6 mg) are very effective, with a lower incidence of side effects, as long as adequate time is allowed for onset of action. Once again, it has been discovered that age is one of the primary determinants of dose requirements with epidural opioids (Table 5–3) (31). The site of the catheter injection in relation to the surgical incision is also a determinant of dose requirement. With a lumbar injection of morphine, a higher dose will be needed to treat a thoracic incision. The ideal

Table 5–3. Epidural Morphine Bolus Doses

Age	Thoracic Incision Thoracic Catheter	Thoracic Incision Lumbar Catheter	Abdominal Incision Lumbar Catheter
<45	4	6	5
45–65	3	5	4
66–75	2	4	3
>75	1	2	2

injection is through a catheter located near the dermatomal site of pain (32). When appropriate doses were used in large series of patients, the incidence of respiratory depression was low. Rawal et al. reported in an extensive survey of Scandinavian practice a very low incidence of depression following epidural morphine (0.09%) (33). The incidence of respiratory depression was somewhat higher (0.3%) when subarachnoid injection of morphine was used (33). Other prospective series suggest an incidence of 0.3 to 0.4% (34). With appropriate dosing, epidural morphine has become much more widely accepted, with a risk of respiratory depression no greater than after intramuscular injection, providing that the significant risk factors associated with respiratorry depression (Table 5–4) are avoided.

The subject of adequate monitoring to protect against respiratory depression has been controversial. Early interest in the use of pulse oximetry, capnography, or apnea (plethysmography) monitoring was frustrating. The incidence of false negatives was high, and the monitors did not seem to provide warning of impending respiratory depression (32). The most reliable indicator of respiratory insufficiency after epidural narcotics seems to be an increasing level of sedation and a decreasing respiratory rate. Current monitoring standards call for hourly monitoring of the patient's level of sedation for the first 12 hours after injection of epidural morphine, with doc-

umentation of the respiratory rate. A rate of less than eight breaths per minute may require treatment, depending on the degree of sedation. Fortunately, narcotic antagonists such as naloxone can be administered systemically to reverse respiratory depression without antagonizing the analgesia at the spinal cord level, as long as the dose is low (35, 36). Immediate treatment of respiratory depression should consist of a bolus of naloxone in a dose of 0.04 to 0.4 mg, as needed. This can be followed by a continuous infusion of 1 to 5 μg/kg per hour of naloxone, with excellent reversal of respiratory depression but maintenance of analgesia. Although respiratory depression is rarely a problem during the PACU stay, it is an issue that must be monitored after discharge to the floor. There seems to be no reason why patients being treated with epidural narcotics cannot be safely observed on surgical wards in most institutions.

Epidural morphine has been shown to be extremely effective for a large number of surgical procedures. It is most effective when used for thoracotomy and abdominal operations (37, 38). Although it provides excellent pain relief for lower abdominal and peripheral surgical procedures, there is no objective evidence supporting its superiority over PCA narcotics for postoperative analgesia in these surgeries (Table 5–5). In fact, after undergoing cesarean section or hysterectomy, patients felt that pain relief was superior with epidural

Table 5–4. Risk Factors for Respiratory Depression

Patient-Controlled Analgesia	Epidural Narcotics
Continuous infusion mode	Thoracic, abdominal incisions
Family interference	Dural puncture
Respiratory disease	Intrathecal vs. epidural
	Thoracic catheter
	ASA status > 3
	Surgery > 4 hrs

Both:

Advanced Age
Overdosage
Other narcotics/sedatives

Table 5-5. Postoperative Analgesic Regimens

Thoracic Incision	Thoracic fentanyl or lumbar morphine, epidural infusion
Upper Abdominal	Lower thoracic or lumbar hydromorphone, morphine epidural infusion
Lower Abdominal	Lumbar hydromorphone, morphine, or patient-controlled analgesia

Table 5-6. Epidural Narcotic Side Effects

	Frequency	Treatment
Respiratory Depression	RARE: < 0.2%	Naloxone bolus followed by infusion
Pruritis	20–60%	Mild — antihistamines Moderate — systemic nalbuphine, 1–3 mg Severe — naloxone infusion Reduced with infusions, lipid-soluble drugs
Nausea	6–50%	Mild — antiemetics Moderate — narcotic antagonist
Urinary retention	4–40%	Indwelling catheter

Table 5-7. Epidural Narcotic Infusions

	Loading dose	Maintenance
Morphine	1–3 mg	0.04 mg/mL, 4–8 mL/hr
Meperidine	20–100 mg	1 mg/mL, 8–12 mL/hr
Hydromorphone	1–2 mg	0.02 mg/mL, 4–10 mL/hr
Fentanyl	75–100 μg	4 μg/mL, 8–16 mL/hr
Sufentanil	50 μg	2 μg/mL, 8–12 mL/hr

morphine; however, they preferred intravenous PCA because of a lower incidence of side effects and a greater perception of control of the analgesic regimen (39).

The issue of other side effects remains a troubling one (Table 5–6). Pruritus occurs in 30 to 60% of patients. Nausea occurs 10 to 20% of the time. Urinary retention has been an issue in the past but is usually resolved by placement of Foley catheters for patients receiving epidural morphine for postoperative pain relief. Several modalities have been attempted to reduce the side effects. The incidence of pruritus can be reduced by 50% if morphine is administered as a continuous infusion, rather than in bolus injection (Table 5–7). Although at first glance, it seems illogical to administer a long-acting drug as a con-

tinuous infusion, this modality avoids the peaks and valleys associated with intermittent bolus injections, just as intravenous PCA maintains a more stable level of systemic analgesia. With lower peak levels of narcotic, side effects are reduced (40). The use of antagonist drugs has also been attempted. As mentioned above, the systemic infusion of naloxone will significantly reverse most of the side effects of epidural morphine without producing antagonism of the analgesia. Agonist antagonists such as nalbuphine and butorphanol have also been mixed with epidural morphine and seem to produce a significant reduction in side effects (34). Administration of a systemic long-acting antagonist drug such as naltrexone has also proven effective. Unfortunately, this drug will also interfere with systemic analgesia, if for some reason the epidural infusion becomes discontinued, and thus may not be a practical alternative for the treatment of side effects. The use of small doses of nalbuphine by the intramuscular or intravenous route are also effective in combating side effects.

There has been an attempt to decrease side effects by the use of more lipid-soluble narcotics. Drugs such as fentanyl and sufentanil are associated with a much lower incidence of pruritis and nausea, and they have become popular as alternative epidural infusions for postoperative analgesia (Table 5–7) (41). Unfortunately, these highly lipid-soluble drugs produce only a narrow band of analgesia and are not as effective in treating pain that is spread over a large number of dermatomes or that is distant from the site of the actual catheter tip. In fact, in these situations, infusion rates of epidural fentanyl have had to be increased to the point at which there is significant systemic absorption of the drug and there is a question of whether the effect is a local one or a systemic one. Loper et al. have shown that for knee surgery, the dose and blood levels of fentanyl were identical, whether it was given through an epidural catheter or intravenously (42). Coda et al. have shown that small doses of the lipid-soluble drugs do produce segmental analgesia but that larger doses (such as 100 μg of fentanyl) actually produce their analgesic effect by a systemic action (43). If fentanyl or sufentanil are used in the epidural space, the catheter tip should be located as close as possible to the actual site of dermatomal pain. Fentanyl infusions are effective for thoracotomy pain if administered through a thoracic catheter, because the narrow band of analgesia is very appropriate for the neural dermatomal distribution of pain (37).

The efficacy of epidural narcotics is increased by the concomitant administration of low-dose bupivacaine. The action of bupivacaine is synergistic with the opioids at the spinal cord level. Low doses (0.05 to 0.1%) are effective in reducing the opioid requirement for both fentanyl and morphine. The lower concentration is as effective as the higher concentration and probably should be used to avoid the potential of sensory blockade associated with the higher rates of local anesthetic infusion, especially when the catheter is placed in the lumbar region. Local anesthetic infusions are also effective in promoting early return of bowel function and may actually be critical in producing rapid return to normal function and early hospital discharge (44–46).

Other alternatives include the use of the intermediate soluble opioids such as hydromorphone and meperidine. Meperidine has the advantage of producing some intrinsic local anesthetic effect and is useful in subarachnoid and epidural injection on its own. Hydromorphone is similar to morphine in its ability to spread in the epidural space and to produce an effect by epidural action rather than systemic effect (47). With these drugs, the incidence of pruritis and nausea is significantly less than after the use of epidural morphine; however, they provide a wider spread of opioid action than drugs of the fentanyl family.

Occasionally, epidural opioid injections will not provide adequate pain relief for postsurgical patients. The two primary causes are an inadequate original loading dose or a nonfunctional epidural catheter. If the catheter position has been previously confirmed, the appropriate first step is to attempt to increase the analgesia. Simply increasing the infusion rate on a continuous infusion mode is not adequate because of the long delay required for the tissue levels to increase after changes in the infusion rate. A bolus injection is needed. Usually 50 to 75 μg of fentanyl as a supplemental bolus is effective in providing additional analgesia within 15 minutes. If the combination of a bolus of fentanyl plus an increase in the infusion rate produces an improvement in analgesia, then the infusion rate should be adjusted accordingly. If pain relief is still not obtained, then the placement of the catheter must be questioned. The most effective way to establish proper epidural placement of the catheter is to inject a sufficient quantity of local anesthesia to produce sensory loss in the incisional area. Usually 6 to 8 mL of 1.5% lidocaine is sufficient. It will provide dense anesthesia within 15 minutes of the time of injection. Such a test dose is effective for two reasons. Not only does it confirm appropriate catheter location, but it also gives the patient the psychological message that pain relief is possible with epidural techniques. The pain-free interval (60 to 90 minutes) should be used to readjust the infusion rate so that when the local anesthetic wears off, the patient should be left with adequate analgesia.

In summary, the epidural narcotics have been shown to be a more effective modality of pain relief in all trials, compared with intramuscular or intravenous use of opioids. The presence of side effects limits the application of this technology. It is most appropriate for thoracotomy and upper abdominal procedures. For thoracotomy analgesia, the use of a fentanyl infusion combined with bupivacaine seems to be very efficacious. For major abdominal procedures, the use of more water-soluble drugs such as morphine or hydromorphone in a continuous infusion mode with the addition of bupivacaine seems to be the most logical choice.

NEW DEVELOPMENT — FUTURE DIRECTIONS

It seems that the use of opioids, particularly through the intravenous route, will remain the mainstay of PACU pain treatment in the near future. The possibility exists, however, that new drugs and new delivery systems will be developed that may have an impact in the PACU. In terms of new drugs, current investigative work is looking into the role of compounds such as meperidine that have dual activity. Specifically, drugs that can act both as opioids and as local anesthetics may prove to be more effective in producing analgesia in the immediate postoperative period and may reduce the side effects usually associated with opioid administration. Another avenue of research is examining the efficacy of combinations of the current drugs available. As noted, the use of nonsteroidal anti-inflammatory drugs can reduce opioid requirements and thus reduce the potential side effects from that class of drug.

Of major interest is the development of alternative delivery systems that avoid the problems of epidural catheter insertion and perhaps provide a more stable blood level of analgesic. One of the newest innovations is the transmucosal delivery of a lipid-soluble opioid such as fentanyl. The drug can be dissolved in a sugar-based "lollipop" that the patient can lick to produce a relatively rapid blood level of the opioid. The current usefulness of this modality is primarily in the pediatric population for presurgical sedation. It has not been evaluated as a potential for postoperative analgesia. It may have limited usefulness because of the unpredictability of the blood levels and the delay of onset of action because of the slow absorption when compared with intravenous administration.

Another novel delivery system is the use of transdermal fentanyl. The drug is available in skin patches that allow a slow release of the drug for a period of up to 3 days. The patches have been used as an attempt to provide postoperative analgesia for several surgical procedures. There are several drawbacks to this system. Again, the increase in blood level is slow, and the patch must be placed before the actual surgical procedure to have adequate analgesia at the end of the operation. Blood levels are unpredictable because of variation in absorption, even though the patches are available in different sizes for different body masses. Most importantly, approximately one-third of the patients treated with the patches do not have adequate analgesia, whereas there have been several reports of overdose resulting in respiratory depression. It seems that this modality, as currently available, is not the answer to most of our PACU analgesia problems. This technique, however, may provide a "baseline" level of analgesia that will allow patients on intravenous PCA to titrate small increments of opioid as needed.

A current trend that seems to be more promising is the application of the patient-controlled administration mode to epidural opioids. This technique has proven effective in the relief of pain in labor and in several studies of postsurgical patients. This technology is similar to intravenous PCA, except that the lockout interval should be longer because of the slower absorption of the epidural opioids. Again, as with intravenous PCA, a bolus injection must be made at the beginning to establish an adequate level of analgesia. This level can be maintained by the self-administration of small boluses by the patient. The epidural route of administration may prove to be much more adaptable to the combination of a low-dose continuous infusion supplemented by patient boluses on an as needed basis, particularly with short-acting lipid-soluble opioids such as fentanyl.

The timing of the insertion of epidural catheters remains controversial. From a practical point of view, it is easier to insert an epidural catheter before the beginning of surgery. Attempting to place the catheter in the recovery room is often far more uncomfortable for the patient because of the incisional pain. Placing an epidural catheter at the end of a surgical procedure while the patient is still under anesthesia is possible, but it carries the risk of unrecognized nerve contact in a patient who is unable to report a paresthesia.

Another strong argument for the placement of epidural catheters preoperatively is the concept of preemptive analgesia. It has been shown in animal models that the injection of epidural opioids before the onset of surgical pain reduces the overall analgesic requirement by blunting the "wind-up" phenomenon of spinal cord excitation (48). A few studies have confirmed this preemptive effect in humans when epidural opioids are injected before surgical incision (49, 50). Other investigations have failed to show the efficacy of preemptive analgesia, but this may be related to the difficulty in showing differences in outcome because of the multiple factors that affect a patient's return to normal function or adequate pain relief. Although this issue remains unresolved currently, it seems a prudent practice to insert epidural catheters in the preoperative period while the patient is still awake and cooperative. This allows the anesthesiologist to use the epidural catheter for surgical anesthesia or supplementation of light general anesthesia during the operation itself. Epidural infusions of opioids/local anesthetic mixtures can then be started in the operating room or on arrival in the PACU.

REFERENCES

1. Mangano DT. Perioperative cardiac morbidity. Anesthesiology 1990;72:153–184.
2. Weissman C. The metabolic response to stress: an overview and update. Anesthesiology 1990;73:308.
3. Kehlet H. Epidural analgesia and the endocrine-metabolic response to surgery: update and perspectives. Acta Anaesthesiol Scand 1984;28:25.
4. Orkin F. What do patients want? Preferences for immediate postoperative recovery. Anesth Analg 1992;74:S225.
5. Dexter F, Tinker JH. Analysis of strategies to decrease postanesthesia care unit costs. Anesthesiology 1995;82:94.
6. Choiniere M, Melzack R, Girard N, et al. Comparisons between patients' and nurses' assessment of pain and medication efficacy in severe burn injuries, Pain 1990;40:143–152.
7. Bonica JJ. Pain terms: a list with definitions and notes on usage. Pain 1979;6:247–252.
8. Bonica JJ, ed. The management of pain. 2nd ed. Philadelphia: Lea and Febiger, 1990;1.
9. Yaksh TL, Hammond DL. Peripheral and central substrates in the rostral transmission of nociceptive information. Pain 1982;13:1.
10. Yaksh TL, Noueihed R. The physiology and pharmacology of spinal opiates. Annu Rev Pharmacol Toxicol 1985;25:433.
11. Cervero F, Iggo A. The substantia gelatinosa of the spinal cord: a critical review. Brain 1980;103:717.
12. Ferrante FM, VadeBoncouer TR, eds. Postoperative pain management. New York: Churchill Livingstone, 1993;48–55.
13. Ferrante FM, VadeBoncouer TR, eds. Postoperative pain management. New York: Churchill Livingstone, 1993;55–59.
14. Donovan M, Dillon P, McGuire L. Incidence and characteristics of pain in a sample of medical-surgical patients. Pain 1987;30:69.
15. Austin KL, Stapelton JV, Mather LE. Relationship between blood meperidine concentrations and analgesic response: a preliminary report. Anesthesiology 1980;53:460.
16. Bellville JW, Forresst WH, Miller E, et al. Influence of age on pain relief from analgesics. JAMA 1971;217:1835.
17. Ready LB. How many acute pain services are there in the United States, and who is managing patient controlled analgesia? (correspondence). Anesthesiology 1995;82:322.
18. White PF. Mishaps with patient-controlled analgesia. Anesthesiology 1987;66:81.
19. Etches RC. Respiratory depression associated with patient-controlled analgesia: a review of eight cases. Can J Anaesth 1994;41:125.
20. Parker RK, Holtmann B, White PF. Effects of a nighttime opioid infusion with PCA therapy on patient comfort and analgesic requirements after abdominal hysterectomy. Anesthesiology 1992;76:362.

21. Brown AR, Weiss R, Greenberg C, et al. Interscalene block for shoulder arthroscopy: comparison with general anesthesia. Arthroscopy 1993;9:295.

22. D'Alessio JG, Rosenblum M, Shea KP, et al. A retrospective comparison of interscalene block and general anesthesia for ambulatory surgery shoulder arthroscopy. Reg Anesth 1995;20:62.

23. Allen HW, Mulroy MF, Fundis K, et al. Regional versus propofol anesthesia for outpatient hand surgery. Anesthesiology 1993;79:A1.

24. Davis WJ, Lennon RL, Wedel DJ. Brachial plexus anesthesia for outpatient surgical procedures on an upper extremity. Mayo Clin Proc 1991; 66(5):470–473.

25. Rorie DK, Nelson DO, Sittipong R, et al. Assessment of block of the sciatic nerve in the popliteal fossa. Anesth Analg 1980;59:37.

26. Flanagan JFK, Edkin B, Spindler K. 3 in 1 femoral nerve block following ACL reconstruction allows predictably earlier discharge and significant cost savings. Anesthesiology 1994;81:A950.

27. Ryan JA, Adye BA, Jolly PC, et al. Outpatient inguinal herniorrhaphy with both regional and local anesthesia. Am J Surg 1984;148:313.

28. Bridenbaugh PO, DuPen SL, Moore DC, et al. Postoperative intercostal nerve block analgesia versus narcotic analgesia. Anesth Analg 1973;52:81.

29. Yaksh TL, Noveihed R. The physiology and pharmacology of spinal opiates. Annu Rev Pharmacol Toxicol 1975;25:443.

30. Camporessi EM, Nielsen CH, Bromage PR, et al. Ventilatory CO_2 sensitivity after intravenous an epidural morphine in volunteers. Anesth Analg 1983;62:633.

31. Ready LB, Chadwick HS, Ross B. Age predicts effective epidural morphine dose after abdominal hysterectomy. Anesth Analg 1987;66:1215.

32. Ready LB, Oden R, Chadwick HS, et al. Development of an anesthesiology-based postoperative pain management service. Anesthesiology 1988;68:100.

33. Rawal N, Arner S, Gustafsson AR. Present state of extradural and intrathecal opioid analgesia in Sweden. Br J Anaesth 1987;59:791.

34. Wittels B, Glosten B, Faure EAM, et al. Opioid antagonist adjuncts to epidural morphine for postcesarean analgesia: maternal outcomes. Anesth Analg 1993;77:925.

35. Rawal N, Schott U, Dahlstrom B, et al. Influence of naloxone infusion on analgesia and respiratory depression following epidural morphine. Anesthesiology 1986;64:194.

36. Thind GS, Wells JCD, Wilkes RG. The effects of continuous intravenous naloxone on epidural morphine analgesia. Anaesthesia 1986;41:582.

37. Kavanaugh BP, Katz J, Sandler AN. Pain control after thoracic surgery: a review of current techniques. Anesthesiology 1994;81:737.

38. Liu SS, Carpenter RL, Neal JM. Epidural anesthesia and analgesia: examining their role in post-operative outcome. Anesthesiology 1995;82:1474.

39. Eisenach JC, Grice SC, Dewan DM. Patient-controlled analgesia following cesarean section: a comparison with epidural and intramuscular narcotics. Anesthesiology 1988;68:444.

40. Rauck RL, Raj PR, Knarr DC, et al. Comparison of the efficacy of epidural morphine given by intermittent injection or continuous infusion for the management of postoperative pain. Reg Anesth 1994;19:316.

41. Fischer RL, Lubenow TR, Liceaga A, et al. Comparison of continuous epidural infusion of fentanyl-bupivacaine and morphine-bupivacaine in the management of postoperative pain. Anesth Analg 1988;67:559–563.

42. Loper KA, Ready LB, Downey M, et al. Epidural and intravenous fentanyl infusions are clinically equivalent and after knee surgery. Anesth Analg 1990;70:72.

43. Coda BA, Brown MC, Schaffer R, et al. Pharmacology of epidural fentanyl, alfentanil, and sufentanil in volunteers. Anesthesiology 1994;81:1149.

44. Kehlet H, Dahl JB. The value of "multimodal" or "balanced analgesia" in postoperative pain treatment. Anesth Analg 1993;77:1048.

45. Wattill M, Thoren T, Hennerdal S, et al. Epidural analgesia with bupivacaine reduces postoperative paralytic ileus after hysterectomy. Anesth Analg 1989;68:353.

46. Hjortso NC, Neumann P, Frosig F, et al. A controlled study on the effect of epidural analgesia with local anaesthetics and morphine on morbidity after abdominal surgery. Acta Anaesth Scand 1985; 29:790.

47. Liu SS, Carpenter RL, Mulroy MF, et al. Intravenous versus epidural administration of hydromorphone: effects on analgesia and recovery after radical retropubic prostatectomy. Anesthesiology 1995;82:682.

48. Woolf CJ, Chong MS. Preemptive analgesia — treating postoperative pain by preventing the establishment of central sensitization. Anesth Analg 1993;77:362.

49. Katz J, Kavanaugh BP, Sandler AN, et al. Preemptive analgesia. Anesthesiology 1992;77:439.

50. Sihr Y, Raja SN, Frank SM. The effect of epidural vs. general anesthesia on postoperative pain and analgesic requirements in patients undergoing radical prostatectomy. Anesthesiology 1994;80:49.

6

NEUROMUSCULAR BLOCKADE

Morris Brown

The use of neuromuscular blocking agents is common in the contemporary management of patients for anesthesia and surgery. The principle use of muscle relaxants in the perioperative period is to provide skeletal muscle relaxation to facilitate intubation of the trachea and provide optimal surgical working conditions. Muscle relaxants are used as adjuncts in providing total anesthesia care and not as a primary anesthetic agent. It is, therefore, essential to appropriately monitor the depth of neuromuscular blockade throughout the intraoperative period and, if necessary, into the postoperative period as well.

PHYSIOLOGY OF THE NEUROMUSCULAR JUNCTION

The neuromuscular junction consists of a prejunctional motor nerve ending separated from a highly folded postjunctional membrane of skeletal muscle by a synaptic cleft (1). Acetylcholine (ACh) is synthesized from choline and acetate and stored in nerve endings in vesicles of the axon for release in response to nerve impulses. The acetylcholine is released in quanta both in response to nerve stimulation and spontaneously at random. The spontaneously released acetylcholine results in a small depolarization of the endplate for a miniature endplate potential, whereas when an action potential invades the nerve terminal, millions of acetylcholine molecules are released into the synaptic cleft with an associated influx of calcium ions (2). Once released, acetylcholine binds to nicotinic cho-

linergic receptors on the postjunctional membranes. These receptors consist of five subunits arranged to form ion channels (3). Sodium ions move inside according to the concentration and electrical gradient depolarizing the cell membrane. Potassium ions tend to move out along their concentration gradient. This change in permeability and movement of ions results in a decrease in the transmembrane potential to a threshold potential, which results in propagation of an action potential over the surface of skeletal muscle fibers resulting in muscular contraction. The postjunctional receptors are generally confined to the area of the endplate across from prejunctional receptors, and extrajunctional receptors are present throughout skeletal muscle. It is, in fact, these postjunctional receptors that are the most important sites of action of muscle relaxants. Extrajunctional receptors may increase with denervation or trauma, including burn injuries. After acetylcholine has been released, it is rapidly hydrolyzed by the enzyme acetylcholinesterase, which results in restoration of membrane permeability. The acetylcholinesterase is located in the folds of the motor endplate and in the basement membrane of the synaptic cleft.

MONITORING NEUROMUSCULAR FUNCTION

Monitoring of neuromuscular function with a peripheral nerve stimulator is essential in contemporary anesthesia practice. The peripheral nerve stimulator permits accurate titration of muscle relaxants intraoperatively to produce the appropriate degree of skeletal muscle relaxation for endotracheal intubation and the surgical procedure. Upon completion of surgery, the peripheral nerve stimulator is used to assess the adequacy of neuromuscular blockade reversal. The most common type of monitoring to detect both the magnitude and type of neuromuscular blockade is stimulation of the ulnar nerve at the wrist or elbow and detection of contraction of the adductor pollicis muscle (4). The peripheral nerve stimulator can assess neuromuscular blockade using a single-twitch train-of-four (TOF) stimulation, a tetanic stimulation, and posttetanic stimulation. The depth of neuromuscular blockade is assessed as the degree of inhibition of the twitch response to peripheral stimulation and the duration of the neuromuscular block determined from the time of neuromuscular block until return of twitch response. The train-of-four stimulation, which delivers four twitches at 2 Hz, is the most common means to assess neuromuscular blockade using nondepolarizing muscle relaxants. After administration of a nondepolarizing muscle relaxant, the height of the fourth twitch diminishes in relation to the first twitch, creating a TOF ratio. This ratio develops because the release of acetylcholine is depleted by each successive stimulation. Recovery of the TOF ratio to higher than 0.7 generally correlates with the return of a single-twitch response. In contradistinction, the TOF ratio remains near 1.0 after administration of a depolarizing muscle relaxant because all responses are decreased to the same extent (Fig. 6–1). When the TOF ratio falls below 0.3 after the administration of succinylcholine, it is indicative of phase II blockade (see following sections on depolarizing muscle relaxants).

Administration of a tetanic stimulus at 50 Hz for 5 seconds results in a reduced but sustained contraction after the administration of succinylcholine. With the administration of nondepolarizing muscle relaxants, the response to a tetanic simulation results in fade, unless the TOF is higher than 0.7. Fade is

constant for frequency stimulation from 2 to 50 Hz (5). Because there is more acetylcholine available at the neuromuscular junction after a tetanic stimulus, there is an enhanced twitch response to subsequent stimulation known as posttetanic facilitation. The intensity and duration of the posttetanic facilitation is dependent on the frequency and duration of the stimulus delivered (6).

In summary, the characteristic response after injection of succinylcholine is reduction in single-twitch height, sustained response to tetanic stimulation, and no TOF fade. The block is antagonized by nondepolarizing agents and potentiated by acetylcholinesterase inhibitors (7). Characteristic responses after injection of a nondepolarizing muscle relaxant include reduced TOF ratio, fade with tetanic stimulation, and posttetanic facilitation. The block is antagonized by anticholinesterase agents and depolarizing muscle relaxants.

PHARMACOLOGY OF DEPOLARIZING MUSCLE RELAXANTS

Succinylcholine is the only depolarizing muscle relaxant with rapid onset and short duration in clinical use. As the name implies, succinylcholine exerts its effect on the neuromuscular junction by depolarizing the postjunctional membrane. It mimics the effect of acetylcholine (8). However, because the hydrolysis of succinylcholine is slow in relation to acetylcholine, there is sustained depolarization. Because the depolarized postjunctional membrane cannot respond to subsequent release of acetylcholine, the skeletal muscle remains paralyzed. Succinylcholine is hydrolyzed to choline and succinylmonocholine by plasma cholinesterase (pseudocholinesterase) (9). Because plasma cholinesterase has an enormous capacity to hydrolyze succinylcholine very rapidly, only a small fraction of the original intravenous dose reaches the neuromuscular junction. The termination of action of succinylcholine results from diffusion of the drug away from the endplate into extracellular

$$T.O.F. \ RATIO = \frac{HT \ OF \ D}{HT \ OF \ A}$$

A B C D

Baseline
T.O.F. ratio = 1.0

A B C D

Nondepolarizing
Neuromuscular Blockade
T.O.F. ratio <1

A B C D

Depolarizing
Neuromuscular Blockade
T.O.F. ratio ~ 1.0

Fig. 6–1. Train-of-four (TOF) ratio after neuromuscular blockade.

fluid. Because pseudocholinesterase exerts its action before succinylcholine reaches the neuromuscular junction, it is the pseudocholinesterase that influences the onset and duration of action of succinylcholine. Prolonged exposure to a depolarizing muscle relaxant such as succinylcholine may result in a lack of responsiveness of the postjunctional membrane. This is known as phase II blockade or desensitization neuromuscular blockade. The characteristics of phase II blockade resemble the neuromuscular blockade produced by nondepolarizing muscle relaxants (10).

Succinylcholine-induced neuromuscular blockade can be prolonged by a reduced quantity of normal plasma cholinesterase or abnormal plasma cholinesterase. Many factors have been described that result in lowered plasma cholinesterase levels, including liver disease, pregnancy, malignancy, chemotherapeutic drugs, insecticides, acetylcholinesterase inhibitors, and metachlorpramide (11–15). However, it has been suggested that even in situations in which the measured pseudocholinesterase levels may be low, it rarely results in clinical problems (16). However, an abnormal genetic variant of plasma cholinesterase may result in a markedly prolonged succinylcholine-induced neuromuscular blockade (17). This atypical plasma cholinesterase is unable to hydrolyze the ester bonds in succinylcholine. This results in prolonged skeletal muscle paralysis. Dibucaine, an amide local anesthetic, has been shown to inhibit normal plasma cholinesterase activity by about 80%. However, the

Table 6–1. Effect of Plasma Cholinesterase on Activity

Plasma Cholinesterase	Dibucaine Number	Duration of Succinylcholine Block
Typical homozygous	80	5–10 minutes
Heterozygous	40–60	16–20 minutes
Atypical homozygous	20	60–180 minutes

atypical enzyme will be inhibited by only 20%. Thus, the dibucaine number reflects the ability of plasma cholinesterase to metabolize succinylcholine. It does not measure levels of the enzyme in the plasma. There are many different genetic variants that result in atypical plasma cholinesterase. Most variants are caused by a single amino acid substitution error or a sequencing error at or near the active site of the enzyme. Table 6–1 reflects the relationship between dibucaine number and duration of neuromuscular blockade with succinylcholine. Any patient with prolonged neuromuscular blockade after administration of succinylcholine should be investigated for atypical plasma cholinesterase.

ADVERSE EFFECTS

Many adverse effects are associated with the use of succinylcholine, which may limit its clinical use.

Cardiovascular Effects

Several cardiac effects have been described with the use of succinylcholine, most notably dysrhythmias including sinus bradycardia, junctional rhythms, and ventricular dysrhythmias. Because succinylcholine is structurally similar to acetylcholine, it mimics the effects of acetylcholine at cardiac postganglionic muscarinic receptors. The resultant parasympathetic activity seems to be more common in children; however, cardiac dysrhythmias may occur in children and adults and are most likely when a second intravenous dose of succinylcholine is administered shortly after the first. Pretreatment with atropine or a subparalyzing dose of a nondepolarizing muscle relaxant before succinylcholine administration reduces the likelihood of these cardiac responses. Other cardiac effects of succinylcholine that have been described include elevation in blood pressure and heart rate resulting from ganglionic stimulation.

Increased Serum Potassium

The normal anticipated elevation in serum potassium after administration of succinylcholine ranges between 0.5 and 1 mEq/L. However, severe life-threatening hyperkalemia may result after the administration of succinylcholine in patients after major denervation injuries, spinal cord transection, peripheral denervation, stroke, trauma, extensive burns, and prolonged immobility. The rise in serum potassium is most probably related to extrajunctional receptor proliferation. Patients with renal failure, however, are not at risk for an exaggerated hyperkalemia response (18).

Increased Intraocular Pressure

Succinylcholine administration results in a predictable transient elevation in intraocular pressure, which cannot be prevented by a pretreatment dose of a nondepolarizing agent (19). Therefore, the use of succinylcholine for patients with increased intraocular pressure should be discouraged.

Increased Intragastric Pressure

The effect of succinylcholine on intragastric pressure is controversial. However, the fasciculations induced by succinylcholine tend to raise intragastric pressure (20). Concomitantly, succinylcholine seems to increase lower esophageal sphincter tone and thus counterbalance the risk for pulmonary aspiration of gastric contents (21).

Increased Intracranial Pressure

Succinylcholine results in transient increases in intracranial pressure that may be attenuated by prior administration of a subparalyzing dose of a nondepolarizing muscle relaxant (22). For patients in whom even a modest and transient increase in intracranial pressure could be detrimental, the use of succinylcholine should be avoided.

Fasciculations and Muscle Pains

Generalized muscle pain after administration of succinylcholine is common, especially following minor surgery in women in an ambulatory setting. It has been speculated that the myalgias are due to fasciculations; however, prevention of fasciculations by prior administration of a subparalyzing dose of a nondepolarizing muscle relaxant does not predictably eliminate the muscle pain after administration of succinylcholine (23).

Masseter Spasm

Administration of succinylcholine occasionally results in masseter muscle spasm, especially in children (24). This may result in a difficult tracheal intubation. Although this may represent an exaggerated response at the neuromuscular junction, consideration must also be given to the diagnosis of malignant hyperthermia.

NONDEPOLARIZING MUSCLE RELAXANTS

Nondepolarizing muscle relaxants compete with acetylcholine for postsynaptic receptors sites. Thus, the nondepolarizing muscle relaxants prevent changes in the permeability of the postjunctional membranes so that depolarization cannot occur. The number of receptors that need to be bound to acetylcholine to produce depolarization of the endplate is only a small fraction of the total number of receptors. Therefore, neuromuscular blockade in a given muscle is not apparent until a certain fixed proportion of receptors is occupied.

Pharmacokinetics

Nondepolarizing muscle relaxants are highly ionized at physiologic pH and, therefore, have a low lipid solubility. Thus, the volume of distribution of this class of drugs is small, approximately equal to the extracellular fluid volume. Because of the low lipid solubility, nondepolarizing muscle relaxants do not produce central nervous system effects. In addition, there is little renal tubular reabsorption, these agents are ineffective given orally, and maternal administration does not result in drug crossing the placenta to the fetus.

Classification

Nondepolarizing neuromuscular blocking agents may be classified by chemical structure or duration of action. The two classes of nondepolarizing muscle relaxants, by chemical structure, are the (a) steroidal compounds, typified by pancuronium, pipecuronium, vecuronium, and rocuronium, and (b) the benzylisoquinoline compounds such as d-tubocurarine, metocurine, doxacurium, atracurium, mivacurium, and cisatracurium. Muscle relaxants may also be divided by duration of action. These include the long-acting muscle relaxants with elimination half-lives longer than 1 hour (e.g., d-tubocurarine, pancuronium, metacurine, gallamine, pipecuronium, and doxacurium), intermediate-acting neuromuscular blocking agents with an intermediate elimination half-life (e.g., atracurium, cisatracurium, and mivacurium), and intermediate-

acting agents with long eliminate half-lives (e.g., vecuronium and rocuronium). Muscle relaxants are classified as long-acting intermediate or short-acting agents based mainly on the pattern of metabolism and elimination of the drug. Long-acting agents show relatively slow onsets to maximum blockade of 3 to 6 minutes after administration of a dose to facilitate tracheal intubation. The clinical duration of action of these agents ranges from 80 to 120 minutes. The drugs in this class of relaxants are primarily excreted unchanged in the urine and require antagonism of residual blockade at the conclusion of surgery. The intermediate-acting relaxants typically have an onset of block of 2 to 3 minutes after administration of a dose sufficient to facilitate tracheal intubation. The clinical duration of action ranges from 30 to 60 minutes. Vecuronium and rocuronium have both hepatic and renal excretory paths, whereas atracurium and cisatracurium undergo Hofmann elimination in the plasma as well as nonspecific esterase hydrolysis. The only nondepolarizing muscle relaxant even considered to be short acting is mivacurium, with an onset for tracheal intubation of 2 to 3 minutes. The clinical duration of action ranges from 12 to 15 minutes because the agent is nearly destroyed by plasma cholinesterase. Less than 5% of the agent is excreted in the urine.

Muscle relaxants may also be classified by chemical structure. The steroidal compounds include pancuronium, pipecuronium, vecuronium, and rocuronium. These agents have the advantage of high potency and lack of histamine release. However, they do generally exhibit vagolytic properties. All steroidal relaxants are excreted by the kidney, although they may also have an alternate path of excretion (e.g., biliary excretion). The steroidal agents are generally not extensively metabolized.

The benzylisoquinoline compounds include d-tubocurarine, metocurine, doxacurine, atracurium, cisatracurium, and mivacurium. Unlike the steroidal compounds, this class of relaxants generally results in histamine release. The benzylisoquinoline compounds are essentially excreted by the kidney. However, with the benzylisoquinoline esters, alternate pathyways for excretion exist, including Hofmann elimination with atracurium and cisatracurium and cholinesterase-catalyzed hydrolysis in the case of mivacurium. Advantages of benzylisoquionoline compounds include high potency and no vagolytic effect.

Commonly Used Nondepolarizing Muscle Relaxants

ATRACURIUM

Atracurium is a benzylisoquinoline compound of intermediate duration. The agent is metabolized by two separate pathways: (*a*) Hofmann elimination or nonenzymatic degradation at body temperature and pH, and (*b*) by ester hydrolysis. Most atracurium is degraded by ester hydrolysis (25). The products of metabolism of atracurium may be toxic and several produce neuromuscular blockade in high doses. In addition, the quaternary monoacrylate, laudanosine, may lead to a decrease in blood pressure and seizure activity in high dose (26). The major untoward effects of atracurium are hypotension and tachycardia as a result of dose-related histamine release (27). This response can be attenuated by a slow injection of the agent or by pretreatment with H_1 and H_2 receptor blockers (28, 29). After administration of a dose sufficient to facilitate endotracheal intubation, the clinical duration of action ranges from 30 to 45 minutes. After administration of a maintenance dose, the duration is reduced to 15 to 20 minutes. Atracurium may be administered by continuous infusion, and prolonged recovery time is not observed, reflecting the unique metabolism and elimination of this drug.

MIVACURIUM

Mivacurium is another of the benzylisoquinoline compounds. The cardiovascular effects of mivacurium are similar to those of atracurium. After rapid injection of large doses of mivacurium, histamine release may result in transient hypotension. After a dose of mivacurium of 0.25 mg/kg, very good intubating conditions can be achieved within 90 seconds. The time to recovery of one palpable twitch on TOF stimulation after this intubating dose of mivacurium is about half the time to full recovery of neuromuscular function. Mivacurium is almost entirely hydrolyzed by plasma cholinesterase. It is this rapid enzymatic hydrolysis that results in the short duration of action of this neuromuscular blocking agent. Indeed, the time to spontaneous recovery to 95% twitch height occurs in approximately 20 to 25 minutes, if the patient is a normal homozygote for plasma cholinesterase. If the interval is 30 to 60 minutes, the patient is probably a heterozygote for the normal and atypical forms of the enzyme. Finally, if the interval is longer than 1 hour, the patient is probably an atypical homozygote for the enzyme. Because of its short duration of action, this agent can also be administered by continuous infusion. The neuromuscular block can be antagonized by anticholinesterases or administration of pseudocholinesterase. However, recent evidence suggests the administration of neostigmine and to a lesser extent edrophonium will temporarily slow the hydrolysis of mivacurium by inhibition of plasma cholinesterase (30–33). However, the enzyme will have recovered much of its activity within 20 to 60 minutes. Thus, anticholinesterase administration will very effectively reverse mivacurium-induced neuromuscular blockade unless low or abnormal enzyme activity is present.

d-TUBOCURARINE

d-tubocurarine is a monoquaternary compound. After administration of a dose sufficient for endotracheal intubation, the clinical duration of action ranges from 60 to 100 minutes. There seems to be no active metabolism of d-tubocurarine; the drug is 30 to 50% protein bound and is excreted in the urine and bile. The major side effect of the drug is the dose-related histamine release, resulting in skin flushing and hypotension. In addition, d-tubocurarine may induce the release of prostacyclin, further potentiating hypotension (34). d-tubocurarine is primarily eliminated through the kidney, and there is no active metabolism.

PANCURONIUM

Pancuronium is a long-acting synthetic nondepolarizing neuromuscular blocking agent. After administration of pancuronium sufficient for endotracheal intubation, the clinical duration of action ranges from 60 to 120 minutes.

Pancuronium does not release histamine but may lead to an increase in heart rate, blood pressure, and cardiac output. These signs seem to be related to the vagolytic effect of pancuronium as well as muscarinic receptor blockade and increase in catecholamine release (35). Pancuronium is metabolized to a 3-OH compound with clinical neuromuscular blocking activity. Both pancuronium and the metabolite are cleared primarily through the kidney. Only a small portion is excreted in the bile.

VECURONIUM

Vecuronium is an intermediate-acting steroid-based neuromuscular blocking agent. After administration of a dose of vecuronium sufficient for endotracheal intubation, the clinical duration of action ranges from 45 to 90 minutes. After administration of a maintenance dose, the clinical duration ranges from 15 to 30 minutes. The cardiovascular profile of vecuronium results in no clinically apparent cardiovascular effects within the clinical dose range. The metabolism and elimination of vecuronium depends both on renal and hepatic function. The short duration of action of this agent makes it suitable for continuous intravenous infusion. It should be noted, however, that the excretion of vecuronium is diminished in the presence of decreased renal or hepatic function and at the extremes of age.

CISATRACURIUM

Cisatracurium is a stereoisomer of atracurium that allows more hemodynamic stability.

It is three to four times more potent than atracurium, with weaker autonomic effects. After a standard dose for endotracheal intubation, the onset is within 5 minutes, with a duration of 40 to 45 minutes. Reversal of 80 to 90% neuromuscular blockade can be accomplished within 10 to 15 minutes (36). Cisatracurium does not result in histamine release. No significant changes in heart rate or blood pressure have been noted in doses up to and including eight times the ED95 (37).

Cisatracurium is broken down by Hofmann elimination with no metabolism by esterases. The half-life of the agent is 22 to 25 minutes. There is little change in the pharmacokinetic and pharmacodynamic profiles of this agent in the presence of renal or hepatic failure.

ROCURONIUM

Rocuronium is a steroid-based intermediate-acting neuromuscular blocking agent. It is less potent than vecuronium, but the onset of action is faster. Good intubating conditions can be achieved in 60 to 90 seconds or sooner if a higher dose is used. However, rocuronium in these higher doses results in a longer duration of action. Rocuronium is not metabolized and is excreted by the liver and kidney. Therefore, as with vecuronium, the duration of action is prolonged in renal and hepatic disease and at the extremes of age.

Antagonism of Neuromuscular Blockade

If residual neuromuscular blockade persists, pharmacologic antagonism of nondepolarizing muscle relaxants can be achieved with the administration of anticholinesterase agents. These agents, edrophonium, neostigmine, and pyridostigmine, inhibit the activity of acetylcholinesterase, resulting in accumulation of acetylcholine at the neuromuscular junction by release of transmitter from the motor nerve terminal and by blockade of neural potassium channels. The depth of neuromuscular blockade at the time of antagonism is a critical factor in the efficacy of reversal of neuromuscular blockade. Indeed, antagonism of nondepolarizing muscle relaxants should not be initiated in the absence of a detectable twitch response by peripheral nerve stimulator. Clearly, the more intense the block at the time of reversal, the longer the recovery time of neuromuscular function. If an anticholinesterase is administered when only the first response in the train-of-four is present or twitch height is less than 5% of control, reversal can be anticipated to require 15 to 30 minutes. In contradistinction, if all four twitches from the train-of-four stimulation are present, reversal of neuromuscular blockade can be anticipated in less than 10 minutes. Other factors affecting the efficacy of reversal of neuromuscular blockade include the (*a*) neuromuscular blocking agent to be reversed, (*b*) age of the patient, (*c*) dose of anticholinesterase administered, (*d*) acid-base balance, (*e*) electrolyte status, (*f*) concomitant drug administration, and (*g*) renal function.

The neuromuscular blocking agent to be reversed is an important determinant in the efficacy of administration of an anticholinesterase. Specifically, recovery of neuromuscular activity after reversal is dependent on the rate of spontaneous recovery as well as the effect of the anticholinesterase administered. Therefore, the reversal of long-acting nondepolarizing neuromuscular blocking agents is more dependent on the action of the anticholinesterase because little drug is removed from the plasma because of the long half-life. The recovery of neuromuscular activity after administration of intermediate-acting agents with a comparable dose of anticholinesterase agent is more rapid because of the faster rate of spontaneous recovery.

The rapidity of reversal of neuromuscular blockade is also dependent on the choice of anticholinesterase. The rapidity of onset of antagonism is greatest with edrophonium and least with pyridostigmine; neostigmine is intermediate between these two. However, the depth of neuromuscular blockade also effects the efficacy of the anticholinesterase adminis-

Table 6–2. Comparison of Anticholinesterases

Anticholinesterase	Dose	Onset of Action
Edrophonium	0.5–1 mg	Rapid
Neostigmine	0.35–0.7 mg	Intermediate
Pyridostigmine	0.15–0.35 mg	Slow

tered. Indeed, neostigmine is more effective than edrophonium in antagonisms of profound blockade. In addition, the onset of action of each of the anticholinesterase agents varies (Table 6–2). The dose of anticholinesterase agent administered affects the time to return of neuromuscular function. However, there is a maximum dose of anticholinesterase agent beyond which additional doses do not produce any greater antagonism. There is no advantage in combining agents or administration of anticholinesterase in divided doses.

Patient age has been postulated as a contributing factor in the recovery of neuromuscular function. Specifically, with advancing age, recovery of neuromuscular activity occurs more slowly than in infants and children. In addition, the clearance of the nondepolarizing neuromuscular blocking agents is decreased with advancing age.

Concomitant administration of other commonly used drugs in the perioperative period may enhance the action of nondepolarizing neuromuscular blockers. Administration of amnioglycosides and magnesium enhance the effect of both depolarizing and nondepolarizing neuromuscular blockade, both at the prejunctional and postjunctional membranes. Similarly, the lincosamines, clindamycin and lincomycin, also can enhance neuromuscular blockade. Similarly, lidocaine, quinidine, and β-antagonist and calcium channel blockers may augment coexisting neuromuscular blockade. These agents also seem to interfere with the prejunctional release of acetylcholine as well as postjunctional stabilization of membrane. Several other agents have also been described to alter the response of neuromuscular blocking agents (38–46).

The patient's acid-base status also influences the reversal of neuromuscular blockade. Respiratory acidosis, but not metabolic acidosis, may augment a nondepolarizing neuromuscular blockade and reduce the efficacy of its antagonism. Metabolic alkalosis also has been reported to inhibit reversal of neuromuscular blockade. Electrolyte disorders may also contribute to an altered response of neuromuscular function after neuromuscular blockade. Hypokalemia enhances the action of neuromuscular blocking agents because of an increase in endplate transmembrane potential. Abnormalities in other electrolytes may further enhance neuromuscular blockade and result in difficulty in reversal. Finally, the clearance of neuromuscular blocking agents may be reduced; renal failure results in marked prolongation of the elimination half-life of these agents, which are dependent on renal excretion.

EFFECTS OF ANTICHOLINESTERASE AGENTS

Cholinesterase inhibitors result in cholinergic stimulation at cholinergic sites throughout the body. These muscarinic effects would result in bradyarrhythmias, atrioventricular nodal block, peripheral vasodilation, excessive salivation, sweating, increased gastrointestinal motility, increased bladder tone, and bronchoconstriction if these agents were administered without concomitant administration of an anticholinergic agent. Specifically, atropine because of the rapid onset of action, and a duration of 30 to 60 minutes is most appropriate for use with edrophonium, whereas glycopyrrolate has a longer onset of action and is more appropriate for use with neostigmine or pyridostigmine. In addition, atropine crosses the blood-brain barrier, whereas glycopyrrolate does not.

Antagonism by Administration of Pseudocholinesterase

Human pseudocholinesterase in a purified form recently has become available for clinical evaluation. It may be administered to antagonize neuromuscular blockade for agents such as mivacurium and succinylcholine (47).

Diseases that Alter Response Neuromuscular Blocking Agents

MYASTHENIA GRAVIS

Myasthenia gravis is an autoimmune disease with circulating antibodies resulting in extreme sensitivity to nondepolarizing muscle relaxants and slight resistance to depolarizing agents (48, 49). It is important to note that not all of the musculature is effected in a similar fashion, so that monitoring at several sites with a nerve stimulator is important. Concomitant administration of pyridostigmine to patients with myasthenia gravis will modify the response to neuromuscular blocking agents, resulting in reduced sensitivity to nondepolarizing agents and prolonged action of succinylcholine and mivacurium. Reversal of neuromuscular blockade may be ineffective, because acetylcholinesterase inhibition already exists with chronic pyridostigmine therapy. Therefore, it is recommended to allow spontaneous recovery from neuromuscular blockade in the postoperative period while continuing mechanical ventilatory support as needed (50, 51).

MYOTONIA

Myotonia is characterized by an abnormal delay in muscle relaxation after contraction. It includes myotonia congenita, myotonia dystrophica, and paramyotonia congenita. Characteristically, patients with myotonia have a sustained dose-related contraction after administration of succinylcholine, making it very difficult to provide adequate ventilatory support (52). In contrast, it seems that the response to nondepolarizing neuromuscular blocking agents is normal. In addition, a myotonic response has been described after reversal with neostigmine (53).

UPPER AND LOWER MOTOR NEURON DISEASE

The potential hazards of administration of succinylcholine to patients with upper or lower motor neuron disease are well described (54, 55). After administration of succinylcholine, hyperkalemia and cardiac arrest have been described. Hyperkalemia usually results 1 week to 6 months after the injury, probably resulting from extrajunctional receptors. Certainly, lower motor neuron denervation results in resistance to nondepolarizing muscle relaxants because of proliferation of acetylcholine receptors (55).

BURNS

There is a significant abnormality in the response to both depolarizing and nondepolarizing neuromuscular blocking agents for patients who have sustained acute, severe burn injuries. Specifically, a life-threatening rise in serum potassium may follow administration of succinylcholine in burned patients. However, succinylcholine has been administered safely in the acute setting within 24 hours of the injury. Nonetheless, it is best to avoid succinylcholine in patients 24 to 48 hours after a burn and for 1 to 2 years thereafter. Similarly, burned patients (56) have an abnormal response to nondepolarizing muscle relaxants (57–60). In general, the dose requirements for most nondepolarizing neuromuscular blocking agents are increased (57, 58, 60). However, there is a variable clinical response to neuromuscular blocking agents with thermal injury so that close monitoring of the depth of neuromuscular blockade with a peripheral nerve stimulator is essential.

PROLONGED NEUROMUSCULAR BLOCKADE IN THE PACU

Several investigators have reported the frequent occurrence of residual neuromuscular blockade in patients in the postanesthesia care unit (PACU) after surgery (61–65). In a study by Viby-Mogensen, 42% of patients given long-acting neuromuscular blocking agents had a TOF ratio lower than 0.7, and more than 20% of patients who were awake were unable to sustain head lift for 5 seconds (61). Subsequent studies with intermediate-acting neuromuscular blocking agents were able to demonstrate a reduction to less than 10% in the incidence of TOF ratio lower than 0.7. Although the introduction of shorter-acting neuromuscular blocking agents has reduced the incidence of residual paralysis in the PACU, it still occurs, and if unrecognized, could be fatal. The clinical presentation of patients arriving in the PACU with residual neuromuscular blockade is shallow respirations and a labored appearance. These patients are at risk for hypercarbia with concomitant acidosis and at risk of aspiration. Mechanical ventilatory support is generally indicated until the neuromuscular blockade resolves.

REFERENCES

1. Ellison MH, Rash JE, Staehelin A, et al. Studies of excitable membranes: II a comparison of specialization at neuromuscular junctions and nonjunctional sarcolemmas of mammalian fast and slow twitch muscle fibers. J Cell Biol 1976;68:752.
2. Bevan DR, Bevan JC, Donati F. Muscle relaxants in clinical anesthesia. Chicago: Year Book Medical Publishers, 1988.
3. Taylor P. Are neuromuscular blocking agents more efficacious in pairs? Anesthesiology 1985;63:1–3.
4. Viby-Mogensen J. Clinical assessment of neuromuscular transmission. Br J Anaesth 1982;54:209–223.
5. Lee C, Katz RL. Fade of neurally evoked compound electromyogram during neuromuscular block by d-tubocurarine. Anesth Analg 1977;56:271.
6. Brull SJ, Connelly NR, O'Connor TZ, et al. Effect of tetanus on subsequent neuromuscular monitoring in patients receiving vecuronium. Anesthesiology 1991;74:64.
7. Lee C. Train-of-four fade and edrophonium antagonism of neuromuscular block by succinylcholine in man. Anesth Analg 1976;55:663.
8. Waud DR. The nature of "depolarization block." Anesthesiology 1968;29:1014.
9. Litwiller RW. Succinylcholine hydrolysis. Anesthesiology 1969;31:356.
10. Lee C. Dose relationship of phase II, tachyphylaxis and train-of-four fade on suxamethonium-induced dual neuromuscular block in man. Br J Anaesth 1975;47:841–845.
11. Foldes FF, Rendell-Baker L, Birch JH. Causes and prevention of prolonged apnea with succinylcholine. Anesth Analg 1956;35:609.
12. Kaniaris P, Fasoulaki A, Tiarmakopoulou K, et al.

Serum cholinesterase levels in patients with cancer. Anesth Analg 1979;58:82.

13. Kopman AF, Strachovsky G, Lichtenstein L. Prolonged response to succinylcholine following physostigmine. Anesthesiology 1978;49:142.

14. Bentz EW, Stoelting RK. Prolonged response to succinylcholine following pancuronium reversal with pyridostimine. Anesthesiology 1976;44:258.

15. Kao YJ, Turner DR. Prolongation of succinylcholine block by metoclopramide. Anesthesiology 1989;70:905.

16. Viby-Mogensen J. Correlation of succinylcholine duration of action with plasma cholinesterase activity in subjects with the genotypically normal enzyme. Anesthesiology 1980;53:517.

17. Pantuck EJ. Plasma cholinesterase: gene and variations. Anesth Analg 1993;77:380.

18. Walton JD, Farman JV. Suxamethonium, potassium and renal failure. Anaesthesia 1973;28:626.

19. Cook JH. The effect of suxamethonium on intraocular pressure. Anaesthesia 1981;36:359.

20. Miller RD, Way WL. Inhibition of succinylcholine-induced increased intragastric pressure by nondepolarizing muscle relaxants and lidocaine. Anesthesiology 1971;34:185.

21. Smith G, Dalling R, Williams TIR. Gastro-oesophageal pressure gradient changes produced by induction of anaesthesia and suxamethonium. Br J Anaesth 1978;50:1137.

22. Stirt JA, Grosslight KR, Bedford RF, et al. Defasciculation "with metocurine prevents succinylcholine-induced increases in intracranial pressure. Anesthesiology 1987;67:50.

23. Brodsky JB, Brock-Urne JG, Samuels SI. Pancuronium pretreatment and post-succinylcholine myalgias. Anesthesiology 1979;51:259.

24. Van Der Spek AFL, Fang WB, Ashton-Miller JA, et al. Increased masticatory muscle stiffness during limb flaccidity associated with succinylcholine administration. Anesthesiology 1988;69:11.

25. Stiller RL, Cook DR, Chakravorti S. In vitro degradation of atracurium in human plasma. Br J Anaesth 1985;57:1085.

26. Hennis PJ, Fahey MR, Canfell PC, et al. Pharmacology of atracurium during isoflurane anesthesia in normal and anephric patients. Anesth Analg 1986;65:743.

27. Savarese JJ, Basta SJ, Ali HH, et al. Neuromuscular and cardiovascular effects of BW 33A (atracurium) in patients under halothane anesthesia. Anesthesiology 1982;57:A262.

28. Basta SJ, Savarese JJ, Ali HH, et al. Histamine releasing potencies of atracurium, dimethyl tubocurarine, and tubocurarine. Br J Anaesth 1983;55:105S.

29. Scott RPF, Savarese JJ, Basta SJ, et al. Atracurium: clinical strategies for preventing histamine release and attenuating the haemodynamic response. Br J Anaesth 1985;57:550.

30. Naguib M, Abdulatif M, Al-Ghamdi A, et al. Dose-response relationships for edrophonium and neostigmine antagonism of mivacurium-induced neuromuscular block. Br J Anaesth 1993;71:709–714.

31. Devcic A, Munshi CA, Gandhi SK, et al. Antagonism of mivacurium neuromuscular block: neo-stigmine versus edrophonium. Anesth Analg 1995;81:1005–1009.

32. Kopman AF, Mallhi MU, Justo MO, et al. Antagonism of mivacurium-induced neuromuscular blockade in humans: edrophonium dose requirements at threshold train-of-four count of 4. Anesthesiology 1994;81:1394–1400.

33. Lien CA, Belmont MR, Wray DL, et al. Pharmacokinetics and dynamics of mivacurium during spontaneous recovery and anticholinesterase-facilitated recovery. Anesthesiology 1995;83:A896.

34. Hatano Y, Arai T, Noda J, et al. Contribution of prostacyclin to d-tubocurarine-induced hypotension in humans. Anesthesiology 1990;72:28.

35. Bowman WC. Pharmacology of neuromuscular function. 2nd ed. London: Wright, 1990.

36. Belmont MR, Lien CA, Abalos A, et al. The clinical neuromuscular pharmacology of 51W89. Anesthesiology 1995;82:1139–1145.

37. Lien CA, Belmont MR, Abalos A, et al. The cardiovascular effects and histamine releasing properties of 51W89 in patients receiving nitrous oxide-opioid-barbiturate anesthesia. Anesthesiology 1995;82:1131–1138.

38. Lee C, deSilva AJC. Acute and subchronic neuromuscular blocking characteristics of streptomycin: a comparison with neomycin. Br J Anaesth 1979;51:431.

39. Sokoll MD, Gergis SD. Antibiotics and neuromuscular function. Anesthesiology 1981;55:148.

40. Kordas M. The effect of procaine on neuromuscular transmission. J Physiol 1970;209:689.

41. Ornstein E, Matteo RS, Weinstein JA, et al. Accelerated recovery from doxacurium-induced neuromuscular blockade in patients receiving chronic anticonvulsant therapy. J Clin Anesth 1991;3:108.

42. Miller RD, Way WL, Katzung BG. The potentiation of neuromuscular blocking agents by quinidine. Anesthesiology 1967;28:1036.

43. Ornstein E, Matteo RS, Schwarts AE, et al. The effects of phenytoin on the magnitude and duration of neuromuscular block following atracurium or vecuronium. Anesthesiology 1987;67:191.

44. Bell PF, Mirakhur RK, Elliott P. Onset and duration of clinical relaxation of atracurium and vecuronium in patients on chronic nifedipine therapy. Eur J Anaesthesiol 1989;6:343.

45. Kanaya N, Sato Y, Tsuchida H, et al. The effects of nicardipine and verapamil on the recovery time of vecuronium-induced neuromuscular blockade. Masui 1991;40:246.

46. Miller RD, Sohn YJ, Matteo RS. Enhancement of d-tubocurarine neuromuscular blockade by diuretics in man. Anesthesiology 1976;45:442.

47. Bownes PB, Hartman GS, Chiscolm D, et al. Antagonism of mivacurium blockade by purified human butyryl cholinesterase in cats. Anesthesiology 1992;77:A909.

48. Buzello W, Noeldge G, Krieg N, et al. Vecuronium for muscle relaxation in patients with myasthenia gravis. Anesthesiology 1986;64:507.

49. Eisenkraft JB, Mann SM, Book WJ, et al. Succinylcholine dose-response in myasthenia gravis. Anesthesiology 1988;69:760.

50. Feldman SA. Muscle relaxants in pathologic states. In: Muscle relaxants. Philadelphia: WB Saunders, 1979;108.

51. Hedley-Whyte J, Burgess GE III, Feeley TW, et al. Respiratory management of peripheral neurologic disease. In: Applied physiology of respiratory care. Boston: Little, Brown & Co., 1976;245.

52. Paterson IS. Generalized myotonia following suxamethonium. Br J Anaesth 1962;34:340.

53. Buzello W, Krieg N, Schlickewei A. Hazards of neostigmine in patients with neuromuscular disorders. Br J Anaesth 1982;54:529.

54. Rosenbaum KJ, Neigh JL, Strobel GE. Sensitivity to nondepolarizing muscle relaxants in amyotrophia lateral sclerosis: report of two cases. Anesthesiology 1971;35:638.

55. Hogue CW, Itani MS, Martyn JAJ. Resistance of d-tubocurarine in lower motor neuron injury is related to increased acetylcholine receptors at the neuromuscular junction (abstract). Anesthesiology 1989;71:A1203.

56. Schaner PJ, Brown RL, Kirksey TD, et al. Succinylcholine-induced hyperkalemia in burned patients. Anesth Analg 1969;48:764.

57. Martyn JAJ, White DA, Gronert GA, et al. Up-and-down regulation of skeletal muscle acetylcholine receptors. Anesthesiology 1992;76:822.

58. Martyn JAJ, Matteo RS, Szyfelbien SK, et al. Unprecedented resistance to neuromuscular blocking effects of metocurine with persistence after complete recovery in a burned patient. Anesth Analg 1982;61:614.

59. Martyn JAJ, Szyfelbein SK, Ali HH, et al. Increased d-tubocurarine requirement following major thermal injury. Anesthesiology 1980;52:352.

60. Mills AK, Martyn JAJ. Neuromuscular blockade with vecuronium in paediatric burned patients. Br J Clin Pharmacol 1989;28:155.

61. Viby-Mogensen J, Jorgensen BC, Ording H. Residual curarization in the recovery room. Anesthesiology 1979;50:539.

62. Lennmarken G, Lofstrom JB. Partial curarization in the postoperative period. Acta Anaesthesiol Scand 1984;28:260.

63. Beemer GH, Rozental P. Postoperative neuromuscular function. Anaesth Intensive Care 1986;14:41.

64. Bevan DR, Smith CE, Donati F. Postoperative neuromuscular blockade: a comparison between atracurium, vecuronium, and pancuronium. Anesthesiology 1988;69:272.

65. Brull SJ, Silverman DG, Ehrenwerth J. Problems of recovery and residual neuromuscular blockade: pancuronium vs. vecuronium. Anesthesiology 1988;69:A473.

7

CARDIOVASCULAR SYSTEM

John R. Moyers, Tanya Oyos

Cardiovascular complications in the postanesthesia care unit (PACU) occur in 0.5 to 4.0% of patients. Hines et al. (1) studied the postoperative complications in 18,473 consecutive patients in the PACU in a university teaching hospital. Hypotension occurred in 2.7% of patients, arrhythmias occurred in 1.4%, and hypertension occurred in 1.1% of the patients studied (Fig. 7–1). Cardiac events, defined as pulmonary edema and myocardial infarction, occurred in 0.1% and 0.3%, respectively. In this study, risk factors for postoperative cardiovascular complications included American Society of Anesthesiologists (ASA) physical class II, duration of anesthesia 2 to 4 hours, general anesthesia, emergency surgery, and orthopedic and abdominal procedures. This investigation suggested that cardiovascular complications were more common in ASA class II patients because many of the ASA class III and IV patients may have been admitted directly to the intensive care unit. The most common reason for unscheduled admission to the intensive care unit (54 of 186 patients) was to rule out myocardial infarction. In a letter to the editor, de Mello et al. (2) described 389 consecutive PACU patients and their complications. They noted hypotension in 8.7% of these patients; occurrence was more common in older and sicker patients. The Australian Incident Monitoring Study (3) reported the occurrence of 2000 untoward incidents in the PACU. Nineteen percent of these cases were cardiovascular in nature and most were detected clinically. Furthermore,

the cardiovascular incidents in the PACU were associated with more adverse outcomes than were the intraoperative incidents. Pedersen (4) investigated complications and death after anesthesia in 7306 surgical patients. Twenty-four (3.3%) of these patients had cardiovascular complications. Those with preoperative congestive heart failure or myocardial infarction were the most likely to have cardiovascular complications in the recovery room.

ROUTINE MANAGEMENT

Patient admission to the PACU involves initial observation, physical examination, and placement and interpretation of appropriate monitoring (5). Important items on physical examination include skin color, mental status, peripheral perfusion, and assessment of capillary refill. Whereas observation and physical examination can be very helpful, most cardiovascular complications require monitoring for either detection or quantification. Monitoring of the cardiovascular system in the recovery room entails assessment of blood pressure, pulse, respiration, pulse oximetry, electrocardiogram, and body temperature. In addition, some patients require measurement of urinary output, blood pressure by intra-arterial catheter, central venous pressure, or pulmonary artery pressure. As in any other setting, one must make certain that the information from the monitors is correct. For example, false or spurious blood pressure measurements can occur

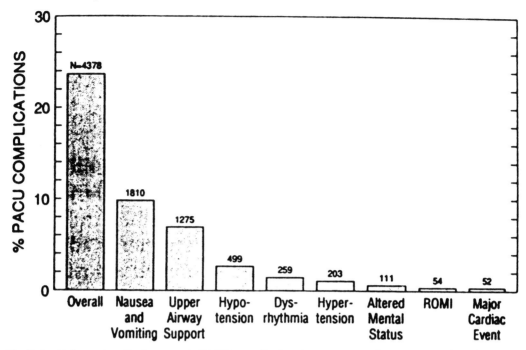

Fig. 7–1. Major postanesthesia care unit (PACU) complications by percentage of occurrence and number (above the bar) of patients experiencing each complication. ROMI = rule out myocardial infarction. (From Hines R, Barash PG, Watrous G, et al. Complications occurring in the postanesthesia care unit: a survey. Anesth Analg 1992;74:503–509.)

in the postoperative setting when a blood pressure cuff different from the cuff used in the operating room is applied. A cuff that is too small will indicate a falsely high blood pressure and a cuff that is too large will record a falsely low pressure. A cuff of improper size may lead to false blood pressure readings and unnecessary or possibly hazardous therapy. There can be problems with intra-arterial lines and transducers. They must be calibrated and zeroed properly. "Overshoot" or resonance can falsely denote hypertension, whereas catheter obstruction or damping of the line can indicate falsely low blood pressure. When taking blood pressure with a cuff and a stethoscope, there may be variance among observers. Pound (6) noted that systolic blood pressure may vary by as much as 40 mm Hg and diastolic pressure may vary by as much as 28 mm Hg when determined by different observers.

Although pulse oximetry gives important information with regard to oxygenation, it may not be valuable as an index of perfusion. The studies by Lawson et al. (7) and Severinghaus et al. (8) lead to the conclusion that presence of pulse oximeter signals should not be used to indicate adequate circulation. Contrarily, the absence of a pulse oximeter signal does not necessarily denote shock (9). Sicker patients, patients undergoing longer surgical procedures, and patients with hypothermia in the recovery room may have adequate circulation but may not have a detectable signal on pulse oximetry.

Although there is potential for the risk of infection from reusable equipment, the risk is very small. For example, Cormican et al. (10) studied the microflora of blood pressure cuffs. Most microorganisms isolated from noninvasive blood pressures holds little threat to healthy patients. However, they did culture bacteria resistant to methicillin and gentamycin in one instance. The microbe was sensitive to vancomycin.

HYPERTENSION

Hypertension is one of the most common cardiovascular events in the PACU (Table 7–1). Its etiology may be multifactorial. Common causes include preoperative hypertension, pain, emergence delirium, arterial blood gas abnormalities (hypoxia or hypercarbia), excessive fluid administration, hypothermia, and the presence of an endotracheal tube. Other causes include withdrawal of antihypertensive medications (especially clonidine and β-blocking drugs), bladder distension, and intracranial hypertension. Elevated blood pressure in the immediate postoperative period is often benign and usually resolves within 3 or 4 hours. However, in some patients, hypertension persists, and in other patients, such as the geriatric age group or those with preexisting cardiovascular disease, untreated hypertension in the recovery room may lead to problems. Untreated increases in blood pressure in these patients can lead to left ventricular failure, myocardial infarction, arrhythmias, pulmonary edema, or cerebral hemorrhage. Hypertension in any patient in the postoperative period can increase the likelihood of bleeding from arterial suture lines.

Gal and Cooperman (11) investigated hypertension in the recovery room in a study published in 1975. Of 1844 admissions, 3.2%

developed hypertension using the blood pressure cuff and the Riva Rocci method of blood pressure determination. Fifty-eight percent of the patients who were hypertensive in the recovery room had preoperative hypertension. Hypertension in the recovery room usually began within 30 minutes of admission (Fig. 7–2) and lasted approximately 2 hours (Fig. 7–3). However, in 20% of patients who became hypertensive in the recovery room, blood pressure remained elevated for longer than 3 hours. Etiologies in their study for hypertension were pain (35%), hypercarbia (15%), and emergence excitement (16%), and in 17% of patients, no demonstrable cause was discovered. Hypertension in the recovery room usually occurred in older patients (mean age, 61 years) with no difference in gender. Hypertensive events were unrelated to either type or duration of surgery. The study by Hines et al. (1) of recovery room events found a 1% incidence of hypertension. The study of hypertensive crisis in the PACU after elective surgery by Carlson and Thornton (12) demonstrated that after pain, hypoxia, bladder distention, and anxiety were excluded as causes, 71 of the 99 hypertensive patients had hypertension preoperatively. Finally, Summers et al. (13) looked at hypertension in the recovery room in previously normotensive, young males. Twenty-three percent of these patients were hypertensive in the recovery room. In their study, hypothermia had the highest correlation with postoperative hypertension.

Hypertension in the immediate postoperative period has been defined as a systolic pressure greater than 180 to 190 mm Hg and diastolic pressure greater than 90 to 110 mm Hg (1, 11, 14). However, the level of blood pressure requiring treatment is arbitrary and will vary among patients depending on concurrent medical problems. Treatment of hypertension in the recovery room is predicated on first treating the underlying cause. Pain must be alleviated with the proper analgesics and blood gas abnormalities, such as hypercapnia and hypoxia, must be addressed. Those with hypervolemia from fluid overload should

Table 7–1. Etiologies of Hypertension in the Postanesthesia Care Unit

Preoperative hypertension
Pain
Emergence excitement
Hypothermia
Presence of endotracheal tube
Excess fluid administration
Blood gas abnormalities
  Hypercarbia
  Hypoxia
Bladder distention
Anxiety
"Rebound" from antihypertensive medication
Increased intracranial pressure
Spurious blood pressure measurement

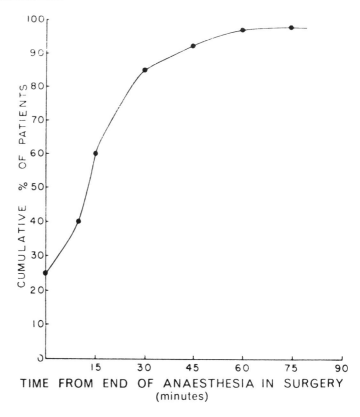

Fig. 7–2. Onset of hypertension following the end of surgery. (From Gal TJ, Cooperman LH. Hypertension in the immediate postoperative period. Br J Anaesth 1975;47:70–74.)

have the head of the bed elevated with consideration given to treatment with diuretics or vasodilators. Those seasoned in recovery room management know that meperidine is superior to morphine in treating shivering and accompanying hypertension postoperatively. The study by Kurz et al. (15) demonstrated this in scientific fashion. Their study showed that meperidine was more effective in treating shivering than equal analgesic doses of morphine in the postoperative period. It indicated that much of meperidine antishivering activity came from nonopioid actions; specifically, stimulation of κ receptors.

After first treating the underlying causes of hypertension, antihypertensive medication may be appropriate. Because immediate postoperative hypertension usually resolves in 4 hours, an antihypertensive drug with the appropriate half-life should be selected (16). Hydralazine is frequently used in the recovery room to lower blood pressure. Increments from 2.5 to 20 mg intravenously or 10 to 40 mg intramuscularly often reduce blood pressure to satisfactory levels within 15 to 20 minutes. β-adrenergic blocking drugs also have a place in the treatment of hypertension in the recovery room, especially if there is accompanying tachycardia. Labetalol, with its combined α- and β-blocking functions, is often therapeutic in 5- to 10-mg increments intravenously (17) (Fig. 7–4). Propranolol (0.5 to 1.0 mg) or metoprolol (1.0 to 5.0 mg) can be given in intravenous boluses, whereas an infusion of esmolol of 25 to 300 mg/kg/minute after a bolus is also possible. An esmolol infusion requires very close blood pressure monitoring. Five to 10 mg of sublingual nifedipine will treat elevations in the blood pressure in the recovery room. However, this method is not titratable and, as with all vasodilators, may lead to an increase in heart rate. When

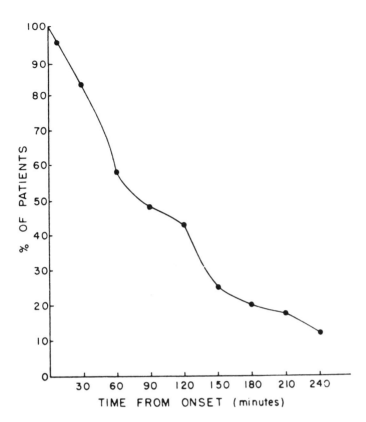

Fig. 7–3. Duration of postoperative hypertension. (From Gal TJ, Cooperman LH. Hypertension in the immediate postoperative period. Br J Anaesth 1975;47:70–74.)

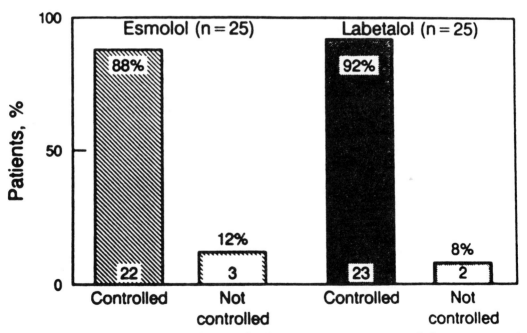

Fig. 7–4.   Efficacy of esmolol and labetalol in controlling hypertension. (From Muzzi DA, Black S, Losasso TJ, et al. Labetalol and esmolol in the control of hypertension after intracranial surgery. Anesth Analg 1990;70:68–71.)

hypertension is otherwise difficult to treat or when precision is needed, infusions of a potent vasodilator such as sodium nitroprusside may be necessary. This usually necessitates the presence of an intra-arterial catheter for blood pressure monitoring and introduces other risks such as cyanide toxicity. Similarly, trimethaphan or nitroglycerine infusions have a place in lowering blood pressure in the recovery room. Less frequently, nimodepine and diazoxide have been employed to produce acceptable levels of blood pressure in the immediate postoperative period.

HYPOTENSION

Hypotension is another common cardiovascular complication in the recovery room (Table 7–2). Etiologies include hypovolemia, ventricular dysfunction, dysrhythmias, and a low systemic vascular resistance. The study by Hines et al. (1) showed an incidence of 2.7% of hypotension in the recovery room. When hypotension occurs, the autonomic system diverts blood to the brain, heart, and kidneys. Despite this mechanism, with severe hypotension, patients may demonstrate a decreased level of consciousness or even confusion, angina pectoris, or oliguria. Hypotension in the recovery room can lead to myocardial infarction, stroke, renal failure, or other injury to vital organs. The lowest acceptable blood pressure postoperatively depends somewhat on the patient's preoperative blood pressure, as well as any concurrent medical problems such as atherosclerotic disease, aortic stenosis, chronic hypertension, or renal failure.

Hypovolemia

Hypovolemia is the most common cause of hypotension in the recovery room. Causes of postoperative hypovolemia include insufficient replacement of preoperative fluid deficit, third space losses, and hemorrhage. Other etiologies include failure to replenish urinary losses (from diuretics, hyperglycemia, or dye studies) drainage of ascites, evaporative losses intraoperatively, sweating, and other insensible loss. One must remember that these losses occur into the postoperative setting and can be masked by vasoconstriction from hypothermia. In the recovery room, mild hypovolemia may be compensated by venoconstriction, tachycardia, and an increase in systemic vascular resistance and may not be accompanied by hypotension. More severe degrees of hypovolemia will lead to a decrease in blood pressure. "Relative hypovolemia" from spinal or epidural can cause hypotension in the recovery room through increases in venous capacitance and the paralysis of compensatory mechanisms. Hypovolemia may be unmasked by taking away the sympathetic stimulation of an endotracheal intubation or from pain relief. Intraoperative medications, such as α blockers may persist in the recovery room. Lastly, intermittent positive pressure ventilation, pneumothorax, or acute pericardial tamponade are remote but real possibilities.

The intravascular volume status of the patient should be assessed on admission to the PACU. Physical examination includes observation of the neck veins and assessment of peripheral pulses and peripheral perfusion. In addition, blood pressure and pulse should be measured and, when available, urine output and central venous and pulmonary artery pressures. One should note the preoperative fluid status, the type and duration of surgery, and intraoperative fluid losses and replacement.

Table 7–2. Etiologies of Hypotension in the Postanethesia Care Unit

Hypovolemia
Regional anesthesia
Ventricular dysfunction
Myocardial ischemia or infarction
Cardiac dysrhythmia
Septic shock
Spurious blood pressure measurement
Intraoperative antihypertensive agents
Increased vagal tone from distended viscus
Pneumothorax
Cardiac tamponade

Urine output during surgery should be reviewed as well.

Ventricular Dysfunction

Ventricular dysfunction can also lead to hypotension in the immediate postoperative period. This usually occurs in patients that have preoperative ventricular dysfunction but may be augmented or produced by intraoperative overhydration. Ventricular dysfunction may also manifest after the resolution of spinal or epidural anesthesia caused by intravenous fluids administered intraoperatively to overcome the venodilating properties of regional anesthesia. In the recovery room, as the venous effects of the regional anesthetics dissipate, increases in preload may produce ventricular dysfunction. Myocardial ischemia or infarction can produce ventricular dysfunction in the PACU (see below). β-adrenergic blocking drugs may exacerbate or even produce ventricular dysfunction. Finally, right ventricular dysfunction may be caused by pulmonary thromboembolism or air embolism. After the diagnosis is made, ventricular dysfunction of any severity usually warrants patient transfer to the intensive care setting.

Myocardial Ischemia and Infarction

Myocardial ischemia or infarction may produce hypotension in the PACU, which is often heralded by perioperative tachycardia or hypotension. However, it may not necessarily be related to any hemodynamic event. In the PACU, hypoxia, hypovolemia, pain, or shivering can produce the hemodynamic events leading to myocardial ischemia. Ischemia may not necessarily be accompanied by chest pain. Mental status changes accompanying emergence from anesthesia may prevent the patient from complaining of chest pain, or analgesics may mask the pain of myocardial ischemia. One must maintain a high index of suspicion for those patients at risk. When myocardial ischemia is suspected, appropriate monitoring, such as a 12-lead electrocardiogram

(ECG), should be instituted along with timely therapy and, when indicated, appropriate consultation.

Cardiac Arrhythmias

Rhythm disturbances can lead to hypotension postoperatively. This is discussed elsewhere within this chapter.

Decrease in Systemic Vascular Resistance

A decrease in systemic vascular resistance is another cause of hypotension in the PACU. A fall in the systemic vascular resistance with regional anesthesia possibly may contribute to hypotension in the recovery room. However, changes in systemic vascular resistance usually are not as important as changes in venous return or heart rate in cardiovascular changes with spinal and epidural anesthesia. α-adrenergic blockers given intraoperatively may have effects in the recovery room that produce hypotension. Examples are hydralazine, droperidol, or labetalol. The hemodynamic effects of rewarming can produce lower peripheral resistance and a lower blood pressure. Sepsis with high cardiac output and low systemic vascular resistance is another cause for hypotension in the recovery room. Less common etiologies include the effects of vasoactive substances from blood component therapy and chronic liver failure.

Treatment of Postoperative Hypotension

The degree of hypotension warranting treatment is arbitrary and varies among patients, depending on concurrent medical problems. Some clinicians use a fall greater than 20 to 30% in systemic blood pressure from the preoperative values, whereas others are guided by evidence of decreased organ prefusion (16). Still other clinicians treat mean systemic blood pressures less than 60 mm Hg (1).

Assessment of the patient necessitates an accurate blood pressure measurement, as well as evaluation of peripheral pulses, heart tones, heart rate and rhythm, and breath sounds. Patient examination should include assessment of the neck veins and peripheral perfusion through capillary refill and temperature of the extremities. When available, there should be quantitation of urine output and assessment of central venous and pulmonary artery pressures and cardiac output. Those at the bedside should be familiar with the anesthesia record and the surgical procedure. The surgical site should be examined with attention to any swelling or oozing. The amount of drainage from the surgical incision should be quantitated. Bleeding in the immediate postoperative period may not be entirely due to surgical causes. It may be related to such medications as aspirin or anticoagulants. Postoperative bleeding can be disease related or a result of disseminated intravascular coagulopathy from massive transfusion. Proper evaluation dictates appropriate laboratory tests such as a 12-lead ECG, arterial blood gases, chest x-ray, and hematocrit and coagulation studies.

Therapy is directed toward the diagnosis. If hypovolemia is suspected, head-down position or elevation of the legs often will restore blood pressure temporarily. Pregnant patients may be moved to the lateral position. Concurrent with the change in position, fluid should be administered. A rapid infusion of the appropriate fluid (crystalloid, colloid, or blood) should be accomplished. Depending on the results of positioning and fluid administration and the urgency of the situation, a sympathomimetic drug can be administered. Commonly, 5 to 20 mg of ephedrine or 50 to 100 μg of Neo-Synephrine is used in this setting. A study by Hines et al. (1) showed that 80% of hypotensive events were treated successfully by volume administration alone. Only 20% of the patients required administration of a vasopressor. Therapy must be assessed and reassessed to make certain that blood pressure and perfusion are restored. If hypotension is not corrected easily with positioning, fluid ad-

ministration, and boluses of vasopressors, one should look for causes other than hypovolemia. One should consider more invasive monitoring with insertion of a central venous pressure catheter for patients with normal ventricular function and a pulmonary artery catheter for patients with abnormal ventricular function. For patients without a urinary catheter, one should be inserted. If the diagnosis of ventricular failure is made, an infusion of inotropes should be begun. Patients with ventricular failure, septic shock, ischemia that is not easily treated, or myocardial infarctions should be transferred to the critical care setting after stabilization.

CARDIAC DYSRHYTHMIAS IN THE PACU

Because the incidence of intraoperative dysrhythmias for patients undergoing anesthesia and surgery is 60% or greater (18–20), it is not uncommon to see cardiac dysrhythmias in the PACU while the patient is recovering from anesthesia and surgery. Even though most of these dysrhythmias will be benign and require no intervention, they may be the first indication of underlying pathology and, if left undetected and uncorrected, may lead to patient decompensation secondary to poor cardiac performance (21). Continuous monitoring of the patient's ECG in the PACU is essential if dysrhythmias, conduction abnormalities, and/or ECG changes consistent with myocardial ischemia are to be detected. Lead II is useful in demonstrating dysrhythmias and lead V5 is useful for myocardial ischemia. Although the electrical changes seen on the monitor will not define the underlying etiology of the irregularity, the type of disturbance seen is an integral part of dysrhythmia management.

Etiologies of Cardiac Dysrhythmias in the PACU

Although dysrhythmias in patients in the recovery room may be secondary to underly-

Table 7–3. Etiologies of Dysrhythmias in the Postanesthesia Care Unit

Hypoxia
Hypercapnia
Electrolyte abnormalities
Metabolic acidosis
Metabolic alkalosis
Myocardial ischemia
Autonomic nervous system imbalances
Preexisting heart disease
Drug effects
Hyperthermia
Hypothermia
Pain
Anxiety
Hypovolemia
Mechanical stimuli
Central nervous system disease
Drug toxicity
Bladder distension
Thyrotoxicosis

ing cardiovascular disease (the incidence of postoperative dysrhythmias correlates with increasing severity of cardiac disease), they commonly are the manifestation of underlying disturbances (Table 7–3) that frequently occur in the postoperative period. The effects of anesthetic agents on the cardiac system do not stop when the anesthetic is terminated at the completion of a surgical procedure, and significant levels of anesthetic drug may be the etiology of dysrhythmias. Halothane, enflurane, and isoflurane exert a depressant effect on the sinoatrial (SA) node (22, 23) as well as prolong the conduction time at the atrioventricular (AV) node and His-Purkinje system (24, 25). These anesthetic alterations in the conduction system can lead to bradycardias, AV junctional rhythms, a wandering atrial pacemaker, and ventricular escape rhythms. Baroreceptor reflex mechanisms to control heart rate are depressed by halothane, enflurane, and isoflurane, resulting in loss of reflex tachycardia during hypovolemia (26). AV junctional rhythms can occur when nitrous oxide is used in conjunction with intravenous narcotics or potent inhalational agents (27). Other anesthetic drugs used in the periopera-

tive setting can result in dysrhythmias seen in the PACU. Fentanyl slows the heart rate, decreases sympathetic tone, and increases vagal efferent tone (28), and morphine has direct depressant effects on the SA and AV nodes (29). Cardiac conduction is affected by pancuronium's ability to inhibit vagus nerve activity directly as well as block cardiac muscarinic receptors (30, 31). The development of dysrhythmias after the use of an anticholinesterase to reverse neuromuscular blockade is quite common, and cardiac conduction is prolonged at both the SA and AV nodes. Whereas most dysrhythmias secondary to anticholinesterase use are transient and benign, deleterious dysrhythmias, including ventricular ectopies and complete heart block, can occur (32). Atropine, commonly administered in conjunction with neostigmine or edrophonium to limit the muscarinic effects of these anticholinesterases, can also precipitate development of dysrhythmias, including tachycardia, AV dissociation, premature ventricular contractions, and junctional premature beats.

Changes in delivered oxygen tension, airway patency, central respiratory drive, and ventilatory mechanics occur following completion of the anesthetic and well into the recovery phase. Hypoxia and/or hypercarbia will result secondary to inadequate delivery of oxygen or poor ventilation and may lead to cardiac dysrhythmias in the PACU. Changes in blood gas values demonstrating acidosis, alkalosis, or hypoxia can be correlated with the onset of new cardiac dysrhythmias (33). Tachycardia and ventricular ectopy may occur in hypercarbic and hypoxic states, particularly if there is a concomitant increase in endogenous catecholamines. Persistent hypoxia will ultimately lead to bradycardia and asystole. Mild conduction abnormalities and atrial dysrhythmias are seen in states of acute respiratory alkalosis.

Electrolyte disturbances are likely to result in cardiac dysrhythmias in the PACU and although alterations in any electrolyte level can potentiate dysrhythmias, potassium abnormalities are associated with the highest incidence of cardiac disturbances. Atrial, ventricular, and junctional dysrhythmias occur with hypokalemia (34) due to delayed or blocked conduction through the AV node (35). Hypokalemia is common in the postoperative setting because of nasogastric suctioning, use of diuretics, intraoperative bleeding, urine output, and aggressive intraoperative volume replacement. Hyperkalemia, seen in renal failure, acidosis, inadvertent exogenous potassium administration, and in association with malignant hyperthermia, will depress AV conduction at levels of 7.5 mEq/L or greater. Extreme alterations in sodium, calcium, and magnesium levels must occur before any discernible effects on cardiac conduction are seen. Very high elevations of calcium can prolong the P-R interval and QRS complex with resultant high-degree AV block (36). Elevated magnesium levels may depress AV conduction.

Patients with hypothermia may exhibit dysrhythmias such as bradycardia, ventricular premature contractions, AV junctional rhythms, and even spontaneous ventricular fibrillation if body temperature falls below 28°C. The direct myocardial depressant effects of hypothermia on rhythm generation and impulse conduction can manifest in the postoperative patient as prolonged P-R, QRS and QT intervals. As the hypothermic patient rewarms in the postoperative period, shivering is commonly seen and metabolic oxygen demand and cardiac output are greatly increased. These increased metabolic demands may place the patient with compromised myocardium at risk as they try to increase cardiac output and development of dysrhythmias is not uncommon (37, 38). Meperidine has been effective for treating postoperative shivering in the awakening patient and causes little hemodynamic trespass in intravenous doses ranging from 12.5 to 50 mg (39, 40).

Certain surgical populations are predisposed to developing cardiac dysrhythmias after surgery and warrant close monitoring in the immediate postoperative period. Radical neck dissections and carotid endarterectomies are associated with repolarization abnormalities. Sinus tachycardia and supraventricular dysrhythmias are common after bronchoscopies and thoracic procedures. Postoperatively, in the neurosurgical patient, a prolonged QT interval may manifest, as well as ventricular dysrhythmias and T-wave inversions and ST segment elevations similar to ECG changes seen with myocardial ischemia (41, 42).

Common PACU Dysrhythmias

Just as there can be many causes for the dysrhythmias seen postoperatively, a multitude of cardiac conduction disturbances and dysrhythmias can be seen in the PACU. Because there are physiologic changes unique to the perioperative and postanesthetic period, certain cardiac dysrhythmias are more likely to be seen in the recovery room (Table 7–4) and have different etiologies than similar dysrhythmias seen in the emergency room or coronary care unit.

SINUS TACHYCARDIA

Sinus tachycardia is the most commonly occurring PACU dysrhythmia. Many stimuli can alter autonomic nervous system balance, and a variety of medications can cause development of sinus tachycardia (Table 7–5). Sinus tachycardia is defined as a heart rate higher than 100 beats per minute and usually not exceeding 180 beats per minute in adults. It is usually harmless and well tolerated by most patients; however, sinus tachycardia can compromise myocardial blood flow in patients with coronary artery disease because of de-

Table 7–4. Commonly Occuring Dysrhythmias in the Postanesthesia Care Unit

Sinus tachycardia
Sinus bradycardia
Ventricular premature beats
Ventricular tachycardia
Supraventricular tachydysrhythmias
Atrioventricular junctional rhythm

Table 7–5. Etiologies of Sinus Tachycardia in the Postanesthesia Care Unit

Increased Sympathetic Activity	Drug Effects
Pain	Ketamine
Anxiety	Isoflurane
Bladder distension	Aminophylline
Presence of ETT	Hydralazine
Hypotension	Ephedrine
Hypercarbia	Nitroprusside
Congestive heart failure	Albuterol
Hypoxia	Terbutaline
Hypovolemia	Dopamine
Increased ICP	Beta agonists
Decreased Parasympathetic Activity	Disease States
Pancuronium	Anemia
Atropine	Thyrotoxicosis
Glycopyrrolate	Sepsis
Gallamine	Guillain-Barré syndrome

creased diastolic filling time, which can precipitate myocardial ischemia. Sinus tachycardia can also compromise cardiac output in patients with stenotic valvular lesions. Therapy should be aimed at decreasing heart rate and blood pressure if elevated. Adequate patient analgesia should be achieved and benzodiazepines used to control patient anxiety. Tachycardia secondary to hypovolemia should be treated with fluid administration, and blood products may be necessary in the face of anemia despite adequate volume replacement. β blockers such as propranolol 0.5 mg to 2.0 mg intravenously, metoprolol 5 mg to 15 mg intravenously, or esmolol 500 μg/kg intravenous bolus followed by a 50 to 300 μg/kg/minute infusion may be useful in controlling heart rate. Verapamil can also be used in doses of 5 to 10 mg intravenously every 10 to 15 minutes.

BRADYCARDIAS

Sinus bradycardia can be precipitated by numerous factors (Table 7–6) and is defined as a heart rate less than 60 beats per minute with normal ECG impulse formation. In healthy patients, hypotension usually does not occur until the heart rate falls below 45 beats per minute. Residual volatile anesthetic effects

and anticholinesterases can produce junctional bradycardias manifest by a heart rate of less than 60 beats per minute and a lack of P waves on the ECG. Junctional bradycardias may decrease cardiac output by 10 to 15%, may result in hypotension, and may occasionally be refractory to treatment. Bradycardia associated with heart block may be seen postoperatively, and preexisting heart block may be aggravated by anesthetic agents that alter AV node conduction or have vagotonic effects. In first-degree AV block, the P-R interval exceeds 0.2 seconds and can progress to second-degree or third-degree heart block. Type I second-degree AV block (Wenckebach) is characterized by successive lengthening of the P-R interval until a nonconducted P wave occurs (Fig. 7–5). In Type II second-degree AV block, the P-R interval is constant before the nonconducted P wave (Fig. 7–6). Third-degree AV block demonstrates complete dissociation of atrial and ventricular pacemakers and may require transvenous pacemaker insertion. Part of the initial management of heart block in the PACU should include consultation and involvement of the cardiology service.

Treatment of bradycardia should begin with a careful assessment of patient condition.

Table 7–6.   Etiologies of Bradycardia in the Postanesthesia Care Unit

Increased Parasympathetic Activity	**Drug Effects**
Vomiting	Neostigmine/edrophonium
Valsalva	Fentanyl
Suctioning the pharynx	Phenylephrine
	β blockade
Decreased Sympathetic Activity	**Disease States**
High spinal/epidural level	Increased intracranial pressure
Hypoxemia	Hypothermia
Local anesthetic agents	Acidosis
Residual general anesthetics	
Ganglionic blockers	
Narcotics/sedatives	
Removal of noxious stimulus	
Extubation	
Emptying bladder	

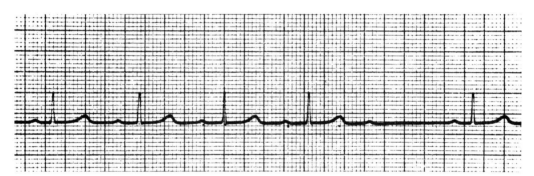

Fig. 7–5.   Type I second-degree AV block (Wenckebach). Successive lengthening of the PR interval is seen until there is a nonconducted P wave. (From Stevenson RL, Rogers MC. Electrocardiographic monitoring and dysrhythmia analysis. In: Blitt CD, ed. Monitoring in anesthesia and critical care medicine. 2nd ed. New York: Churchill Livingstone, 1990;157.)

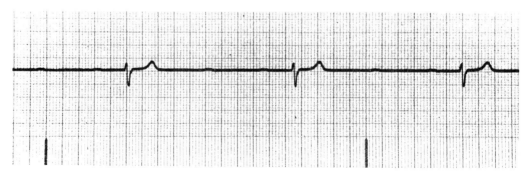

Fig. 7–6.   Type II second-degree AV block. A constant PR interval is seen prior to the nonconducted P wave. (From Stevenson RL, Rogers MC. Electrocardiographic monitoring and dysrhythmia analysis. In: Blitt CD, ed. Monitoring in anesthesia and critical care medicine. 2nd ed. New York: Churchill Livingstone, 1990;157.)

If normal blood pressure and evidence of adequate perfusion are present, the underlying cause of the bradycardia should be sought and corrected. Bradycardia associated with hypotension, poor perfusion, decreased urine output, or ventricular premature contractions requires immediate intervention. If the bradycardia is caused by increased parasympathetic nervous system tone, atropine (0.4 to 1.0 mg intravenous) or glycopyrrolate (0.2 mg intravenous) can produce adequate muscarinic blockade and restore sinus rhythm. Bradycardias resulting from loss of sympathetic nervous system tone can be successfully treated with β-agonist drugs such as isoproterenol (2 to 20 μg/kg/minute). Calcium chloride (500 mg intravenous) can be useful in treating junctional bradycardias. Although effective, pharmacologic treatment of bradycardia may result in unstable escape beats or malignant tachydysrhythmias. A temporary transvenous pacing wire should be placed for refractory, compromising bradycardias, and consultation with a cardiologist should be obtained.

PREMATURE VENTRICULAR CONTRACTIONS

Premature ventricular contraction (PVC) is the second most common dysrhythmia seen in the PACU, and most of these beats do not reflect serious pathology. PVCs commonly manifest as wide, large-amplitude, abnormal QRS complexes that occur at varying intervals from a previously normal QRS complex (Fig. 7–7). In the postoperative patient, PVCs can result from excessive parasympathetic nervous system activity, as diminished depolarization in supraventricular pacemakers will allow ventricular escape beats or from excessive sympathetic nervous system activity. Other common causes of PVCs are found in Table 7–7. Patient morbidity may increase when PVCs occur more frequently than 5 beats per minute, when PVCs occur in runs of two or more, or when PVCs are multifocal in nature. Multifocal PVCs occur when more than one aberrant pacemaker focus fires. The danger in this is an R wave occurring during a T wave and

development of ventricular tachycardia or ventricular fibrillation. Goals of treatment for premature ventricular contractions include assuring adequate oxygenation and ventilation and normal electrolyte levels. For patients on digoxin, the level should be evaluated because digoxin toxicity can lead to PVCs. Pharmacologic therapy should be aimed at controlling ventricular automaticity and lidocaine, procainamide, or bretylium may be used to control premature ventricular activity.

VENTRICULAR TACHYCARDIA

Ventricular tachycardia occurs when three or more sequential ventricular complexes occur at a heart rate greater than 100 beats per minute (Fig. 7–8). These beats may be regular or irregular and may occur intermittently or in sustained runs. Episodes of ventricular tachycardia are frequently associated with acidosis, hypoxia, and myocardial ischemia or infarction. A patient experiencing intermittent ventricular tachycardia who has pulses and stable hemodynamics can be treated with lidocaine, procainamide, or bretylium. Ventricular tachycardia associated with pulselessness, poor perfusion, and unstable hemodynamics should be treated with direct current (DC) synchronized countershock as well as achieving adequate oxygenation, ventilation, and correction of acid/base abnormalities. β-agonist drugs such as epinephrine may be useful, and refractory ventricular tachycardia may require overdrive pacing.

SUPRAVENTRICULAR TACHYCARDIA

Reentrant or aberrant loops of conduction can result in conduction of supraventricular complexes in the PACU patient. A rapid, narrow complex is seen on the ECG and the rapid ventricular rate may compromise cardiac output because of inadequate ventricular filling time (Fig. 7–9). Numerous treatment modalities can be used to slow conduction and interrupt reentrant loops (Table 7–8). Adenosine is useful in diagnosing and treating supraventricular tachycardia (SVT) (43). Six milli-

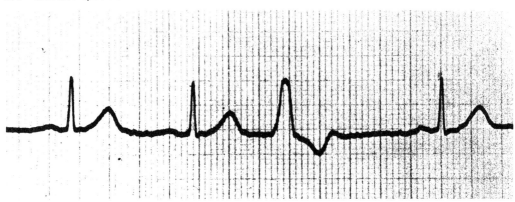

Fig. 7–7. Premature ventricular contraction. A wide, large amplitude abnormal QRS complex is seen surrounded by normal QRS complexes. (From Stevenson RL, Rogers MC. Electrocardiographic monitoring and dysrhythmia analysis. In: Blitt CD, ed. Monitoring in anesthesia and critical care medicine. 2nd ed. New York: Churchill Livingstone, 1990;154.)

Table 7–7. Etiologies of Premature Ventricular Contractions in the Postanesthia Care Unit

Digitalis toxicity
Mechanical stimuli from central catheters
Hypocalcemia
Hypokalemia
Hypomagnesemia
Hypoxia
Hypercarbia
Metabolic acidosis
Myocardial ischemia
Hypertension
Congestive heart failure

grams of adenosine is given initially, and if SVT recurs, 12 mg of adenosine should be administered (Fig. 7–10). A second 12-mg dose may be used if necessary. Antidysrhythmic agents such as lidocaine are most often ineffective in treating supraventricular dysrhythmias.

PREMATURE ATRIAL CONTRACTIONS

Premature atrial contractions (PACs) appear as an early but normal QRS complex and frequently without a preceding P wave on the ECG. PACs arise from abnormal impulse gen-

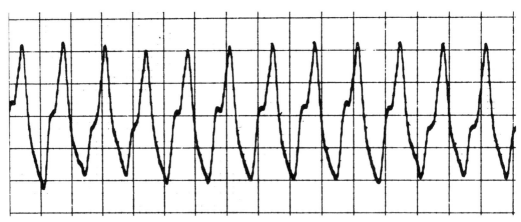

Fig. 7–8.   Ventricular tachycardia. (From Stevenson RL, Rogers MC. Electrocardiographic monitoring and dysrhythmia analysis. In: Blitt CD, ed. Monitoring in anesthesia and critical care medicine. 2nd ed. New York: Churchill Livingstone, 1990;156.)

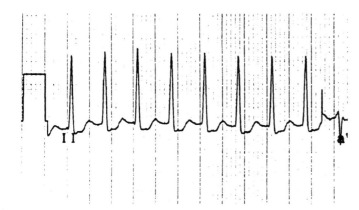

Fig. 7–9. Supraventricular tachycardia. A narrow complex rhythm at a rate of 197 beats per minute is seen on ECG.

Table 7–8. Treatment Modalities for Supraventricular Tachycardia

Vagal stimulation
Carotid massage
Anticholinesterases
   Neostigmine (0.5 to 1.0 mg i.v.)
   Edrophonium (5 to 10 mg i.v.)
Phenylephrine
β blockade
Calcium channel blocker
Digitalis
Adenosine
   Initial dose: 6 mg i.v.
   Second dose: 12 mg i.v. (may be repeated once)
Cardioversion

eration in the atria, AV node, or bundle of His and usually are not associated with hemodynamic changes. PACs frequently are seen when sympathetic nervous system activity is increased postoperatively and require no intervention other than treating the underlying etiology. Rarely, PACs can progress to paroxysmal supraventricular tachycardia or atrial fibrillation. In patients on digoxin, PACs may be indicative of right heart failure and a digoxin level should be checked. A low digoxin level should be treated, and if PACs are recurrent, β blockade may be useful.

ATRIAL FIBRILLATION

There is an increased incidence of atrial fibrillation in patients with mitral valve disease, patients with preexisting atrial fibrillation, and patients recovering from thoracic procedures. New-onset atrial fibrillation can also occur

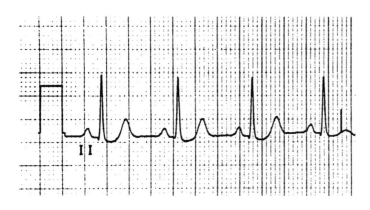

Fig. 7–10. Resolution of supraventricular tachycardia. Normal sinus rhythm has been restored in the patient with paroxysmal supraventricular tachycardia (Fig. 9) after treatment with adenosine.

postoperatively in settings of acute left atrial failure. Atrial fibrillation without a rapid ventricular response usually exhibits no hemodynamic instability and can be treated with digoxin. Beta blockade or calcium channel blockers may be added because of the slow peak effect of digoxin. Atrial fibrillation associated with a rapid ventricular response frequently results in hemodynamic instability and ischemia from poor cardiac filling and decreased cardiac output. In these cases, digoxin loading should be initiated and DC cardioversion should be undertaken to avoid further hemodynamic decline. New-onset atrial fibrillation in patients in the PACU warrants cardiology consultation.

ST SEGMENT AND T-WAVE CHANGES

New T-wave changes frequently are seen in patients in the PACU, and these abnormalities are not commonly associated with myocardial ischemia. Postoperative T-wave changes are more common after intra-abdominal procedures and rarely require further evaluation (44). Further evaluation of new ST-segment changes postoperatively either with or without symptoms of myocardial ischemia is needed. ST segment depression is frequently seen in subendocardial ischemia, and ST segment elevation indicates transmural involvement of the myocardium and is also associated with coronary artery vasospasm. The occurrence of T-wave changes in conjunction with dysrhythmias, angina, or poor perfusion should be evaluated further for myocardial ischemia.

Dysrhythmias occurring in the PACU may develop into real sources of patient morbidity and mortality. Although most cardiac dysrhythmias seen in the PACU are benign and require no pharmacologic intervention, their existence should serve as a reminder to the anesthesiologist that the patient has some physiologic or pharmacologic abnormality that is being manifest as cardiac dysrhythmia. Proper identification of the dysrhythmia is essential to management, and attempts to correct any underlying cause(s) should be made. If the precipitating etiology cannot be cor-

rected, tissue perfusion and/or myocardial performance are compromised, the dysrhythmia persists despite normalizing underlying etiologies, or the potential for developing increasingly malignant rhythms is present, specific drug and/or electrical therapies should be instituted. When diagnosis and/or treatment modalities are elusive and questions arise regarding postoperative dysrhythmias, the expertise of a cardiologist should be sought to assist in patient care.

DISCHARGE CRITERIA

With regard to the cardiovascular system, patients may be discharged from the PACU when their intravascular volume status is assessed as normal and blood pressure is within approximately 20% of resting preoperative values. Heart rate and rhythm should be stable. There should have been simple resolution of any new dysrhythmias or ischemic changes on the electrocardiogram.

ACKNOWLEDGMENT

The authors thank Joyce Jones for assistance in preparing this chapter.

REFERENCES

1. Hines R, Barash PG, Watrous G, et al. Complications occurring in the postanesthesia care unit: a survery. Anesth Analg 1992;74:503–509.
2. de Mello WF, Tully A, Restall J. Morbidity in the postanesthesia care unit [letter]. Anesth Analg 1992;75:633–646.
3. Van der Walt JH, Webb RK, Osborne GA, et al. The Australian incident monitoring study. Recovery room incidents in the first 2000 incident reports. Anaesth Intensive Care 1993;21(5):650–652.
4. Pedersen T. Complications and death following anaesthesia. Dan Med Bull 1994;41:319–331.
5. Orkin LR, Shapiro G. Admission assessment and general monitoring. Int Anesthesiol Clin 1983; 21(1):3–12.
6. Pound JL. Consistency in measurement of blood pressure in postanesthesia care unit. J Post Anesth Nurs 1987;2:78–83.
7. Lawson D, Norley I, Korbon G, et al. Blood flow limits and pulse oximeter signal detection. Anesthesiology 1987;67:599–603.
8. Severinghaus JW, Spellman MJ. Pulse oximeter failure thresholds in hypotension and vasoconstriction. Anesthesiology 1990;73(3):532–537.

9. Gillies BS, Posner K, Freund P, et al. Failure rate of pulse oximetry in the postanesthesia care unit. J Clin Monit 1993;9:326–329.
10. Cormican MGM, Lowe DJ, Keane P, et al. The microbial flora of in-use blood pressure cuffs. Br J Med Sci 1991;160:112–113.
11. Gal TJ, Cooperman LH. Hypertension in the immediate postoperative period. Br J Anaesth 1975; 47:70–74.
12. Carlson CW, Thorton S. Hypertensive crisis in the postanesthesia care unit. J Post Anesth Nurs 1986;1:157–160.
13. Summers S, Dudgsen N, Dubin JS. Postanesthesia care unit hypertension in normotensive young adult males: a pilot study. J Post Anesth Nurs 1988;3:324–331.
14. Prys-Roberts C. Cardiovascular action: too much, too little, or irregular. In: Frost EAM, ed. Post anesthesia care unit. 2nd ed. St. Louis: Mosby, 1990;31–43.
15. Kurz M, Belani KG, Sessler DI, et al. Naloxone, meperidine, and shivering. Anesthesiology 1993; 79(6):1193–1201.
16. Klein P, Rosenbaum SH, Greenberg C. Emergency diagnosis and treatment. In: Israel JS, DeKarnfeld TJ. Recovery room care. 2nd ed. Chicago: Year Book, 1987.
17. Muzzi DA, Black S, Losasso TJ, et al. Labetalol and esmolol in the control of hypertension after intracranial surgery. Anesth Analg 1990;70:68–71.
18. Kuner J, Enescu V, Utsu F, et al. Cardiac arrhythmias during anesthesia. Dis Chest 1967;52:580–587.
19. Bertrand CA, Steiner NV, Jameson AG, et al. Disturbances of cardiac rhythm during anesthesia and surgery. JAMA 1971;216:1615–1617.
20. Atlee JL. Perioperative cardiac dysrhythmias: mechanisms, recognition and management. 2nd ed. Chicago: Year Book Medical Publishers, 1990;1–13.
21. Atlee JL, Zeljko JB. Mechanism for dysrhythmias during anesthesia. Anesthesiology 1990;72:347–374.
22. Atlee JL. Anaesthesia and cardiac electrophysiology. Eur J Anaesthesiol 1985;2(3):215–256.
23. Bosnjak ZJ, Kampine JP. Effects of halothane, enflurane and isoflurane on the SA node. Anesthesiology 1983;58:314–321.
24. Atlee JL, Alexander SC. Halothane effects on conductivity of the AV node and HIS-purkinje system in the dog. Anesth Analg 1977;56:378–386.
25. Atlee JL, Rusy BF. Atrioventricular conduction times and atrioventricular nodal conduction during enflurane anesthesia in dogs. Anesthesiology 1977; 47:498–508.
26. Kotorly KJ, Ebert TJ, Vucins E, et al. Baroreceptor reflex control of heart rate during isoflurane anesthesia in humans. Anesthesiology 1984;60:173–179.
27. Roizen MF, Plummer GO, Lichtor JL. Nitrous oxide and dysrhythmias. Anesthesiology 1987;66:427–431.
28. Daskalopoulos N, Laubie M, Schmitt H. Localization of the central sympatho-inhibitory effects of a narcotic analgesic agent — fentanyl — in cats. Eur J Pharmacol 1975;33:91–97.
29. DeSilva RA, Verrier RL, Lown B. Protective effect of vagotonic action of morphine sulfate on ventricular vulnerability. Cardiovasc Res 1978;12:167–172.
30. Son SL, Waud BE. Potencies of neuromuscular blocking agents at the receptors of the atrial pacemaker and the motor endplate of the guinea pig. Anesthesiology 1977;47:34–36.
31. Son SL, Waud DR. A vagolytic action of neuromuscular blocking agents at the pacemaker of the isolated guinea pig atrium. Anesthesiology 1978;48:191–194.
32. Pratila MG, Pratila V. Anesthetic agents and cardiac electromechanical activity. Anesthesiology 1978; 49:338–360.
33. Braman S, Dunn S, Amico C, et al. Complications of intrahospital transport in critically ill patients. Ann Intern Med 1987;107:469–473.
34. Davidson S, Surawicz B. Ectopic beats and atrioventricular conduction disturbances in patients with hypopotassemia. Arch Intern Med 1967;120:280–285.
35. Fisch C. Relation of electrolyte disturbances to cardiac arrhythmias. Circulation 1973;47:408–419.
36. Voss DM, Drake EH. Cardiac manifestations of hyperparathyroidism with presentation of a previously unreported arrhythmia. Am Heart J 1967;72:235–239.
37. Guffin A, Girard D, Kaplan JA, et al. Shivering following cardiac surgery: hemodynamic changes and reversal. J Cardiothorac Anesth 1987;1:24–28.
38. Bay J, Nunn JF, Prys-Roberts C. Factors influencing arterial PO_2 during recovery from anesthesia. Br J Anaesth 1968;40:398–407.
39. Claybon LE, Hirsh RA. Meperidine arrests post-anesthesia shivering. Anesthesiology 1980;53:S180.
40. Pauca AH, Savage RT, Simpson S, et al. Effect of pethidine, fentanyl, and morphine on postoperative shivering in man. Acta Anaesthesiol Scand 1984;28:138–143.
41. Prys-Roberts C. Cardiovascular action: too much, too little, or irregular. In: Frost EAM, ed. Post anesthesia care unit: current practices. 2nd ed. St. Louis: CV Mosby, 1990;31–43.
42. Cropp GJ, Manning GW. Electrocardiographic changes simulating myocardial ischemia and infarction associated with spontaneous intracranial hemorrhage. Circulation 1960;22:25–38.
43. Dimich I, Singh PP, Herschmann A, et al. Role of adenosine in the diagnosis and treatment of postoperative supraventricular tachy-arrhythmias. J Clin Anesth 1993;5:325–328.
44. Breslow MJ, Miller CF, Parker SD, et al. Changes in T-wave morphology following anesthesia and surgery — a common recovery room phenomenon. Anesthesiology 1986;64:398–402.

8

THE RESPIRATORY SYSTEM

Thomas W. Feeley

POSTOPERATIVE CHANGES

The postoperative changes in respiration can be divided into three categories: changes in lung mechanics, changes in oxygenation, and changes in carbon dioxide elimination. These changes have been described extensively in the literature and in other texts (1).

Changes in Lung Mechanics

The vital capacity of a postoperative patient is reduced to the greatest extent after upper abdominal surgery and to the least extent after peripheral surgery and neurosurgery; lower abdominal and thoracic surgeries fall between these extremes. Decreases in postoperative vital capacity impair the patient's ability to take deep breaths, cough, and clear pulmonary secretions.

The other important lung volume change in the postoperative patient is a reduction in the functional residual capacity (FRC). Reductions in the FRC place patients at risk for hypoxemia due to the development of atelectasis leading to an intrapulmonary right-to-left shunt.

Changes in Oxygenation

Hypoxemia is a common postoperative change. The usual reason for postoperative hypoxemia is an increased intrapulmonary right to left shunt. Patients with chronic obstructive lung disease maybe hypoxemic because of areas of lung with low ventilation-to-

perfusion ratios. Patients with increased intrapulmonary shunts can become more hypoxemia when physiologic changes decrease the mixed venous oxygen saturation. The two postoperative changes that may produce this effect are shivering and reduced cardiac output. Shivering increases oxygen consumption by as much as 400%, thereby reducing the mixed venous oxygen saturation. In the presence of a shunt, this venous blood mixes with the arterial blood, thereby reducing the arterial oxygen saturation. Similarly, reduced cardiac output decreases the venous oxygen saturation and, in the presence of a shunt, decreases the arterial oxygen saturation.

Postoperative causes of increased shunt are atelectasis, aspiration, pulmonary edema, pneumothorax, hemothorax, pneumonia, pulmonary hemorrhage, and pulmonary embolism. In patients with severe hypoxemia in the PACU, these etiologies must be sought by chest x-ray so that specific therapy can be instituted promptly.

Changes in Carbon ioxide Elimination

The most frequent abnormality in carbon dioxide elimination is hypoventilation. Hypoventilation can occur as a consequence of excessive sedation and can be exacerbated by the changes in lung mechanics mentioned above. Narcotics can lead to hypoventilation by direct suppression of ventilation. Narcotics also alter the response to a rising carbon dioxide tension. Normally, as the carbon dioxide tension rises, alveolar ventilation increases. In the presence of narcotics, the increase alveolar ventilation is attenuated, leading to eventual carbon dioxide retention. This effect is commonly referred to as suppression of the carbon dioxide response curve.

Alveolar hyperventilation is less commonly seen in the PACU and is less dangerous than hypoventilation because acidemia is far more dangerous than an alkalemic state. Reasons for hyperventilation include pain, agitation, and direct stimulation from the central nervous system.

MONITORING RESPIRATORY FUNCTION

Monitoring respiration is a major component in the evaluation of patients in the PACU. Observational skills are important and provide information about the rate and pattern of ventilation. Observation of airway patency is especially important in evaluating obtunded patients. The obstructed airway should be quickly recognized before other respiratory monitors warn of a problem. Observations of the patient's color and hemodynamic status also describe important factors concerning respiratory function.

In the PACU, unrecognized respiratory failure can lead to circulatory failure and cardiac arrest. For this reason, respiratory monitoring is designed to provide early recognition of respiratory compromise. To that end, respiratory monitoring focuses on the assessment of oxygenation and CO_2 elimination and, to a lesser degree, measurement of lung volume and function.

Oxygen

Oxygen measurement techniques have been advanced by the development of the pulse oximeter, allowing for continuous assessment of arterial oxygenation in the PACU (2). For many years, direct measurement of the arterial oxygen tension from sampled blood using the Clark electrode was the only method of accurately determining the level of arterial oxygenation. A major disadvantage of the technique is that it is intermittent. The oxygen tension is known only at the time it is sampled and therefore cannot provide a warning of a changing situation unless samples are taken frequently. In addition, this technique usually is not performed at the bedside, resulting in a delay in obtaining results. Pulse oximetry provides a continuous assessment of the hemoglobin oxygen saturation (SpO_2) immediately at the bedside. Artificial measurements can often be detected by simultaneous observation of the pulses signal from the oximeter with the electrocardiogram (ECG). Pulse oximetry can provide a warning of deteriorating oxygenation on a real-time basis and can help evaluate the effectiveness of therapeutic interventions. A major disadvantage of pulse oximetry is that it is dependent on good perfusion for an accurate signal. Another disadvantage is that because it measures saturation, it does not provide information regarding the level of arterial oxygen tension after the arterial blood is fully saturated.

It is standard practice to monitor the SpO_2 of all patients in the PACU after general anesthesia as well as patients requiring mechanical support for ventilation. Oximetry monitoring should be considered during transport from the operating room to the PACU because of the frequency of decreased SpO_2 during transport, especially in children (3). During the patient's stay in the recovery room, decreased SpO_2 is also not an uncommon event. For children, wakefulness does not seem to correlate with hypoxemia (4). For adults, the risk factors for hypoxemia are age, obesity, length of surgery, and American Society of Anesthesiologists (ASA) physical status. One study found that the most common time for hypoxemia to occur is just before PACU discharge, when supplemental oxygen is often discontinued (5). SpO_2 should be monitored continuously in all patients before induction of anesthesia through discharge from the PACU. Patients who are being transferred to the ward without supplemental oxygen should have an

SpO_2 of higher than 95% on room air before discharge.

All patients receiving positive-pressure ventilation should be monitored with a pulse oximeter. For those patients, the device can be used not only as a warning of an acute problem with oxygenation but also to titrate alterations in the patient's oxygen therapy.

Transcutaneous measurement of oxygen tension ($PtcO_2$) has been used in the PACU and ICU, but it is not yet popular among clinicians for several reasons. Although the transcutaneous technique measures oxygen tension and not saturation, it does so by heating an area of skin. When first applied, it takes time to establish a reading, and burns are a potential problem (6). Once it is working, the major disadvantage is that its response time in detecting hypoxemia is slower than that of the pulse oximeter (7). The transcutaneous technique has achieved wider use in pediatrics than in adults. Both techniques work poorly when there is poor peripheral perfusion.

Other forms of oxygen monitoring involve the assessment of oxygen supply. Although monitoring the inspired oxygen concentration has been standard practice in the operating room for many years, only recently manufactured ventilators have provided the ability to monitor the inspired concentration of oxygen and alarm when there is a deviation from the desired concentration. Most rely on paramagnetic analyzers. The use of the mass spectrometer in some ICUs and PACUs has resulted in an ability to evaluate inspired and expired oxygen concentrations. Whenever possible, patients whose lungs are being mechanically ventilated should have their inspired oxygen concentration continuously monitored.

Carbon Dioxide

Attempts to measure or estimate the arterial CO_2 tension noninvasively have been used less widely in the PACU than the methods of measuring arterial oxygen tension. The directly measured tension from an arterial sample measured with a Severinghaus electrode remains the gold standard for CO_2 measurement. Results, however, are neither immediate nor continuous.

Capnography, or the measurement of CO_2 in the expired gas, can be achieved in the PACU by the use of a freestanding infrared analyzer or a mass spectrometer. The end-tidal CO_2 concentration correlates well with the arterial tension in the absence of increases in dead-space ventilation. The technique is less reliable for patients with lung disease but can provide information about trends. Capnography is most effective when the patient's trachea is intubated, although several authors have described methods of obtaining a capnogram from spontaneously breathing patients with a mask or nasal prongs. Capnography can be combined with oximetry for evaluation of patients who are being separated from mechanical ventilation. A simple, nonquantitative colorimetric device can rapidly confirm tracheal intubation in the PACU (8).

Transcutaneous methods of CO_2 measurement are available but infrequently used because of problems similar to those with the transcutaneous oxygen technique. Whenever an abnormality of CO_2 elimination is suspected or detected by another technique, a sample of arterial blood should be analyzed.

Lung Volumes and Pressures

Measurement of lung volumes can be useful for managing PACU patients. Measuring tidal volume, vital capacity, and minute ventilation can provide important information about the ability of a ventilated patient to breathe spontaneously. These volumes can be measured using simple spirometers. The newest generation of ventilators are frequently equipped with a pneumotachometer, which can, by integrating flow rate, provide continuous measurement of tidal volume and minute ventilation with alarms for abnormal or dangerous values. The adequacy of alveolar ventilation can be determined by examining the arterial CO_2 tension. Dead space can be monitored by intermittently measuring the ratio of dead space to tidal volume using the Enghoff modification of the Bohr equation, which requires simultaneous measurement of the arterial and mixed expired CO_2 tension.

$$VD/VT = \frac{PaCO_2 - PeCO_2}{PaCO_2}$$

where VD/VT = dead space/tidal volume ratio; $PaCO_2$ = arterial CO_2; and $PeCO_2$ = mixed expired CO_2. Examination of the gradient between arterial and end-tidal CO_2 tensions may also be used to follow changes in dead-space ventilation. A direct correlation between VD/VT and this gradient has been documented in patients with respiratory insufficiency (9).

The FRC is an extremely important determinant of arterial oxygen tension. It is frequently reduced in postsurgical patients and in patients with many forms of acute lung disease. Although various washout techniques have been evaluated for measuring FRC, most are technically demanding and not easily applied at the bedside in the PACU. Monitoring the FRC is therefore not a routine clinical practice.

Measurement of inspiratory pressure is also important in the monitoring of respiratory function of patients who remain intubated in the PACU. The peak inspiratory pressure generated during a positive-pressure inflation is a nonspecific guide to the level of airway resistance and total respiratory compliance. Patients with high peak inspiratory pressures are at increased risk of developing pulmonary barotrauma. The plateau pressure, or the pressure generated when a tidal volume is held in the lungs, can be used to monitor pulmonary static compliance. The plateau pressure can be used to help distinguish high peak inspiratory pressures caused by poor compliance from that caused by a high airway resistance. Peak pressure and plateau pressure will be similar if the increase is due to poor compliance. Plateau pressure will be considerably lower than the peak pressure if the cause of the high pressure is increased airway resistance. The calculation requires monitoring of baseline pressure, plateau pressure, and exhaled tidal volume as follows:

$$C = \frac{V}{Ppl \ PB}$$

where C = compliance; V = exhaled tidal volume; Ppl = inspiratory plateau pressure; and PB = baseline pressure.

Negative pressure generated during attempted inspiration through an obstructed airway is often used as a guide to the ability of a patient to breathe spontaneously. The maximum inspiratory force (MIF) is the negative pressure generated as a patient attempts to breathe against an occluded airway. This bedside test can be performed daily to assess the strength of the respiratory muscles. It is also affected by restrictive lung disease and by poor or impaired central neural output. Respiratory drive can be monitored, using techniques such as the occlusion pressure, although the clinical usefulness of such techniques remains unproven (10).

Other calculated measures of respiratory function are the alveolar-to-arterial oxygen tension gradient, the shunt fraction, and the oxygenation index (PaO_2/FIO_2). Calculating and monitoring these indices have no clinical advantage over simpler methods of assessing oxygen requirement.

RESPIRATORY COMPLICATIONS IN THE PACU

Incidence

The major respiratory complications encountered in the PACU are airway obstruction, hypoxemia, hypercapnia, and aspiration. Prompt recognition and treatment of these life-threatening problems are crucial to good postanesthesia care.

Until recently, studies of complications in the PACU were rare in the anesthesia literature. A recent survey from Yale has provided the most comprehensive assessment of complications occurring in the PACU (11). Hines et al. studied 18,473 PACU admissions in a university hospital. They found that the incidence of PACU complications was high, with significant events occurring in nearly 24% of all patients. The most common events were nausea and vomiting (9.8%), need for airway support (6.9%), hypotension (2.7%), dysrhythmia (1.4%), hypertension (1.1%), altered mental status (0.6%), possible myocardial infarction (0.3%), and major cardiac events (0.3%). The factors that seemed to have the greatest influence on the complication rate were ASA Physical Status 2, a duration of anesthesia between 2 and 4 hours, emergency procedures, and the type of surgical procedure; abdominal and orthopedic procedures had the highest incidence of complications. In another study on recovery, a history of smoking also resulted in longer stays in the PACU (12).

Hypoventilation

Hypoventilation is defined as reduced alveolar ventilation resulting in an increase in the arterial carbon dioxide tension ($PaCO_2$). During the postoperative period, hypoventilation occurs as a result of poor respiratory drive, poor respiratory muscle function, or as the direct result of acute or chronic lung disease.

Central respiratory depression occurs with any anesthetic. Narcotic anesthetics produce a respiratory depression that is detectable by a shift of the carbon dioxide response curve downward and to the right. Neuroleptic anesthetic techniques can produce a biphasic respiratory depression with respiratory depression intraoperatively, which dissipates on arrival in the recovery room, only to be followed by a second period of respiratory depression (13). Narcotic-induced respiratory depression can be reversed by use of narcotic antagonists (14). When small doses are used, these agents can reverse the narcotic-induced respiratory depression without altering pain relief; however, the duration of action of currently available antagonists is shorter than most narcotics and the dose must be repeated at least once. Larger doses of these agents reverse the anal-

gesic effects of the narcotics and result in severe pain and often profound increases in heart rate (HR) and blood pressure. These increases in rate pressure product (HR × systolic blood pressure) signify large increases in myocardial oxygen consumption and can result in ischemia in patients with coronary artery disease. An inadequate central respiratory drive can also be seen after certain neurosurgical procedures such as cervical cordotomy.

Poor respiratory muscle function occurs after surgery and often contributes to hypoventilation. The site of the incision affects the ability to take a large breath as measured by the vital capacity. Nearly all patients have reductions in vital capacity that are the greatest on the day of surgery. Patients undergoing upper abdominal surgery have the greatest reduction in vital capacity, demonstrating as much as a 60% reduction on the day of surgery (15). This reduction in vital capacity, secondary to diaphragmatic impairment, results in problems with both carbon dioxide elimination and oxygenation (16).

Inadequate respiratory muscle function may result from inadequate reversal of neuromuscular blocking agents or neuromuscular disease (17–19). Obesity, gastric dilation, tight dressings, and body casts also inhibit respiratory muscle function and can predispose CO_2 retention. A high level of CO_2 production from sepsis or shivering can result in CO_2 retention, especially if the patient cannot increase minute ventilation (20).

Bronchospasm can lead to hypoventilation. Patients who develop postoperative wheezing should be evaluated to determine the etiology. Patients with preexisting asthma or chronic obstructive pulmonary disease can certainly wheeze after surgery; however, pulmonary edema and aspiration can also present as wheezing in the PACU. Only after the etiology has been determined can definitive therapy be provided. Treatment of pulmonary edema involves diuresis. Treatment of wheezing from chronic lung disorders is best approached by first administering inhaled bronchodilators. If bronchodilators are not effective, then intravenous corticosteroids are given. Aminophylline can be used in severely refractory cases.

The direct measurement of $PaCO_2$ is the best method of detecting hypoventilation in the postoperative period. Although hypertension and tachycardia commonly occur during CO_2 retention, these signs may not be seen in postsurgical patients and in elderly patients, who have an attenuated response to increased levels of CO_2. Measurement of the vital capacity and maximum inspiratory force are good guides to the ability of the postsurgical patient to breathe spontaneously in the postoperative period. The vital capacity should be at least 10 mL/kg body weight, and the inspiratory force should be numerically greater than –20 cm H_2O (20). If these minimum values cannot be maintained, the patient should receive controlled mechanical ventilation until he or she is awake enough to generate adequate respiratory muscle function.

Airway Obstruction

The most common cause of postoperative airway obstruction is pharyngeal obstruction from a sagging tongue in the unconscious patient (21). Laryngeal obstruction can also occur secondary to laryngeal spasm or direct airway injury (22–24). The most effective method of dealing with airway obstruction due to pharyngeal obstruction is a combination of backward tilt of the head and some degree of anterior displacement of the mandible. The proper position for each patient will depend to some degree on trial and error until one has a completely patent airway. If the obstruction is not immediately reversible, a nasal or oral airway can be inserted. The nasal airway is preferred because it is much better tolerated by patients as they emerge from general anesthesia. Also, the oral airway may stimulate gagging and vomiting as well as laryngeal spasm. If the airway obstruction is caused by laryngospasm, it may be relieved by administering 100% oxygen under gentle positive pressure. If the spasm cannot be relieved by

this maneuver, the administration of a small dose of succinylcholine (0.1 to 0.2 mg/Kg^{-1}) may be necessary. If succinylcholine is given, assisted ventilation with 100% oxygen should be continued for at least 5 to 10 minutes, even if the obstruction has been relieved and the patient is breathing spontaneously (20). For all cases of airway obstruction, if an adequate airway cannot be established by simple physical or pharmacological means, one must be established via orotracheal intubation using direct laryngoscopy. In the very rare case in which the trachea cannot be intubated, an emergency cricothyroidotomy will relieve the obstruction. This procedure is probably safer than emergency tracheostomy, because excessive bleeding is common when the latter procedure is performed under emergency conditions. Prompt action is crucial in airway obstruction because the $PaCO_2$ increases 6 mm Hg during the first minute of total obstruction and then at a rate of 3 to 4 mm Hg per minute thereafter. In such cases, there is also a progressive fall in PaO_2, owing to the continuously falling alveolar PO_2.

Hypoxemia

Hypoxemia is a common and potentially serious postoperative complication (25–27). The pulse oximeter has allowed for more careful evaluations of the incidence of postoperative hypoxemia than ever before in the history of the PACU. In a recent survey performed in Denmark, 55% of patients had one or more episodes of hypoxemia (SaO_2<90%), often despite the presence of routine supplemental oxygen. Ninety-five percent of those episodes went unrecognized by the PACU staff. Factors predisposing these incidents were duration of anesthesia, use of general anesthesia, and a history of smoking (28).

Hypoxemia after anesthesia and surgery can be caused by many factors. Evaluation of the hypoxemic postoperative patient should include consideration of each of the classic causes of hypoxemia: (*a*) low inspired concentration of oxygen, (*b*) hypoventilation, (*c*) areas of low ventilation-to-perfusion relations, and (*d*) an increased intrapulmonary right-to-left shunt. Situations such as increased age, postanesthetic shivering, and a lowered cardiac output may worsen the degree of hypoxemia in postsurgical patients when an intrapulmonary shunt is present (29–31).

Low inspired concentrations of oxygen ($FIO_2 < 0.21$) are, fortunately, rare causes of significant postoperative hypoxemia; however, the delivery of hypoxic gas mixtures to postoperative patients is possible. Crossing of nitrous oxide and oxygen pipelines during hospital construction resulted in the loss of more than 30 lives in a Canadian hospital. Pipelines have been crossed during hospital modernization projects. Switching of all adapters can also lead to delivery of the wrong gas as can purging the system with nitrogen for pipeline repairs (32).

The most common cause of postoperative hypoxemia is an increase in right-to-left intrapulmonary shunt. Increases in intrapulmonary shunt can be caused by many processes. Atelectasis is the most common cause of an increased right-to-left shunt. Atelectasis occurs as the result of collapse of an entire lung, lobe, or lung segment or it can occur in a diffuse pattern. Bronchial obstruction from secretion or blood is a frequent cause of atelectasis. Lobar and segmental collapses often result from bronchial obstruction with secretions and are best managed by providing adequate humidification of the inspired gases, coughing, deep breathing, and postural drainage. Endobronchial intubation with collapse of the opposite lung is a serious complication and should be avoided. Pneumothorax is a cause of hypoxemia that can have serious sequelae. Pneumothorax causes hypoxemia due to atelectasis and an intrapulmonary shunt. Pneumothorax occurs as a result of direct lung or airway injury from trauma, rib fractures, or attempts at percutaneous vascular cannulation. Pneumothoraces resulting from mechanical ventilation per se are rare unless airway pressures are high (33, 34). Treatment depends on the size of the pneumothorax and the patient's condition. A 10 to 20% pneumothorax in a spontaneously breathing patient can be observed with frequent upright chest roentgenograms. A pneumothorax of more than 20% in a spontaneously breathing patient or any pneumothorax in a mechanically ventilated patient should be treated by insertion of a chest tube for drainage. This is usually performed in the second intercostal space in the midclavicular line. A tension pneumothorax occurs when the pleural cavity fills with air and compresses the mediastinum, resulting in circulatory compromise. Tension pneumothorax is treated in the same manner; however, one should not await roentgenographic confirmation of the diagnosis if tension pneumothorax with circulatory depression is diagnosed. A 14-gauge needle inserted into the second intercostal space can relieve the tension before chest-tube insertion.

Arterial hypoxemia may be present in postoperative patients who have no discernible change in the chest roentgenogram. Perhaps these patients have an increased right-to-left intrapulmonary shunt due to diffuse airway collapse. The relationship between the FRC of the lung and closing capacity is a prime determinant of this effect (35, 36). When the closing capacity exceeds FRC, airways collapse during tidal breathing and an intrapulmonary shunt develops. Any situation that results in either an increased closing capacity (e.g., increasing age) or reduced FRC (pulmonary edema, infection, aspiration, obesity) will place the patient at increased risk for hypoxemia. Difficulties in interpreting the true meaning of what is believed to be the closing capacity has led some investigators to question this FRC: closing capacity relationship as being the sole determinant of impaired gas exchange during the perioperative period (37).

Pulmonary edema is another process that can result in hypoxemia in the postoperative period. Although pulmonary edema has been well studied in patients with left ventricular failure (38, 39), studies of this process in the immediate postoperative period are rare. Cooperman and Price examined 40 cases of perioperative pulmonary edema and found one-half the patients to have preoperative evidence of cardiovascular disease (40). The most common time of appearance of pulmonary edema was observed within 60 minutes of completion of surgery. More than one-half of these cases were preceded by hypertension, suggesting that this problem may be related to the high pulmonary vascular pressures seen in acute, postoperative hypertension. Detection was made frequently by the presence of wheezing. Elevation of the central venous pressure and neck vein distention were not common findings. Patients develop pulmonary edema postoperatively because of high hydrostatic pressure in the pulmonary capillaries, an increased capillary permeability, or after sustained reductions in the interstitial hydrostatic pressure. The last-named type of pulmonary edema is seen after prolonged airway obstruction (41, 42). Patients with a permeability injury can have their pulmonary edema exacerbated by increases in hydrostatic pressure. High-pressure pulmonary edema is usually caused by ischemic or valvular heart disease. Pulmonary edema characterized by a permeability injury is seen after a wide variety of serious clinical situations, such as disseminated intravascular coagulation, shock, trauma, massive transfusion, sepsis, and anaphylaxis. This type of pulmonary edema is frequently called "adult respiratory distress syndrome" and is characterized by hypoxemia, diffuse pulmonary infiltrates on roentgenogram, and reduced lung compliance. A common early pathologic finding is neutrophil accumulation in the lung vasculature and tissue. There is increasing evidence that activation of arachidonic acid metabolites, the prostaglandins and the leukotrienes, may be responsible for the permeability injury seen in humans (43). Experimentally, leukotriene D_4 increases pulmonary permeability (44). Because more is being learned about these substances, future breakthroughs in the adult respiratory distress syndrome probably will center on the use of naturally occurring inhibitor substances of key reactions.

Current treatment of both forms of pulmonary edema centers on lowering the hydrostatic pressure in the lungs to the lowest possible level consistent with adequate perfusion of all organ systems. Hydrostatic pressure may be lowered with diuretics, fluid restriction, vasodilators, or dialysis if there is associated renal failure. Positive-pressure ventilation is useful if there is severe hypoxemia or respiratory acidosis. Ventilation with end-expiratory pressure improves oxygenation by increasing lung volume, not by decreasing lung water (45). Monitoring with a pulmonary artery catheter is often helpful. Monitors of extravascular lung water employing double-indication dilution techniques are available and accurate but are probably too technically demanding for routine clinical use (46, 47). Respiratory support with oxygen and mechanical ventilation are frequently necessary while the patient receives definitive treatment. Vomiting and aspiration of gastric contents during and after anesthesia can produce a severe permeability injury, resulting in pulmonary edema and hypoxemia.

Pulmonary embolism occurring in the immediate postoperative period is a serious event that can lead to profound hypoxemia. The exact physiologic explanation of the hypoxemia is unclear. Patients on bedrest for prolonged periods before surgery are very susceptible to emboli. The diagnosis is suspected in a patient with sudden pleuritic chest pain, shortness of breath, pleural effusion, or tachypnea. Evidence of right heart strain can sometimes be seen on the ECG. Massive emboli result in hypotension, pulmonary hypertension, and an elevated central venous pressure. Because the treatment of choice is anticoagulation, the establishment of an accurate diagnosis is imperative so that patients in the immediate postsurgical period are not needlessly exposed to the risks of anticoagulation. Thrombolytic therapy has been used very successfully for patients with massive emboli; however, it is rare to be secure enough about potential bleeding to use thrombolytic therapy in the PACU.

The only certain way to make the diagnosis is pulmonary angiography. This is often the procedure of choice for this type of patient. Once the diagnosis is made, heparin is given via continuous intravenous infusion to keep the patient's partial thromboplastin time two to 2.5 times the control. If emboli recur or bleeding develops with heparinization, vena caval obstruction by percutaneously placed umbrella may be indicated.

Posthyperventilation hypoxemia and diffusion hypoxemia can occur but are rarely seen in clinical practice because oxygen administration prevents the clinical manifestations of the events. After anesthetic techniques that use hyperventilation, the body's supplies of carbon dioxide are restored from endogenous CO_2 production and ventilation. Alveolar oxygen tension (PAO_2) is reduced accordingly. Diffusion hypoxia occurs when N_2O is replaced with air at the end of the anesthetic. Because N_2O is 31 times more soluble than nitrogen, there is dilution of the inspired air with N_2O and the PAO_2 falls (31).

The type of anesthetic and the site of operation influence the reduction in arterial oxygen tension (PaO_2) seen after anesthesia and surgery. Abdominal operations are associated with the most prolonged reductions in PaO_2. Although the PaO_2 may be normal during the immediate postoperative period, abdominal operations under regional anesthesia are associated with the greatest reduction in PaO_2 after 24 hours (29). This reduction in PaO_2 is likely due to the reduced vital capacity seen after upper abdominal surgery. A shift from diaphragmatic to rib-cage breathing probably accounts for this well-recognized decrease in postoperative vital capacity (16).

Reductions in cardiac output can contribute to large decreases in PaO_2 in patients with existing intrapulmonary shunts. This is because of the effect of the lowered mixed venous PO_2, which is added directly to the arterial circulation through the right-to-left shunt (31). Postoperative shivering can result in increases in oxygen consumption of as much as 500%, but this only rarely contributes to arterial hypoxemia (30). Shivering also reduces the arterial oxygen tension in patients with an intrapulmonary shunt by lowering of the mixed venous oxygen tension. Significant increases in postoperative oxygen consumption also occur after anesthesia for burn treatment leading to inadequate oxygen delivery (48).

Recognition of hypoxemia can be difficult during the recovery from anesthesia if pulse oximetry is not used. Lowered hemoglobin concentrations may prevent the detection of peripheral cyanosis. The ventilatory and circulatory responses to hypoxemia may also be attenuated for elderly patients. Currently, the best method of assessing hypoxemia during anesthetic recovery is use of a pulse oximeter (49).

Treatment of hypoxemia by face-mask oxygen is effective in restoring the PaO_2 in many cases. The PaO_2 response to oxygen breathing depends on the degree of intrapulmonary shunt. Increasing the FIO_2 from room air to 100% results in a large increase in PaO_2 when the shunt fraction is small; however, oxygen will have little effect on the PaO_2 in patients with a large shunt fraction (50). If hypoxemia persists ($PaO_2 < 60$ mm Hg) despite maximal oxygen therapy (FIO_2, 1.0), tracheal intubation and mechanical ventilation should be initiated. In such patients, ventilation with positive end-expiratory pressure (PEEP) will increase the functional residual capacity and result in an improvement in arterial oxygenation. Ventilation with PEEP eventually permits a reduction in FIO_2 without a fall in PaO_2.

POSTOPERATIVE VENTILATORY SUPPORT

Classification of Ventilating Devices

The tremendous explosion of medical technology during the past 20 years has resulted in the availability of many different types of mechanical ventilating devices throughout the country. Although the underlying principles of operation are similar from device to device, the actual operation of these devices may vary remarkably. A clear understanding of the basic principles of ventilating devices is therefore necessary to properly select and apply a ventilator to a patient with respiratory insufficiency. A simple system of ventilator classification allows one to examine the similarities and differences among devices and rationally apply them patient management. All ventilators fall into one of two basic types: negative pressure ventilators and positive-pressure ventilators.

NEGATIVE-PRESSURE VENTILATORS

Negative-pressure devices create a negative pressure around the chest to result in airflow into the lung. These devices are still used today but have no use in the PACU. They are most effective in the management of patients with chronic respiratory insufficiency due to neuromuscular disorders. They are of no use intraoperatively or for patients with acute lung disease.

POSITIVE-PRESSURE VENTILATORS

Positive-pressure devices create a positive pressure in the airway and result in mass airflow into the lung. Positive-pressure devices can be divided into two groups: devices that deliver the gas with a high volume, high pressure, and slow rate (conventional ventilators) and devices that deliver low volume and low pressure using a high rate (high-frequency devices).

Subclassification of Ventilating Devices

Most ventilators available in the PACU are the conventional positive-pressure devices. These devices are further classified by a system in which the function of any mechanical ventilator is described by how it works in each of four phases: inspiration, transition from inspiration to expiration, expiration, and the transition from expiration to inspiration.

INSPIRATION

During the inspiratory phase, the ventilator can deliver gas to the lungs in several ways. Ventilators can deliver gas at a certain flow rate.

These are called flow generators. The flow can be constant (square wave), accelerative, or decelerative. Decelerative flow is probably associated with a better distribution of ventilation than either accelerative or constant flow. Other types of ventilators do not deliver a constant-flow rate pattern but rather deliver a constant pressure or pressure pattern. These are called "pressure generators."

In addition to the flow and pressure characteristics during inspiration, many devices provide a brief inspiratory hold at the end of the delivery of the tidal volume. This extra time in inspiration may possibly improve the distribution of ventilation but convincing evidence is minimal. The major disadvantage of inspiratory hold is that it raises mean intrathoracic pressure and can interfere with venous return to the heart. This is especially true for hypovolemic patients.

TRANSITION FROM INSPIRATION TO EXPIRATION

The transition from inspiration to expiration provides a type of classification that is familiar to most physicians. Ventilators stop delivering gas when either a certain volume, pressure, or time is reached. Ventilators that stop delivering gas after a preset volume is delivered are termed "volume-cycled ventilators."

Volume-cycled ventilators are the most common type of ventilators used for postoperative ventilation and for the treatment of acute respiratory failure. They deliver the same volume into the breathing circuit irrespective of the pressure it takes to achieve that volume within certain limits. A volume-cycled ventilator will deliver a nearly constant tidal volume in the face of changing airway resistance or lung compliance. Most common volume-cycled ventilators have a pressure-limiting device that is designed to protect the patient from extremely high pressures. Such high pressures could occur if the patient coughs or strains during inspiration. When a certain preset pressure is reached, the ventilator stops delivering the tidal volume and an alarm sounds. When this occurs, the actual tidal volume is reduced and minute ventilation will be reduced if the process continues. Another important consideration is that although a volume-cycled ventilator will deliver a constant volume in the face of falling compliance, the distribution of that volume will be compressed into the circuit and less volume may actually reach the lungs. Both of these situations can result in alveolar hypoventilation.

Pressure-cycled ventilators are devices that make the transition from inspiration to expiration after the preset pressure is reached. These ventilators are simple, small, lightweight, and often less expensive than volume-cycled ventilators. Their major problem is that they will not deliver a constant tidal volume in the face of changing airway resistance or compliance. Their use may result in marked changes in alveolar ventilation in those circumstances. These devices are best suited for use in the patient who has minimal lung disease when changes in airway resistance or total respiratory compliance are unlikely. They can be used for brief postoperative ventilation. Monitoring of the expired volume is an important method of ensuring that the patient's minute ventilation remains constant.

Timed-cycled ventilators terminate inspiration after a preset time is reached. Tidal volume is determined altering both the time of inspiration and the flow rate of the inspired gas. Many ventilators designed for operating room use employ this mechanism. Although pressure and volume vary a bit from breath to breath, these ventilators are reliable, are safe, and can perform as well as most volume-cycled ventilators. There are no time-cycled ventilators for postoperative ventilation of adults.

EXPIRATION

The expiratory phase provides time for passive exhalation. Ventilators can provide two basic alterations to the flow of the expired gas. They can slow the rate of escape of gas by providing a resistance to flow. This is sometimes called expiratory retard. This is useful for patients with chronic obstructive pulmonary disease (COPD), who require more time to allow for an even exit of gas from the lungs and it is believed to be analogous to the "purse-lipped" breathing of a patient with COPD. When using expiratory retard, the airway pressure returns to atmospheric pressure at the end of expiration. This is in contrast to the other expiratory maneuver that can be applied, which is positive end-expiratory pressure (PEEP). PEEP keeps the airway pressure positive with respect to the atmospheric pressure during the entire expiratory phase. PEEP improves arterial oxygenation in patients with an increased right-to-left intrapulmonary shunt by increasing the functional residual capacity and providing a better matching of ventilation and perfusion.

TRANSITION FROM EXPIRATION TO INSPIRATION

The transition from expiration to inspiration is the final way ventilators are classified. Ventilators can be described as controllers, assistors, or ventilators that deliver intermittent mandatory ventilation (IMV). The current generation of ventilators also can provide pressure support during the IMV mode. With pressure support, the IMV breaths are volume-limited and occur at a preset time. The spontaneous breaths are assisted in that the ventilator delivers flow into the system until a preset pressure is reached, thus augmenting the tidal volume of a patient during the spontaneous breaths. This classification was useful when the commonly available ventilators provided only one method of starting inspiration. Most modern ventilators provide all of these methods of starting inspiration.

Controllers, or ventilators operating in the control mode, do so by providing constant tidal volumes at a preset rate. They do not use the patient's spontaneous ventilatory efforts. Controlled mechanical ventilation (CMV) is best suited for use when anesthetics and muscle relaxants suppress spontaneous ventilation. The development of IMV has made the need for long-term CMV less common.

Assistors are ventilators that begin inspiration only after a spontaneous breath by the patient reduces the airway pressure and initiates the ventilator cycle. The tidal volume is set by the operator, and the patient determines the rate. Alveolar ventilation becomes normal after a brief period of alveolar hyperventilation. Pure assist devices are not available because of the danger of a patient's becoming apneic and not receiving any breaths from the ventilator. For that reason, most devices provide what is called assist-control. During assist-control, the patient initiates each breath; however, if apnea develops, a predetermined rate is delivered from the machine. This backup system avoids the major potential harm of assisted ventilation.

IMV is a system in which the patient is allowed to take breaths of oxygenated, humidified gas, spontaneously between ventilator-delivered breaths. The ventilator-delivered breaths occur at a fixed, preset time with IMV. Ventilator-delivered breaths occur at the start of the patient's inspiration with intermittent demand ventilation (IDV, or synchronized IMV). Although theoretically appealing, there is no evidence that IDV is safer or produces less physiologic disruption than IMV.

IMV was originally introduced as a method of weaning patients from mechanical ventilation. It became quickly obvious, however, that IMV weaning can be as difficult as conventional weaning, and it is now commonly used as an alternative to assisted or controlled ventilation. By allowing some spontaneous breathing, IMV offers the following advantages: (*a*) there is less need for sedation and the use of relaxants can be avoided completely; (*b*) spontaneous breathing allows a slower ventilator rate and therefore potentially less chance of barotrauma; and (*c*) spontaneous breathing results in augmentation of venous return via the thoracic pump mechanism (hence, IMV results in less depression of cardiac output than controlled or assisted ventilation and allows for the use of higher levels of PEEP when necessary); and (*d*) the IMV mechanism allows for smoother transition from ventilatory assistance to complete, spontaneous breathing. The latter is due, in part, to the

fact that the respiratory muscles are put at rest and atrophy during paralysis, sedation, and starvation. IMV allows these muscles to work, thereby maintaining muscular function at a higher level.

The addition of pressure support to IMV has been useful in providing patients comfort during ventilation with low IMV rates. The higher the preset pressure, the greater the augmentation in tidal volume. If the pressure is set at the peak pressure that is generated during the IMV breaths, then the tidal volume during the "spontaneous breaths" will be close to the tidal volume during the IMV breaths. In that situation, the patient is effectively receiving assisted respiration. It is important during weaning with IMV and pressure support that the level of pressure support be reduced after the IMV rate has been reduced to ensure that the patient is indeed breathing spontaneously without major assistance from the ventilator.

High-Frequency Ventilators

High-frequency ventilators deliver small tidal volumes at high rates. High-frequency, positive-pressure ventilation (HFPPV) was originally developed by a group of investigators who needed a system of ventilation that did not interfere with cardiac output to study blood pressure control. By delivery of gas at a high rate, minimal pressure is used. The technique has been successfully applied for bronchoscopy, laryngoscopy, and neonatal ventilation. The major use has been for patients with bronchopleural fistulas.

Indications for Mechanical Ventilation

The goal of using any mechanical ventilator is to normalize oxygen delivery and carbon dioxide elimination. There are a wide variety of clinical situations in which mechanical ventilation is now routinely used. The three basic situations include: (*a*) intraoperative ventilation; (*b*) prophylactic postoperative ventilation; and (*c*) ventilation for the treatment of acute respiratory failure.

PROPHYLACTIC VENTILATION

Prophylactic postoperative ventilation is used for many patients undergoing major surgery. All patients selected have a high likelihood of developing respiratory failure if not ventilated prophylactically.

Prophylactic ventilation is especially helpful after cardiac valve replacement surgery, for patients who have had long periods of cardiopulmonary bypass, for patients with preexisting lung disease or congestive failure, and after repair of most congenital defects. Nearly all patients who have had high-dose narcotic anesthetic techniques will require at least several hours of mechanical ventilation. There is some evidence that otherwise healthy coronary bypass patients who have an inhalation anesthetic have fewer cardiopulmonary complications when extubated early after surgery than if they are reanesthetized for prophylactic ventilation. Because these types of patients now constitute an increasing percentage of cardiac cases, one must carefully consider which patients truly need prophylactic postsurgical ventilation.

Patients having prolonged aortofemoral bypass procedures, renovascular reconstruction, and splenorenal shunt all will have a need for intravenous fluids postoperatively. As a result, many of these patients develop abdominal distention, which interferes with spontaneous breathing. This factor makes many of these patients candidates for developing respiratory failure if they are not ventilated prophylactically.

For some patients, relaxants will not be reversed after gastrointestinal surgery. Other patients will have incomplete reversal because of many factors, such as hypothermia, acidemia, or the presence of drugs, such as gentamycin, which potentiate neuromuscular blockade. The best guide to whether such a patient should be ventilated lies in a simple examination of two tests of respiratory function: (*a*) the maximum inspiratory pressure should be

at least −20 cm H_2O before extubation; and (*b*) the vital capacity should be at least 10 mL/kg of body weight. Both of these tests are simple to perform in the operating room or recovery room and are good guides to the ability of patients with muscle weakness to breathe spontaneously.

Patients with severe chronic or acute respiratory disease who have undergone a major operative procedure are good candidates for prophylactic ventilation. Upper abdominal operations reduce the vital capacity to 20 to 25% of the preoperative value. Lower abdominal and lateral thoracic procedures reduce the vital capacity to 40 to 60% of the preoperative value. Patients with borderline respiratory function preoperatively may not tolerate further impairment in vital capacity.

The decision to employ postoperative ventilatory support should be made as early as possible. It is advisable to discuss the possibility of ventilatory support with the patient preoperatively so the patient understands the reason for continued intubated on awakening. Ventilatory support, properly carried out, is much safer than a sequence of extubation, followed by hypoxemia and hypercapnia leading to emergency reintubation.

RESPIRATORY FAILURE

Acute respiratory failure is a common indication for mechanical ventilation in the postoperative period. In the assessment of these patients, there are a number of very clear indications for providing ventilatory support.

Hypoxemia

When the PaO_2 falls below 60 torr despite maximal FIO_2 being delivered from a well-fitted face mask, intubation and ventilation are necessary. Patients such as these are at great risk for sudden arterial desaturation if they even briefly remove their oxygen supply.

Hypercapnia

When the $PaCO_2$ increases acutely, resulting in an arterial pH of less than 7.25, there is a great risk of developing arrhythmias and circulatory instability. Patients with chronic hypercapnia due to chronic lung disease may tolerate $PaCO_2$ in the 70s or 80s without noticeable mental changes or acidemia. For those patients, close observation is necessary and intubation should be performed when the patient becomes fatigued or the mental status begins to deteriorate.

Decreased Vital Capacity

The vital capacity is an excellent guide to the need for postoperative ventilatory support. Patients usually cannot tolerate spontaneous respiration when the vital capacity is less than 10 mL/kg of body weight.

Respiratory Distress

The patient who develops respiratory failure will often go through a phase of respiratory distress manifested by tachypnea, tachycardia, and sometimes agitation before there are noticeable blood gas changes. The period of time that a patient will be able to breathe effectively in this manner varies considerably, depending on the nature and severity of the acute lung disease as well as the patient's premorbid status. A young, previously healthy person with acute pulmonary edema may tolerate breathing at spontaneous rates of 30 to 40 per minute for several days, whereas an elderly, debilitated person with the same process will be able to breathe spontaneously at those rates for only minutes or hours. We will often employ intubation and mechanical ventilation in such patients when respiratory failure seems likely but before the blood gases deteriorate. The decision to ventilate the lungs in this setting depends on the degree of distress, the degree of fatigue, and the reversibility of the acute lung disorder. Obviously, this is a clinical decision but one that is often easy to make. An elective, planned intubation in this setting is usually better for the patient than an emergency intubation.

Tracheal Intubation

Treatment of serious respiratory failure necessitates emergency tracheal intubation. The need to perform reintubation in the PACU is rare, occurring in 0.2% of about 13,000 patients in a recent study (51). In that series of patients, 77% of the reintubations occurred within the first hour in the PACU and reintubation was more common in children and elderly patients. Many of the cases were believed to be preventable and related to excessive anesthetic and sedative drugs, excessive fluid administration, persistent effects of muscle relaxants, and upper airway obstruction.

When reintubation is necessary in the PACU, all necessary equipment should be available. For emergency situations, it is best to use as few drugs as possible because the patient's spontaneous respirations are frequently life-sustaining. Topical anesthesia is often all that is necessary. However, under certain circumstances, sedatives such as midazelam and induction agents such as etomidate can facilitate the procedure. Muscle relaxants such as succinylcholine can be used if there is no contraindication; however, one must be certain that the patient can be ventilated with a face mask before paralyzing the patient. For situations in which there is no ability to ventilate and the patient cannot be intubated, an emergency carothyroidotomy must be performed.

Setting the Ventilator

The ventilator settings are, in general, the same irrespective of the particular ventilating device chosen. Because most modern ventilators allow selection of controlled, assist-control, IMV, or IDV modes, this is the first setting made. One must then select the inspired concentration of oxygen (FIO_2), rate, tidal volume, inspiratory flow rate, and inspiratory-to-expiratory ratio (I:E ratio).

INSPIRED OXYGEN CONCENTRATION

The initial FIO_2 should be 1.0 in nearly all cases and especially after emergency intubation in the PACU. The use of 100% oxygen initially will provide some margin of safety for patients who are already hypoxemic. It will also give a rough idea of the magnitude of the intrapulmonary right-to-left shunt. This is especially helpful for patients with COPD who develop postoperative respiratory failure. A large alveolar-to-arterial oxygen tension difference in such a patient suggests new, acute lung disease such as pneumonia or pulmonary edema. A low or normal alveolar-to-arterial oxygen tension difference suggests that there may be little acute reversible lung disease.

TIDAL VOLUME

The tidal volume selected should be 10 to 15 mL/kg of body weight. This large volume will prevent the progressive atelectasis that may develop with mechanical ventilation delivered at tidal volumes similar to spontaneous ventilation (5 to 6 mL/kg). This is true both during anesthesia and for patients with respiratory failure.

RATE

If the assist-control mode is used, the sensitivity is set so the patient can easily get a breath and a backup control rate of approximately 8/minute is used. If IMV or controlled ventilation is used, the rate is selected based on an approximation of the patient's total minute ventilation (VE; VE = tidal volume × rate). A rough guide is that a normal healthy person requires a minute ventilation of approximately 100 mL/kg/minute to maintain normal alveolar ventilation (a normal $PaCO_2$). In the presence of a large dead space or a high carbon dioxide production rate, that estimate will have to be increased. I usually employ controlled ventilation initially to rest a fatigued patient and then proceed to use IMV at a slower rate after the first 12 hours of ventilatory assistance. Usually, a rate of 8 to 10 is then necessary to control ventilation completely. The level of alveolar ventilation obtained is easily checked by sampling the arterial blood and measuring the carbon dioxide ten-

sion. During general anesthesia with inhalation agents, the peripheral venous blood is arterialized and can be used to estimate the carbon dioxide tension if an arterial puncture cannot be performed.

INSPIRATORY FLOW RATE

The inspiratory flow rate is the mean rate of flow of the inspired gases. High flow rates (>40 L/minute) result in a short time for inspiration, a high peak inspiratory pressure, and a poor distribution of ventilation. The slower the flow rate, the better the distribution of ventilation. However, as the rate of flow slows, the time spent in inspiration increases. More time in inspiration results in an increase in the I:E ratio, which means that there will be a higher mean intrathoracic pressure and a greater reduction in cardiac output. Set the inspiratory flow rate as slow as possible to deliver an I:E ratio of 1:2. This is the ratio of time spent by the ventilator delivering gas to the lung compared to the time available for expiration. Increasing the I:E ratio to 1:1 or 2:1 results in a progressive reduction in cardiac output. Although we strive to get a ratio of 1:2, some patients will need more time for expiration. These are usually patients with COPD who, because of air trapping in diseased lungs, may need ratios as small as 1:3.

PRESSURE LIMIT

Finally, on most volume ventilators, the pressure limit must be set. The limit is set to approximately 10 cm H_2O above the patient's peak inspiratory pressure. If obstruction develops, volume will be delivered only until the pressure limit value is attained and further volume will not be delivered. This is a safety device to prevent a volume ventilator from delivering very high pressures.

The above limits constitute the basic settings needed to initiate ventilation. An arterial blood gas should be checked in most patients 15 minutes after the final settings. Additionally, a chest x-ray should be obtained immediately to assess the position of the tracheal tube with respect to the carina. The tip of the tube should lie 3 to 4 cm above the carina to prevent selective ventilation of one lung. In addition to the basic settings, others are available, such as the humidifier temperature, sighs, inspiratory hold, retard, and PEEP. The FIO_2 will need to be reduced according to the level of the arterial oxygenation. We usually aim to keep the arterial oxygen tension between 60 and 80 mm Hg.

HUMIDITY

Humidification of gases is important because the tracheal tube bypasses the normal humidification mechanism. Most humidifiers have uncalibrated scales for adjusting the heat of the inspired gas. This should be set to deliver a gas mixture that has a temperature of 32 to 36°C when measured at the patient's airway. Higher temperatures may burn the airway, and lower temperatures will result in the drying of secretions. The line temperature should be continuously monitored as close to the airway as possible.

SIGHS

Sighs were originally advocated to prevent the alveolar collapse that develops during controlled ventilation in the operating room when low (5 mL/kg) tidal volumes were used. There is no evidence that using sighs helps the lung in any way when large tidal volumes are used (10 to 15 mL/kg). Because sighs result in higher airway pressures, they also present the risk of barotrauma. For those reasons, we and many other centers no longer routinely use sighs.

INSPIRATORY HOLD

Inspiratory hold devices retain the gas in the lungs for up to 1 second after the end of the delivery of the tidal volume to produce a better distribution of ventilation. There are, however, no convincing studies demonstrating any beneficial effect. They do increase

mean intrathoracic pressure and can reduce cardiac output by prolonging the I:E ratio.

EXPIRATORY RETARD

Expiratory retard is a method of prolonging the patient's expiration by narrowing the orifice through which the expired gases travel. This allows for a more complete exit of gas from patients during mechanical ventilation. The airway pressure returns to atmospheric at the end of each breath in contrast to positive and end-expiratory pressure.

POSITIVE END-EXPIRATORY PRESSURE

PEEP is commonly employed in the management of patients with hypoxemia due to an increased intrapulmonary shunt. PEEP increases the arterial oxygen tension quickly by increasing the functional residual capacity. Collapsed lung is reinflated, thereby providing a better matching of ventilation and perfusion. PEEP's major mechanism of action is lung expansion and it does not decrease lung water. There are two major indications for PEEP: (*a*) to increase the arterial oxygen tension in patients with hypoxemia despite 100% oxygen; and (*b*) to increase the arterial oxygen tension so that the FIO_2 can be reduced. The second indication is by far the most common reason for using PEEP. There is a danger of oxygen toxicity if more than 50% oxygen is used for a prolonged period (>24 hours). PEEP should be used if a patient needs more than 50% oxygen to achieve an arterial oxygen tension of 65 mm Hg or greater. PEEP is used by some "prophylactically" during mechanical ventilation because it will nearly always improve the oxygen tension. There is no evidence, however, that the "prophylactic" use of PEEP alters the course of acute lung disease.

Although often helpful, PEEP has a number of complications related to its increase in intrathoracic pressure. PEEP is contraindicated for patients who have a pneumothorax. It should also be used with caution for patients with a bronchopleural fistula or for patients with other forms of preexisting barotrauma. One should exercise caution in applying PEEP to patients after recent lung surgery. PEEP will sometimes increase intracranial pressure in patients with intracranial hypertension. PEEP reduces cardiac output by decreasing venous return to the heart. It may also interfere with ventricular contraction by displacing the ventricular septum of the heart.

When applying PEEP, one should increase the PEEP by 3 to 5 cm H_2O increments until the desired goal is reached. For most patients, that goal is a level of PEEP at which the arterial oxygen tension is >65 mm Hg with an FIO_2 of 0.5 or less. One must be aware, however, that as the level of PEEP is increased, a progressive fall in cardiac output will result. It is important to remember that oxygen delivery to the tissues is a function of both the arterial oxygen content (CaO_2) and the cardiac output (O_2 transport = CaO_2 × CO). If PEEP improves oxygen content but reduces cardiac output, the net result could be decreased oxygen delivery. It is, therefore, important to monitor both arterial oxygenation and cardiac output when PEEP is applied. We routinely monitor cardiac output via a thermodilution pulmonary artery catheter in any patient who requires more than 8 cm of PEEP. Blood pressure is, unfortunately, an imprecise guide to cardiac output. If a patient does suffer a decrease in cardiac output before the desired level of arterial oxygenation is achieved, one can maintain cardiac output by increasing ventricular preload. Inotropic agents should be avoided if possible, because they will markedly increase myocardial work. Although survival of patients with respiratory failure treated with high levels of PEEP is similar to patients for whom more conventional PEEP levels are used, there is a higher incidence of barotrauma in patients with high levels of PEEP. Most patients can be managed easily with less than 20 cm H_2O of PEEP, and the need to employ higher levels of PEEP is quite uncommon.

ALARMS

Alarms have become an integral part of most ventilating devices. Alarms should be used for the following situations.

Oxygen

Both supply pressure and FIO_2 should be monitored.

Pressure

A low-pressure alarm activated by low pressure at the patient's airway will signify a circuit leak or failure of the machine to cycle. Usually, a delay of 20 to 30 seconds is set to allow temporary disconnection.

Volume

Expired-volume alarms are activated, on a breath-to-breath basis, if the desired exhaled volume is not achieved. This gives information about disconnection or circuit leak as well as a failure to cycle.

Pressure Limit

An alarm should provide notification that a patient's pressure limit is being exceeded and that the tidal volume is being lost. Most ventilator alarms should be impossible to shut off by nursing or medical staff. One of the greatest causes of alarm failure is that the device was turned off and never turned back on. Alarms should be able to be delayed by the operator but should not be able to completely stop their function. Many newer ventilators not only alarm for pressure and volume but will give a continuous digital display of expired volume, rate, I:E ratio, as well as peak inspiratory pressure.

When a tracheal tube is present, patients are unable to cough and clear pulmonary secretions. Some form of artificial coughing is necessary to prevent atelectasis. The simplest and most effective method is to provide chest physical therapy for all mechanically ventilated patients. This includes a change in position every 1 to 2 hours, as well as percussion, vibration, and postural drainage with airway suction at least three times daily. Chest therapy is especially important for patients who produce sputum. It is also very effective in the treatment of segmental, lobar, or lung collapse. Chest therapy is usually of little or no benefit to patients who are not intubated.

Weaning and Extubation

The process of weaning the patient from the ventilator should begin as soon as mechanical ventilation is begun. Care is taken to quickly reverse the etiology of the acute lung disorder. This may involve antibiotics for an infection, diuretics or dialysis for pulmonary edema, chest physical therapy or bronchoscopy for atelectasis or readjustment of steroids, and bronchodilators for the asthmatic.

WEANING WITH INTERMITTENT MANDATORY VENTILATION AND PRESSURE SUPPORT

IMV weaning is currently the most popular method and involves minimal additional equipment. The ventilator rate is slowly reduced, allowing the patient to increase spontaneous breathing between ventilator-delivered breaths. The patient's level of respiratory work, respiratory rate, and blood gases are followed after each reduction in rate. The patient is allowed to continue to wean if there is no large increase in respiratory distress and as long as there is no significant alteration in blood gases. If the patient does become noticeably fatigued or if the $PaCO_2$ rises or the PaO^2 falls, the patient's rate is returned to the prior level. This is continued daily until the patient can comfortably tolerate spontaneous ventilation. The more severe the acute lung disease, the longer the period of observation. In the long-term ventilator-dependent patient, weaning is performed in the daytime only to prevent sleep deprivation and severe fatigue. We routinely return patients to a rate of 6 to 8 overnight to allow natural rest.

This form of weaning is simple, well tolerated by patients, and easy to employ. Although it has many seemingly apparent benefits, there is, to date, no scientific evidence to show that IMV weaning alters the outcome of patients treated for respiratory failure. IMV weaning is well suited for use in both postsurgical patients and medical patients. IMV weaning may, however, delay the extubation process in prophylactically ventilated patients who are awake, are alert, and have good lung mechanics. Those types of patients are probably better off with prompt T-tube or continuous positive airway pressure (CPAP) weaning.

The relatively recent introduction of pressure support ventilation has added a new but unproven aspect to ventilator weaning. When pressure support is used, the clinician must be aware that higher levels of pressure support provide significant augmentation to the patient's tidal volume and so, after the IMV rate has been weaned down, it is very important to wean the level of pressure support down to 5 cm of water before assuming that the patient is ready for extubation.

T-TUBE WEANING

T-tube weaning consists of abruptly stopping the ventilator and allowing the patient to breathe through a T-tube with humidified oxygen. T-tube weaning requires more preweaning assessment and closer observation during weaning. Before a T-tube trial a vital capacity greater than 10 mL/kg and a maximum inspiratory pressure greater than –20 cm H_2O. The patient should be hemodynamically stable and have a normal acid-base status. The patient is informed of the procedure, placed in the sitting position, and connected to the T-tube. Vital signs are monitored closely during the first 30 minutes and the blood gases are checked. Patients doing well after 30 minutes without fatigue, tachycardia, hypoxemia, or carbon dioxide retention can be extubated and administered oxygen by face mask. Patients who develop circulatory instability, arrhythmias, carbon dioxide retention, or hypoxemia should be returned to mechanical ventilation. With this type of weaning, there is usually a slight rise in $PaCO_2$, even in patients who have been successfully weaned. There is also a variable fall in oxygen tension in most patients. The fall in oxygen tension occurs because of alveolar collapse. This fall in PaO_2 can be overcome usually by increasing the FIO_2 during weaning by 10 to 20% of what was required during ventilation (52).

In a recent study examining the various weaning modalities available in the 1990s, it was concluded that T-tube weaning resulted in better patient outcome as demonstrated by more rapid weaning. A once-a-day trial of spontaneous breathing resulted in extubation three times more quickly than IMV and twice as fast as pressure support (53). The problem is that T-tube weaning is more labor intensive in the ICU because it ties up one nurse with the patient being weaned. In the PACU, however, T-tube or CPAP weaning is probably the most efficacious and allows for a prompt assessment of the patient's ability to breathe spontaneously.

CONTINUOUS POSITIVE AIRWAY PRESSURE

CPAP has been advocated as an alternative to T-tube weaning. It is especially helpful for patients who develop a profound fall in oxygen tension during T-tube weaning. CPAP keeps the lung expanded during weaning by increasing the functional residual capacity in the same way that PEEP helps during controlled, assisted, or IMV ventilation. Although commonly used, there is no evidence that CPAP weaning applied to everyone is clearly beneficial. It is helpful, however, for patients with unstable airways, low lung volumes, and a tendency for alveolar collapse.

EXTUBATION

Tracheal extubation is considered when the patient tolerates 30 to 60 minutes of spontaneous breathing without tachypnea, respiratory distress, hypercapnia, or hypoxemia. This is true whether the patient has been on IMV, T

tube, or receiving CPAP. In addition to being able to exchange gas, the patient must also demonstrate the ability to protect and clear the airway. The patient should be awake and able to follow simple commands. There should be a good gag reflex and cough reflex. The patient should be able to cough spontaneously and clear secretions. If all of these factors are acceptable, the trachea is extubated and humidified oxygen is delivered by a face mask. Nasal prongs deliver dry gas and a low FIO_2 and are, therefore, rarely useful in caring for critically ill patients. Blood gases should be examined after extubation and periodically to ensure that adequate blood gas exchange continues.

OTHER RESPIRATORY CARE MODALITIES

The use of CPAP by an external mask (mask or nasal CPAP) is increasing for treatment of patients with severe hypoxemia who have adequate carbon dioxide elimination (54). Certainly, patients have avoided tracheal intubation because of the use of mask or nasal CPAP. However, many patients who have a trial of mask or nasal CPAP fail that trial and need tracheal intubation and mechanical ventilation. Good candidates for mask or nasal CPAP are patients with severe hypoxemia requiring more than 80% oxygen to attain a PaO_2 above 60 mm Hg. They must have a normal or low $PaCO_2$ and must not have severe respiratory distress. They must be awake and alert. Mask or nasal CPAP is most useful when the cause of hypoxemia can be quickly corrected, such as cardiogenic pulmonary edema, because the mask becomes very uncomfortable for the patient, even after several hours of use. Newer mask designs have improved on this problem, but they have not eliminated it.

Other oxygen delivery systems in the PACU are face masks and nasal prongs. Nasal prongs are very effective in reversing the hypoxemia seen in most PACU patients. Nasal prongs do not require the patient to be a nose breather, because they work by filling the nasopharyngeal space with oxygen. A flow rate of greater than 5 L per minute does not increase the inspired concentration of oxygen, which rarely exceeds 35% when nasal prongs are used. If a higher concentration of oxygen is needed, a face mask can be employed. The maximal inspired concentration can be reached by using a tight-fitting mask with a reservoir. Such systems provide 80 to 90% inspired oxygen.

SPECIAL CONSIDERATIONS AFTER THORACIC SURGERY

After major lung resections, several surgical complications must be watched for in the PACU. Bronchial disruption can eventually lead to a bronchopleural fistula; however, immediate bronchial disruption may put the patient at risk for pneumothorax and respiratory failure if the chest tube does not function. Postoperative hemorrhage can lead to shock and usually requires reoperation. Reexpansion pulmonary edema can occur, even after the short period during which the lung is collapsed for thoracic surgery. Respiratory failure can certainly present in the PACU and careful respiratory monitoring of these patients is required. Other less frequent complications are cardiac herniation, pulmonary torsion, right heart failure, and neural injuries to the phrenic and recurrent laryngeal nerves (55).

After thoracic surgery, the major goal is to avoid positive-pressure ventilation if at all possible. Positive-pressure ventilation can lead to the development of a bronchopleural fistula in patients who have had a lung resection and should therefore be avoided unless clearly indicated by the patient's condition.

Pain is a serious problem for these patients because a lateral thoracotomy is one of the most painful procedures. Narcotics can suppress ventilation and lead to the need for postoperative ventilation. This is the reason why many feel that epidural narcotics are indicated for thoracotomy patients. The site of the epidural is controversial, however; the lumbar route is safer than the thoracic route, but

slightly higher doses of narcotics are needed (56).

All of these patients require careful monitoring of their respiratory function using the modalities previously described.

REFERENCES

1. Hedley-Whyte J, Burgess GE, Feeley TW, et al. Applied physiology of respiratory care. Boston: Little Brown & Co., 1976.
2. Yelderman M, New W. Evaluation of pulse oximetry. Anesthesiology 1983;59:349–352.
3. Tyler IC, Tantisira B, Winter PM, et al. Continuous monitoring of arterial oxygen saturation with pulse oximetry during transfer to the recovery room. Anesth Analg 1985;64:1108–1112.
4. Soliman IE, Patel RI, Ehronpreis MB, et al. Recovery scores do not correlate with post operative hypoxemia in children. Anesth Analg 1988;67:53–56.
5. Morris RW, Buchmann A, Warren DL, et al. The prevalence of hypoxemia during recovery from anesthesia. J Clin Monit 1988;4:16–20.
6. Shapiro BA, Cane RD. Blood gas monitoring: yesterday, today, and tomorrow. Crit Care Med 1989;17:573–580.
7. Eberhard P, Mindt W, Schafer R. Cutaneous blood gas monitoring in the adult. Crit Care Med 1981;9:702–705.
8. Zehnder JL, Sladen RL. Colorimetric end-tidal carbon dioxide monitoring for tracheal intubation. Anesth Analg 1990;70:1991–1994.
9. Yamanaka MK, Sue DY. Comparison of arterial-end-tidal P difference and deadspace/tidal volume ratio in respiratory failure. Chest 1987;92:832–835.
10. Tobin MJ. Respiratory monitoring in the intensive care unit. Am Rev Respir Dis 1988;138:1625–1642.
11. Hines R, Barash PG, Watrous G, et al. Complications occurring in the postanesthesia care unit: a survey. Anesth Analg 1992;74:503–509.
12. Handlin DS, Baker T. The effects of smoking on postoperative recovery. Am J Med 1992;93:32S–37S.
13. Becker LD, Paulson BA, Miller RD, et al. Biphasic respiratory depression after fentanyl-droperidol or fentanyl alone used to supplement nitrous oxide anesthesia. Anesthesiology 1976;44:291–296.
14. Longnecker DE, Grazis PA, Eggers GWN. Naloxone for antagonism of morphine induced respiratory depression. Anesth Analg 1973;52:447–453.
15. Ali J, Weisel RD, Layug AB, et al. Consequences of postoperative alterations in respiratory mechanics. Am J Surg 1974;128:376–382.
16. Ford GT, Whitelaw WA, Rosenal TW, et al. Diaphragm function after upper abdominal surgery in humans. Am Rev Respir Dis 1983;127:431–436.
17. Miller RD, Cullen DJ. Renal failure and postoperative respiratory failure: recurarization? Br J Anaesth 1976;48:253–256.
18. Fogdall RP, Miller RD. Prolongation of pancuronium-induced neuromuscular blockade by clindamycin. Anesthesiology 1974;41:407–408.
19. Miller RD. Antagonism of neuromuscular blockade. Anesthesiology 1976;44:318–329.

20. Cullen DJ, Cullen BL. Postanesthetic complications. Surg Clin North Am 1975;55:987–998.
21. Morikawa S, Safer P, De Carlo J. Influence of head-jaw position on upper airway patency. Anesthesiology 1961;22:265–270.
22. Ruben HM, Elam JO, Ruben AM, et al. Investigation of upper airway problems in resuscitation. Anesthesiology 1961;22:271–279.
23. Komorn RM, Smith CP, Irwin JR. Acute laryngeal injury with short-term endotracheal anesthesia. Laryngoscope 1973;82:683–690.
24. Jaffe BF. Postoperative hoarseness. Am J Surg 1972;123:432–437.
25. Parfrey PS, Harte PI, Quinlan JP. Pulmonary function in the early postoperative period. Br J Surg 1977;64:384–389.
26. Nunn JF, Payne JP. Hypoxia after general anesthesia. Lancet 1962;2:631–632.
27. Katamur AH, Sawa T, Ikezono E. Postoperative hypoxemia: the contribution of age to the mal-distribution of ventilation. Anesthesiology 1972;36:244–252.
28. Moller JT, Wittrup M, Johansen SH. Hypoxemia in the postanesthesia care unit: an observer study. Anesthesiology 1990;73:890–895.
29. Marshall BE, Wyche MQ. Hypoxemia during and after anesthesia. Anesthesiology 1972;37:178–209.
30. Bay I, Nunn JF, Prys-Roberts C. Factors influencing arterial PO_2 during recovery from anesthesia. Br J Anaesth 1968;40:398–407.
31. Philbin DM, Sullivan SF, Bowman FOR, et al. Postoperative hypoxemia: contribution of cardiac output. Anesthesiology 1970;32:136–142.
32. Feeley TW, Hedley-Whyte J. Bulk oxygen and nitrous oxide delivery system. Anesthesiology 1976;44:301–305.
33. Cullen DJ, Caldera DL. The incidence of ventilator-induced pulmonary barotrauma in critically ill patients. Anesthesiology 1979;50:185–190.
34. Hamilton WK. Atelectasis, pneumothorax, and aspiration as postoperative complications. Anesthesiology 1961;22:708–722.
35. Don HF, Wahba WM, Craig DB. Airway closure, gas trapping, and the functional residual capacity during anesthesia. Anesthesiology 1972;36:533–539.
36. Alexander JI, Horton PA, Miller WT, et al. The effect of upper abdominal surgery on the relationship of airway closing point to end-tidal position. Clin Sci 1972;43:137–141.
37. Rehder K, Marsh HM, Rodarte JR, et al. Airway closure. Anesthesiology 1977;47:40–52.
38. Robin ED, Cross CE, Zelis R. Pulmonary edema (part 1). N Engl J Med 1973;288:239–246.
39. Robin ED, Cross CE, Zelis R. Pulmonary edema (part 2). N Engl J Med 1973;288:292–304.
40. Cooperman LH, Price HR. Pulmonary edema in the operative and postoperative period: review of 40 cases. Ann Surg 1970;172:833–891.
41. Weissman C, Damask MC, Yang J. Noncardiogenic pulmonary edema following laryngeal obstruction. Anesthesiology 1984;60:163–165.
42. Jackson FN, Rowland V, Corssen G. Laryngospasm induced pulmonary edema. Chest 1980;78:819–821.
43. Crandall ED, Staub NC, Goldberg HS, et al. Recent developments in pulmonary edema. Ann Intern Med 1983;99:808–822.
44. Shapiro JM, Mihm FG, Trudell JR, et al. Leukotriene D_4 increases extravascular lung water in the dog. Circ Shock 1987;21:121–128.
45. Saul GM, Feeley TW, Mihm FG. Effect of graded administration of PEEP on lung water in noncardiogenic pulmonary edema. Crit Care Med 1982;10:667–669.
46. Mihm FG, Feeley TW, Rosenthal MH, et al. Measurement of extravascular lung water in dogs using the thermal-green dye indicator dilution method. Anesthesiology 1982;57:116–122.
47. Lewis FR, Elings VB, Hill SL, et al. The measurement of extravascular lung water by thermal-green dye indicator dilution. Ann N Y Acad Sci 1982;384:394–410.
48. Demling RH, Lalonde C. Oxygen consumption is increased in the postanesthesia period after burn excision. J Burn Care Rehabil 1989;10:381–387.
49. Tremper KK, Barker SJ. Pulse oximetry. Anesthesiology 1989;70:98–108.
50. Pontoppidan H, Laver MB, Geffin B. Acute respiratory failure in the surgical patient. Adv Surg 1970;4:163–254.
51. Mathew JP, Rosenbaum SE, O'Connor T, et al. Emergency tracheal intubation in the postanesthesia care unit: physician error or patient disease? Anesth Analg 1990;71:691–697.
52. Feeley TW, Hedley-Whyte J. Weaning from controlled ventilation and supplemental oxygen. N Engl J Med 1975;292:903–906.
53. Esteban A, Frutos F, Tobin M, et al. A comparison of four methods of weaning patients from mechanical ventilation. N Engl J Med 1995;332:345–350.
54. Smith RA, Kirby RR, Gooding JM, et al. Continuous positive airway pressure (CPAP) by face mask. Crit Care Med 1980;8:483–485.
55. Benumoff JL, Alfrey DD. Anesthesia for thoracic surgery. In: Miller RD, ed. Anesthesia. 4th ed. New York: Churchill-Livingstone, 1994;1717–1719.
56. Steidl LJ, Fromme GA, Danielson DR. Lumbar versus thoracic epidural morphine for post-thoracotomy pain. Anesth Analg 1985;64:454–455.

9

THE RENAL SYSTEM

Karen S. Sibert, Robert N. Sladen

No matter how successful the surgical procedure, renal dysfunction in the perioperative period may pose a perilous threat to the final outcome. Acute renal failure, defined as the abrupt reduction in renal function that results in a rise in blood levels of nitrogenous waste products, continues to carry a mortality risk of up to 75%, although treatment with dialysis has been available for more than 30 years (1–5). It has been estimated that perioperative renal failure accounts for up to 50% of all patients who require acute dialysis (6). Failure to manage hemodynamic parameters or oxygen delivery in the postanesthesia care unit (PACU) may jeopardize renal perfusion, especially for high-risk patients with atherosclerotic disease or diabetes mellitus. On the other hand, careful perioperative management may help ensure a successful surgical outcome, even for patients with chronic renal failure who, in past years, would not have been considered candidates for major surgery.

RENAL PROTECTIVE MECHANISMS

The kidney receives approximately 20% of the cardiac output, which is a larger blood volume than it needs to satisfy its oxygen requirements. Thus, the normal renal venous oxygen saturation is higher than the total body mixed venous oxygen saturation, and the arterial-venous oxygen difference across the renal circulation is only 1 to 2 vol.% compared with 4 to 5 vol.% in most other organs. This high-flow state confers an important measure of protection to the kidney and helps ensure adequate renal perfusion in the face of external insult. However, the benefit of abundant oxygenation is not shared equally by all portions of the kidney. The nephrons that occupy the outer and middle renal cortex are far more numerous, have short loops of Henle, and receive about 85% of the renal blood flow (RBF). In contrast, the nephrons that occupy the juxtamedullary renal cortex receive only about 10% of the RBF and have larger glomeruli and long loops of Henle, which penetrate deeply into the inner medulla. A steep gradient of oxygen exists between the renal cortex and medulla, because of the countercurrent exchange of oxygen within the inner medulla (Fig. 9–1). Even under circumstances of normal renal blood flow, medullary cells exist with a tissue PO_2 as low as 8 to 10 mm Hg and are therefore predisposed to anoxic injury. Severe hypoxia may develop in the medulla despite apparently normal RBF (7). In particular, the tubular cells of the medullary thick ascending limbs seem to be especially vulnerable to ischemic injury because of their high rate of metabolism and their special location with limited oxygen supply (8), giving rise to the clinical lesion known as acute tubular necrosis (ATN).

Renal autoregulation is a second protective mechanism for the kidney that is familiar to most anesthesiologists because of the classic studies undertaken in dogs by Shipley and Study in 1951 (9). Their work demonstrated that the kidney maintains a constant renal blood flow and glomerular filtration rate (GFR) through mean arterial pressure rates of

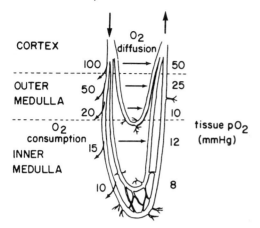

Fig. 9–1. Countercurrent exchange of oxygen within the inner medulla by the vasa recta. The high oxygen consumption of the inner medulla keeps medullary PO_2 low and is almost undisturbed by high total renal blood flow. (From Byrick RJ, Rose DK. Pathophysiology and prevention of acute renal failure: the role of the anaesthetist. Can J Anaesth 1990;37:457–467, reproduced with permission from the Canadian Anaesthetist Society.)

80 to 180 mm Hg (Fig. 9–2), although the precise mechanism for renal autoregulation has yet to be defined. The modification of renal vascular resistance seems to be mediated by variations in the degree of constriction and dilation of the preglomerular afferent arteriole. As mean arterial pressure (MAP) decreases, the resistance within the afferent arteriole decreases and RBF is maintained. One likely mechanism responsible for this phenomenon is a myogenic response that causes the arterioles to constrict in response to increased MAP and dilate in response to hypotension. There may also be a feedback mechanism arising from the juxtaglomerular apparatus, in which increased MAP enhances delivery of sodium chloride to the cells of the macula densa, which induces afferent arteriolar constriction with consequent declines in RBF and GFR. The net effect of autoregulation, regardless of the underlying mechanisms, is to enable the kidney to maintain solute and volume regulation even in the face of wide fluctuations of arterial blood pressure. However, the protective effect of autoregulation is lost under con-

ditions of severe stress to the organism and is affected adversely also by chronic conditions including atherosclerotic vascular disease and hypertension, which are believed to raise the lower limit of MAP under which RBF and GFR will remain steady (7).

VASOACTIVE REGULATION OF RENAL FUNCTION

Sympathetic and Adrenergic Effects

When a decrease in arterial blood pressure is sensed by baroreceptors in the aortic arch, carotid sinus, and afferent arterioles, impulses are transmitted via the vagus nerve to the mediating centers in the hypothalamus, which increase adrenergic nerve activity. Circulating epinephrine increases and norepinephrine is released from the plexus of autonomic nerve fibers in the renal cortex. The effects of these substances on the α-adrenergic receptor are directly dose-related. Mild α-adrenergic stimulation preferentially causes the efferent arteriole to constrict, which will preserve filtration fraction and GFR in the event of decreased

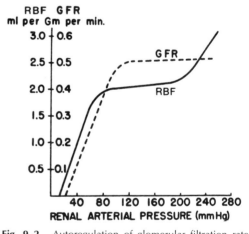

Fig. 9–2. Autoregulation of glomerular filtration rate (GFR) and renal blood flow (RBF), based on the original work of Shipley and Study (9). GFR and RBF remain constant between renal arterial pressures of 80 and 180 mm Hg. (With permission from Pitts RF. Physiology of the kidney and body fluids, 3rd ed. St. Louis, MO: Mosby-Year Book, 1974;168.)

RBF. In contrast, severe α-adrenergic stimulation causes constriction of the afferent arteriole, which results in the decline of RBF and GFR. Further, adrenergic stimulation releases renin from the juxtaglomerular apparatus and activates the renin-angiotensin system (see below). Adrenergic stimulation and vasoconstriction may be blocked either by direct-acting α-adrenergic blockers such as prazosin and phentolamine or by angiotensin-converting enzyme (ACE) inhibitors such as captopril and enalapril.

Exogenous adrenergic medications affect the kidney just as the endogenous pressors do, depending on the dose and the degree of agonist activity. Drugs with predominantly α-adrenergic effects, such as norepinephrine, epinephrine, phenylephrine, and dopamine at ≥10 μg/kg/minute, exacerbate the vasoconstriction of the afferent arteriole in response to hypotension, with the possibility of deleterious effects on RBF and GFR. Dobutamine and isoproterenol, with predominant β activity, cause increases in cardiac output that may augment RBF. The dopaminergic agonists, including dopamine at ≤3 μg/kg/minute, dopexamine, and fenoldopam, selectively increase RBF and may act to oppose sympathetically mediated renal vasoconstriction (10). The dopaminergic agonists will be discussed separately below.

Controversy has existed for many years among clinicians regarding whether the increase in urine output that typically follows dopamine infusion is caused by the improved cardiac output or the specific renal effects of dopamine. Investigations in dogs demonstrated that dopamine causes direct vasodilation in the renal vascular bed by action on specific dopaminergic receptors, and in humans, dopamine was shown to produce sodium diuresis in patients with congestive heart failure (11). It has been difficult, however, to determine whether the effects of dopamine on the kidney are caused solely by renal dopaminergic activity or hemodynamic alterations initiated by dopamine's α and β stimulation. This issue was addressed in a 1984 study by Hilberman et al. (12), who infused either dopamine or dobutamine into patients undergoing cardiac operation. With cardiac output maintained at the same level in both groups, dopamine at 5 μg/kg/minute produced significantly greater diuresis, natriuresis, and kaliuresis (12). The marked diuretic effect also suggested a direct tubular action of dopamine because RBF was equally increased by both drugs. This study reinforced the widespread clinical practice of infusing dopamine in the range of 1 to 3 μg/kg/minute as part of the management protocol for oliguria or prophylaxis against acute tubular necrosis.

The Renin-Angiotensin System

Any decrease in renal artery perfusion pressure triggers baroreceptor responses in the afferent arterioles, which contain β-receptors in addition to specialized fenestrated endothelial cells that produce renin. Thus, renin secretion is stimulated either by actual hypovolemia (diuresis, hemorrhage, acute sodium loss) or by clinical conditions that simulate hypovolemia, including congestive heart failure, positive pressure ventilation, sepsis, and end-stage cirrhosis with ascites. Renin, in turn, is the rate-limiting enzyme that acts on angiotensinogen, a large glycoprotein that is released by the liver into the general circulation and cleaves it to produce angiotensin I. Angiotensin-converting enzyme (ACE) present in the kidney and lung further modifies angiotensin I to form angiotensin II, which is a potent vasoconstrictor. Angiotensin II in turn inhibits renin secretion by a negative feedback mechanism.

Angiotensin II, even in small amounts, is capable of provoking renal cortical vasoconstriction, but initially, this occurs predominantly at the level of the efferent arterioles. Thus, this action is directly comparable to small amounts of α-adrenergic stimulation because it supports the maintenance of glomerular filtration pressure in the face of mild to moderate hypotension and decline in RBF. The importance of this beneficial effect of angiotensin II became apparent clinically during the early clinical experience with the ACE inhibitor captopril. Although it was believed initially that captopril would be very useful in the treatment of renal artery stenosis and renovascular hypertension by decreasing the activity of the renin-angiotensin system, what actually occurred was that a number of these patients experienced deterioration in renal function leading in some cases to complete renal failure (13, 14). Presumably the unopposed dilation of the efferent arteriole in these patients served to decrease glomerular filtration rather than to improve overall renal perfusion. In contrast, patients with conditions such as congestive heart failure and extracellular-fluid volume depletion develop an excessively high local level of angiotensin II, which is believed to cause profound afferent as well as efferent arteriolar constriction and cause a fall in the glomerular plasma flow rate. Under these circumstances, blockade of angiotensin II actions may be expected to dilate the constricted afferent arterioles, increasing intraglomerular capillary pressure and augmenting GFR (15). The benefit experienced by patients with congestive heart failure who begin treatment with ACE inhibitors is believed to be due to two mechanisms: the improvement in cardiac performance resulting from afterload reduction and the renal effect of dilating the afferent arterioles and improving glomerular blood flow.

Antidiuretic Hormone

Antidiuretic hormone (ADH) is synonymous with the neuropeptide 8-arginine-vasopressin (AVP), which is synthesized in the anterior hypothalamus and stored in granules in the posterior pituitary gland. Its overall action, through activation of cyclic adenosine monophosphate (cAMP), is to produce a decreased flow of concentrated urine (16). Tubular conservation of water in the presence of ADH secretion leads to increased urine osmolality, decreased plasma osmolality, and negative free water clearance without significant alteration in solute excretion.

The sensation of thirst and the secretion of ADH are stimulated by small increases in osmolality. Osmoreceptors in the hypothalamus are exquisitely sensitive to any deviation and can sense alterations in serum osmolality of as little as 1% from normal. The threshold for ADH secretion is 280 to 290 mOsm/kg, and even mild dehydration will lead rapidly to antidiuresis. Of major importance to the PACU setting is the fact that surgical stress is a major stimulus to ADH secretion, and this stress response lasts at least 2 to 3 days after the surgical procedure. ADH secretion is also stimulated by stretch receptors in the left atrium and pulmonary veins, which respond to decreases in intravascular volume, and by aortic and carotid baroreceptors, which react to any drop in arterial blood pressure. The hypovolemia-induced secretion of ADH takes precedence over osmolar responses and, in turn, will be overridden by the onset of hypotension. ADH secretion inappropriate to osmolar requirements thus occurs as a common perioperative problem, in which the clinical complication of hypotension may be addressed by administration of hypotonic solutions, which then exacerbate the problem by decreasing serum osmolality. The resulting inevitable ADH secretion will then produce further fluid retention, hypo-osmolality, and hyponatremia (17).

Prostaglandins

Factors such as ischemia and hypotension, which mediate stress responses, also simultaneously activate prostaglandins to defend the kidney against their actions. Vasodilator prostaglandins that are synthesized in the kidney are important not so much to sustain normal renal function as to preserve it during the ischemic insults of acute trauma and surgery. These vasodilator renal prostaglandins (PGD_2, PGE_2, and PGI_2 or prostacyclin) oppose the actions of norepinephrine and angiotensin II, antagonize ADH, and block distal tubule sodium reabsorption. They may play a critical role in decreasing the vasoconstrictor activity of angiotensin II on the afferent arteriole and glomerular mesangial cells (18). The production of these prostaglandins promotes renal vasodilation, maintains intrarenal hemodynamics, and enhances sodium and water excretion. The exogenous infusion of synthetic prostaglandins prevents the induction of acute renal failure by ischemia in animal models and may mediate the renal vasodilator response to mannitol during hypoperfusion states (19, 20).

Prostaglandins are synthesized in the kidney by the action of a key enzyme, phospholipase A_2, which is stimulated by ischemia, norepinephrine, and angiotensin II. This enzyme cleaves arachidonic acid, which in turn is acted upon by cyclo-oxygenase and converted to the precursors of the vasodilator prostaglandins. The action of cyclo-oxygenase is reversibly inhibited for 8 to 24 hours by nonsteroidal anti-inflammatory drugs (NSAIDs) such as indomethacin, ibuprofen, and ketorolac and it is irreversibly acetylated by a single dose of aspirin. In platelets, the ability to resynthesize cyclo-oxygenase is lost for the lifetime of the cells (7 to 10 days), but the kidney is able to restart cyclo-oxygenase production within 24 to 48 hours.

The beneficial effect of prostaglandins has been demonstrated superbly by the fact that NSAIDs cause nephrotoxicity in ischemic kidneys but not in normal ones. During conditions of stress to the organism, in which afferent arteriolar vasoconstriction may be provoked by high angiotensin II levels, NSAIDs or aspirin compromise prostaglandin-dependent renal vasodilation, resulting in decreased RBF and GFR and increased vascular resistance. Even in the presence of diuretic therapy, sodium excretion is diminished and hyperkalemia may ensue. The adverse effects of NSAIDs, including aspirin, have been demonstrated in animal models of hemorrhage, endotoxemia, and low cardiac output. It is now well recognized clinically that patients with mild underlying renal dysfunction, especially with additional risk factors such as congestive heart failure, ascites, or systemic lupus erythematosis, are susceptible to worsening renal function if therapy with NSAIDs is initiated (21). This raises the question of whether the prevalent practice today of using ketorolac and other NSAIDs for the treatment of mild postoperative pain in the PACU setting should be tempered, at least in certain patient groups. Further long-term follow-up will be required to elucidate whether brief therapy with NSAIDs poses any serious threat to renal function in the perioperative period.

EFFECTS OF ANESTHESIA ON RENAL FUNCTION

The Halogenated Vapors

Because halothane has the longest history of clinical use in anesthesiology, it is not surprising that more information is available about it than about enflurane or isoflurane. There is no evidence for any fluoride-related nephrotoxic effect of halothane, because it is not metabolized to inorganic fluoride under the usual conditions of clinical anesthesia (22). The studies in the literature are not in complete agreement with one another regarding the effect of halothane on RBF, because of differences in animal models and in whether para-amino-hippurate (PAH) clearance or flow-probe techniques were used to measure RBF. However, it seems that halothane causes, at most, only a mild decrease in RBF at anesthetic depths of 1 to 1.5 MAC, primarily owing to the anticipated depression of myocardial function and fall in systemic blood pressure (23). GFR undergoes a more significant change; halothane uniformly decreases GFR and urine output because of altered hydrostatic gradients in the peritubular capillaries in the setting of lowered blood pressure. Studies in isolated preparations and intact animals demonstrate that halothane does not alter renal autoregulation, lending support to the conclusion that the primary effect of halothane is on systemic hemodynamics rather than specifically on the kidney (24).

Enflurane causes a decrease in GFR and urine output again because of its effects on systemic arterial pressure and renal vascular resistance but, like halothane, shows no specific deleterious effect on renal blood flow. Concern has been raised in the past over a potential nephrotoxic effect of enflurane because it is defluorinated approximately one-third as much as methoxyflurane. Mazze et al. reported that a group of patients with mild preoperative renal insufficiency (preoperative serum creatinine 1.5 to 3.0 mg/dL) showed no decline in postoperative renal function regardless of whether enflurane or halothane was used as the primary inhaled anesthetic (25). The patients who received enflurane showed a peak rise in serum fluoride levels to $19.0 \pm 3.0 \mu M$ at 4 hours after surgery, significantly less than the levels of 80 μM and higher, which were associated with overt clinical nephrotoxicity with methoxyflurane (22).

Because isoflurane causes less effect on myocardial stroke volume than halothane or enflurane, it is logical that it minimally alters renal blood flow at levels of anesthesia up to 1 MAC (26, 27). As the level of anesthesia with isoflurane is deepened, the decrease in systemic blood pressure comes to exceed the decrease in renal vascular resistance and GFR and urine output fall. Isoflurane, although it is also a fluorinated ether, is biotransformed to inorganic fluoride to a much lesser extent than either methoxyflurane or enflurane, and there is no evidence for any direct nephrotoxic effect of this vapor.

Sevoflurane is a new halogenated agent that undergoes hepatic biotransformation to fluoride ion. However, although serum fluoride levels occasionally exceed those considered to be nephrotoxic with methoxyflurane (50 $\mu M/L$), in studies to date, sevoflurane-induced nephrotoxicity has not been encountered. Recently, Kharasch et al. found that both methoxyflurane and sevoflurane undergo in situ metabolism in the kidney but that methoxyflurane is metabolized to fluoride to a much greater extent than sevoflurane (27a). They postulated that this may account for the lack of sevoflurane nephrotoxicity despite occasionally elevated serum fluoride levels.

Intravenous Anesthetic Medications

Priano compared alterations in renal hemodynamics by thiopental, diazepam, and ketamine in dogs (28). Thiopental and diazepam both decrease GFR and urine output; renal blood flow seems to remain unchanged with thiopental (despite decreases in systemic vascular resistance, arterial pressure, and cardiac output) because of the concomitant decrease in renal vascular resistance. Diazepam decreases renal blood flow to a mild degree, about 10 to 15% from control. Ketamine also minimally affects renal blood flow and may even increase it in some circumstances, despite significantly increased renal vascular resistance. It seems possible that this finding could indicate a breakthrough, or a leftward shift, of the autoregulation curve in the presence of ketamine. The increase in systolic blood pressure in adults receiving clinical doses of ketamine is usually 20 to 40 mm Hg, which normally would not exceed the range of autoregulatory MAP (80 to 180 mm Hg) and therefore should not lead to increased renal blood flow if autoregulation is unchanged. However, in the setting of hemorrhagic hypovolemia in dogs, ketamine administration did not improve renal blood flow (29) and it is known that ketamine decreases urine flow rate, probably through adrenergic activation. Because greater increases in arterial lactate concentrations occur in animals anesthetized with ketamine than in animals with lower arterial pressure anesthetized with a volatile anesthetic (30), it may be that ketamine maintains blood pressure at the expense of tissue perfusion, which would be expected eventually to produce deleterious effects on the kidney.

Etomidate, a nonbarbiturate imidazole compound, has been used widely in anesthesiology over the past decade because its administration evokes minimal changes in heart rate, stroke volume, or cardiac output. It is now the agent of choice in the hands of many clinicians for the patient who is unstable hemodynamically because of either hypovolemia or cardiovascular disease, although MAP may decrease up to 15% because of reduction in systemic vascular resistance (SVR). There has been no report of renal function abnormality, as measured by serum creatinine rise, after administration of etomidate (31). The drug is known to cause adrenocortical suppression by inhibiting the enzymatic conversion of cholesterol to cortisol in a dose-dependent manner. This effect was first reported in intensive care unit (ICU) patients who received prolonged infusions of etomidate (32), and it was found subsequently that this enzyme inhibition lasts 4 to 8 hours after a single anesthetic induction dose (33). Although it might be supposed that the suppression of "stress" responses to surgery might benefit the kidney by reducing adrenergic stimuli for reflex vasoconstriction, the plasma concentrations of epinephrine and norepinephrine did not differ in healthy surgical patients who received etomidate compared with a group receiving thiopental (34). Because etomidate lacks analgesic effect and does not blunt the hemodynamic responses of tachycardia and hypertension after direct laryngoscopy and intubation, there is no reason to assume that the renal function of patients who receive etomidate is protected from adrenergic vasoconstriction in response to surgical and anesthetic stress.

Propofol, a substituted isopropylphenol compound, is chemically unrelated to barbiturates, benzodiazepines, or other intravenous anesthetic agents and has been in widespread use in the United States only since 1989. Like thiopental, propofol produces a dose-dependent reduction in systemic blood pressure because of a reduction in SVR. However, whereas thiopental produces a reflex tachycardia that may temper its hypotensive effect, propofol tends to produce a stable or slightly slower heart rate and thus seems to cause a greater reduction in blood pressure than thiopental or other intravenous induction agents (35). Controversy exists in the literature as to whether propofol affects myocardial contrac-

tility directly or produces its hypotensive effect by altering arterial compliance and sympathetic tone. Azari and Cork compared the direct myocardial effects of thiopental and propofol in an isolated guinea pig left atrial preparation and concluded that thiopental is a more potent myocardial depressant than propofol (36). As with etomidate, propofol has not been shown to affect renal function adversely as reflected by measurement of creatinine concentration (31). However, the clinical profile of propofol suggests that it should be used with caution in the setting of hypovolemia, preexisting renal insufficiency, or compromised left ventricular function, so that exaggerated decreases in arterial pressure do not lead to prolonged reduction in renal blood flow and GFR.

Of the pure narcotic agonists, morphine has been used longest clinically although it is seldom used today as a primary anesthetic technique. Morphine has been shown in one study to significantly increase renal blood flow (37) but clinically is associated with decreased urine output because of its stimulation of ADH secretion. High-dose opioid techniques today most commonly employ fentanyl or sufentanil, which do not depress myocardial contractility and have minimal effect on RBF and GFR. Fentanyl and sufentanil are more effective in suppressing the release of catecholamines, angiotensin II, aldosterone, and ADH during surgery than are volatile agents, although during cardiopulmonary bypass both ADH and catecholamine levels rise significantly (38–40).

Regional Anesthesia

Major conduction blockade, such as epidural or spinal anesthesia, has no effect on the innervation of the kidney unless the sympathetic fibers are blocked from the 11th thoracic through the first lumbar spinal segments (41). It is noteworthy, however, that even when the kidney is completely denervated — either by surgery, by ganglionic blocking agents, or by spinal anesthesia — there is little or no change in renal blood flow as long as arterial pressure remains in a normal range. Sartorius and Burlington in 1956 studied acute renal denervation in dogs and found that both GFR and urine output were greater in a denervated kidney than in a normally innervated one at the same mean arterial pressure (42). Although the comparable experiment cannot be performed on humans, patients with congestive heart failure have been observed to demonstrate improvement in GFR and renal plasma flow under high spinal anesthesia (43), suggesting that the afferent arteriolar constriction characteristic of congestive heart failure (CHF) was reversed by the sympathetic blockade. However, it is conceivable that improved renal function was simply the result of increased cardiac output in response to decreased systemic vascular resistance.

The phenomenon of autoregulation keeps RBF and GFR relatively constant between mean arterial pressures of 80 and 180 mm Hg. However, autoregulation does not maintain urine flow, which is likely to decrease as blood pressure decreases because of altered tubular hemodynamics. It is therefore to be expected that spinal anesthesia would produce little effect as long as the blood pressure and cardiac output remain within normal physiologic range. In normal patients, there seems to be a critical MAP of approximately 80 to 85 mm Hg, below which any further reduction in pressure is associated with a decline in RBF and urine output (41).

In a study of T_1 levels of spinal anesthesia in Rhesus monkeys, Sivarajan et al. found that the percentage of cardiac output perfusing the kidneys remained constant at about 15%, and that any significant decrease in cardiac output resulted in a concomitant decrease in RBF (44). GFR (like RBF) remains constant during spinal anesthesia through a wide range of arterial pressures, but it has been demonstrated consistently to fall once MAP is less than 100 mm Hg; Greene and Brull have observed that diminished GFR and urinary flow "may be considered a characteristic of spinal anesthesia" (41).

Even if GFR and urine output show a temporary decline during major regional blockade, the expectation of clinicians is that adequate hydration will result in the prompt return of normal urine production and that no increase in the blood urea nitrogen (BUN) level will result postoperatively. The sympathetic blockade and mild to moderate hypotension that often occur during spinal and epidural anesthesia, whereas not sufficient to support a completely normal GFR, are adequate nonetheless to maintain adequate RBF and normal renal cellular metabolism. Extreme degrees of hypotension are another issue, however. Because the pressures within renal capillaries average 13 to 18 mm Hg (45), it has been assumed that mean arterial pressures below 35 mm Hg are ill advised and may ultimately result in parenchymal renal damage secondary to inadequate RBF if allowed to persist. Patients of advanced age, with atherosclerotic disease or chronic hypertension, may be susceptible to renal damage at arterial pressures considerably above this level. If the preservation of RBF is held as a key objective, the question of how best to manage clinical hypotension during major regional blockade comes to the forefront and has occasioned much lively debate among clinicians. On one hand, many clinicians advocate the use of phenylephrine, a pure α-agonist, on the grounds that the hypotension is caused by decreased SVR, which this drug will reverse, and because they believe that the reflex slowing of the heart rate will benefit coronary artery perfusion. The other school of thought argues that the hypotension is caused more specifically by venodilation and decreased preload, which may be reversed better by a mixed-adrenergic agent such as ephedrine, with redirection of blood flow to the heart, brain, and kidney by the β-adrenergic component of its activity. Although the definitive study to settle this question has yet to be conducted, Butterworth et al. demonstrated recently in anesthetized dogs that ephedrine corrected the noncardiac circulatory effects of spinal anesthesia more effectively than either phenylephrine or a pure β-agonist (isoproterenol) because ephedrine alone produced both an increase in MAP and a decrease in venous capacitance (46).

CAUSES OF ACUTE RENAL FAILURE

Prerenal, Intrarenal, and Postrenal Factors

Azotemia with or without reduction in urine output is the final result of acute renal failure, whatever the cause. However, consideration of possible causes is the key to understanding the pathophysiology of the renal dysfunction and determining the best possible treatment. Classically, the initial step in the evaluation of acute renal failure is to determine whether prerenal factors, intrinsic renal disease or damage, or postrenal factors are predominant.

Prerenal azotemia implies that a rise in serum creatinine is directly caused by decreased renal perfusion and may be reversed by correcting inadequate volume or pressure to restore renal blood flow. Prerenal azotemia most commonly is seen in the setting either of hypovolemia or congestive heart failure, both of which compromise cardiac output and activate the sympathetic nervous system, causing a state of avid salt and water retention by the renal tubules in an effort to maintain volume homeostasis. The term "prerenal failure" is a misnomer, because by very definition, tubular function is intact. Nonetheless, prerenal factors such as hypovolemia and sepsis are very important in the causation of preoperative acute renal failure. In the PACU, hypovolemia is frequent because of intraoperative blood loss or insensible fluid losses; a fluid challenge is the best initial step in the management of oliguria, which will be discussed in more detail later in this chapter.

Postrenal obstruction also may be seen and identified in the PACU because of a variety of factors that may cause urinary tract obstruction: urinary catheters kinked or occluded by blood clot; intraoperative surgical disruption or ligation of ureters; dislodgment of renal stones into the urinary tract; or inability to void because of urethral edema or loss of sensation from regional anesthesia. Ellenbogen et al. recommended the use of ultrasonography as a reliable means of detecting urinary tract obstruction in cases of postoperative oliguria (47), especially for patients with preexisting renal insufficiency or allergy to contrast material.

Most cases (80 to 90%) of perioperative renal failure are due to acute tubular necrosis (ATN), which may be caused by an ischemic or nephrotoxic insult (which frequently coexist and exacerbate each other). Acute or chronic renal insufficiency and vascular injury are also important causes of renal failure, but acute glomerular disease is rarely encountered in the perioperative period.

Nephrotoxic Injury

The chance of nephrotoxic injury in the perioperative period is not insignificant because a surgical patient may be exposed to 20 or more different drugs within the span of a few hours. Direct tubular toxicity may result from the aminoglycoside antibiotics. In one study of hospital-acquired renal insufficiency, nine of 129 patients developed renal toxicity from gentamicin or amikacin therapy and one death was attributed to renal failure (2). Risk factors for aminoglycoside-induced renal failure included advanced age, inadequate volume status, sepsis, and concurrent administration of other nephrotoxic drugs such as cyclosporine. Immunologic (hypersensitivity) reactions may be provoked by penicillins or diuretics, which are commonly given in the perioperative setting, and may lead rarely to vasculitis or acute interstitial nephritis. Radiographic contrast material is administered frequently to patients before vascular surgery and has been linked to high risk for the development of renal failure, especially in diabetic patients with preexisting renal insufficiency (1). As previously noted, nonsteroidal anti-inflammatory agents are linked to a functional reduction in glomerular filtration rate, which may lead to renal failure in susceptible patients. Other causes of drug-induced acute renal failure are listed in Table 9–1. Drug-induced nephrotoxicity may not necessarily lead to complete renal failure and may occur without oliguria. However, iatrogenic nephrotoxicity

Table 9–1.   Drug induced acute renal failure

Acute tubular necrosis
  Aminoglycosides
  Amphotericin B
  Polymyxins
  Cephaloridine, cephalothin (?)

Hypersensitivity reaction
  Vasculitis-glomerulonephritis
    Penicillin
    Sulfonamides
    Penicillamine
  Acute (allergic) interstitial nephritis
    Penicillins (especially semisynthetic agents)
    Sulfonamides
    Rifampin
    Diuretics (furosemide, thiazides)
    Allopurinol
    Anticonvulsants
    Nonsteroidal anti-inflammatory agents

Obstructive nephropathy
  Intratubular precipitation of drug
    Sulfonamides
    Methotrexate
  Intratubular precipitation of organic acids
    Uric acid (tumor-lysis syndrome)
    Oxalic acid (methoxyflurane)

Functional reduction in glomerular filtration rate
  Nonsteroidal anti-inflammatory agents
  Captopril

Pseudorenal failure
  Increased urea production
    Tetracycline
    Corticosteroids
  Decreased renal secretion of creatinine
    Trimethoprim
    Cimetidine

From Gornick et al., reproduced with permission from Carter Publishing.

is estimated to account for 20 to 30% of the cases of acute renal failure observed in teaching hospitals (48).

Renal Ischemia

Renal ischemia may occur at virtually any point in the perioperative period when patients may be exposed to dehydration, blood loss, hypotension, or iatrogenic insults such as vasoconstrictor drugs, aortic cross-clamping, or cardiopulmonary bypass. Certainly, the victims of major trauma, hemorrhage, myoglobinuria, or cardiopulmonary arrest are at extremely high risk for renal ischemia and the development of ATN.

Renal injury may be considered as a continuum between prerenal dysfunction, in which all compensatory tubular functions are preserved, and ATN, in which tubular function is lost, renal failure is established, and simple interventions such as volume infusion are not adequate to reverse the functional and anatomic lesions (15, 49). The development of the nonoliguric form of acute renal failure is relatively common in current clinical practice because multiple small insults occur in a "protected" milieu (i.e., in the setting of aggressive fluid administration, vasodilator therapy, dopamine, etc.).

Anderson et al. studied the clinical outcome of 92 patients with acute renal failure, 54 of whom were nonoliguric, and found that the nonoliguric group had a shorter hospital stay, fewer complications, and lower mortality (26% mortality among nonoliguric patients versus 50% in the oliguric patient group) (3). However, this study examined mostly patients with isolated nephrotoxic ATN; patients with ischemic ATN were specifically excluded. When nonoliguric ATN occurs after cardiac surgery, the prognosis is much worse, probably because it exists in the setting of poor cardiac function and multiorgan system failure.

The common pathway in the development of ATN is the fact that ischemic and toxic insults, carried far enough, lead to renal tubu-

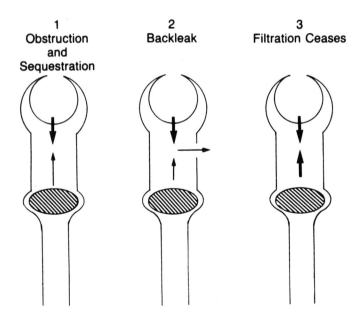

1
Obstruction and Sequestration

2
Backleak

3
Filtration Ceases

Fig. 9–3. Maintenance phase of acute renal failure illustrating obstruction of tubules with necrotic cellular debris causing 1) proximal tubular dilatation and sequestration of ultrafiltrate, 2) leakage into the interstitium, and 3) rising intratubular pressure to cause cessation of ultrafiltration. (From Byrick RJ, Rose DK. Pathophysiology and prevention of acute renal failure: the role of the anaesthetist. Can J Anaesth 1990;37:457–467, reproduced with permission from the Canadian Anaesthetist Society.)

lar cell necrosis. The primary role of tubular injury is emphasized by the fact that GFR is reduced to less than 10% of normal, although RBF may be decreased by only 40 to 50%, and GFR remains low despite restoration of RBF. Damage to the tubules may be patchy, and all nephrons are unlikely to be affected equally. However, two tubule mechanisms are responsible for the loss of glomerular filtration: obstruction of the tubular lumen by cellular or pigment debris, and backleak of filtrate through disrupted tubular cells (49, 50). As the cells sustain damage, they slough and obstruct at the narrowed portion of the descending loop of Henle (pars recta). Tubular pressure increases and impedes glomerular filtration. The filtrate that does form leaks back through the damaged tubular membrane into the renal interstitium (Fig. 9–3). If abnormal material within the tubule, such as myoglobin, becomes inspissated, the flow of filtrate through the nephron ultimately must cease because backpressure is transmitted to Bowman's space and exceeds filtration pressure. These initial events are perpetuated by tubuloglomerular feedback in which increased chloride delivery to the macula densa triggers renin activation and excessive angiotensin

elaboration causes arteriolar constriction and further loss of perfusion. If protective maneuvers are to work, they must be given early enough in the cycle to lessen the severity of the tubular lesion. Experimentally, the presence of any of several renal protective agents (volume loading with saline, osmotic diuresis with mannitol, vasodilation with dopamine, furosemide, PGE_1) prevents tubular obstruction and backleak so that oliguria does not occur and recovery is rapid.

The concept of "renal angina" is closely related to the development of tubular damage. In an elegant model of isolated rat kidneys, Brezis et al. demonstrated that cells of the medullary thick ascending limbs (mTAL) exist normally at a very low tissue pO_2 of 8 to 10 mm Hg and are especially susceptible to mitochondrial swelling, nuclear pyknosis, and cell death when exposed to mild hypoxic perfusion (8). Severely hypoxic perfusion exaggerated the cellular lesions, wiping out all gradations of damage, whereas O_2-enriched perfusion completely eliminated the lesion. The same authors demonstrated also that complete vascular occlusion, which reduced GFR to zero, is associated with less cellular damage than is hypoxic perfusion. Just as the familiar concept of oxygen supply and demand is understood in relation to the myocardial and cerebral circulations, this evidence suggests that renal tubular cells also are more susceptible to injury when the metabolic work demanded of them exceeds their oxygenated blood supply. Because the normal kidney's response to hypoperfusion (prerenal compensation) is to initiate active mTAL sodium and chloride reabsorption, the work of the mTAL cells is increased, along with their oxygen demand at exactly the time when they are most likely to become hypoxic and vulnerable to "renal angina" (51).

Risk Factors for Renal Injury

Every experienced clinician recognizes that certain groups of surgical patients, such as trauma victims (52) and patients with long-standing diabetes (53), are at higher risk for perioperative renal dysfunction than are healthy patients presenting for elective procedures. However, attempts to quantify this risk are more difficult than might be anticipated. An excellent review article published in 1993 by Novis' group at the University of Chicago reviewed 28 studies of preoperative risk factors for postoperative renal failure (54). Although more than 10,000 patients were encompassed in the 28 studies, the authors concluded that formal meta-analysis of the data was not possible because no two of the studies used the same criteria to define acute renal failure, and consistent criteria for the presence or absence of risk factors were also lacking. Of the 30 variables considered in this review article, only preoperative renal risk factors (such as the preexistence of increased serum creatinine and BUN) consistently predicted postoperative renal dysfunction. Advanced age and a history of cardiac failure also were predictive, although the studies did not agree on a definition or limit for advanced age or on specific diagnostic criteria for congestive heart failure. Despite the inconclusiveness of the literature, it is worth examining some of the data on preexisting medical conditions, as well as intraoperative risk factors, in more detail.

DIABETES MELLITUS

Patients with diabetes mellitus have such a high incidence of comorbid disease that any study of their perioperative risk is in danger of confounding its variables. MacKenzie and Charlson addressed this problem by reviewing retrospectively the records of 282 diabetic patients to analyze in detail their preoperative medical condition and incidence of postsurgical complications (53). The preoperative presence of nephropathy was documented in the same category as other diabetic end-organ diseases: retinopathy and neuropathy. Postoperative renal insufficiency was reported to occur in 7% of the entire patient group. However, the incidence of postoperative renal insufficiency rose to 30% in the setting of preexisting infection and peripheral vascular disease and 22% in patients with preexisting end-organ damage. The incidence of any major noncardiac complication was only 4% in patients with no comorbid disease. Noncardiac as well as cardiac complications were common in patients with congestive heart failure or valvular heart disease; the incidence of noncardiac complication (defined as infection, renal insufficiency, and/or cerebrovascular ischemic event) was 29% in this group, and the incidence of postoperative myocardial infarction or CHF was 27%.

In a subsequent study, Charlson et al. prospectively studied a cohort of 254 surgical patients with a history of diabetes and hypertension and found that 23 (9%) demonstrated a postoperative rise in serum creatinine of more than 20% of the baseline value; one patient developed acute renal failure (55). Fifty percent of the patients with postoperative renal dysfunction failed to recover to their preoperative serum creatinine level. Analysis of these patients' intraoperative anesthesia records revealed that either hypotension or hypertension during surgery heightened the risk of postoperative renal dysfunction. Specifically, either an increase in MAP ≥20 mm Hg over the baseline for 30 minutes or more, or a decrease in MAP ≥20 mm Hg below baseline for 60 minutes or more, was predictive of postoperative renal dysfunction regardless of the type of anesthesia used. This information may be of use to the PACU physician who is interested in identifying patients who may need particularly close observation for urine output and filling pressure during the immediate postoperative period. Other predictors identified in this study were inadequate volume replacement (defined as ≤300 cc/hour of intravenous fluid), intraoperative cardiac arrest, drainage of massive ascites, and preoperative CHF.

OBSTRUCTIVE JAUNDICE

For more than 50 years, a clinical association has been recognized between acute renal failure and obstructive jaundice. The term "hepatorenal syndrome" is still used to describe the coexistence of hepatic and renal failure, which carries a bleak prognosis. Little known today is the fact that this term was originally used to describe the deaths caused by renal failure after operation on the biliary tract. Wait and Kahng recently reviewed the literature on renal failure complicating obstructive jaundice and noted that renal failure occurs in approximately 9% of patients who undergo surgery, which is a 76% mortality rate (56). The clinical observation that jaundiced patients seem predisposed to intraoperative hypotension has been substantiated by animal studies that demonstrated worsened hypotension and mortality after hemorrhage in bile duct-ligated animals than in sham-operated ones. Hemodynamic measurements typically indicate decreased peripheral vascular resistance and normal or high cardiac output, similar to the findings in acute sepsis. The most likely etiology is that bile salts, which bind and detoxify endotoxin, are not secreted into the gut. Portal endotoxemia has been demonstrated in patients with a preoperative serum bilirubin of greater than 8 mg/dL; postoperative renal dysfunction can be prevented by the preoperative administration of bile salts (e.g., sodium taurocholate).

The clinical management of patients who have undergone surgery for obstructive jaundice should include restoration of blood volume, vigilant attention to fluid status and cardiac performance, and the strict avoidance of nonsteroidal anti-inflammatory drugs. Mannitol administration has been advocated either preoperatively or intraoperatively for renal protection. However, if the large osmotic diuresis induced is not adequately replaced by fluids, the risk of nephrotoxicty may actually be increased.

AORTIC CROSS-CLAMP

The patient who must undergo major vascular surgery involving aortic cross-clamp is rarely free of underlying medical disease such as hypertension, diabetes, and/or coronary artery disease. However, it is well recognized that major vascular surgery confers additional risk to the postoperative renal function of these patients, which already may be tenuous. Gamulin et al. measured renal clearance before, during, and after infrarenal aortic cross-clamping in 12 patients undergoing elective aortic surgery (57). Although cardiac output and systemic vascular resistance did not undergo significant change, profound alteration in renal hemodynamics was observed. Renal vascular resistance increased by 75%, RBF declined by 38%, and these changes persisted for more than 1 hour after release of the aortic clamp. The authors speculated that these changes might have been more profound if mannitol had not been administered for renal protection throughout the study, because mannitol has been shown to preserve renal perfusion during infrarenal aortic cross-clamping in animals.

The practice of giving mannitol, furosemide, or large volumes of crystalloid for renal protection during aortic surgery is predicated on the assumption that it will prevent oliguria and that oliguria is the precursor of renal insufficiency or failure. This assumption is not always accurate. Just as renal failure may exist without oliguria, the development of oliguria may not be predictive of postoperative renal dysfunction. This hypothesis was tested in a study that examined the mean and the lowest

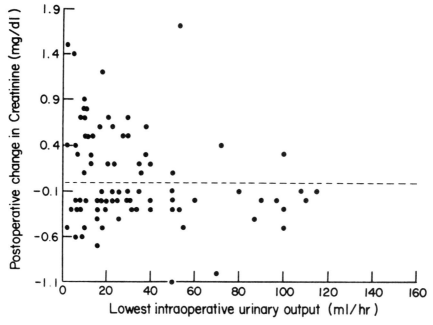

Fig. 9–4. For 137 patients, no significant correlation ($r = 0.21$) existed between the lowest hourly urinary output during the operation and the greatest change in each patient's creatinine level on postoperative days 1, 3, or 7. (From Alpert RA, Roizen MF, Hamilton WK, et al. Intraoperative urinary output does not predict renal function in patients undergoing abdominal aortic revascularization. Surg 1984;95:707–711, reproduced with permission from Mosby-Year Book.)

hourly intraoperative urine output in 137 patients who underwent aortic reconstruction; the aim of the study was to correlate urine output with postoperative serum creatinine and BUN levels up to 1 week postoperatively. New renal insufficiency was defined as an increase in creatinine level of 0.5 mg/dL or more above the preoperative level. No significant correlation was found between intraoperative oliguria and the development of postoperative renal insufficiency (Fig. 9–4). The presence of preoperative renal disease, however, was strongly predictive; 17 of the 21 patients whose creatinine rose postoperatively had evidence of preoperative renal disease (58).

Preoperative renal dysfunction was identified as a major factor contributing to postoperative ATN after aortic aneurysm repair in a 15-year retrospective review by Gornick and Kjellstrand (59). Of the 47 patients who developed ATN requiring dialysis, only 10 survived (Fig. 9–5); there were no survivors with a preoperative serum creatinine greater than 1.5 mg/dL. This study included both ruptured aneurysm cases requiring emergency surgery (64%) as well as elective cases. The incidence of prior cardiovascular history (angina, previous myocardial infarction, or CHF) — about 40% — was similar in survivors and nonsurvivors. There was a significant association between hypotension in the perioperative period and the development of postoperative ATN, although whether the surgery was emergency or elective had no influence on survival if acute renal failure developed. Hypotension was believed to be the most common cause of renal failure in 31 of the 37 patients who died, whereas the remaining six patients died from renal failure attributed to a combination of insults, including hypotension, nephrotoxic antibiotics, and sepsis.

Another retrospective review in 1986 examined the postoperative course of 25 patients

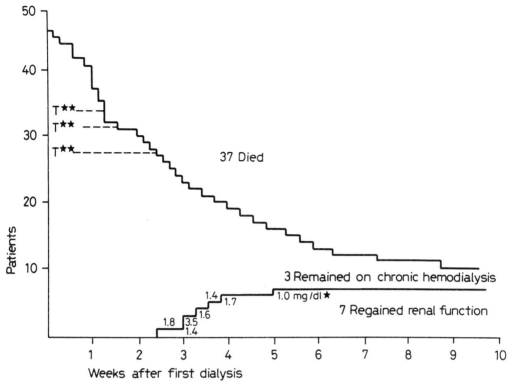

Fig. 9–5. Curves describing time of death, time of recovery with ultimate renal function, and need for chronic hemodialysis in 47 patients dialyzed at day 1 for acute tubular necrosis after aortic aneurysm surgery. * ultimate creatinine level; ** renal function regained at time (T) before ultimate death. (From Gornick CC, Kjellstrand CM. Acute renal failure complicating aortic aneurysm surgery. Nephron 1983;35:145–157, reproduced with permission from Carter Publishing.)

who underwent aortic aneurysm repair with preoperative serum creatinine levels greater than 2 mg/dL (60). Of the 16 patients with preoperative serum creatinine values between 2 and 4 mg/dL, only one patient developed renal failure, which was nonoliguric and resolved before hospital discharge. Six patients had preoperative serum creatinine values greater than 4 mg/dL but were not receiving dialysis; four of these (66%) required acute hemodialysis after operation, and none survived longer than 9 months after hospital discharge. An additional four patients had preoperative serum creatinine values greater than 4 mg/dL but were on chronic hemodialysis, which was performed on the day before surgery. All four patients survived surgery without major complications, although one ulti-

mately died with ischemia of the left colon. This study makes the point that it is actually safer to operate on patients in chronic renal failure who are on a stable dialysis regimen, than patients at risk for developing new-onset postoperative acute renal failure.

MONITORING RENAL FUNCTION

Clearance Measurement

Assessment of renal function has long been conducted by clearance techniques, but these provide, at best, an indirect estimate of the renal function measured. Clearance (C) is defined as the virtual volume of plasma cleared of substance x per unit time (in mL/minute). For the kidney, clearance is expressed as

$C_x = U_x V / P_x$, where U_x is the concentration of substance x in the urine in mg/dL, V is the urine flow rate in mL/minute, and P_x is the concentration of substance x in the plasma. Note that $U_x V$ (urine concentration times flow rate) represents the urine excretion rate of substance x. It is generally accepted that the most accurate determination of GFR (the "gold standard") is provided by the clearance of inulin, an inert sugar that is completely filtered by the glomerulus and neither secreted nor absorbed by the renal tubules; thus, that volume in milliliters of plasma cleared of inulin per minute represents the GFR. In other words, the renal excretion rate of inulin is determined solely by GFR and by the plasma concentration of inulin. However, accurate measurement of inulin clearance is laborious and requires meticulous attention to detail. An indwelling intravenous cannula and urinary catheter are placed, and a loading dose plus infusion of inulin are given to establish a steady-state plasma concentration. Then, a very carefully timed urine collection is made, and inulin clearance is calculated from the equation above. However, inulin itself is in short supply, and inulin clearance thus remains a largely investigational tool that has not become part of clinical practice even in the intensive care setting (61).

Accurate assessment of GFR nonetheless is desirable in critically ill patients for many reasons. As noted earlier, the mortality rate from postoperative and posttraumatic acute renal failure may exceed 60 to 75% and increases dramatically as other organ systems fail. Early detection of impairment in GFR is essential for the prevention of further nephrotoxic and ischemic insults that may ultimately result in tubular necrosis. Estimation of GFR also is crucial for the appropriate dosing of medications such as aminoglycoside antibiotics that are dependent on renal clearance, to avoid the vicious cycle of impaired drug elimination and accumulation to more toxic levels. In another example, the major hepatic metabolite of procainamide, N-acetyl procainamide, is neurotoxic rather than nephrotoxic but ac-cumulates so rapidly in renal dysfunction that the use of procainamide is contraindicated.

Creatinine is an endogenous end product of creatine phosphate metabolism that is normally generated from muscle at a uniform rate. Because creatinine is handled by the kidney in a manner similar to inulin, the measurement of creatinine clearance is a simple, inexpensive method of estimating GFR. It requires only a single blood sample, usually drawn at the midpoint of a carefully timed urine collection. To reduce errors caused by residual urine in the bladder, urine for creatinine clearance has traditionally been collected over a 24-hour period. However, a long collection introduces greater opportunity for collection errors, disrupts other diagnostic tests, curtails the frequency with which the test is performed, and delays the availability of the information for clinical decisions. In addition, a long urine collection is matched to a single serum sample during a period when serum creatinine may be rapidly changing (0.5 to 1.5 mg/dL/day in oliguric acute renal failure). The direct reciprocal relationship between serum creatinine and GFR as measured by creatinine clearance is illustrated in Figure 9–6.

In modern ICU practice, the presence of an indwelling urinary catheter reduces the error caused by residual urine and, as long as the urine collection is carefully timed, the duration of collection is immaterial to the principle of clearance studies. To identify deteriorating renal function at an early stage, the use of serial creatinine clearance estimations at shorter time intervals may be expected to be more useful than a single isolated measurement. Sladen et al. prospectively compared creatinine clearance values obtained from 2-hour or 22-hour collections in catheterized patients in the ICU who had a variety of serious clinical problems, differing renal function, and urine flow rates of at least 15 mL/hour (62). Paired values of 2-hour versus 22-hour creatinine clearance demonstrated a high positive correlation with a correlation coefficient $r = 0.95$ (Fig. 9–7). The 2-hour and 22-hour creatinine clearance values in fact correlated

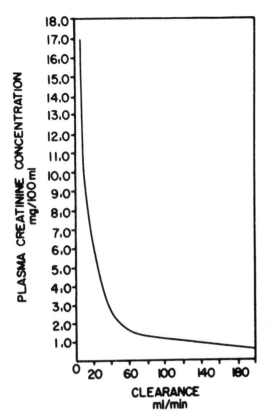

Fig. 9–6. The relationship between serum creatinine and glomerular filtration rate (GFR) as measured by creatinine clearance is reciprocal and exponential. Doubling of the serum creatinine corresponds to halving of the GFR. Declines in GFR from normal are associated relatively with small increases in serum creatinine until GFR decreases below 60 mL/minute; further decrements are associated with large increases in serum creatinine. (From Alfrey et al., reproduced with permission from Little Brown Publishing Company.)

Unfortunately, apart from collection errors, there are a number of limitations with even carefully performed creatinine clearance determinations. Creatinine generation rate may vary with physical activity, protein intake, and catabolism. In cachectic patients with depleted lean body mass, creatinine production is so low that the serum creatinine concentration, which is frequently less than 1.0 mg/dL, underestimates the true GFR. There is an intrinsic error in serum creatinine measurement of about 10%. Barbiturates and cephalosporin antibiotics, which are ubiquitous in the perioperative period, may artifactually increase the serum creatinine concentration by as much as 100%, thereby falsely decreasing creatinine clearance. Unlike inulin, creatinine undergoes a variable amount of proximal tubular secretion, so that creatinine clearance predictably tends to overestimate GFR. Some widely used drugs, such as trimethoprim, histamine-2-receptor antagonists, and salicylates, may block tubular secretion of creatinine, increase the serum creatinine value, and decrease the measured creatinine clearance.

best when creatinine clearance was less than 50 mL/minute, when the information is the most critical. In another study, a 1-hour creatinine clearance of less than 25 mL/minute performed within 6 hours of surgery was shown to be a reliable prognosticator of subsequent posttraumatic renal dysfunction or failure (63). These studies would indicate that wider adoption of the time-limited creatinine clearance measurement is warranted in the PACU setting, particularly for the at-risk patient who stands to benefit most from the early detection and aggressive therapy of postoperative renal deterioration.

Tubular Function Tests

Tests of renal tubular function may serve to distinguish reversible states of inadequate perfusion (prerenal azotemia) from established ATN. In the former, tubular function is preserved; in the latter, it is lost. It is the hope of clinicians that early diagnosis of prerenal azotemia may prompt appropriate therapeutic intervention and prevent the progression to ATN and complete renal failure. The full range of predictive and diagnostic tests was recently discussed in an excellent review by Kellen et al. (6).

Prerenal azotemia is characterized by diminished GFR with intact tubular function. The most useful test is tubular conservation of sodium. In prerenal syndromes, the tubules avidly conserve sodium to restore the intravascular volume. Urine sodium diminishes to very low values, usually less than 10 mEq/L. In ATN, the kidneys can no longer conserve

Fig. 9–7. Correlation between 2-h (CC02) and 22-h (CC22) creatinine clearance in mL/minute. The line of regression is shown. (From Sladen RN, Endo E, Harrison T. Two-hour versus 22-hour creatinine clearance in critically ill patients. Anesthesiology 1987;67:1013–1016, reproduced with permission from J.B. Lippincott Company.)

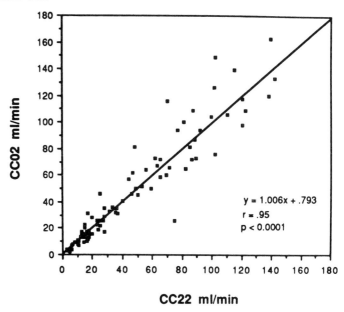

sodium and urine sodium is usually greater than 50 mEq/L. This phenomenon may be also be described by the fractional excretion of sodium (FENa), which is the sodium clearance expressed as a percentage of creatinine clearance. The test is relatively simple, requiring a paired blood and urine sample:

$$FENa = \text{Na clearance} \,/\, \text{Cr clearance}$$
$$= (U_{Na}V \,/\, P_{Na} \div U_{Cr}V \,/\, P_{Cr}) \times 100\%$$
$$= (U_{Na} \,/\, P_{Na} \div U_{Cr} \,/\, P_{Cr}) \times 100\%$$

where Na = sodium, Cr = creatinine, U = urine concentration, V = urine flow rate and P = serum concentration. In prerenal states, FENa is less than 1%; in ATN, it increases to more than 3%.

Tubular concentrating ability is a sensitive test of tubular function. In prerenal states, the ratio of urine to serum osmolality is markedly increased (>1.5). In ATN, concentrating ability is lost and urine and serum osmolality approach unity. Loss of concentrating ability may precede elevations in BUN and creatinine by 24 to 48 hours. Water conservation is reflected by the urine:plasma creatinine ratio (U/P_{cr}); in prerenal azotemia it is high (>40),

but in patients with ATN it decreases to less than 20.

In practice, tubular function tests are helpful only in the evaluation of oliguria. If urine flow is normal, these indices are usually equivocal. Patients of advanced age may have impaired ability to concentrate urine as a baseline, and in some patients, the pathophysiology of ATN includes patchy or heterogeneous tubular damage, which makes tubular function testing unreliable. For many patients in whom the diagnosis is mostly in doubt, tubular indices will be in the indeterminate middle range and values may overlap significantly in as many as 33% of patients (1, 6). A false profile of ATN may result from tubular function tests if saluresis is induced by diuretics such as furosemide or mannitol or by dopamine infusion. Nonetheless, a prerenal profile despite diuretic therapy is a firm indication of severe hypovolemia and reversible renal dysfunction; the one exception is in the hepatorenal syndrome, a vasomotor nephropathy in which an intensely prerenal state is induced by liver failure and circulating endotoxemia. The prerenal state is usually irreversible unless liver function improves.

MANAGEMENT OF ABNORMAL URINE OUTPUT

Oliguria

Oliguria is a relative term; it does not necessarily indicate impaired renal function, nor does a normal or high urine output guarantee perfectly functioning kidneys. Intraoperative urine flow is frequently decreased in the presence of hypotension and improves toward the end of the case when blood pressure returns to normal levels. The only conclusion that may be reached with certainty is that a kidney that is producing urine must be receiving some blood flow, because without renal perfusion, there can be no glomerular filtration and urine cannot be formed. Oliguria or anuria is expected during suprarenal aortic cross-clamping, and oliguria represents the normal renal response to hypovolemia.

Functional perioperative oliguria generally is defined as a urine output of less than 0.5 to 1.0 mL/kg/hr. Acute renal failure is defined as oliguric when the urine flow is less than 15 mL/hr. In the PACU setting, oliguria must be assumed to be hemodynamically mediated and potentially reversible until proven otherwise, and aggressive evaluation and management to optimize cardiac output and renal blood flow are expected as the standard of care. Complete cessation of urine output in the postoperative period should prompt an immediate search for causes of mechanical obstruction such as a kinked urinary catheter; rarely, anuria may result from extravasation of urine from the bladder into the abdominal cavity.

Initial evaluation of the PACU patient with inadequate urine output should focus on a thorough review of the patient's medical history, preoperative medication intake, surgical procedure, and anesthetic management (Table 9–2). An appreciation of preexisting renal impairment or poor left ventricular function is critical, because either will interfere with the patient's ability to self-regulate fluid balance. Untreated hypertension usually implies that

Table 9–2. Management of Oliguria

Anuria:
  Exclude problem with urine collecting system
History:
  Preoperative, intraoperative fluid losses
Examination:
  Mucus membranes, vital signs
Fluid challenge:
  Crystalloid, colloid, or red blood cells

Response:
  ECF deficit 25%—increase maintenance fluids

No response:
  Repeat fluid challenge
No response:
  Place central venous pressure and/or pulmonary artery catheter

Repeat fluid challenges until:
  Urine flow increases, or
  filling pressures are moderately elevated, or
  CO no longer increases or heart rate slows, or
  evidence of fluid overload, lung dysfunction

No response, normal cardiac function:
  Dopamine 1–3 μg/kg/min
No response, impaired cardiac function
  Inotropic support (dopamine, dobutamine)
  Afterload reduction, if indicated

No response:
  Furosemide 10–20 mg i.v., repeat p.r.n.

the patient has a baseline status of vasoconstriction and volume depletion and may be prone to extremes of blood pressure lability both intraoperatively and postoperatively. If the patient has had preoperative bowel cleansing with potent laxatives, the resulting fluid losses may produce a volume deficit of a liter or more, which may not have been adequately replaced during surgery and must be addressed during postanesthesia care. Information must be obtained about intraoperative blood loss, hemodynamic function, and specific renal insults (dye studies, aortic cross-clamping, transfusion reaction, etc.) and treatment given (e.g., dopamine, Lasix, mannitol, etc.) Extensive surgical procedures such as bowel resection or burn eschar removal and grafting commonly result in considerable insensible fluid losses and third-spacing of fluid, so oliguria in a patient who has undergone such operation should be assumed a priority to result from volume deficit, which must be corrected. Intraoperative hemorrhage or another untoward event resulting in a prolonged period of hypotension may lead to renal ischemia especially in the high-risk patient with hypertension, diabetes, or cardiac disease. Trauma, surgical stress, and number of drugs used during anesthesia, including morphine, barbiturates, and phenothiazines, stimulate the release of antidiuretic hormone (ADH). Inappropriate ADH secretion may result in oliguria, retention of ingested water, and hyponatremia and volume overexpansion.

Physical examination of the oliguric patient should focus first on heart rate and blood pressure, because hypotension and tachycardia are the normal physiologic responses to hypovolemia. The degree of skin turgor and the moisture or dryness of mucous membranes are also valuable signs. Even if these are within normal limits, however, the first intervention is to give the patient a fluid challenge. Packed red cells should be used if indicated by intraoperative blood loss or preexisting anemia, because they will correct volume deficit as well as enhance oxygen delivery to the kidneys and other tissues. If the patient's hemoglobin level is considered adequate, crystalloid or colloid should be given. The choice of crystalloid or colloid solution is not critical, although each school of thought has its passionate adherents; the most important point is that a sufficient volume challenge must be given. This should consist of a rapid infusion of 250 to 500 mL crystalloid, such as Ringer's lactate solution, or the osmotic equivalent of a colloid, such as hetastarch. (It should be noted that the difference in cost among solutions is significant; in our institution, a liter of Ringer's lactate solution costs $0.90, whereas one-half liter of hetastarch costs $37.50.) Loop diuretics should be used as first-line therapy only if there are unequivocal signs of fluid overload or CHF or as an adjunct to osmotic diuresis in rhabdomyolysis or intravascular hemolysis.

If urine flow increases after the first fluid challenge, an extracellular fluid deficit of at least 25% exists, and the rate of the patient's maintenance intravenous infusion should be increased accordingly. If there is no response, the fluid challenge should be repeated once. At this stage, careful reevaluation of the patient's physical status should be performed, and the placement of invasive monitors such as a central venous pressure (CVP) or pulmonary artery (PA) catheter should be seriously considered. If the patient still seems clinically to be volume depleted on the basis of the history and physical examination, a CVP catheter may be placed initially. A low CVP measurement (<5 mm Hg) will confirm the diagnosis of hypovolemia, and further fluid challenges may be given to raise the CVP without fear of excess. If the patient seems clinically euvolemic, it is still reasonable to begin evaluation with a CVP catheter or a PA introducer sheath, which carries less risk to the patient than full PA catheterization. A low CVP will support a trial of further volume infusion, whereas a high CVP (>12 mm Hg) suggests the need for diuretic therapy and/or PA catheterization. High filling pressures accompanied by oliguria and clinical signs of hypervolemia suggest either cardiac dysfunction (pump failure) with failure to perfuse the kidneys or severe primary renal dysfunction. Either may necessitate intracardiac monitoring to track the success of interventions designed to improve cardiac output. Maximization of cardiac output with measures such as dopamine infusion at "renal doses" (3 to 5 µg/kg/minute), will improve renal perfusion because of dopamine's β-adrenergic and dopaminergic effects, as noted above. Simultaneous afterload reduction with agents such as nitroglycerin or nitroprusside will reduce systemic vascular resistance and improve cardiac output further. Once preload and cardiac output are optimal, or if obvious signs of hypervolemia such as pulmonary edema are present, a trial of diuretic therapy may be indicated.

Patients who have been on chronic diuretic therapy before operation may indeed require a diuretic stimulus to initiate urine output after a period of oliguria. Great care should be taken, however, to avoid the error of administering a potent diuretic to any patient whose volume replacement is inadequate, because this could worsen the volume depletion, possibly precipitate hypotension, and compound the ischemic insult to the kidneys.

Patients with low GFR (creatinine clearance <50 mL/minute) are relatively resistant to diuretic therapy because of decreased excretion into the renal tubules. Strategies to enhance diuresis in these patients include the use of furosemide infusion or combination of furosemide with a loop diuretic (ethacrynic acid) or thiazide-type (bumetanide). The attempted conversion of established oliguric to nonoliguric ATN with aggressive furosemide therapy is successful sometimes in patients with simple aminoglycoside-induced ATN. However, when nonoliguric renal failure occurs after cardiac surgery or in the setting of multisystem organ failure, the mortality is no better than oliguric renal failure and ranges from 60 to 90% (64). High-dose furosemide (2 to 10 mg/kg) may cause acute hypotension and permanent deafness. Although induction of diuresis may facilitate nutritional support, high-dose furosemide does not seem to alter the natural history of established acute renal failure. Patients who respond to furosemide probably had less impairment of renal function at the outset. There is some evidence that the addition of low-dose dopamine to furosemide may enhance renal function in oliguric patients with renal insufficiency and failure, depending on the severity of the renal insult.

Polyuria

Polyuria is a relatively uncommon problem in the PACU setting, certainly relative to oliguria. Review of the anesthetic record may reveal the intraoperative administration of mannitol as the culprit, most often in a neurosurgical or aortic aneurysm case. Furosemide may be administered intraoperatively along with methylene blue in cases such as hysterectomy in which definitive identification of patent ureters becomes necessary. Dextran solutions may be used in plastic surgery cases to improve perfusion to free flaps and may cause osmotic diuresis and prolific urine output. If one of these drugs is believed to be the cause of the increased urine output, care should be taken in the postoperative management to replace volume adequately, because withholding intravenous fluid will not halt the diuresis and could lead to hypotension. In the absence of an obvious iatrogenic cause of polyuria, glucose should be considered as the next most likely cause of an osmotic, or solute, diuresis. Diabetic ketoacidosis and hyperglycemic nonketotic states may result in polyuria with isotonic urine formation and unresponsiveness to vasopressin (65).

Pituitary diabetes insipidus causes polyuria that results from a lack of sufficient ADH, usually because of destruction of ADH-synthesizing cells in the neurohypophysis. This condition is occasionally seen in the postpartum patient who has suffered hemorrhagic shock and sustained necrosis of the anterior pituitary; the panhypopituitarism that results is known as Sheehan's syndrome. Traumatic destruction of the posterior pituitary may occur with intracranial injury, although polyuria does not usually develop until several days later (66). Intracranial neoplasms may cause diabetes insipidus, either as primary tumors such as craniopharyngioma, or secondary metastases, most commonly from carcinoma of the breast. Diabetes insipidus may develop abruptly in the PACU after pituitary gland surgery but is generally transient and reversible. The high output of poorly concentrated urine from any of these causes persists despite high serum osmolarity and may become so severe that hypernatremia and hypovolemia reach dangerous levels. Medical management initially involves intravenous infusion of electrolyte solutions with close monitoring of serum sodium levels; normal saline solution should be used because hypotonic solutions given too rapidly may result in cerebral edema and seizures. A synthetic analog of ADH, DDAVP (1-deamino, 8-D-arginine vasopressin), is available as a nasal spray or subcutaneous injection, 0.5 to 1.0 μg, and provides antidiuretic activity for 12 or more hours with little or no pressor activity.

The volatile anesthetic gas methoxyflurane, which is no longer currently used, has been the cause in the past of nephrogenic diabetes insipidus (the failure of the renal tubules to respond to ADH) because of its nephrotoxic metabolic products, fluoride and oxalic acid. The polyuric state is related to the increased serum concentration and urinary excretion of inorganic fluoride. Depending on the duration of administration of methoxyflurane, a full spectrum of renal injury may occur, ranging from a loss of urine concentrating ability to full ATN (22). The antibiotic demeclocycline has been associated with a reversible urine concentrating defect. Lithium, even at normal therapeutic serum concentration, may produce nephrogenic diabetes insipidus in up to 30% of patients who receive it (usually for affective disorders), but the urine concentrating ability returns to normal when treatment is discontinued (65). Fluid management is the same for nephrogenic diabetes insipidus as for the pituitary-related disease, but therapy with DDAVP is not indicated because of the inability of the kidneys to respond.

Chronic Renal Failure

Postanesthesia care of the patient with chronic renal failure is a frequent event in hospitals today, because these patients may come to surgery on a number of occasions for the placement of vascular access catheters or arteriovenous fistulae for hemodialysis, as well as for other procedures. The patient with little or no urine output who is dependent on hemodialysis requires very careful perioperative fluid management, because there is little margin of safety between insufficient and excessive intravenous fluid delivery. As a rule, these patients should undergo hemodialysis during the 24 hours before surgery and have a potassium level checked after dialysis is completed to ensure that it is less than 6 mEq/L. No potassium-containing fluids should be administered to anuric patients. For noninvasive surgical procedures, patients should receive fluid replacement with 5% dextrose in water, consisting of the amount necessary to replace insensible losses in the intraoperative and postoperative period. More invasive operations will require more vigorous administration of fluid and blood products; in many cases, a CVP catheter will be used to guide intraoperative replacement and should be used as well during PACU care. No monitoring devices or intravenous lines should be placed in an extremity that has an arteriovenous fistula.

The placement of an arterial catheter will assist in the close monitoring of electrolyte status, which may undergo serious disturbance during the postoperative period. The appearance of peaked T waves or QRS widening on the electrocardiogram should prompt the immediate suspicion of hyperkalemia. If succinylcholine was used during the patient's anesthetic, the potassium level may be expected to rise by approximately 0.5 mEq/L from the preoperative value. Serum potassium levels may be lowered acutely by hyperventilation in the patient who is still intubated, or by the infusion of glucose and insulin. The intravenous administration of calcium may be indicated if cardiac conduction disturbances are appreciated. Other electrolyte abnormalities, such as hypermagnesemia and hypocalcemia, routinely accompany chronic renal failure. Hypermagnesemia in the postoperative period can lead to hypotension, inadequate ventilation, and CNS depression to the point of coma. Increased magnesium levels will also potentiate the actions of muscle relaxants such as vecuronium and pancuronium, which may have been administered as a component of general anesthesia, and the presence of residual paralysis may lead to hypoventilation and worsening acidosis (67). Even if drugs such as neostigmine were given to reverse the actions of muscle relaxants at the end of surgery, it is possible for muscle relaxation to recur because the kidneys are unable to contribute to the metabolism of these drugs. Antibiotics such as gentamicin and vancomycin may contribute to the potentiation of the muscle relaxant actions. Mechanical ventilation may be necessary to support the patient until the effects of the muscle relaxants have dissipated; dialysis also may be used to effect their removal. Chronic hypocalcemia is commonly seen in renal failure because of hyperphosphatemia and decreased activity of vitamin D; the bone decalcification that occurs in renal osteodystrophy makes these patients vulnerable to pathologic fractures during perioperative positioning and transport.

Patients with chronic renal failure develop a number of medical problems that affect postanesthesia care. Normochromic, normocytic anemia occurs in almost all patients with serum creatinine levels higher than 3.5 mg/dL, and hemoglobin levels typically range between 5 and 8 g/dL. The mechanism for the anemia is believed to be caused by decreased production of erythropoietin in the presence of elevated BUN levels and by the fact that survival time for erythrocytes is shortened by chronic uremia. The anemia is usually well tolerated because of an increase in 2,3-diphosphoglycerate (2,3-DPG) and increased cardiac output. Release of oxygen from hemoglobin is facilitated in chronic renal failure, because the usual metabolic acidosis seen in these patients shifts the oxyhemoglobin dissociation curve to the right. Alkalosis and/or hypophosphatemia may therefore be harmful for patients with coronary artery disease. A patient who complains of chest pain or is suspected to have ischemia due to coronary artery disease in the postoperative period may benefit from transfusion of packed red cells to augment oxygen-carrying capacity and improve the oxygen supply to the myocardium.

Uremic coagulopathy is characterized by a thrombocytopathy — i.e., abnormal platelet function, without thrombocytopenia. In severe cases, the Ivy bleeding time (normal 3 to 8 minutes) may be prolonged beyond 20 minutes. The mechanism is suppression of the release of factor VIII-von Willebrand complex (VIII-vWF) from the endothelium, essential for normal platelet aggregation. Bleeding time may be corrected by the administration of cryoprecipitate, which contains VIII-vWF, or DDAVP (see above) in a dose of 0.3 µg/kg. DDAVP seems to stimulate the release of VIII-vWF from capillary endothelium. It should be infused slowly, over 20 to 30 minutes, to avoid hypotension. Onset of action occurs in about 30 minutes and may last as long as 12 hours. However, repeat administration is usually associated with tachyphylaxis, presumably because VIII-vWF stores become depleted. Prothrombin time and partial thromboplastin time are usually within normal limits. Uremic coagulopathy may contribute to problems such as menorrhagia and gastrointestinal bleeding, which will worsen the patient's anemia.

Longstanding hypertension may lead to the development of chronic renal failure or may complicate renal failure that was originally caused by other disease processes such as diabetes or systemic lupus. Over time, hypertension frequently results in left ventricular hypertrophy, cardiomegaly, and in some cases, CHF. Arteriovenous fistulae for hemodialysis produce a high-output state that may worsen CHF in susceptible individuals, and pericardial effusions due to chronic uremia may compromise cardiac output further. Patients with renal failure are likely to be taking one or more antihypertensive drugs before surgery and should be instructed to take medications on schedule beforehand. Clonidine, in particular, should not be withdrawn abruptly because of possible rebound hypertensive effect.

Management of acute hypertension in the PACU depends on the hemodynamic state of the patient. After pain is excluded, tachycardia (heart rate greater than 100 beats/minute) suggests the use of β blockers such as esmolol (50 to 300 µg/kg/minute) or metoprolol, or the mixed α-β blocker, labetalol (5 to 20 mg p.r.n.). However, β blockade may increase extracellular potassium concentration and should be used with caution in the presence of hyperkalemia. In this situation, calcium blockers may be preferred. Dihydropyridine derivatives have a pure vasodilator action and are useful especially in the absence of tachycardia. Nifedipine 10 to 20 mg can be given sublingually to patients who cannot yet take oral medications. Alternatively, nicardipine may be given by continuous infusion with a loading dose of 10 to 15 mg/hour for 10 minutes, followed by a maintenance infusion of 3 mg/hour. If tachycardia is a problem, intravenous diltiazem, which has substantial negative chronotropic effects, can be used. The patient is loaded with 5-mg increments every 5 minutes up to a total of 20 mg; thereafter, an infusion of 5 to 20 mg/hour may be given. More severe postoperative hypertension may necessitate the use of sodium nitroprusside (SNP) infusion, which should be started at approximately 0.25 µg/kg/minute and titrated to effect. Esmolol or labetalol may be added to suppress reflex tachycardia and resistance to SNP. Interestingly, patients with renal failure may be less likely to develop cyanide toxicity from nitroprusside, because they do not excrete thiosulfate via the kidney and thus have more thiosulfate available to convert cyanide to thiocyanate (68). However, thiocyanate, a neurotoxin, is dependent on renal elimination and may accumulate.

Renal Transplantation

Postanesthesia care of the patient who has undergone renal transplantation must include consideration of the underlying problems that are likely to accompany chronic renal failure: electrolyte disturbances (especially hyperkalemia), anemia, coagulopathy, hypertension with or without CHF, and lowered resistance to infection. Many patients undergo renal transplantation because of juvenile-onset diabetes, and some of these will require special attention to airway management because of stiff joints, which make intubation difficult. Most kidney transplants are performed under general anesthesia, which commonly includes the use of isoflurane, as the volatile agent that undergoes least metabolism, and atracurium, a muscle relaxant that is not dependent on the kidney for elimination. CVP monitoring is frequently used because generous fluid replacement is indicated after anastomoses of the donor kidney has been completed, and a CVP of 12 to 14 mm Hg is the goal to ensure optimal perfusion. In our institution, mannitol, cyclosporine, and methylprednisolone are given intraoperatively as part of the standard protocol, and steroid therapy is continued in the postoperative period. Unless the patient has underlying pulmonary disease, mechanical ventilation is not usually necessary in the postoperative period, and most patients arrive in the PACU awake and extubated.

An important consideration in the PACU management of patients with chronic renal insufficiency and failure (including successful renal transplantation) is the presence of chronic metabolic acidosis. The acidosis may be caused by hyperchloremia (renal tubular acidosis with failure of bicarbonate excretion is a constant feature of renal insufficiency) or accumulation of nonvolatile acid (phosphates, sulfates, etc). Thus, in the patient just extubated with residual narcosis, even mild to moderate degrees of hypercarbia (e.g., $PaCO_2$ 42 to 44 mm Hg) may lead to substantial acidemia (e.g., pH < 7.25). This in turn could exacerbate hyperkalemia (potassium may rise as much as 0.5 mEg/L with a 0.1 decrease in pH) or cause recurarization after reversal of nondepolarizing muscle relaxants.

Recovery care should include fluid replacement sufficient to maintain a high-normal CVP and close attention to electrolyte levels, remembering that mannitol if it has been given intraoperatively may produce a brisk diuresis. Many patients receive transfusions before or during surgery, both to correct chronic anemia and because blood transfusion has been demonstrated to increase the chance of the transplanted kidney's survival. With adequate volume replacement and a successful transplantation result, urine output in the recovery period should be normal to high, with adequate excretion both of waste products and drugs. A somewhat less successful result may produce a high rate of urine flow but less elimination of toxic waste products; this situation is reminiscent of nonoliguric renal failure but may correct itself if the transplanted kidney is not rejected. Serial 2-hour creatinine clearance estimations may be very helpful in determining the state of function of the transplanted kidney and distinguish between established ATN (less than 12 mL/minute) and a prerenal syndrome or more minor degree of insult (15 to 25 mL/minute). In the former case, aggressive fluid administration should be curtailed, whereas in the latter it may promote renal recovery.

Treatment of hypertension should continue in the postanesthesia period, although it is better to err on the side of higher rather than lower pressure to ensure perfusion of the new kidney. Blood glucose levels may be more difficult to control in diabetic patients because of the glucose intolerance caused by steroid therapy. Although intravenous lines and an indwelling urinary catheter will be necessary for the first 1 to 2 days after transplantation, the goal should be to discontinue them as soon as it is reasonable to do so, because of the risk of infection that may be masked by the administration of steroids.

Transplantation with a kidney from a living related donor usually involves negligible ischemic time and a very high rate of successful graft function. In contrast, cadaveric kidney transplantation commonly involves some degree of transport and donor kidney preservation. A prolonged ischemic interval, especially if longer than 24 hours, may be followed by ATN in the transplanted kidney. A variable period of anuria or oliguria (days or weeks) is usually followed by a diuretic phase that leads to full recovery if the transplant is successful. However, the survival time is decreased by about one-third in grafted kidneys that have undergone ATN.

The most important considerations in patients with oliguria or anuria after renal transplantation are fluid overload (particularly be-

Table 9–3. Management of Acute Hyperkalemia

Antagonize K⁺ at membrane
   Calcium chloride, 1 g over 15–20 minutes

Shift K⁺ into cell
   Hyperventilation
   Sodium bicarbonate, 25–50 mEq
      pH increase of 0.1 can decrease serum K⁺ by
         0.5 mEq/L
   Insulin 5 u + dextrose 25 g infused over 10–15 minutes
   β2 agonists (epinephrine, albuterol)
      [Avoid β blockade]

Na⁺-K⁺ exchange
   Sodium polystyrene resin (Kayexalate) 30 g by enema

Remove K from body
   Hemodialysis
   Peritoneal dialysis
   Continuous venovenous hemodialysis
   Continuous arteriovenous hemodialysis

cause the patient will have been kept very well hydrated intraoperatively) and hyperkalemia. The management of acute hyperkalemia is summarized in Table 9–3. Fluid overload that results in pulmonary congestion or edema that does not respond to diuresis requires urgent dialysis, usually by the same mode used by the patient before surgery. Oliguria associated with a low creatinine clearance may be evaluated by a renal ultrasound (which may reveal urinary tract obstruction), Doppler renal artery flow studies (which can define the sufficiency of arterial supply), and/or radioisotopic scan (which can distinguish between ATN, where perfusion is intact, and cortical necrosis, where perfusion is absent).

GENITOURINARY SURGERY

TURP Syndrome

Transurethral resection of the prostate (TURP), a surgical procedure commonly performed on elderly men with prostatic hypertrophy, is associated with a constellation of intraoperative and postoperative problems that result from the absorption of large amounts of nonelectrolyte irrigating fluid. Circulatory overload, hyponatremia, and serum hypo-osmolality may ensue. The so-called "TURP syndrome" consists of CNS aberrations, including visual disturbances, excessive sedation, and coma, and cardiovascular compromise, including hemodynamic instability and occasional cardiovascular collapse (69–75). It is necessary to use nonelectrolyte solutions as irrigants during TURP because ionized solutions like Ringer's lactate will promote dispersion of high current from the resectoscope; distilled water cannot be used because it would lead to hemolysis of red blood cells. The most common solutions used contain either sorbital and mannitol or glycine 1.5%. The amount of irrigating fluid absorbed may be several liters and is generally believed to be related to the duration of resection although one case report documented a seizure resulting from a serum sodium of 104 mEq/L after a resection time of only 15 minutes (73). Irrigant absorption is also related to the number of opened venous sinuses, which may be greater if the gland is infected, and to the hydrostatic pressure of the irrigating fluid.

The classic case of water intoxication and hyponatremia includes hypertension, bradycardia, agitation, nausea, obtundation, and pulmonary edema. Seizures may occur after the serum sodium falls below 110 mEq/L, and ventricular tachycardia or fibrillation may follow if the level is below 100 mEq/L. The mental confusion and coma are the result of cerebral edema and electrophysiologic disturbances. There are other parts of the picture, however, that are incompletely explained by hyponatremia alone. A direct correlation between the amount of fluid absorbed and the serum sodium level has not, in fact, been demonstrated (70). Some of the CNS symptomatology, most notably the visual disturbances, have been attributed to elevated blood concentrations of ammonia, which is a metabolite of glycine (72). Most recently, Wang et al. measured the serum biochemical profiles of patients undergoing TURP and correlated changes in concentrations of sodium, glycine, and ammonia with abnormalities of vision by changes in visual evoked potentials and electroretinogram (74). They found a significant correlation of both high serum glycine levels and low serum sodium levels in patients who demonstrated electrophysiologic visual abnormalities, but no correlation with increased serum ammonia. One patient with significant visual changes had a high glycine level but a serum sodium nearly normal at 132 mEq/L. These authors concluded that serum sodium and glycine levels both contribute to the manifestations of the TURP syndrome, although glycine seems to have a more specific effect on retinal electrophysiology and probably is responsible for the visual symptoms and occasional transient blindness reported.

Spinal anesthesia frequently is used for TURP because it provides good surgical conditions, is well tolerated by elderly patients who may have coexisting medical problems, and because it allows the anesthesiologist to remain in verbal contact with the patient to recognize early any changes in sensorium that might herald the onset of TURP syndrome. Nonetheless, it is possible for TURP syndrome to present in the PACU. Some patients undergo TURP under general anesthesia because of contraindications to spinal anesthesia (e.g., sepsis, coagulopathy) or because they are averse to spinal anesthesia. If hyponatremia has developed during the resection, it may present as delayed awakening or altered mental status during the recovery period. Any failure to emerge promptly from general anesthesia, or an atypical response to sedation during spinal anesthesia, should lead the PACU physician to evaluate the patient's electrolytes to rule out hyponatremia and to check a serum ammonia level to rule out the less likely alternative of encephalopathy from ammonia toxicity. Mild levels of hyponatremia may be treated by intravenous infusion of normal saline and loop diuretics, with careful follow-up of sodium levels. More severe hyponatremia (<120 mEq/L) may be treated with hypertonic saline as a 3 to 5% solution. Caution must be exercised in the administration of hypertonic saline, which may provoke congestive failure in susceptible patients who are already volume-expanded. It may also be hazardous to raise serum sodium rapidly to levels higher than 120 to 125 mEq/L, which can result in acute shrinkage of brain cells and cause permanent CNS damage. With appropriate management, even patients who are hyponatremic to the point of coma may enjoy complete recovery, but intubation, ventilatory support, and aggressive hemodynamic monitoring may be necessary in the acute phase of the illness.

ACKNOWLEDGMENT

We thank Ms. Kathleen Barbee for her expert assistance in the preparation of the manuscript.

REFERENCES

1. Hou SH, Cohen JJ. Diagnosis and management of acute renal failure. Acute Care 1985;11:59–83.
2. Hou SH, Bushinsky DA, Wish JB, et al. Hospital-acquired renal insufficiency: a prospective study. Am J Med 1983;74:243–248.
3. Anderson RJ, Linas SL, Berns AS, et al. Nonoliguric acute renal failure. N Engl J Med 1977;296:1134–1138.
4. Wilkins RG, Faragher EB. Acute renal failure in an intensive care unit: incidence, prediction and outcome. Anesthesiology 1983;38:628–634.
5. Cioffi WG, Ashikaga T, Gamelli RL. Probability of surveying postoperative acute renal failure: development of a prognostic index. Ann Surg 1984;200:205–211.
6. Kellen M, Aronson S, Roizen MF, Barnard J, Thisted RA. Predictive and diagnostic tests of renal failure: a review. Anesth Analg 1994;78:134–142.
7. Sladen RN. Renal physiology. In: Miller R, ed. Anesthesia, 4th ed. New York: Churchill Livingstone, 1994;663–688.
8. Brezis M, Rosen S, Silva P, et al. Selective vulnerability of the medullary thick ascending limb to anoxia in the isolated perfused rat kidney. J Clin Invest 1984;74:182–190.
9. Shipley RE, Study RS. Changes in renal blood flow, extraction of inulin glomerular filtration rate, tissue pressure and urine flow with acute alterations of renal artery pressure. Am J Physiol 1951;167:676.
10. Schaer GL, Fink MP, Parrillo JE. Norepinephrine alone versus norepinephrine plus low-dose dopamine: enhance renal blood flow with combination pressor therapy. Crit Care Med 1985;13:492.
11. Miller ED. Renal effects of dopamine (editorial views). Anesthesiology 1984;61:487–488.
12. Hilberman M, Maseda J, Stinson EB, et al. The diuretic properties of dopamine in patients after open heart operation. Anesthesiology 1984;61:489–494.
13. Hricik D, Browning P, Kopelman R, et al. Captopril-induced functional renal insufficiency in patients with bilateral renal-artery stenoses or renal-artery stenosis in a solitary kidney. N Engl J Med 1983;308:373.
14. Bender W, La France N, Walker W. Mechanism of deterioration of renal function in patients with renovascular hypertension treated with epalapril. Hypertension 1984;1(Suppl 6):I193.
15. Badr KF, Ichikawa I. Prerenal failure: a deleterious shift from renal compensation to decompression. N Engl J Med 1988;319:623–629.
16. Hays RM. Cell biology in vasopressin. In: Brenner BM, Rector FCJ, eds. The kidney. 4th ed. Philadelphia: WB Saunders, 1991;424.
17. Bartter FC, Schwartz WB. The syndrome of inappropriate secretion of antidiuretic hormone. Am J Med 1967;42:790.
18. Ballerman BJ, Zeidel ML, Gunning ME, et al. Vasoactive peptides and the kidney. In: Brenner BM, Rector FCJ, eds. The kidney. 4th ed. Philadelphia: WB Saunders, 1991;520.
19. Tobimatsu M, Konomi K, Saito S, et al. Protective effect of prostaglandin E₁ on ischemia-induced acute renal failure in dogs. Surgery 1985;98:45.
20. Johnston P, Bernard D, Perrin N, et al. Prostaglandins mediate the vasodilatory effect of mannitol in the hypoperfused rat kidney. J Clin Invest 1981;68:127.
21. Clive D, Stoff J. Renal syndromes associated with nonsteriodal antiinflammatory drugs. N Engl J Med 1984;310:563.
22. Mazze RI, Calvery RK, Smith NT. Inorganic fluoride nephrotoxicity: prolonged enflurane and halothane anesthesia in volunteers. Anesthesiology 1977;46:265–271.
23. Priano LL. The effects of anesthesia on renal blood flow and function. In: Barash PG, ed. Refresher courses in anesthesiology. Park Ridge, IL: American Society of Anesthesiologists, 1985;143–156.
24. Bastron RD, Perkins FM, Pyne JL. Autoregulation of renal blood flow during halothane anesthesia. Anesthesiology 1977;46:142–144.
25. Mazze RI, Sievenpiper TS, Stevenson J. Renal effects of enflurane and halothane in patients with abnormal renal function. Anesthesiology 1984;60:161–163.
26. Mazze RI, Cousins MJ, Barr GA. Renal effects and metabolism of isoflurane in man. Anesthesiology 1974;40:536–542.
27. Lundeen G, Manohar M, Parks C. Systemic distribution of blood flow in swine while awake and during 1–1.5 MAC isoflurane anesthesia with or without 50% nitrous oxide. Anesth Analg 1983;62:499–512.
27a. Kharasch ED, Hankins DC, Thummel KE. Human kidney methoxyflurane and sevoflurane metabolism: intrarenal fluoride production as a possible mechanism of methoxyflurane nephrotoxicity. Anesthesiology 1995;82:689–699.
28. Priano LL. Alteration of renal hymodynamics by thiopental, diazepam, and ketamine in conscious dogs. Anesth Analg 1982;61:853–862.
29. Priano LL. Renal hemodynamic alterations following administration of thiopental, diazepam and ketamine

in conscious hypovolemic dogs. Adv Shock Res 1983;9:173–188.

30. Weiskopf RB, Townley MI, Riordan KK, et al. Comparison of cardiopulmonary responses to graded hemorrhage during enflurane, halothane, isoflurane and ketamine anesthesia. Anesth Analg 1981; 60:481–492.

31. Stoelting RK. Nonbarbiturate induction drugs. In: Stoelting RK, ed. Pharmacology and physiology in anesthetic practice. 2nd ed. Philadelphia: JB Lippincott Company, 1991;142–145.

32. Ledingham IMcA, Watt I. Influence of sedation on mortality in critically ill multiple trauma patients. Lancet 1983;1:1270.

33. Wagner RL, White PF. Etomidate inhibits adrenocortical function in surgical patients. Anesthesiology 1984;61:647–651.

34. Fragen RJ, Shanks CA, Molteni A, et al. Effects of etomidate on hormonal responses to surgical stress. Anesthesiology 1984;61:652–656.

35. Sebel PS, Lowdon JD. Propofol: a new intravenous anesthetic. Anesthesiology 1989;71:260–277.

36. Azari DM, Cork RC. Comparative myocardial depressive effects of propofol and thiopental. Anesth Analg 1993;77:324–329.

37. Priano LL, Vatner SF. Morphine effects on cardiac output and regional blood flow distribution in conscious dogs. Anesthesiology 1981;55:236–243.

38. Kono K, Philbin DM, Coggins CH, et al. Renal function and stress response during halothane or fentanyl anesthesia. Anesth Analg 1981;60:522.

39. Stanley TH, Philbin DM, Coggins CH. Fentanyl-oxygen anesthesia for coronary artery surgery: cardiovascular and antidiuretic hormone responses. Can J Anaesth 1979;26:168.

40. Stanley TH, Berman L, Green O, et al. Plasma catecholamine responses to fentanyl-oxygen anesthesia for coronary artery operation. Anesthesiology 1980;53:250.

41. Greene NM, Brull SJ. Renal function. In: Greene NM, Brull SJ, eds. Physiology of spinal anesthesia. 4th ed. Baltimore: Williams & Wilkins, 1993;263–279.

42. Sartorius OW, Burlington H. Acute effects of denervation on kidney function in the dog. Am J Physiol 1956;185:407.

43. Mokotoff R, Ross G. Effect of spinal anesthesia on the renal ischemia in congestive heart failure. J Clin Invest 1948;27:335.

44. Sivarajan M, Amory DW, Lindbloom LE, et al. Systematic and regional blood-flow changes during spinal anesthesia in the Rhesus monkey. Anesthesiology 1975;43:78.

45. Brun C, Crone C, Davidsen HG, et al. Renal interstitial pressure in normal and in anuric man based on wedged renal vein pressure. Proc Soc Exp Biol Med 1956;91:199.

46. Butterworth JF, Piccione W, Berrizbeitia LD, et al. Augmentation of venous return by adrenergic agonists during spinal anesthesia. Anesth Analg 1986;65:612.

47. Ellenbogen PH, Scheible FW, Talner LB, Leopold GR. Sensitivity of gray ultrasound in detecting urinary tract obstruction. Am J Roentgenol 1978;130:731–733.

48. Bennett W, Plamp C, Porter G. Drug related syndromes in clinical nephrology. Ann Intern Med 1977;87:582–590.

49. Wilkes BM, Mailloux LU. Acute renal failure: pathogenesis and prevention. Am J Med 1986;80:1129–1136.

50. Myers BD, Moran SM. Hemodynamically mediated acute renal failure. N Engl J Med 1986;314:97–105.

51. Byrick RJ, Rose DK. Pathophysiology and prevention of acute renal failure: the role of the anaesthetist. Can J Anaesth 1990;37:457–467.

52. Shin B, Mackenzie CF, McAslan TC, et al. Postoperative renal failure in trauma patients. Anesthesiology 1979;51:218–221.

53. MacKenzie CR, Charlson ME. Assessment of perioperative risk in the patient with diabetes mellitus. Surg Gynecol Obstet 1988;167:293–299.

54. Novis BK, Roizen MF, Aronson S, Thisted RA. Association of preoperative risk factors with postoperative acute renal failure. Anesth Analg 1994;78:143–149.

55. Charlson ME, MacKenzie R, Gold JP, et al. Postoperative renal dysfunction can be predicted. Surg Gynecol Obstet 1989;169:303–309.

56. Wait RB, Kahng KU. Renal failure complicating obstructive jaundice. Am J Surg 1989;157:256–263.

57. Gamulin Z, Forster A, Morel D, et al. Effects of infrarenal aortic cross-clamping on renal hemodynamics in humans. Anesthesiology 1984;61:394–399.

58. Alpert RA, Roizen MF, Hamilton WK, et al. Intraoperative urinary output does not predict renal function in patients undergoing abdominal aortic revascularization. Surgery 1984;95:707–711.

59. Gornick CC, Kjellstrand CM. Acute renal failure complicating aortic aneurysm surgery. Nephron 1983;35:145–157.

60. Cohen JR, Mannick JA, Couch NP, Whittemore AD. Abdominal aortic aneurysm repair in patients with preoperative renal failure. J Vasc Surg 1986;3:867–870.

61. Sladen RN. Accurate estimation of glomerular filtration in the intensive care unit: another holy grail? Crit Care Med 1993;21:1424–1427.

62. Sladen RN, Endo E, Harrison T. Two-hour versus 22-hour creatinine clearance in critically ill patients. Anesthesiology 1987;67:1013–1016.

63. Shin B, Mackenzie C, Helrich M. Creatinine clearance for early detection of postraumatic renal dysfunction. Anesthesiology 1986;64:605–609.

64. Sladen RN. Perioperative renal protection. ASA Annual Refresher Course Lectures, Lecture 213. Chicago: American Society of Anesthesiologists, 1994.

65. Andreoli TE. The posterior pituitary. In: Wyngaarden JB, Smith LH, eds. Cecil textbook of medicine. Philadelphia: WB Saunders, 1985;1266–1273.

66. Stoelting RK, Dierdorf SF, McCammon RL. Anesthesia and co-existing disease. New York: Churchill Livingstone, 1988;473–515.

67. Maddern PJ. Anaesthesia for the patient with impaired renal function Anaesth Intens Care 1983;11:321.

68. Stoelting RK, Dierdorf SF, McCammon RL. Anesthesia and co-existing disease. New York: Churchill Livingstone, 1988;409–444.
69. Wong KC. Transurethral resection of the prostate: anesthetic implications. Cleveland, OH: International Anesthesia Research Society, 1984;191–197.
70. Zucker JR, Bull AP. Independent plasma levels of sodium and glycine during transurethral resection of the prostate. Can Anaesth Soc J 1984;31:307–313.
71. Still JA, Modell JH. Acute water intoxication during transurethral resection of the prostate, using glycine solution for irrigation. Anesthesiology 1973;38:98–99.
72. Roesch RP, Stoelting RK, Lingeman JE, et al. Ammonia toxicity resulting from glycine absorption during a transurethral resection of the prostate. Anesthesiology 1983;58:577–579.
73. Hurlbert BJ, Wingard DW. Water intoxication after 15 minutes of transurethral resection of the prostate. Anesthesiology 1979;50:355–356.
74. Wang JM, Creel DJ, Wong KC. Transurethral resection of the prostate, serum glycine levels, and ocular evoked potentials. Anesthesiology 1989;70:36–41.
75. Marx GF, Orkin LR. Complications associated with transurethral surgery. Anesthesiology 1962;23:802–813.

10
NEUROLOGIC SYSTEM

Deborah Culley, Gregory Crosby

Central nervous system (CNS) dysfunction is a fundamental characteristic of the anesthetic state. In fact, general anesthesia would not occur without it. Because some degree of transient postoperative CNS impairment is a natural consequence of most forms of anesthesia, it is sometimes a challenge to identify, let alone treat, the rare but potentially devastating neurologic complications that do occur infrequently in anesthetized patients. Accordingly, the first part of this chapter focuses on perioperative CNS complications of anesthesia and surgery, including cognitive and psychologic consequences of anesthesia, new neurologic deficits after "routine" procedures, and neurologic risks inherent in carotid and cardiac procedures. The second part of this chapter deals with the neurologic complications of spinal and epidural anesthesia as well as perioperative peripheral nerve injury.

However, a few words of caution are warranted. Most data on neurologic dysfunction in the perioperative period are epidemiologic in nature; rarely have cause: effect relationships been established directly. Nevertheless, the information presented aims to help the clinician develop a rational and realistic approach to anticipating, identifying, and managing neurologic dysfunction in the perioperative period.

COGNITIVE AND NEUROLOGIC DYSFUNCTION AFTER "ROUTINE" SURGERY

Cognitive and Psychomotor Dysfunction as a Part of Normal Recovery

It is not possible to administer a general anesthetic without also producing postoperative CNS dysfunction. This is because CNS dysfunction is the goal of general anesthesia, and drugs used for premedication, induction, and maintenance have some lingering CNS effects. Even drugs such as midazolam and methohexital, which are generally regarded to have a short duration of action, may produce relatively long-lasting CNS dysfunction (1–3). In contrast, volunteers who have induction of anesthesia with propofol return to baseline psychomotor function within 1 hour, but if propofol is combined with other drugs or is used for maintenance of anesthesia, the duration of cognitive dysfunction is longer (4, 5). Inhalation anesthetics, of course, also have prolonged effects on mental function. In fact, psychomotor performance is worsened significantly for 5 hours following only 3–1/2 minutes of anesthesia with halothane or enflurane in normal volunteers (6). In contrast, psychomotor performance after desflurane seems to return to baseline within about 60 minutes of discontinuation of the anesthetic (7) and allows earlier recovery of cognitive functions than isoflurane (8). All of these sequelae of general anesthesia are transient, however, and there is no evidence for permanent changes in memory and cognitive ability (9–12). Even in elderly patients, careful neuropsychologic testing yields no evidence to suggest a decrement in performance 1 to several months after anesthesia relative to preanesthesia scores (13, 14). Interestingly, the short- and longer-term psychologic and cognitive effects of general and regional anesthesia are similar, particularly if intravenous sedation is used to supplement a regional technique (10–12, 15–17). Almost by definition, however, these changes are considered side effects — the "cost of doing business" — rather than complications of anesthesia and are fundamentally benign and self-limited. The more worrisome types of postoperative CNS dysfunction begin with delirium and include permanent structural or functional damage to the nervous system.

Postoperative Delirium

Delirium is not simply an exaggerated form of "normal" postoperative CNS dysfunction (14). The differential diagnosis is extensive (18–20) and of more than academic interest because postoperative delirium can be a warning of serious but treatable underlying pathology. Many causes of postoperative delirium are not treatable, however (18–23). Preexisting organic brain disease, psychiatric disorders, the extremes of age (14, 15, 24, 25), and the type of surgery — particularly cardiac (14, 15, 25–27), ophthalmologic (25, 28), and hip repair (17, 25, 29) — as well as prolonged ICU care (14) all increase the risk of postoperative delirium. On emergence, delirium also may be a manifestation of awareness during anesthesia (30, 31) and is presumably a response to stress. Of most clinical interest are the potentially treatable causes of postoperative delirium. In particular, conditions that result in an imbalance of the normally close relationship between cerebral oxygen supply and demand are the most ominous and important to recognize. Thus, cerebral hypoxia (14,

18, 22, 25, 29, 32–34) must be considered immediately in any patient who presents with delirium in the perioperative period. Only after the possibility of cerebral hypoxia has been excluded should one consider other treatable causes of delirium such as endocrine or ionic imbalances, postoperative pain, bowel or bladder distension, language difficulties, the porphyrias (acute intermittent and variegata), sepsis, and drugs (14, 15, 19–22, 25).

Medication history is an important component in the evaluation of the patient with delirium. High-dose steroids may produce an acute psychotic reaction (35) and delirium may occur during withdrawal from drugs of abuse such as alcohol, opiates, and hallucinogens (24). Certain anesthetic agents and adjuvants have also been implicated in postoperative confusional states. Ketamine, a derivative of phencyclidine (PCP), has hallucinogenic and convulsive properties that are related primarily to the negative stereoisomer in the racemic clinical preparation; emergence delirium, as well as vivid unpleasant dreams, perceptual distortion, disorientation, agitation, and nightmares, may occur (35). The incidence of psychologic disturbances associated with ketamine can be reduced by administration of benzodiazepines (36–38) and, possibly, the newer agent, dexmedetomidine (39). For unknown reasons, elderly persons and young children are less likely to experience the troublesome CNS effects of ketamine (40). Anticholinergic medications such as atropine and scopolamine are another classic pharmacologic cause of postoperative confusion, particularly in elderly patients (14, 15, 34, 41–43). Glycopyrrolate, however, has essentially no CNS effects because its quaternary ammonium structure prevents it from crossing the blood-brain barrier (41). In some situations, the psychotropic or neurologic effects of other anesthetic agents and adjuvants could be mistaken for a perioperative confusional state. Droperidol, a butyrophenone, has psychotropic effects characterized by severe dysphoria and ill-defined anxiety (44) and may also produce extrapyramidal reactions (45) that respond well to treatment with diphenhydramine. Propofol also has been implicated in a variety of unusual perioperative behaviors and symptoms, including hallucinations (46), bad dreams, muscular hypotonus (47, 48), abnormal posturing (49), amorous behavior (50), difficulty with eye opening (51), and possibly seizures (48, 52–56). The etiology of these problems is unknown and treatment is supportive. Because the pharmacologic causes of postanesthetic delirium are fundamentally benign and self-limited, it is most important to be certain that delirium is not attributed mistakenly to a drug effect when cerebral hypoxia or some other correctable metabolic disturbance is actually the cause.

New Neurologic Impairment

In contrast to the ubiquitous but essentially benign consequences of general anesthesia, major neurologic complications such as stroke, seizures, or hypoxia after nonneurologic, noncardiac surgery are rare but very serious. In a prospective, randomized study (57) of outcome after anesthesia in 17,201 patients, only 7 patients (0.04%) had a stroke and a retrospective study (58) reported an even lower incidence of new focal deficits upon emergence from anesthesia. Elderly patients (59) and those undergoing peripheral vascular surgical procedures (60, 61) are at higher risk for perioperative stroke, presumably because of coexisting cerebral or carotid vascular disease. Seizures and hypoxic brain injury also occur, but these events are even less frequent than stroke (62). From the perspective of a patient recovering from anesthesia, the central questions are how does one distinguish between cerebral pathology and "normal" CNS dysfunction and, if a neurologic event is identified, what, if anything, can be done?

PERIOPERATIVE STROKE

Development of a new focal neurologic deficit during the perioperative period is un-common and unpredictable but perhaps not random (58, 63, 64). Moreover, predisposing factors are not always obvious. An asymptomatic carotid bruit, which is present in about 14% of surgical patients 55 years of age or older and in about 20% of vascular surgical patients, is not a risk factor for perioperative stroke (65, 66), even though carotid endarterectomy improves long-term outcome in patients with high-grade carotid stenosis (67–69). The relationship between symptomatic cerebrovascular disease and perioperative stroke is controversial. A few studies (70, 71) have indicated that patients with transient ischemic attacks (TIAs) or amaurosis fugax have a significantly higher incidence of stroke in the perioperative period than asymptomatic individuals, but others refute any such relationship (72, 73). However, because carotid endarterectomy improves long-term neurologic outcome in symptomatic patients with high-grade stenosis (74–76), it would be prudent in this situation to consider repairing the carotid lesion before undertaking elective surgery. Finally, the surgical patient who has had a recent stroke seems to be at greater risk for cerebral reinfarction (77), but because the vulnerability to reinfarction does not seem to decrease with time, there is uncertainty regarding whether elective surgery should be delayed. Intraoperative hypotension is another time-honored explanation for perioperative stroke, but studies indicate that many patients who suffer a postoperative stroke experienced and survived intraoperative hypotension without neurologic sequelae (63, 71, 72). More direct evidence regarding hypotension as a cause of stroke comes from a study (78) of 37 patients with TIAs deliberately exposed to nearly a 60% decrease in systolic blood pressure. Such profound hypotension recreated a true TIA in only one individual; some patients developed unrelated focal signs, but 17 had no focal findings at all. Nevertheless, no one would suggest that hypotension is benign; if severe enough and sustained, it certainly can produce irreversible neurologic injury (79). Thrombotic and embolic events, which are common causes of stroke in nonhospitalized patients with cerebrovascular disease (80), are probably also responsible for most perioperative strokes. Cardiogenic embolism was considered the most common mechanism of cerebral infarction in a retrospective review (63), accounting for 5 of 12 (42%) perioperative strokes, whereas only one stroke was attributed to hypotension. Similarly, among three recently reported cases of new focal neurologic deficits detected upon emergence from anesthesia, two were attributed to embolism (one cardiogenic, the other paradoxic embolism of CO_2) and one was caused by a cerebral hemorrhage (58).

PERIOPERATIVE SEIZURES

Perioperative seizures may be idiopathic or related to hypoxia, metabolic disorders such as hypocalcemia and hypoglycemia, fever, occult concomitant CNS diseases (e.g., cerebrovascular diseases, brain tumor) (81) or anesthetic agents (82, 83). Enflurane, for instance, produces epileptiform EEG activity, with maximal EEG spiking at end-tidal concentrations of 2–3% and grand mal seizure patterns at 3–6% (84, 85). Hyperventilation increases enflurane-induced seizure activity and hypoventilation decreases it such that the minimum epileptogenic concentration is approximately 1% lower at $PaCO_2$ of 20 mm Hg and 1% higher at $PaCO_2$ of 60 mm Hg than it is at 40 mm Hg (84, 85). Even though seizures have been reported hours to days after enflurane anesthesia in nonepileptic patients (86–91), EEG documentation of postoperative seizure activity is rare (86, 91, 92). In volunteers followed for 6–30 days with surface electroencephalogram (EEG) recordings after receiving 9.6 MAC hours of enflurane, only nonepileptiform changes were noted even though one-half of the volunteers had clinical and EEG evidence of seizures during anesthesia (93). It is also interesting that enflurane, like most anesthetics, has anticonvulsant properties (94). Halothane (95, 96), isoflurane (97–99), and nitrous oxide (95) also have been the subject of isolated case reports of seizure-like

activity during exposure, but none are believed to cause postoperative seizures.

Seizure activity also has been associated with certain intravenous anesthetics. Etomidate produces involuntary myoclonic movements that occasionally persist into the recovery period (100–102), but this myoclonic activity is not associated with EEG spikes in nonepileptic patients (100, 103, 104). Etomidate does provoke seizures in a large percentage of epileptic patients (94, 105–107), but there is no good evidence that such intraoperative events increase the risk of postoperative seizures. Similarly, ketamine and propofol activate epileptogenic foci (53, 108, 109) but do not produce electroencephalographic seizures in nonepileptic patients (54, 83, 110–115). In fact, propofol reduces seizure duration during electroconvulsive therapy (116–118) and has been used successfully to treat status epilepticus (119). In contrast, methohexital, well known to produce excitatory phenomena such as tremor and muscle movements, has not been demonstrated to precipitate clinical or EEG seizures in patients with generalized convulsive disorders but is epileptogenic in patients with psychomotor epilepsy (120–122).

There has been some concern about the seizure potential of narcotic analgesics as well. Meperidine, or more accurately, its metabolite normeperidine, may produce tremulousness, myoclonus, and seizures (123–125). Because normeperidine has a long half-life (14–21 hours), this effect may persist into the postoperative period, particularly in patients with reduced clearance caused by renal failure (126) or in those receiving very large doses of meperidine for chronic pain (126, 127). Morphine, on the other hand, has no documented seizure activity in humans (83). There are reports of grand-mal seizure-like behavior after administration of fentanyl, sufentanil, and alfentanil (128–136). However, whereas most studies have failed to document abnormal EEG patterns in patients treated with fentanyl or its analogs (137–142), some report isolated sharp wave activity (137, 138). In one study, epileptiform discharges were observed in 19 of 20 patients within 3 minutes of the administration of fentanyl or sufentanil (143). Nonetheless, evidence that intraoperative seizure activity increases the risk of postoperative seizures, even in seizure-prone patients, is weak.

CLINICAL EVALUATION OF PERIOPERATIVE CNS DYSFUNCTION

Emergence from anesthesia may be neurologically unsatisfactory because of prolonged drowsiness, delirium, a focal neurologic deficit, or even true coma (i.e., unresponsiveness to painful stimuli). The most important diagnostic question in such a situation is whether the problem is caused by exaggerated anesthetic-induced dysfunction or a neurologic event.

Data specifically concerning neurologic recovery after anesthesia are surprisingly few. In one study (57) involving more than 17,000 patients randomized to receive one of four anesthetic agents (enflurane, halothane, isoflurane, and fentanyl), 6% and 3% were scored as "not recovered" at 60 and 90 minutes after anesthesia, respectively. Because the incidence of stroke and other major CNS events in this population was only 0.04%, one can safely assume that non-CNS problems (e.g., protracted vomiting, pain, hemodynamic or respiratory instability) accounted for low recovery scores in most patients. Outpatients who received about 1 hour of propofol or thiopental-isoflurane anesthesia responded to commands, opened their eyes, and were oriented within about 10 minutes of discontinuing nitrous oxide (144). However, a prospective study involving all surgical patients admitted to the recovery room during a single month reported that 41 of 443 patients (9%) were unarousable for as long as 15–90 minutes after entering the recovery room even though none had a neurologic event (145). This illustrates two features of postanesthesia neurologic recovery: (a) most patients awaken promptly after anesthesia, but the variability is quite large; and (b) delayed arousal is much more commonly due to drug effects than neurologic events.

The first step in evaluating a patient whose emergence from anesthesia is abnormal or delayed is to perform a neurologic examination. It is essential to recognize that even neurologically normal patients awakening from anesthesia frequently have abnormal eye signs and "pathologic" reflexes (146). Indeed, 40–100% of neurologically normal patients have an absent pupillary response to light 20 minutes after anesthesia and in 10% of patients, the pupillary and lid responses can be depressed for 40 minutes (146). Bicep and quadricep hyperreflexia, sustained and unsustained ankle clonus, and a plantar (Babinski) reflex occur in a large percentage of neurologically intact patients recovering from anesthesia and, in many cases, abnormalities are present even when patients are fully awake (146). The type of anesthesia influences the incidence of transient neurologic abnormalities. Abnormal reflexes occur more commonly in patients recovering from enflurane or halothane than from nitrous-oxide-narcotic anesthesia (146) and in those who receive thiopental or diazepam (147). Age is also a factor; younger patients seem to be more likely to exhibit abnormal reflexes on emergence than the elderly (147). A variety of other transient neurologic abnormalities have been reported during recovery from anesthesia; opisthotonus (49) and difficulty with eye opening have been associated with propofol, extrapyramidal reaction has been associated with droperidol, (45) and seizures have been associated with several agents (82, 83). Attention to eye signs is important because ophthalmoplegia may signal thrombosis of the basilar artery (148) and visual disturbances may not be immediately apparent in a somnolent patient. Surprisingly, transient neurologic abnormalities that occur in normal patients emerging from general anesthesia are not always bilateral. Thus, unilateral reflex changes, which are always a worrisome finding but are particularly so in a unresponsive patient, can occur in the course of normal neurologic recovery from anesthesia (147). In most cases, however, these drug-induced changes resolve shortly after anesthesia is discontinued. As such, persistence of these neurologic abnormalities, particularly if the patient's level of consciousness remains depressed, is most worrisome.

Another issue to be considered when evaluating CNS dysfunction in the immediate postanesthetic period is that centrally acting drugs can exacerbate or unmask occult CNS pathology. For example, small dosages of sedating drugs such as fentanyl and midazolam can, sometimes dramatically, worsen an existing or recently resolved focal motor deficit (149). Like the reflex abnormalities one sees in otherwise normal patients recovering from anesthesia, this unmasking of underlying neurologic disease is transient and benign. Thus, in the case of a patient awakening from anesthesia with seemingly new focal motor weakness, a history of a focal motor deficit involving the same region of the body should be sought and the diagnosis of anesthetic-induced exacerbation or unmasking of this occult problem should be considered.

Because CNS dysfunction is produced deliberately with induction of general anesthesia, an exaggerated drug effect or response is the most likely cause of delayed emergence. However, only by excluding the possibility of an exaggerated drug effect can one be sure that a prolonged deficit is not due to a neurologic event. Since an individual patient may have received several drugs capable of obtunding consciousness, identifying a pharmacologic cause of delayed or abnormal arousal may not be easy. A relative narcotic overdosage might be suspected clinically in a patient with slow, deep inspirations and pinpoint pupils, whereas midposition pupils and rapid shallow breathing may suggest a lingering inhalation agent. The possibility of continuing neuromuscular blockade, which might limit patient cooperation but does not explain drowsiness or un-

consciousness, can be evaluated in standard fashion by hand grasp strength, ability to sustain a head lift, or by train-of-four testing (see Chapter 6). More often than not, a combination of drugs, rather than a single agent, is the cause of delayed emergence. This situation is further complicated by the fact that only a few anesthetic agents and adjuvants have pharmacologic antagonists. In this context, pharmacologic antagonists such as naloxone, flumazenil, and physostigmine should be viewed as diagnostic aids, not therapy. Considering the limited selection of antagonists and the multiplicity of drugs a patient may have received, one must be pragmatic; if in doubt, reverse what can be reversed. The goal of this approach is to permit a brief period of arousal during which clinical neurologic evaluation can be performed (150, 151).

Residual drug-induced paralysis is usually corrected easily with an anticholinesterase and antimuscarinic agent such as atropine or glycopyrrolate. If narcotics have been administered, a very small dose of naloxone (40–80 μg intravenously) typically will reverse respiratory depression and awaken the patient transiently without intensifying incisional pain or producing nausea and vomiting (150). Some caution should be exercised when using naloxone, however, because on rare occasions even small doses may produce severe hypertension and arrythmias (152, 153). An attempt to reverse the CNS effects of an inhalational agent with a nonspecific analeptic such as physostigmine should be considered. Physostigmine (2 mg intravenously) produces transient EEG arousal and few side effects, but clinical arousal is unreliable and short-lived. Physostigmine is the antagonist of choice for CNS depression caused by scopolamine or atropine (154) and may produce improvement in postoperative somnolence caused by benzodiazepines (155). Flumazenil produces prompt recovery from benzodiazepine sedation with minimal side effects and is useful for the postoperative patient whose emergence is believed to be delayed or clouded by the lingering effects of diazepam or midazolam (156, 157). The underlying assumption of this approach is simple: if a patient is arousable (even if only transiently) by pharmacologic means and is neurologically intact, no further evaluation is necessary and recovery from anesthesia can proceed naturally. Judgments regarding the need for continued support such as intubation and mechanical ventilation in such patients should be made according to the usual criteria, recognizing that the clinical effects of anesthetic antagonists are typically brief.

Failure to awaken sufficiently to assess alterations in level of consciousness and motor function despite passing of a reasonable period of time requires an active search for other causes of prolonged coma. A careful review of the history, particularly with respect to previous transient ischemic attacks, subarachnoid hemmorrhage, seizures, or medical conditions that are associated with coma — e.g., diabetes (158), porphyria (159) — is essential (160). Hypothermia may delay awakening (161, 162), particularly in elderly patients, but coma does not occur unless body temperature is 18–21°C (73). Chronic medications, such as cimetidine (163), may slow metabolism or elimination of anesthetic drugs and adjuvants. Severe hyperglycemia (158), hyperosmolarity, and illicit drug usage also should be considered at this stage. An active seizure focus can depress consciousness, but in the absence of gross tonic-clonic movements, the diagnosis requires EEG documentation. Finally, an unrecognized preexisting intracranial mass lesion such as a meningioma or new intracerebral hemorrhage may delay emergence from anesthesia (164).

If a new and persistent focal neurologic deficit is identified, both additional diagnostic procedures and neurologic consultation are required. The history should be reviewed carefully for cardiac conditions such as arrhythmias, recent myocardial infarction, and intracardiac shunts that could predispose to emboli (58, 63). A thorough auscultatory examination of the heart should be performed with the same objective. Considering the high incidence of embolic causes of stroke (58, 63), an echocardiogram can be diagnostically helpful and is essential whenever the history or physical examination is suggestive of an intracardiac source for emboli. A precordial echocardiogram is not reliable for detecting a patent foramen ovale, however, and so a negative study does not eliminate the possibility of a paradoxic embolism (165). A computed tomography (CT) scan is required to identify an intracranial mass lesion such as tumor or hemorrhage and, if contrast is used, may help identify a vascular anomaly (such as arteriovenous malformation) as well. Until recently, ischemic areas were not identifiable radiographically for hours to days after the event (166). However, newer diagnostic modalities such as perfusion-weighted magnetic resonance imaging (MRI) (167) and perfusion imaging (168) permit the detection of ischemic zones within the brain in as few as 3 hours after the onset of neurologic symptoms.

Early detection becomes important as promising new therapeutic modalities to reverse or minimize the permanent consequences of injury are tested. Some strategies to ameliorate ischemic neuronal injury are based on improved understanding of the pathophysiology of cerebral ischemia, particularly with respect to the neurotoxic potential of calcium and excitatory amino acid neurotransmitters (169, 170). The results in this regard are conflicting, however. One prospective, randomized, placebo-controlled, double-blinded study (171) indicated that nimodipine improved neurologic outcome and reduced mortality in patients suffering an acute ischemic stroke, whereas a more recent study (172) failed to confirm these results. Interest in the use of thrombolytic agents to decrease morbidity and mortality after stroke has increased. Investigations are ongoing to evaluate the use of intra-arterial thrombolytics in the setting of acute stroke (173–175). Intravenous thrombolysis with tissue plasminogen activator has provided mixed results; in one study, improvement in neurologic outcome was identified in only one subgroup of patients (176), whereas another study reported improved clinical outcomes at 3 months (177). Finally, subcutaneous low-molecular-weight heparin seems to be effective in improving outcome from acute ischemic stroke at 6 months (178). A new area of interest concerns the potential for a variety of commonly used drugs to adversely affect neurologic outcome from stroke. A recent retrospective review (179) identified a direct correlation between poor outcome and the use of benzodiazepines, dopamine antagonists, α_2 agonists, α_1 antagonists, and phenytoin or phenobarbitol in the first 28 days after stroke. The authors freely admit that there is no proof that the drugs cause the poor outcome, but it suggests that common drugs can have unanticipated neurologic consequences for patients with ischemia.

NEUROLOGIC DYSFUNCTION AFTER "HIGH RISK" SURGERY

Carotid Endarterectomy

The most common cause of neurologic dysfunction after carotid endarterectomy (CEA) is stroke. This is not surprising, considering that CEA is the clinical prototype of transient focal cerebral ischemia with reperfusion (180–182). Based on several large recent prospective studies of CEA, the overall risk of stroke and death for the procedure must be 5–6% or less (183) to be considered acceptable (184). Indeed, inasmuch as prospective, randomized studies of both asymptomatic (67) and symptomatic patients with severe carotid stenosis (greater than 60%) (74–76) have documented improved neurologic outcome with surgery as compared to medical management, one can anticipate a growing number of these cases.

Stroke in the perioperative period of CEA may be caused by hypoperfusion because of carotid cross-clamping, emboli occurring during shunt insertion or reperfusion of the carotid, (185) or reperfusion cerebral hyperemia (186). Contrary to the common perception, many strokes during CEA are probably not related to cerebral hypoperfusion caused by carotid cross-clamping. In fact, studies of CEA performed under local anesthesia in awake patients (187–190) or with EEG monitoring in anesthetized patients (191) indicate that stroke is commonly embolic in origin because neurologic events often occur at the moment of clamping or reperfusion of the carotid. Transcranial doppler studies support this idea; there is an increase in high-intensity transient signals compatible with microembolism in the middle cerebral artery at the time of shunting and unclamping (192). Furthermore, strokes commonly occur postoperatively (190, 193). Thus, because many strokes associated with CEA are related to surgical technique and occur postoperatively (190, 193–197), the degree to which it is possible to prevent neurologic complications during CEA by meticulous intraoperative management may be limited.

Nevertheless, intraoperative physiologic and anesthetic management may be important in terms of reducing the risk of cerebral ischemic events. A goal of management, therefore, is to prevent ischemia by maintaining an acceptable balance between cerebral metabolic demand and blood supply or, alternatively, to minimize the consequences of cerebral ischemia before it becomes severe enough to produce permanent CNS injury. In practice, this requires following neurologic status in awake patients under local anesthesia or using an index of cerebral ischemia such as EEG or, possibly, transcranial doppler (TCD) in anesthetized patients, because stump pressure (181, 198) and transconjunctival oxygen tension (199) correlate poorly with regional cerebral flood flow. Routine shunting without EEG monitoring, selective shunting with EEG (200), surgery under superficial cervical plexus block (201), and evaluation using TCD each has proponents (202, 203), but whether one approach leads to improved neurologic outcome remains controversial. EEG changes are not necessarily indicative of irreversible neuronal injury and direct comparison of EEG and neurologic examination during CEA performed under local anesthesia indicates that both false-positive and false-negative EEGs occur (204). However, agreement between the two is usually good. Whether EEG monitoring positively influences neurologic outcome from CEA remains a matter of speculation. Although no prospective, controlled studies have yet been performed, major, untreated, cross-clamp-associated EEG changes are predictive of stroke in some patients (191, 205) and, in large centers, the incidence of stroke without new, persistent EEG changes is less than 0.5%. Moreover, EEG monitoring permits selective shunting, which itself may reduce the incidence of major neurologic morbidity (200). TCD is another monitoring modality that is gaining in popularity because of its ability to detect cerebral microembolism and to provide an index of cerebral blood flow (CBF) velocity (202, 203). In fact, TCD monitoring of patients undergoing Carotid Endarterectomy shows that microemboli occur postoperatively, perhaps explaining some postoperative strokes in these patients (206). However, there is as yet no good evidence that TCD monitoring improves neurologic outcome from CEA.

Other measures intended to reduce the risk of stroke during CEA include shunt insertion, careful blood pressure management, control of blood glucose, and possibly selection of anesthetic agents. Routine shunt insertion remains controversial because the shunt itself may cause cerebral emboli and increase neurologic morbidity (194, 200); therefore, many surgeons perform a shunt selectively. Because vessels in ischemic areas are maximally dilated due to tissue acidosis and, therefore, are incapable of autoregulating normally (207, 208), a decrease in arterial pressure may reduce CBF in ischemic areas, whereas moderate induced hypertension may improve flow to marginal regions (209, 210). Accordingly, moderate induced hypertension is used occasionally during the period of carotid cross-clamping in an attempt to improve CBF (190). Another

physiologic consideration that may be important in patients at risk for cerebral ischemia is the plasma glucose concentration. Studies in animals (211–213) and humans (214, 215) demonstrate that hyperglycemia worsens neurologic outcome from transient, focal incomplete cerebral ischemia (169). However, not all data are consistent in this regard (216), and the blood glucose threshold for increased risk of injury is controversial. Nonetheless, it seems reasonable to avoid administering glucose-containing solutions to nondiabetic patients undergoing CEA or to maintain plasma glucose within broadly normal limits in diabetics. Insofar as the potential of anesthetic agents to prevent cerebral ischemia during CEA is concerned, some retrospective data suggest that intraoperative cerebral ischemia, as determined by EEG criteria, is significantly less common during anesthesia with isoflurane than either enflurane or halothane (217), but there was no difference in neurologic outcome among the three groups (217). Although the "critical" CBF (i.e., the CBF below which ischemic EEG changes are likely during carotid cross-clamping) is also lower with isoflurane than either halothane or enflurane anesthesia (218, 219), several other studies (220, 221) report no meaningful protection with isoflurane. Barbiturates also have been used to protect the brain during CEA (208, 222–224), but no controlled clinical trials have been performed and issues related to optimal timing, dose, and duration of therapy must be resolved before such therapy confidently can be considered protective during CEA.

Despite meticulous intraoperative management, some patients will awaken from CEA with a neurologic deficit. In this situation, the first step is to rule out anesthetic-induced neurologic dysfunction in the manner described previously. Of particular note in these patients is the widely held view that an otherwise clinically mild focal neurologic deficit may be worsened transiently by anesthesia (148, 149, 225, 226). This possibility, therefore, should be seriously considered in the stroke-prone CEA population. The only surgically remediable cause of stroke after CEA is carotid occlusion (185, 190). Thus, the patient awakening from CEA with a dense hemiplegia or other major focal deficit that persists without improvement despite attempts to antagonize anesthetic agents as described earlier should be evaluated promptly with carotid noninvasive studies or angiography because surgical reexploration may be indicated. Even if there is no surgically correctable reason for stroke, newer therapeutic modalities such as thrombolysis or low-molecular-weight heparin should be considered, because they may be able to reverse or minimize the permanent consequences of injury (see New Neurologic Impairment After Routine Surgery).

Cardiac Surgery and Cardiopulmonary Bypass

Despite numerous technical advances in the field, neurologic and neuropsychologic dysfunction continues to be a significant and undeniable risk of cardiac surgery. Fatal cerebral damage occurs in as many as 2% of patients undergoing cardiac procedures (227–230) and the reported incidence of gross neurologic deficits such as stroke averages about 4% (231, 232). Such obvious neurologic injury, although certainly very important because of the emotional and economic costs (233), is only one small subset of all CNS dysfunction associated with cardiac surgery; subtle deterioration of cognitive or neuropsychologic function is much more common. In one study (232), careful testing revealed impaired neuropsychiatric function in 70% of 312 patients undergoing coronary artery bypass surgery (CABG); in 24% of patients, the deterioration was judged to be moderate or severe. In contrast, none of a simultaneously studied control group of patients undergoing major peripheral vascular surgery had a moderate or severe neuropsychologic deficit. Other studies (230, 232, 235) of cardiac surgical patients confirm substantial decrements in performance on neuropsychologic tests in

the perioperative period. Although most of the deterioration in cognitive and neuropsychologic performance resolves over a period of months or years (230, 235), as many as 11–35% of patients are still impaired 12 months later (230, 236).

The potential causes of cerebral dysfunction during cardiac surgery fall into two general categories: cerebral hypoperfusion or embolic phenomena. Global cerebral hypoperfusion (or hypoxia) and massive embolism of air or debris can certainly cause catastrophic cerebral injury in cardiac surgical procedures complicated by cardiac arrest, equipment malfunction, or human error. However, most studies argue convincingly that during hypothermic cardiopulmonary bypass perfusion pressure is not a major determinant of CNS dysfunction (229, 234, 237–239), but this may not be true during "warm" bypass or in all age groups (240). The prevailing opinion is that microemboli, consisting of air, fat, plastic, or aggregates of cellular elements (241), are responsible for most neurologic and neuropsychologic deficits associated with CPB. Microemboli have been documented in the left ventricle (242) and aortic arch (243) by echocardiography and in the middle cerebral artery by transcranial doppler (244, 245). Furthermore, evidence that arterial filtration reduces both the embolic load as well as the incidence of CNS dysfunction (244–247), although still controversial, provides additional support for the microemboli theory.

Other factors that add to the intrinsic risks of cardiac surgery include the duration of CPB (227–229, 238, 248–252), coexisting symptomatic cerebrovascular disease (73, 253), advancing age (229, 230, 251, 252, 254–256), and especially atherosclerosis of the ascending aorta. Although not proven, the common link between these factors may be an association with progressive cerebral embolization.

Efforts to reduce the risk of CNS complications during cardiac surgery make the reasonable assumption that various technical or physiologic details of CPB are important determinants of neurologic outcome. Thus, some suggest that membrane oxygenators are preferable to bubble oxygenators (257), that a higher perfusion pressure is critical (258, 259), and that arterial filtration is beneficial (244, 246). The optimal CO_2 management strategy during CPB is an ongoing debate. Basically, there are two approaches: "alpha-stat" management, which aims for normal pH and $PaCO_2$ values as measured in the blood-gas machine at 37°C, and "pH-stat," which corrects the measured values for body temperature and requires addition of CO_2 to the pump to maintain pH. In practical terms, the pH-stat method is associated with higher cerebral blood flow, uncoupling of CBF and metabolism, and impaired autoregulation (260, 261), whereas alpha-stat management preserves autoregulation and global CBF still exceeds metabolic demand (260, 261). Thus, those concerned that hypercarbia could increase CBF and thereby predispose cerebral microembolism favor alpha-stat management, whereas those who fear that hypocarbia might result in cerebral hypoperfusion favor the pH-stat method. A few studies have addressed this question, but the results are mixed. One prospective, randomized study of neuropsychologic function in patients undergoing CPB failed to identify differences in outcome based on the two CO_2 management strategies (234), whereas others have found that neurologic dysfunction and cognitive deficits occur more often in pH-stat-managed patients (262, 263). However, in one study, the difference was only apparent when CPB lasted more than 90 minutes (251). Thus, there seems to be no neurologic disadvantage to alpha-stat management and a possible advantage exists.

Brain "protection" probably is used more commonly in cardiac surgery than in any other place in the operating room. Hypothermia, widely regarded to protect the brain from anoxic or ischemic events (237, 264–266), has been a mainstay of CPB protocol in many institutions. However, the value of hypothermia in the setting of cardiopulmonary bypass recently has been questioned as techniques

such as retrograde cardioplegia decrease the need of hypothermia for cardiac protection (267) and as the role of microemboli and their occurrence at times when hypothermia is impractical are noted (243, 268, 269). Randomized prospective studies in this regard are conflicting, and in some cases of poor quality because investigators were not blinded and evaluations of perioperative stroke rates rather than neuropsychologic testing were used as the outcome measure (267, 270). In one study involving 1,001 patients, warm CPB (35° and higher) was associated with a statistically significant increase in the incidence of neurologic events when compared to systemic hypothermia (28° or lower) (267), whereas other investigators found no such difference in the incidence of perioperative stroke (270, 271). Evidence that even mild hypothermia may have some neuroprotective effects (272), combined with the fact that cerebral emboli in the setting of CPB frequently occur at times when hypothermia is impractical, may explain these differences (243, 273).

The high incidence of post-CPB CNS dysfunction combined with conflicting reports about the neuroprotective effects of hypothermia in this setting is adequate justification to search for supplementary efforts to protect the brain during CPB. Thiopental may have potential benefit in this regard. In a prospective, controlled study (274) of patients undergoing open ventricle procedures during normothermic CPB, which stands as the only valid demonstration of barbiturate protection in humans (275), thiopental, administered as a bolus before aortic cannulation, was shown to reduce the frequency of persistent neuropsychiatric deficits. The disadvantage of high-dose thiopental treatment (e.g., longer period of postoperative intubation; more inotropic support) (274) as well as questions regarding its applicability to other cardiac surgical centers evidently have discouraged its widespread use. There is, however, some recent evidence from an uncontrolled clinical trial (231) that thiopental, administered by continuous infusion before aortic cannulation or as a bolus before weaning from CBP, is associated with a low incidence of gross neurologic deficits. Nevertheless, the role of thiopental in brain protecting during CPB continues to be controversial (276). Other strategies of cerebral protection, including retrograde cerebral perfusion during circulatory arrest, may hold promise in some patient populations (277–279) but currently is still controversial (280).

Treatment of a patient with a post-CPB neurologic deficit is primarily supportive and aimed to prevent a secondary neurologic insult due to hyopoxia, hypoventilation, or hypoperfusion. However, one unique and rare cause of post-CPB CNS injury, namely cerebral embolization of large amounts of air, lends itself to an unusual and specific form of treatment. Hyperbaric therapy capitalizes on the fact that a gas-filled space will decrease in size as pressure surrounding it increases (281). Thus, hyperbaric therapy is believed to reduce the size of cerebral air emboli and speed reabsorption. Comparatively few patients have been treated in this manner (282–284), probably reflecting the limited number of such chambers and the practical difficulties encountered in caring for critically ill patients in such a device (281). Results have nonetheless been encouraging (285), even when treatment is begun hours after the embolic event.

NEUROLOGIC COMPLICATIONS OF SPINAL AND EPIDURAL ANESTHESIA

Neurologic complications after regional anesthesia can result from the anesthetic or its contaminants, surgery, positioning, or exacerbation of preexisting diseases (286–289). The regional anesthetic is always suspect (290); sometimes, a regional anesthetic is blamed for a neurologic complication when none was used (286).

Most large studies and reviews evaluating postoperative neurologic dysfunction after spinal and epidural anesthesia have found complications limited to postdural puncture headaches and minor sensory deficits such as numbness and paresthesia. The latter usually resolves spontaneously over a period of 6 months (288, 289, 291, 292). Devastating neurologic complications of spinal and epidural anesthesia are believed to be rare, but a recent review suggests that the incidence of such complications may be higher than previously reported (286). Thirteen cases of permanent neurologic dysfunction were reported among 17,733 central neural blocks for an incidence of 0.07%. Of these permanent neurologic disorders, most involved residual sensory deficits; however, among those with motor deficits, four were wheelchair-bound because of their lesions and two could walk only with assistance. This is compared to an incidence of permanent neurologic dysfunction of 0.006–0.02% after epidural anesthesia (293) and an even lower incidence among patients who received spinal anesthesia (294), as well as with older studies (295) (289), which failed to find a single case of major neurologic dysfunction among a combined total of 21,900 patients who underwent spinal anesthesia. For the most part, descriptions of temporary and permanent paralysis after central neural blockade come from case reports (296, 297).

The most serious neurologic complications of spinal or epidural anesthesia is paraplegia or paraparesis due to ischemia, infection, or drug toxicity. Spinal cord ischemia or infarction may be caused by arterial hypotension (294) or compromise of the blood supply to the cord by an expanding mass, such as an epidural hematoma (286) or epidural abscess (298). Alternatively, paraplegia may be secondary to the administration of toxic chemicals, including anesthetic agents such as intrathecal 2-chloroprocaine (299–301), 5% lidocaine (302–305), preservatives such as sodium bisulfite (306), or chemical contamination of anesthetic agents (287, 307). These complications usually present as myelopathy, infection, peridural hematomas, aseptic meningitis, cauda equina syndrome, or adhesive arachnoiditis (287, 294). Myelopathy of spinal cord and nerve roots presents as an immediate, severe nonprogressive paraplegia in which it seems the anesthetic agent never wore off. Treatment is supportive and recovery of function is unlikely.

Aseptic meningitis usually presents with high fever, headache, nuchal rigidity, and photophobia in the setting of an elevated cerebrospinal fluid (CSF) pressure with leukocytosis and negative CSF culture (308, 309). Complete spontaneous recovery is expected during the course of a week (308, 309). Chemical contamination often has been questioned (309) and epidemic cases have been reported (308).

Infectious complications of peridural blockade include meningitis (310) and epidural abscess formation (311). With septic meningitis, peripheral neurologic findings are infrequent and the development of permanent damage depends on the tendency of the organism to produce arachnoiditis (312). Conditions associated with epidural abscess include old age, trauma, debilitating disease, and immunocompromised states such as cancer, human immunodeficiency virus (HIV), steroid administration, and diabetes (313). With meticulous technique and careful patient selection, the risk of epidural abscesses seems to be small after peridural blockade (313); most are documented only as case reports (298, 311, 314). An epidural abscess may present with symptoms of acute spinal cord compression such as paresthesia, motor weakness, bladder and bowel dysfunction or as disorientation, fever, headache, back pain, and neck stiffness. Culture of the CSF may be positive (311, 314, 315). An epidural abscess can manifest acutely after the block but, in some cases, may not be noted for weeks after the procedure (298, 314, 316). The key to treatment of the problem is early diagnosis. After an epidural abscess is suspected, radiologic evaluation (MRI) should follow immediately (311). A positive finding is treated with surgical decompression and/or antibiotic therapy directed toward the offending organism (usually Staphylococcus) (311, 315). The prognosis is usually good; most patients with neurologic dysfunction preoperatively have partial or total return of function if the neurologic changes were not chronic (298, 311, 314, 315).

Most clinicians would avoid spinal or epidural anesthesia in untreated patients with overt untreated sepsis. However, there is controversy about the contraindications to these anesthetic techniques in other infectious situations (317). It has been argued that placement of a block before the development of an anticipated transient low-grade intraoperative bacteremia is safe and that antibiotic therapy before needle placement may decrease the risk of meningitis and epidural abscesses, (318) whereas others suggest that the insertion site may create an area of decreased resistance, which increases the likelihood of subsequent infection (319). The data are inconclusive.

Cauda equina syndrome is another rare complication of peridural anesthesia. This syndrome is characterized by urinary and fecal incontinence, sensory loss in the perineal area, and leg weakness. The problem usually presents immediately after the effects of the local anesthetic have worn off; recovery of function is often partial and generally occurs over weeks to years (294, 296, 304). Furthermore, cauda equina syndrome may be followed by adhesive arachnoiditis (320) and its presentation may be delayed for some time after the administration of a peridural anesthetic (321). Toxic effects of anesthetic agents (301, 303) such as 2-chloroprocaine (320) or lidocaine (304, 321) concentrated in a small area (296, 305) are proposed to explain some cases of cauda equina syndrome in patients with spinal tumors (296) or after continuous spinal anesthesia (321). Treatment is primarily supportive.

Adhesive arachnoiditis is characterized by a gradual progressive motor weakness and sensory loss involving the lower extremities, which occurs several weeks to months after intentional or inadvertent administration of spinal anesthetics (320) and may lead to complete paraplegia or death (294, 307, 312), and is characterized by anarachnoid that is thickened and replaced by collagenous fibrous tissue in association with arteritis (312). The etiology may include reactions to local anesthesthetics (301), such as 2-chloroprocaine (299, 300, 320, 321) and lidocaine (303, 321) in high concentrations, or nonanesthetic drugs such as preservatives (306) and sterilizing detergents (307, 312). Again, treatment is mainly supportive, but steroids have been used to decrease the inflammatory response (320).

Spinal hematoma is a rare and potentially catastrophic complication of spinal and epidural anesthesia. Fortunately, the incidence of neurologic dysfunction from peridural hematomas in the anesthetic setting is probably small (292, 295) but may be as high as 0.02% (286). Leukemia, blood dyscrasias, alcoholism, thrombocytopenia, antiplatelet therapy, anticoagulation, and traumatic or difficult lumbar puncture are all considered predisposing factors to peridural hematomas (322–325). However, evidence for a relationship between peridural hematoma and these predisposing factors is derived mostly from case reports (322, 323, 326). In addition, a number of these factors have been challenged recently. Abnormal coagulation studies and bleeding times do not always identify patients at risk for peridural hematomas and there are many cases of difficult and bloody epidural placements without subsequent neurologic sequelae (327, 328).

There has been much discussion in the literature about the risks of peridural anesthetic administration in an anticoagulated patient (329). Case reports of peridural hematomas in patients who have undergone peridural anesthesia after receiving antiplatelet drugs have caused some authors to propose a relationship between the two (330). However, neither recent retrospective (327) nor prospective (331) studies demonstrate a relationship between preoperative administration of antiplatelet drugs and the subsequent development of a peridural hematoma. The role of anticoagulation is another controversial issue. Inasmuch as spontaneous epidural hematoma formation is a well recognized complication of anticoagulation therapy (332), few would advocate peridural needle insertion or catheter placement in a fully anticoagulated patient. However, is peridural anesthesia safe when anticoagulation will occur after peridural anesthesia is established or in the setting of mild anticoagulation (333, 334)? Although some clinicians may avoid peridural manipulation whenever anticoagulation is likely in the perioperative period, several retrospective studies fail to demonstrate an association between peridural hematoma and monitored postinsertion heparin (324, 325, 335) or coumadin (328) therapy. Similarly, there is no conclusive evidence concerning whether anticoagulants should be reversed before removal of an epidural catheter postoperatively (324).

With respect to the risk of mini "prophylactic" doses of heparin (326, 334), a recent meta-analysis involving 9,013 patients who underwent spinal or epidural anesthesia while receiving low-molecular-weight heparin for DVT prophylaxis identified no case of peridural hematoma (336). Thus, the risk of neurologic complications due to a peridural hematoma after spinal or epidural anesthesia in the setting of antiplatelet medications, low-dose prophylactic heparin therapy, or postinsertion monitored anticoagulation seems to be low. However, one cannot assume that there is no risk involved (325, 328, 331, 336).

The diagnosis of peridural hematoma should be considered whenever the sequence of back pain, urinary incontinence, sensory changes, and muscle weakness progressing toward paralysis occurs over the course of hours to days (330, 332, 334). Backache may be the first sign of this complication (324, 325). If peridural hematoma is suspected, immediate neurologic and radiographic (CT, MRI, myelogram) evaluation should be performed, followed by emergent decompressive laminectomy if the studies are positive (327, 330). Although immediate surgical intervention minimizes the likelihood of permanent neurological sequelae, spinal cord ischemia may leave many patients paraplegic even after laminectomy (286, 329, 330, 332–334, 337), but there are case reports in which documented epidural hematomas underwent spontaneous resolution without surgical therapy (286, 323, 334).

Central neural blockade may also unmask known and unknown preexisting CNS pathology (292, 294, 296, 338). This has led to the suggestion, which is not uniformly accepted, that peridural blockade should be avoided for patients with neurologic disorders (286, 296, 312, 338).

Inadvertent administration of agents into the peridural region can also produce paraplegia (339). Proposed treatments for this type of mishap include flushing the catheter with normal saline (340) and local anesthetic agents (341) and infusing steroids into the epidural space to minimize inflammation (342, 343). However, it is not clear whether such treatment is necessary or helpful; prevention is obviously preferable.

An association between paresthesias and radiating pain on injection of local anesthetics and postoperative neurologic complications has been proposed. Indeed, it has been suggested to stop the injection if paresthesia develops (286, 289, 296). In contrast, many patients have transient paresthesia during needle placement with no subsequent neurologic problems if the needle is redirected and no anesthetic is administered at the site of a paresthesia (289, 295). If the injury is due to trauma, the injury will be discrete and limited to the specific nerve roots involved with paralysis if the motor root is involved and pain/paresthesias if the sensory root is involved. In either case, spontaneous regression is the rule (312).

Postdural puncture headache (PDPH) is probably the most common minor neurologic complication of peridural blockade. The presentation of PDPH remains as eloquently described by Bier in 1899 (344). Classically, patients experience a bifrontal, temporal, or occipital headache that may extend to the neck

and shoulders; this headache is usually aggravated by assuming the upright position, coughing, or sudden movements and is relieved by assuming a recumbent position (338, 345, 346). Associated symptoms include nausea and vomiting, changes in hearing, tinnitus, vertigo, and occasionally diplopia due to traction on the cranial nerves (344–347). The syndrome typically occurs hours to days after the dural puncture (345, 346) but may take weeks to develop (338). The syndrome usually resolves with conservative therapy over a few days but may persist for more than 1 year (346, 348). The etiology of PDPH is unknown (347), although substantial but indirect evidence supports the leakage theory first hypothesized by MacRoberts in 1918 (349). In general, PDPH is believed to result when the rate of CSF leakage is greater than the rate of production, with the leakage rate being determined by the size of the hole and the pressure differential across the dura (345, 348). However, it has been suggested recently that the drug mixture may also play a role, particularly as it relates to the development of symptoms in the first 36 hours (350). Regardless of the precise etiology of PDPHs, the cure seems to involve the sealing of the dural hole (347).

Many treatments have been proposed for PDPH; the general strategy is to increase the production or decrease the loss of CSF until the dural hole is sealed. Unfortunately, most treatments have failed to prove effective in randomized studies. Caffeine, administered either intravenously (351) or orally (352), may be an exception to this rule. It is effective in 70% of patients (352) and is believed to work via temporary cerebral vasoconstriction (351). More effective still is an epidural blood patch, which is successful in 80–98% of patients who have failed more conservative treatment (345, 353–355) and can be used safely in an outpatient setting (353, 356). Nevertheless, initially a conservative approach involving bedrest, hydration, caffeine, and mild analgesics is recommended, followed by epidural blood patch within 24–48 hours if the PDPH does not resolve (345). The blood patch is believed to work via two mechanisms: both by increasing CSF pressure and thus the cushioning provided to the intracranial pain sensitive structures (348, 357, 358), and by sealing the hole in the dura and thus preventing further CSF leakage (358). Major complications are rare after epidural blood patch (345, 354, 355), but minor complications lasting less than 24 hours such as transient tinnitus (354), radicular pain (345), neck ache (354, 355), the sensation of abdominal fullness (355), and backache (345, 354, 355) do occur. Transient bradycardia also has been noted during epidural blood patch administration, suggesting that the electrocardiogram should be monitored during placement, particularly for patients with preexisting cardiac disease (359). Overall, however, epidural blood patch placement is a safe and effective treatment for PDPH.

Other rare neurologic complications of spinal or epidural anesthesia include a subdural hematomas, which is associated with an atypical postprocedure headache followed a few weeks later by symptoms of increased intracranial pressure (360–362), transient hearing changes (363–365), visual disturbances due to a transient lateral rectus muscle palsy (289, 366), and self-limited radicular back pain (286). Of recent interest has been the association of 5% lidocaine and transient radicular irritation after spinal anesthesia, which occurs in up to 37% of patients (367–369). Although these symptoms are transient with spontaneous resolution over 2–3 days, it raises the question of potential neurotoxicity with this concentrated solution of lidocaine (303). Except for a subdural hematoma, treatment of these conditions is supportive because most resolve spontaneously.

Although it generally does not produce a neurologic complication, an issue arises when a spiral or epidural catheter breaks off and remains in the patient's back. The data are limited, but because removing the catheter fragment may create more problems than it alone (293, 370), it is likely that the best approach is to inform the patient and leave the catheter in place if the patient is asymptomatic.

PERIPHERAL NERVOUS SYSTEM COMPLICATIONS

Peripheral nerve injuries are rare after anesthesia and surgery (371, 372). When they occur, complete recovery can usually be anticipated, but permanent disability has been reported (371, 373). The most common causes of anesthesia-related nerve injury are probably poor patient positioning and needle trauma during the performance of a block (374). Most cases of postoperative peripheral nerve lesions involve the brachial plexus and ulnar nerve (371, 372).

Brachial Plexus Injury

Because of the long fixed course of the brachial plexus and its proximity to many bony structures, the brachial plexus is perhaps most vulnerable to injury (371, 372) and is the second most likely site of peripheral nerve injury in closed malpractice claims (375). Nevertheless, the incidence of brachial plexus injury postoperatively is believed to be less than 0.02% (376). The etiology of brachial plexus injury is believed to be caused by stretching the plexus (377, 378). This can occur with abduction of the arm (379), especially when combined with external rotation and turning of the head contralaterally; simultaneous abduction of both arms also increases the stretch and tension on the plexus (378, 380). Additional etiologic factors associated with brachial plexus injury in the operating room include the use of shoulder braces with the Trendelenberg position and suspension of the patient's arm on an arm bar (372, 375, 379). Patients who undergo cardiac surgery seem to be at increased risk for postoperative brachial plexus injury (371), typically involving the lower rather than upper trunks of the plexus. Compression of the plexus in the neck by hemorrhage on the side of internal jugular cannulation is one mechanism proposed (381–383); similarly, it has been argued that internal mammary artery dissection may stretch the plexus in some patients (384), but at least one study found an increased incidence of brachial plexus lesions in cardiac surgery patients even when the arms were tucked next to the patient rather than abducted (385). The optimal positioning of the arms seems to involve abduction limited to 90° with careful prevention of posterior displacement by elevation of the elbows above the level of the shoulder (378, 379).

The clinical picture of brachial plexus injury due to improper positioning is that of a motor or sensory deficit of the muscles and nerves supplied by the roots involved (frequently the upper roots) (371). Pain is not a prominent finding. The prognosis of postoperative brachial plexus palsy is good and recovery occurs spontaneously (377, 380). Most patients recover within 3 months, although in some recovery may take as long as 1 year (372, 378, 379, 381, 382, 386, 387). Electrophysiologic studies are often useful to evaluate the extent and location of the lesions. However, inasmuch as acute changes are usually not evident within the first 1–3 weeks, it is important to perform both an early examination to document any preexisting lesions and a repeat test 2–3 weeks later to evaluate the damage inflicted by the acute incident (371, 388). As is the case with most nerve lesions, prevention seems to be the best treatment for postoperative brachial plexus injuries.

Ulnar Neuropathy

Ulnar neuropathy is among the most common neuropathies in the perioperative period. Although perioperative ulnar neuropathy seems to be rare (371, 372, 389), it is the leading cause of peripheral nerve injury malpractice claims related to anesthesia (375). Ulnar neuropathy is more common after general than regional anesthesia (389), but it also can occur spontaneously (390), suggesting that some postoperative ulnar neuropathies may simply represent an untimely manifestation or exacerbation of a preexisting disease state.

The signs and symptoms of ulnar neuropathy include tingling, numbness, pain, loss of sensation, "pins and needles" sensations, muscle cramps, and weakness. Of course, these signs and symptoms are limited to areas innervated by the ulnar nerve, especially the fourth and fifth fingers (389–392), and electrophysiologic evidence of a pure ulnar neuropathy is present (390, 392, 393).

The first symptoms of ulnar neuropathy may present anywhere from the time of anesthesia to more than 48 hours later (375, 389, 391), perhaps because the initial symptoms are ignored by physicians or not noted by the patient because of perioperative sedation (389). Events that occur outside the operating room, such as patient positioning, may also contribute and participate in the delayed presentation (375, 389, 394, 395).

Risk factors hypothesized to be involved include male gender (375, 389, 391), extremes of body habitus (389), as well as nerve subluxation (395, 396). Associated factors may include preexisting subclinical neuropathies caused by diabetes mellitus, vitamin deficiency, increasing age, alcoholism, cancer, and chronic subclinical compression of the ulnar nerve in the cubital tunnel (388, 389, 391, 392, 396, 397). Occupations that require repeated movements of the hands with the elbows in the flexed position may also lead to chronic subclinical nerve compression (390). It is noteworthy that patients who develop postoperative ulnar neuropathy uniformly have abnormalities of nerve conduction in both arms (398); likewise, patients with preexisting ulnar neuropathies are at increased risk for exacerbation of the neuropathy in the involved arm or for development of symptoms in the contralateral arm even when appropriately positioned and padded (389, 399). This suggests that intraoperative and postoperative factors may exacerbate chronic subclinical ulnar compression at the elbow rather than produce injury de novo (396).

Despite the fact that the mechanism of injury to the ulnar nerve is unknown (396, 400), patient positioning is suspect (389, 391) and anesthesiologists are often identified for litigation purposes when injuries occur (375).

Certainly, careful patient positioning is important but, for reasons already mentioned, unlikely to prevent all ulnar nerve injuries during anesthesia. Conversely, improper positioning can lead to injury. The ulnar nerve passes through the cubital tunnel at the elbow. The capacity of the tunnel is maximal with elbow extension, but when the elbow is flexed to 90°, the arcuate ligament, which forms the roof of the cubital tunnel, becomes tight and compresses the nerve (395–397). This anatomic configuration renders the ulnar nerve vulnerable to compression injury both from extreme flexion of the arm and direct injury because of its superficial course by automated blood pressure cuffs (401) or compression of the ulnar groove on the edge of an armboard or operating table (391, 395, 396, 402, 403). Suggestions for patient positioning during anesthesia, such as supination of the arm while in the supine position, avoidance of elbow contact with hard surfaces while in the flexed position, and protection of the nerve by placement of soft pads to prevent injury, follow directly from these anatomic considerations (396, 397, 401, 403, 404). However, additional factors are involved because ulnar neuropathy has occurred despite appropriate padding and positioning (375, 392, 396, 405).

The prognosis for recovery from a postoperative ulnar neuropathy is poor, (391) with only 53% of patients having complete recovery over the course of a year (389). Sensory deficits seem to be more likely to resolve than motor deficits (389). Unfortunately, no therapeutic maneuvers seem to enhance recovery (389), but decompression of the nerve at the cubital tunnel may lead to some improvement (390, 405). Again the best treatment for any nerve injury is prevention (391). But postoperative ulnar neuropathy may not always be a preventable complication (389, 396).

REFERENCES

1. Skelly AM, Boscoe MJ, Dawling S, et al. A comparison of diazepam and midazolam as sedatives for minor oral surgery. Eur J Anaesthesiol 1984;1:253.
2. Korttila K, Linnoila M, Ertama P, et al. Recovery and simulated driving after intravenous anesthesia with thiopental, methohexital, propanidid, or alphadione. Anesthesiology 1975;43:291.
3. Korttila K, Nuotto EJ, Lichtor JL, et al. Clinical recovery and psychomotor function after brief anesthesia with propofol or thiopental. Anesthesiology 1992;76:676–681.
4. Larsen LE, Gupta A, Ledin T, et al. Psychomotor recovery following propofol or isoflurane anaesthesia for day-care surgery. Acta Anaesthesiol Scand 1992;36:276–282.
5. Milligan KR, O'Tolle DP, Howe JP, et al. Recovery from out patient anaesthesia: a comparison of incremental propofol and propofol-isoflurane. Br J Anaesth 1987;59:1111–1114.
6. Korttila K, Tammisto T, Ertama P, et al. Recovery, psychomotor skills, and simulated driving after brief inhalational anesthesia with halothane or enflurane combined with nitrous oxide and oxygen. Anesthesiology 1977;46:20.
7. Lebenbom-Mansour MH, Pandit AK, Kothary SP, et al. Desflurane versus propofol anesthesia: a comparative analysis in outpatients. Anesth Analg 1993;76:936–941.
8. Tsai SK, Lee C, Kwan WF, et al. Recovery of cognitive functions after anaesthesia with desflurane or isoflurane and nitrous oxide. Br J Anaesth 1992;69:255–258.
9. Chung F, Seyone C, Dyck B, et al. Age-related cognitive recovery after general anesthesia. Anesth Analg 1990;71:217–224.
10. Chung FF, Chung A, Meir RH, et al. Comparison of perioperative mental function after general anaesthesia and spinal anesthesia with intravenous sedation. Can J Anaesth 1989;36:381–387.
11. Ghoneim MM, Hinrichs JV, OÆhara MW, et al. Comparison of psychologic and cognitive functions after general or regional anesthesia. Anesthesiology 1988;69:507–515.
12. Riis J, Haxholdt O, Kehlet H, et al. Immediate and long-term mental recovery from general versus epidural anesthesia in elderly patients. Acta Anaesthesiol Scand 1983;27:44–49.
13. Williams-Russo P, Urquhart BL, Sharrock NE, et al. Post-operative delirium: predictors and prognosis in elderly orthopedic patients. J Am Geriatr Soc 1992;40:759–767.
14. O'Keeffe ST, Chonchubhair AN. Postoperative delirium in the elderly. Br J Anaesth 1994;73:673–687.
15. Dyer CB, Ashton CM, Teasdale TA. Postoperative delirium: a review of 80 primary data-collection studies. Arch Intern Med 1995;155:461–465.
16. Williams-Russo P, Sharrock NE, Mattis S, et al. Cognitive effects after epidural vs general anesthesia in older adults: a randomized trial. JAMA 1995;274:44–50.
17. Chung F, Meier R, Lautenschlaeger E, et al. General or spinal anesthesia: which is better in the elderly? Anesthesiology 1987;67:422–427.
18. Seibert CP. Recognition, management, and prevention of neuropsychological dysfunction after operation. Int Anesthesiol Clin 1986;24:39–58.
19. Lipowski ZJ. Delirium in the elderly patient. N Engl J Med 1989;320:578–582.

20. Weigner MB, Swedlow NR, Nillar WL. Acute post-operative delirium and extrapyramidal signs in a previously healthy parturient. Anesth Analg 1988;67:291–295.

21. Titchener JL, Zwerling I, Gottschalk I, et al. Psychosis in surgical patients. Surg Gynecol Obstet 1956;102:59–65.

22. Eckenhoff JE, Kneale DH, Dripps RD. The incidence and etiology of postanesthetic excitement. Anesthesiology 1961;22:667–673.

23. Tune L, Folstein MF. Post-operative delirium. In: Guggenheim FG, ed. Psychological aspects of surgery. Basel: S Karger AG, 1986.

24. Marcantonio ER, Goldman L, Mangione CM, et al. A clinical prediction rule for delirium after elective noncardiac surgery. JAMA 1994;271;134–139.

25. Parikh SS, Chung F. Postoperative delirium in the elderly. Anesth Analg 1995;80:1223–1232.

26. Svensson IS. Postoperative psychosis after heart surgery. J Thorac Cardiovasc Surg 1975;70:717.

27. Heller SS, Franj KA, Kornfeld DS, et al. Psychological outcome following openheart surgery. Arch Intern Med 1974;134:908.

28. Summers WK, Reich TC. Delirium after cataract surgery: review and two cases. Am J Psychiatry 1979;136:386.

29. Hole A, Terjesen T, Breivk H. Epidural versus general anesthesia for total hip arthroplasty in elderly patients. Acta Anaesthesiol Scand 1980;24:279–287.

30. Hutchinson R. Awareness during surgery: a study of its incidence. Br J Anaesth 1960;33:463.

31. McIntyre JWR. Awareness during general anesthesia: preliminary observations. Can Anaesth Soc J 1966;13:495.

32. Aackerlund LP, Rosenberg J. Postoperative delirium: treatment with supplementary oxygen. Br J Anaesth 1994;72:286–290.

33. Kehlet H, Rosenberg J. Late post-operative hypoxia and organ dysfunction. Eur J Anaesthesiol 1995;10(Suppl):31–34.

34. Berggren D, Gustafson Y, Eriksson B, et al. Postoperative confusion after anesthesia in elderly patients with femoral neck fractures. Anesth Analg 1987;66:497–504.

35. Lewis DA, Smith RE. Steroid-induced psychiatric syndromes: a report of 14 cases and a review of the literature. J Affect Disord 1983;5:319.

36. White PF, Way WL, Trevor AJ. Ketamine – its pharmacology and therapeutic uses. Anesthesiology 1982;56:119–136.

37. Kothary SP, Zsingmond EK. A double-blinded study of the effective antihallucinatory doses of diazepam prior to ketamine anesthesia. Clin Pharmacol Ther 1977;21:108–109.

38. Lilburn JK, Dundee JW, Nair SG, et al. Ketamine sequelae: evaluation of the ability of various premedicants to attenuate its psychic actions. Anaesthesia 1978;33:307–311.

39. Levanen J, Makela ML, Sheinin H. Dexmedetomidine premedication attenuates ketamine-induced cardiostimulatory effects and postanesthetic delirium. Anesthesiology 1995;82:1117–1125.

40. Sussman DR. A comparative evaluation of ketamine anesthesia in children and adults. Anesthesiology 1974;40:459–464.

41. Smith DA, Orkin FK, Gardner SM, et al. Prolonged sedation in the elderly after intraoperative atropine administration. Anesthesiology 1979;51:348.

42. Tune LE, Holland A, Folstein MF, et al. Association of postoperative delirium with raised serum levels of anticholinergic drugs. Lancet 1981;26:651.

43. Simpson KH, Smith RJ, Davies LF. Comparison of the effects of atropine and glycopyrrolate on cognitive function following general anesthesia. Br J Anaesth 1987;59:966–969.

44. Lee CM, Yeakel AE. Patient refusal of surgery following Innovar premedication. Anesth Analg 1975;54:224–226.

45. Melnick BM. Extrapyramidal reactions to low-dose droperidol. Anesthesiology 1988;69:424–426.

46. Nelson VM. Hallucinations after propofol. Anesthesia 1988;43:170.

47. Celleno D, Capogana G, Tomasetti M, et al. Neurobehavorial effects of propofol on the neonate following elective caesarean section. Br J Anaesth 1989;62:649–654.

48. Sutherland MJ, Bart P. Propofol and seizures. Anaesth Intensive Care 1994;22:733–737.

49. Laycock GJA. Opisthotonus and propofol: a possible association. Anaesthesia 1988;43:257.

50. Hunter DN, Thornily A, Whitburn R. Arousal from propofol. Anaesthesia 1988;42:1128–1129.

51. Marsh SCU, Schaefer HG. Problems with eye opening after propofol anesthesia. Anesth Analg 1990;70:127–128.

52. Defriez CB, Wong HC. Seizures and opisthotonos after propofol anesthesia. Anesth Analg 1992;75:630–632.

53. Hodkinson BP, Frith RW, Mee EW. Propofol and the electroencephalogram. Lancet 1987;2:1518.

54. Yate PM, Maynard DE, Major E, et al. Anaesthesia with ICI 35,868 monitored by the cerebral function analyzing monitor (CFAM). Eur J Anaesthesiol 1986;3:159–166.

55. Nowack WJ, Jordan R. Propofol, seizures and generalized paroxysmal fast activity in the EEG. Clin Electroencephalogr 1994;25:110–114.

56. Finley GA, MacManus B, Sampson SE, et al. Delayed seizures following sedation with propofol. Can J Anaesth 1993;40:863–865.

57. Forrest JB, Cahalan MK, Rehder K, et al. Multicenter study of general anesthesia. II. Results. Anesthesiology 1990;72:262–268.

58. Oliver SB, Cucchiara RF, Warner MA, et al. Unexpected focal neurologic deficit on emergence from anesthesia: a report of three cases. Anesthesiology 1987;67:823–826.

59. Wilder AJ, Fishbein RH. Operative experience with patients over 80 years of age. Surg Gynecol Obstet 1961;113:205–212.

60. Turnipseed WD, Berkoff HA, Belzer FO. Postoperative stroke in cardiac and peripheral vascular disease. Ann Surg 1980;192:365–367.

61. Barnes RW, Leibman PR, Marzalek PB, et al. The natural history of asymptomatic carotid disease in patients undergoing cardiovascular surgery. Surgery 1981;90:1075–1081.

62. Eichhorn JH. Prevention of intraoperative anesthesia accidents and related severe injury through safety monitoring. Anesthesiology 1989;70:572–577.
63. Hart R, Hindman B. Mechanisms of perioperative cerebral infarction. Stroke 1982;13:766–773.
64. Warner MA, Shields SE, Chute CG. Major morbidity and mortality within 1 month of ambulatory surgery and anesthesia. JAMA 1993;270:1437–1441.
65. Roper AH, Wechsler LR, Wilson LS. Carotid bruit and risk of stroke in elective surgery. N Engl J Med 1982;307:1388.
66. Van Ruiswyk J, Noble H, Sigmann P. The natural history of carotid bruits in elderly persons. Ann Intern Med 1990;112:340–343.
67. Executive Committee for the Asymptomatic Carotid Atherosclerosis Study. Endarterectomy for asymptomatic carotid artery stenosis. JAMA 1995;273:1421–1428.
68. CASANOVA Study Group. Carotid surgery versus medical therapy in asymptomatic carotid stenosis. Stroke 1991;22:1229–1235.
69. Hobson RWII, Weis DG, Fields WS, et al., for the Veterans Affairs Cooperative study group. Efficacy of carotid endarterectomy for asymptomatic carotid stenosis. N Engl J Med 1993;328:221–227.
70. Hertzer NR, Beven EG, Young JR, et al. Incidental asymptomatic bruits in patients scheduled for peripheral vascular reconstruction: results of cerebral and coronary angiography. Surgery 1984;96:535.
71. Carney WI, Stewart WB, DePinto DJ, et al. Carotid bruit as a risk factor in aorto-iliac reconstruction. Surgery 1977;81:567.
72. Treiman RL, Foran RF, Cohen JL, et al. Carotid bruit: a follow-up report on its significance in patients undergoing an abdominal aortic operation. Arch Surg 1979;114:1138.
73. Kartchner MM, McRae LP. Carotid occlusive disease as a risk factor in major cardiovascular surgery. Arch Surg 1982;117:1086.
74. European Carotid Surgery Trialists' Collaborative Group. European carotid surgery trial: interim results for symptomatic patients with severe (70–99%) or with mild (0–29%) carotid stenosis. Lancet 1991;337:1235–1243.
75. North American Symptomatic Carotid Endarterectomy Trial Collaborators. Beneficial effect of carotid endarterectomy in symptomatic patients with high-grade stenosis. N Engl J Med 1991;325:445–453.
76. Mayberg MR, Wilson SE, Yatsu F, et al., for the Veterans Affairs Cooperative Studies Program 309. Carotid endarterectomy and prevention of cerebral ischemia in asymptomatic carotid stenosis. JAMA 1991;266:3289–3294.
77. Landercasper J, Merz BJ, Cogbill TH, et al. Perioperative stroke risk in 173 consecutive patients with a past history of stroke. Arch Surg 1990;125:986–989.
78. Kendell RE, Marshall J. Role of hypotension in the genesis of transient focal cerebral ischemic attacks. Br Med J 1963;2:344–348.
79. Bladin CF, Chambers BR. Frequency and pathogenesis of hemodynamic stroke. Stroke 1994;25:2179–2182.
80. Kistler JP, Ropper AH, Heros RC. Therapy of ischemic cerebral vascular disease due to atherothrombosis. N Engl J Med 1984;311:27.
81. Manner JM, Wills A. Post-operative convulsions: a review based on a case report. Anaesthesia 1971;26:66–77.
82. Modica PA, Tempelhoff R, White PF. Pro- and anticonvulsant effects of anesthetics (part I). Anesth Analg 1990;70:303–315.
83. Modica PA, Tempelhoff R, White PF. Pro- and anticonvulsant effects of anesthetics (part II). Anesth Analg 1990;70:433–444.
84. Lebowitz MH, Blitt CD, Dillon JB. Enflurane-induced central nervous system excitation and its relation to carbon dioxide tension. Anesth Analg 1972;51:355–363.
85. Burchiel KJ, Stockard JJ, Myers RR, et al. Metabolic and electrophysiologic mechanisms in the initiation and termination of enflurane-induced seizures in man and cats. Electroencephalogr Clin Neurophysiol 1975;38:55.
86. Kruczek M, Albin MS, Wolf S, et al. Postoperative seizure activity following enflurane anesthesia. Anesthesiology 1980;53:175–176.
87. Allan NS. Convulsions after enflurane. Anesthesia 1984;39:605–606.
88. Yazji NS, Seed RF. Convulsive reaction following enflurane anesthesia. Anesthesia 1984;39:1249.
89. Nicoll JMV. Status epilepticus following enflurane anesthesia. Anesthesia 1986;41:927–930.
90. Grant IS. Delayed convulsions following enflurane anesthesia. Anesthesia 1986;41:1024–1025.
91. Ohm WW, Cullen BF, Amory DW, et al. Delayed seizure activity following enflurane anesthesia. Anesthesiology 1975;42:367–368.
92. Fariello RG. Epileptogenic properties of enflurane and their clinical interpretation. Electroencephalogr Clin Neurophysiol 1980;48:595–598.
93. Burchiel KJ, Stockard JJ, Calverly RK, et al. Relationship of pre- and postanesthetic EEG abnormalities to enflurane-induced seizure activity. Anesth Analg 1977;56:509–514.
94. Opitz A, Marschall M, Degan R, et al. General anesthesia in patients with epilepsy and status epilepticus. In: Delgado-Escueta AV, Wasterlain CG, Treiman DM, Porter RJ, eds. Status epilepticus: mechanisms of brain damage and treatment. New York: Raven, 1983;531–535.
95. Krenn J, Porges P, Steinbereithner K. Case of anesthesia convulsions under nitrous oxide-halothane anesthesia. Anesthetist 1967;16:83–85.
96. Smith PA, McDonald TR, Jones CS. Convulsions associated with halothane anesthesia. Anesthesia 1966;21:229–233.
97. Hymes JA. Seizure activity during isoflurane anesthesia. Anesth Analg 1985;64:367–368.
98. Harrison JL. Postoperative seizures after isoflurane anesthesia. Anesth Analg 1986;65:1235–1236.
99. Poulton TJ, Ellingson RJ. Seizure associated with induction of anesthesia with isoflurane. Anesthesiology 1984;61:471–476.
100. Meinck H, Molenhof O, Kettler D. Neurophysiologic effects of etomidate, a new short acting hypno-

tic. Electroencephalogr Clin Neurophysiol 1980; 50:515–522.

101. Laughlin TP, Newberg LA. Prolonged myoclonus after etomidate anesthesia. Anesth Analg 1985;64:80–82.

103. Grant IS, Hutchinson G. Epileptiform seizures during prolonged etomidate sedation (letter). Lancet 1983;2:511–512.

104. Doenicke A, Loffler B, Kugler J, et al. Plasma concentration and EEG after various regimens of etomidate. Br J Anesth 1982;54:393–399.

105. Krieger W, Copperman J, Laxer KD. Seizures with etomidate anesthesia (letter). Anesth Analg 1985;64:1226–1227.

106. Gancher S, Laxer KD, Krieger W. Activation of epileptogenic foci by etomidate. Anesthesiology 1984;61:616–618.

107. Ebrahim ZY, DeBoer GE, Lauders H, et al. Effect of etomidate on the electroencephalogram of patients with epilepsy. Anesth Analg 1986;65:1004–1006.

108. Ferrer-Allado T, Brechner VL, Daymond A, et al. Ketamine-induced electro-convulsive phenomena in the human limbic and thalamic regions. Anesthesiology 1973;38:333–344.

109. Bennett DR, Madssen JA, Jordan WS, et al. Ketamine anesthesia in brain-damaged epileptics: electroencephalographic and clinical observations. Neurology 1973;23:449–460.

110. Thompson CE. Ketamine-induced convulsions (letter). Anesthesiology 1972;37:662–663.

111. Wyant GM. Intramuscular Ketalar (CI-581) in paediatric anesthesia. Can J Anaesth 1971;18:72–83.

112. Elliott E, Hanid TK, Arthur LJH, et al. Ketamine anesthesia for medical procedures in children. Arch Dis Child 1976;51:56–59.

113. Page P, Morgan M, Loh L. Ketamine anesthesia in paediatric procedures. Acta Anaesthesiol Scand 1972;16:155–160.

114. White PF. Propofol: pharmacokinetics and pharmacodynamics. Sem Anesth 1988;7(Suppl):4–20.

115. Stephen H, Sonntag H, Schenk HD, et al. Effects of Disoprivan (propofol) on cerebral blood flow, cerebral oxygen consumption, and cerebral vascular reactivity. Anesthetist 1987;36:60–65.

116. Simpson KH, Halsall PJ, Carr CME, et al. Propofol reduces seizure duration in patients having anesthesia for electroconvulsive therapy. Br J Anaesth 1988;61:343–344.

117. Rampton AJ, Griffin RM, Stuart CS, et al. Comparison of methohexital and propofol for electroconvulsive therapy: effects on hemodynamic responses and seizure duration. Anesthesiology 1989;70:412–417.

118. Fredman B, d'Etienne J, Smith I, et al. Anesthesia for electroconvulsive therapy: effects of propofol and nethohexital on seizure activity and recovery. Anesth Analg 1994;79:75–79.

119. Wood PR, Browne GPR, Pugh S. Propofol infusion for the treatment of status epilepticus (letter). Lancet 1988;1:480–481.

120. Gumpert J, Paul R. Activation of the electroencephalogram with intravenous brietal (methohexitone): the findings in 100 cases. J Neurol Neurosurg Psychiatry 1971;34:646–648.

121. Musella L, Wilder BJ, Schmidt RP. Electroencephalographic activation with intravenous methohexital in psychomotor epilepsy. Neurology 1971;21:594–602.

122. Ryder W. Methohexitone and epilepsy. Br Dent J 1969;126:343.

123. Goetting MG, Thirman MJ. Neurotoxicity of meperidine. Ann Emerg Med 1985;14:1007–1009.

124. Andrews HL. Cortical effects of Demerol. J Pharmacol Exp Ther 1942;76:89–94.

125. Hagmeyer KO, Mauro LS, Mauro VF. Meperidine-related seizures associated with patient-controlled analgesia pumps. Ann Pharmacother 1993; 27:29–31.

126. Szeto HH, Inturrisi CE, Houde R, et al. Accumulation of normeperidine, an active metabolite of meperidine in patients with renal failure and cancer. Ann Intern Med 1977;86:738–741.

127. Kaiko RF, Foley KM, Grabinski PY. Central nervous system excitatory effects of meperidine in cancer patients. Ann Neurol 1983;13:180–185.

128. Rao TLK, Mummaneni N, El-Etr AA. Convulsion: an unusual response to intravenous fentanyl administration. Anesth Analg 1982;61:1020–1021.

129. Safwat AM, Daniel D. Grand mal seizure after fentanyl administration (letter). Anesthesiology 1983;59:78.

130. Hoien AO. Another case of grand mal seizure after fentanyl administration (letter). Anesthesiology 1984;60:387–388.

131. Goroszeniuk T, Albin M, Jones RM. Generalized grand mal seizure after recovery from uncomplicated fentanyl-etomidate anesthesia. Anesth Analg 1986;65:979–981.

132. Rosenberg M, Lisman SR. Major seizure after fentanyl administration: two case reports. J Oral Maxillofac Surg 1986;44:577–579.

133. Bailey PL, Wilbrink J, Zanikken P, et al. Anesthetic induction with fentanyl. Anesth Analg 1985; 64:48–53.

134. Molbegott LP, Flashburg MH, Karasic L, et al. Probable seizures after sufentanil. Anesth Analg 1987;66:91–93.

135. Katz RI, Eide TR, Hartman A, et al. Two instances of seizure-like activity in the same patient associated with two different narcotics. Anesth Analg 1988;67:289–290.

136. Strong WE, Matson M. Probable seizure after alfentanil. Anesth Analg 1989;68:692–293.

137. Sebel PS, Bovill JG, Wauquier A, et al. Effects of high-dose fentanyl anesthesia on the electroencephalogram. Anesthesiology 1982;55:203–211.

138. Wauquier A, Bovill JG, Sebel PS. Electroencephalographic effects of fentanyl-, sufentanil-, and alfentanil anesthesia in man. Neuropsychobiology 1984;11:203–206.

139. Smith NT, Dec-Silver H, Sanford TJ, et al. EEGs during high dose fentany-, sufentanil-, or morphine-oxygen anesthesia. Anesth Analg 1984;63:386–393.

140. Murkin JM, Moldenhauer CC, Hug CC Jr, et al. Absence of seizures during induction of anesthesia with high-dose fentanyl. Anesth Analg 1984;63: 489–494.

141. Bovill JG, Sebel PS, Wauquier A, et al. Electroencephalographic effects of sufentanil anesthesia in man. Br J Anaesth 1982;54:45–52.

142. Bovill JG, Sebel PS, Wauquier A, et al. The influence of high-dose alfentanil anesthesia on the electroencephalogram: correlation with plasma levels. Br J Anaesth 1983;55:1995–2005.

143. Kearse LA, Koski G, Husain MV, et al. Epileptiform activity during opioid anesthesia. Electroencephalogr Clin Neurophysiol 1993;87:374–379.

144. Korttila K, Faure E, Apfelbaum J, et al. Recovery from propofol versus thiopental-isoflurane in patients undergoing outpatient anesthesia. Anesthesiology 1988;69:A–564.

145. Zelcer J, Wells DG. Anesthetic-related recovery room complications. Anesth Intensive Care 1987; 15:168.

146. Rosenberg H, Clofine R, Bialik O. Neurologic changes during awakening from anesthesia. Anesthesiology 1981;54:125–130.

147. Thal G, Szabo MD, Lopez-Bresnahan M, Crosby G. Neurologic changes during emergence from general anesthesia in neurologically normal patients. Anesthesiology 1993;79:A–192.

148. Ropper AH, Kennedy SK. Postoperative neurosurgical care. In: Roper AH, Kennedy SK, eds. Neurological and neurosurgical intensive care. Rockville, MD: Aspen Publishers, 1988;159–164.

149. Thal G, Szabo MD, Lopez-Bresnahan M, Crosby G. Exacerbation or unmasking of focal neurologic deficits by sedative medication. Anesthesiology 1996, in press.

150. Finck AD, Salcman M, Balis E. Alleviation of prolonged postoperative central nervous system depression after treatment with naloxone. Anesthesiology 1977;47:392.

151. Artru AA, Hui GS. Physostigmine reversal of general anesthesia for intra-operative neurological testing: associated EEG changes. Anesth Analg 1986;65:1059–1062.

152. Azar I, Turndorf H. Severe hypertension and multiple atrial premature contractions following naloxone administration. Anesth Analg 1979;58:524–525.

153. Prough DS, Roy R, Bumgarner J, et al. Acute pulmonary edema in healthy teenagers following conservative doses of naloxone. Anesthesiology 1984;60:485–486.

154. Holzgrafe RE, Vondrell JJ, Mintz SM. Reversal of postoperative reaction to scopalamine with physostigmine. Anesth Analg 1973;52:921.

155. Bidwai AV, Stanley TH, Rogers C, et al. Reversal of diazepam-induced post-anesthetic somnolence with physostigmine. Anesthesiology 1979;51:256.

156. Dodgson MS, Skeie B, Emhjellen S, et al. Antagonism of diazepam-induced sedative effects by RO15-1788 in patients after surgery under lumbar epidural block. Acta Anesthesiol Scand 1987; 31:629.

157. Darragh A, Lambe R, Brick I, et al. Reversal of benzodiazepine-induced sedation by intravenous RO15-1788. Lancet 1981;2:1042.

158. Toker P. Hyperosmolar hyperglycemic nonketotic coma, a cause of delayed recovery from anesthesia. Anesthesiology 1974;41:284.

159. Mustajoki P, Heinonen J. General anesthesia in "inducible" porphyrias. Anesthesiology 1980; 53:15.

160. Seibert CP. Recognition, management, and prevention of neuropsychological dysfunction after operation. Int Anesthesiol Clin 1986;24:39–58.

161. Johnston KR, Vaughan RS. Delayed recovery from general anesthesia. Anaesthesia 1988;43:1024.

162. Regan MJ, Eger EI II. Effect of hypothermia in dogs on anesthetizing and apneic doses of inhalational agent. Determination of the anesthetic index (apnea/MAC). Anesthesiology 1967;28:689.

163. Lam AM, Parkin JA. Cimetidine and prolonged postoperative somnolence. Can J Anaesth 1981; 28:450.

164. Fraser AC, Goat VA. Unrecognized presentation of a meningioma. Delayed recovery after general anesthesia presenting as a sign of intracranial pathology. Anaesthesia 1983;38:128.

165. Blake SB, Muzzi DA, Nishimura RA, et al. Preoperative and intraoperative echocardiography to detect right-to-left shunt in patients undergoing neurosurgical procedures in the sitting position. Anesthesiology 72:436–438.

166. Davis O, Kobrine A. Computed tomography. In: Youmans JR, ed. Neurological surgery. Philadelphia: WB Saunders Co., 1982;111–142.

167. Warach S, Gaa J, Siewert B, et al. Acute human stroke studied by whole brain echo planar diffusion-weighted magnetic resonance imaging. Ann Neurol 1995;37:231–241.

168. Fisher M, Prichard JW, Warach S. New magnetic resonance techniques for acute ischemic stroke. JAMA 1995;274:908–911.

169. Raichle ME. The pathophysiology of brain ischemia. Ann Neurol 1983;13:2.

170. Rothman S, Olney JW. Glutamate and the pathophysiology of hypoxicischemic brain damage. Ann Neurol 1986;19:105.

171. Gelmers HJ, Gorter K, de Weerdt CJ, et al. A controlled trial of nimodipine in acute ischemic stroke. N Engl J Med 1988;318:203–207.

172. Kaste M, Fogelholm R, Erila T, et al. A randomized, double-blind, placebo-controlled trial of nimodipine in acute ischemic hemispheric stroke. Stroke 1994;25:1348–1353.

173. Jansen O, Kummer RV, Forsting M, et al. Thrombolytic therapy in acute occlusion of the intracranial internal carotid artery bifurcation. AJNR 1995; 16:1977–1986.

174. Barnwell SL, Clark WM, Nguyen TT, et al. Safety and efficacy of delayed intraarterial urokinase therapy with mechanical clot disruption for thromboembolic stroke. AJNR 1994;15:1817–1822.

175. Ferguson RDG, Ferguson JG. Cerebral intraarterial fibrinolysis at the crossroads: is a phase III trial advisable at this time? AJNR 1994;15:1201–1216.

176. The European Cooperative Acute Stroke Study. Intravenous thrombolysis with recombinant tissue plasminogen activator for acute hemispheric stroke. JAMA 1995;274:1017–1025.

177. National Institute of Neurological Disorders and

Stroke rt-PA Stroke Study Group. Tissue plasminogen activator for acute ischemic stroke. N Engl J Med 1995;333:1581–1587.

178. Kay R, Wong KS, Yu Yl, et al. Low-molecular-weight heparin for the treatment of acute ischemic stroke. N Engl J Med 1995;333:1588–1593.

179. Goldstein LB, the Sygen in Acute Stroke Study Investigators. Common drugs may influence motor recovery after stroke. Neurology 1995;45:865–871.

180. Fode NC, Sundt TM Jr, Robertson JT, et al. Multicenter retrospective review of results and complications of carotid endarterectomy in 1981. Stroke 1986;17:370–376.

181. Harada RN, Comerota AJ, Good GM, et al. Stump pressure, electroencephalographic changes, and the contralateral carotid artery: another look at selective shunting. Am J Surg 1995;170:148–153.

182. Toronto Cerebrovascular Study Group. Risks of carotid endarterectomy, Stroke 1986;17:848–852.

183. Rothwell PM, Slattery J. A systematic review of the risks of stroke and death due to endarterectomy for symptomatic carotid stenosis. Stroke 1996;27:260–265.

184. Ad Hoc Committee, American Heart Association. Guidelines for carotid endarterectomy. Stroke 1995;26:188–201.

185. Warlow C. Carotid endarterectomy: does it work? Stroke 1984;15:1068–1076.

186. Reigel MM, Hollier LH, Sundt TM Jr, et al. Cerebral hyperperfusion syndrome: a cause of neurologic dysfunction after carotid endarterectomy. J Vasc Surg 1982;5:628.

187. Peitzman AB, Webster MW, Loubeau J-M, et al. Carotid endarterectomy under regional (conductive) anesthesia. Ann Surg 1982;196:59.

188. Grundy BL, Webster MW, Richey ET, et al. EEG changes during carotid endarterectomy: drug effect and embolism. Br J Anaesth 1985;57:445.

189. Evans WE, Hayes JP, Waltke EA, et al. Optimal cerebral monitoring during carotid endarterectomy: neurologic response under local anesthesia. J Vasc Surg 1985;2:775.

190. Walleck P, Becquemin JP, Desgranges P, et al. Are neurologic events occuring during carotid artery surgery predictive of postoperative neurologic complications. Acta Anaesthesiol Scand 1996;40:167–170.

191. Chiappa KH, Burke SR, Young RR. Results of electroencephalographic monitoring during 367 carotid endarterectomies: use of a dedicated minicomputer. Stroke 1979;10:381.

192. Gravrilescu T, Babikian VL, Cantelmo NL, et al. Cerebral microembolism during carotid endarterectomy. Am J Surg 1995;170:159–164.

193. Riles TS, Imparato AM, Jacobowitz GR, et al. The cause of perioperative stroke after carotid endarterectomy. J Vasc Surg 1994;19:206–216.

194. Prioleau WH Jr, Aiken AF, Hairston P. Carotid endarterectomy: neurological complications as related to surgical techniques. Ann Surg 1977;185;678–681.

195. Perkins WJ, Weglinski MR, Meyer FB, et al. Timing and etiology of perioperative stroke following carotid endarterectomy. Anesthesiology 1995;83:A180.

196. Sieber FE, Toung TJ, Diringer NM, et al. Factors influencing stroke outcome following carotid endarterectomy. Anesth Analg 1990;70:s–370.

197. Asiddao C, Donegan JH, Whitesell R, et al. Factors associated with perioperative complications during carotid endarterectomy. Anesth Analg 1982;61:631.

198. McKay Rd, Sundt RM Jr, Michenfelder JD, et al. Internal carotid artery stump pressure and cerebral blood flow during carotid endarterectomy: modification by halothane, enflurane, and Innovar. Anesthesiology 1976;45:390.

199. Gibson BE, McMichan JG, Cuchiara RF. Lack of correlation between transconjunctibval O_2 and cerebral blood flow during carotid artery occlusion. Anesthesiology 1986;64:277.

200. Cho I, Smullens SN, Streletz LJ, et al. The value of intraoperative EEG monitoring during carotid endarterectomy. Ann Neurol 1986; 203(17):96508.

201. Allen BT, Anderson CB, Rubin BG, et al. The influence of anesthetic technique on perioperative complications after carotid endarterectomy. J Vasc Surg 1994;19:834–843.

202. Jansen C, Vriens EM, Eikelboom BC, et al. Carotid endarterectomy with transcranial doppler and electroencephalographic monitoring: a prospective study in 130 patients. Stroke 1993;24:665–669.

203. Jansen C, Ramos LMP, van Heesewijk JPM, et al. Impact of microembolism and hemodynamic changes in th brain during crotid endarterectomy. Stroke 1994;25:992–997.

204. Astrup J, Siesjo Bk, Lymon L. Thresholds in cerebral ischemia: the ischemic penumbra. Stroke 1981;12:723.

205. Blume WT, Ferguson GG, McNeill DK. Significance of EEG changes at carotid endarterectomy. Stroke 1986;17:891.

206. van Zuilen EV, Noll FL, Vermeulen FEE, et al. Detection of cerebral microemboli by means of transcranial doppler monitoring before and after carotid endarterectomy. Stroke 1995;26:210–213.

207. Harper AM. Autoregulation of cerebral blood flow: influence of arterial blood pressure on the blood flow through the cerebral cortex. J Neurol Neurosurg Psychiatry 1966;29:398.

208. Hoedt-Rasmussen K, Skinhoj E, Paulson OB, et al. Regional cerebral blood flow in acute apoplexy: the "luxury perfusion syndrome" of brain tissue. Arch Neurol 1967;17:271.

209. Gross CE, Adams HP Jr, Sokoll MD, et al. Use of anticoagulants electroencephalographic monitoring, and barbiturate cerebral protection in carotid endarterectomy. Neurosurgery 1981;9:1.

210. Drummond JC, Yong-Seok O, Cole DJ, et al. Phenylepherine-induced hypertension reduces ischemia following middle cerebral artery occlusion in rats. Stroke 1989;20:1538.

211. Myers RE, Yamaguchi T. Nervous system effects of cardiac arrest in monkeys. Arch Neurol 1974;34:65.

212. Pulsinelli WA, Waldman S, Rawlinson D, et al. Moderate hyperglycemia augments ischemic brain

damage: a neuropathologic study in the rat. Neurology 1982;32:1239.

213. Lanier WE, Strangland KJ, Scheithauer BW, et al. The effects of dextrose infusion and head position on neurologic outcome after complet cerebral ischemia in primates: examination of a model. Anesthesiology 1987;66:39.

214. Pulsinelli WA, Levy DE, Sigsbee B, et al. Increased damage after ischemic stroke in patients with ischemic stroke in patients with hyperglycemia with or without established diabetes mellitus. Am J Med 1986;74:540.

215. Candelize L, Landi G, Orazio EN, et al. Prognostic significance of hyperglycemia in stroke. Arch Neurol 1985;42:661.

216. Ginsberg MD, Prado R, Dietrich WD, et al. Hyperglycemia reduces the extent of cerebral infarction in rats. Stroke 1987;18:570.

217. Michenfelder JD, Sundt TM Jr, Fode N, et al. Isoflurane when compared to enflurane and halothane decreases the frequency of cerebral ischemia during carotid endarterectomy. Anesthesiology 1987;67:336–340.

218. Sharbrough FW, Messick JM Jr, Sundt TM. Correlation of continuous electroencephalograms with cerebral blood flow measurements during carotid endarterectomy. Stroke 1973;4:674–683.

219. Messick JM, Casement B, Sharbrough FW, et al. Correlation of regional cerebral blood flow (rCBF) with EEG changes during isoflurane anesthesia for carotid endarterectomy: critical rCBF. Anesthesiology 1987;66:344–349.

220. Nehls DG, Todd MM, Spetzler RF, et al. A comparison of the cerebral protective effects of isoflurane and barbiturates during temporary focal ischemia in primates. Anesthesiology 1987;66:453–464.

221. Gelb AW, Boisvert DP, Tang C, et al. Primate brain tolerance to temporary focal cerebral ischemia during isoflurane or sodium nitroprusside-induced hypotension. Anesthesiology 1989;70:678.

222. Spetzler RF, Martin N, Hadley MN, et al. Microsurgical endarterectomy under barbiturate protection: a prospective study. J Neurosurg 1986;65:63.

223. McMeniman WJ, Fletcher JP, Little JM. Experience with barbiturate therapy for cerebral protection during carotid endarterectomy. Ann R Coll Surg Engl 1984;66:361.

224. Gelb AW, Floyd R, Lok P, et al. A prophylactic bolus of thiopental does not protect against prolonged focal cerebral ischemia. Can J Anaesth 1986;33:173.

225. Miller RA, Crosby G, Sundaram P. Exacerbated spinal neurologic deficit during sedation of a patient with cervical spondylosis. Anesthesiology 1987;67:844.

226. Bensel EC, Hadden TA, Mossaman BD, et al. Does sufentanil exacerbate marginal neurological dysfunction? J Neurosurg Anesthesiol 1990;2:50.

227. Branthwaite MA. Prevention of neurological damage during open heart surgery. Thorax 1975;30:258.

228. Sotaniemi KA. Brain damage and neurological outcome after open heart surgery. J Neurol Neurosurg Psychiatry 1980;43:127.

229. Slogoff S, Girgis KZ, Keats AS. Etiologic factors in neuropsychiatric complication associated with cardiopulmonary bypass. Anesth Analg 1982;61:903–911.

230. Townes BD, Bashien G, Hornbein TF, et al. Neurobehavioral outcomes in cardiac operations. J Thorac Cardiovasc Surg 1989;98:774–782.

231. Metz S, Slogoff S. Thiepental sodium by single bolus dose compared to infusion for cerebral protection during cardiopulmonary bypass. J Clin Anesth 1990;2:226–231.

232. Shaw PJ, Bates D, Cartlidge NEF, et al. Neurologic and neuropsychological morbidity following major surgery: comparison of coronary artery bypass and peripheral vascular surgery. Stroke 1987;18:700–707.

233. Weintraub WS, Jones EL, Craver J, et al. Determinants of prolonged length of hospital stay after coronary bypass surgery. Circulation 1989;80:276–284.

234. Bashein G, Townes BD, Nessly ML, et al. A randomized study of carbon dioxide management during hypothermic cardiopulmonary bypass. Anesthesiology 1990;72:7–15.

235. Klonoff H, Clark C, Kavanagh-Gray D, et al. Two-year follow-up study of coronary artery bypass surgery. J Thorac Cardiovasc Surg 1989;97:78–85.

236. Venn G, Klinger L, Smith P, et al. Neuro-psychologic sequelae of bypass twelve months after coronary artery surgery. Br Heart J 1987;57:565.

237. Ellis RJ, Wisniewski A, Potts R, et al. Reduction of flow rate and arterial pressure at moderate hypothermia does not result in cerebral dysfunction. J Thorac Cardiovasc Surg 1980;79:173–180.

238. Kolkka R, Hilberman M. Neurologic dysfunction following cardiac operation with low-flow, low-pressure cardiopulmonary bypass. J Thorac Cardiovasc Surg 1980;79:432–437.

239. Fish KJ, Helms KN, Sarnquist FH, et al. A prospective, randomized study of the effects of prostacyclin on neuropsychologic dysfunction after coronary artery operation. J Thorac Cardiovasc Surg 1987;93:609–615.

240. Newman MF, Kramer D, Croughwell MD, et al. Differential age effects of mean arterial pressure and rewarming on cognitive dysfunction after cardiac surgery. Anesth Analg 1995;81:236–242.

241. Solis RT, Noon GP, Beall AC, et al. Particulate microembolism during cardiac surgery. Ann Thorac Surg 1974;17:332–344.

242. Roigas PC, Meyer FJ, Haasler CB, et al. Intraoperative 2-dimensional echocardiography: ejection of microbubbles from the left ventricle after cardiac surgery. Am J Cardiol 1982;50:1130–1132.

243. Yao FS, Barbut D, Hager DN, et al. Detection of aortic emboli by transesophageal echocardiography during coronary bypass surgery. Anesthesiology 1995;83:A126.

244. Pugsley W, Klinger L, Paschalis C, et al. The impact of microemboli during cardiopulmonary bypass on neuropsychological functioning. Stroke 1994;25:1393–1399.

245. Barbut D, Hinton RB, Szatrowski TP, et al. Cerebral emboli detected during bypass surgery are asso-

ciated with clamp removal. Stroke 1994; 25:2398–2402.

246. Aris A, Solanes H, Camara ML, et al. Arterial line filtration during cardiopulmonary bypass. Neurologic, neuropsychologic, and hematologic studies. J Thorac Cardiovasc Surg 1986;91:526–533.

247. Stump DA, Kon NA, Rogers AT, et al. Emboli and neuropsychological deficits after cardiac valve replacement surgery. Anesthesiology 1995; 83:A132.

248. Aberg T, Ronquist G, Tyden H, et al. Adverse effects on the brain in cardiac operations as assessed by biochemical, psychometric, and radiologic methods. J Thorac Cardiovasc Surg 1984;87:99–105.

249. Tufo HM, Ostfeld AM, Shekelle R. Central nervous system dysfunction following open-heart surgery. JAMA 1970;212:1333.

250. Smith PLC, Newman S, Treasure T, et al. Cerebral consequences of cardiopulmonary bypass. Lancet 1986;1:823–824.

251. Murkin JM, Martzke JS, Buchan AM, et al. A randomized study of the influence of perfusion technique and pH management strategy in 316 patients undergoing coronary artery bypass surgery. J Thorac Cardiovasc Surg 1995;110:349–362.

252. Kuroda Y, Uchimoto R, Kaieda R, et al. Central nervous system complications after cardiac surgery: a comparison between coronary artery bypass grafting and valve surgery. Anesth Analg 1993;76:222–227.

253. Jones EL, Craver JM, Michalik RA, et al. Combined carotid and coronary operations: when are they necessary? J Thorac Cardiovasc Surg 1984;87:7.

254. Gardner TJ, Horneffer PJ, Manolio TA, et al. Stroke following coronary artery bypass grafting: a ten-year study. Ann Thorac Surg 1985;40:574–581.

255. Tuman KF, McCarthy RJ, Najafi H, et al. Differential effects of advanced age on neurologic and cardiac risks of coronary artery operations. J Thorac Cardiovasc Surg 1992;104:1510–1517.

256. Stump DA, Newman SP, Coker LH, et al. The effect of age on neurologic outcome after cardiac surgery. Anesth Analg 1992;74:S310.

257. Blauth CI, Smith PL, Arnold JV, et al. Influence of oxygenator type on the prevalence and extent of microembolic retinal ischemia during cardiopulmonary bypass. Assessment by digital image analysis. J Thorac Cardiovasc Surg 1990;99:61–69.

258. Stockard JJ, Bickford RG, Schauble JF. Pressure dependent cerebral ischemia during cardiopulmonary bypass. Neurology 1973;23:321–329.

259. Newman MF, Kramer D, Croughwell, ND et al. Differential age effects of mean arterial pressure and rewarming on cognitive dysfunction after cardiac surgery. Anesth Analg 1995;81:236–242.

260. Martin JM, Farrar JK, Tweed WA, et al. Cerebral auto-regulation and flow/metabolism coupling during cardiopulmonary bypass: the influence of $PaCO_2$. Anesth Analg 1987;66:825–832.

261. Roger AT, Stump DA, Gravlee GP, et al. Response of cerebral blood flow to phenylephrine infusion during hypothermic cardiopulmonary bypass: influence of $PaCO_2$. management. Anesthesiology 1988;69:547–551.

262. Stephan H, Weyland A, Kazmaier S, et al. Acid-base management during hypothermic cardiopulmonary bypass does not affect cerebral metabolism but does affect blood flow and neurological outcome. Br J Anaesth 1992;69:51–57.

263. Venn GE, Patel RL, Chambers DJ. Cardiopulmonary bypass: perioperative cerebral blood flow and postoperative cognitive deficit. Ann Thorac Surg 1995;59:1331–1335.

264. Wolfe KB. Effect of hypothermia on cerebral damage resulting from cardiac arrest. Am J Cardiol 1960;6:809.

265. Norwood WJ, Norwood CR, Casteneda AR. Cerebral anoxia: effect of deep hypothermia and pH. Surgery 1979;86:203.

266. Molina JE, Einzig S, Mastri AR, et al. Brain damage in profound hypothermia. J Thorac Cardiovasc Surg 1984;87:596.

267. Martin TD, Craver JM, Gott JP, et al. Prospective, randomized trial of retrograde warm blood cardioplegia: myocardial benefit and neurologic threat. Ann Thorac Surg 1994;57:298–304.

268. Barzilai B, Marshall WG Jr, Saffitz JE, et al. Avoidance of embolic complications by ultrasonic characterization of the ascending aorta. Circulation 1989;80:1275–1279.

269. Newman M, Croughwell N, Lowry E, et al. Emboli detection in warm and cold cardiopulmonary bypass. Anesthesiology 1995;83:A130.

270. The Warm Heart Investigators. Randomised trial of normothermic versus hypothermic coronary bypass surgery. Lancet 1994;343;559–563.

271. McLean RF, Wong BI, Naylor D, et al. Cardiopulmonary bypass, temperature, and central nervous system dysfunction. Circulation 1994;90:II250–II255.

272. Wass CT, Lanier WL, Hofer RE, et al. Temperature changes of >1 degree C alter functional neurologic outcome and histopathology in a canine model of complete cerebral ischemia. Anesthesiology 1995;83:325–335.

273. Barzilai B, Marshall WG Jr, Saffitz JE, et al. Avoidance of embolic complications by ultrasonic characterization of the ascending aorta. Circulation 1989;80:1275–1279.

274. Nussmeier NA, Arlund C, Slogoff S. Neuropsychiatric complications after cardiopulmonary bypass: cerebral protection by a barbiturate. Anesthesiology 1986;64:165–170.

275. Michenfelder JD. A valid demonstration of barbiturate-induced cerebral protection in man – at last. Anesthesiology 1986;64:140–142.

276. Prough DS, Mills SA. Should thiopental sodium administration be a standard of care for open cardiac procedures? J Clin Anesth 1990;2:221–225.

277. Deeb GM, Jenkins E, Bolling SF, et al. Retrograde cerebral perfusion during hypothermic circulatory arrest reduces neurologic morbidity. J Thorac Cardiovasc Surg 1995;109:259–268.

278. Lytle BW, McCarthy PM, Meaney KM, et al. Systemic hypothermia and circulatory arrest combined with arterial perfusion of the superior vena cava: effective intraoperative cerebral protection. J Thorac Cardiovasc Surg 1995;109:738–743.

279. Lin PJ, Chang CH, Tan PPC, et al. Protection of the brain by retrograde cerebral perfusion during circulatory arrest. J Thorac Cardiovasc Surg 1994;108:969–974.

280. Alamanni F, Agrifoglio M, Pompilio G, et al. Aortic arch surgery: pros and cons of selective cerebral perfusion: a multivariate analysis for cerebral injury during hypothermic circulatory arrest. J Cardiovasc Surg 1995;36:31–37.

281. Moon RE, Camporeai EM. Clinical care in the hyperbaric environment. In: Miller RE, ed. Anesthesia. New York: Churchill Livingstone, 1990;2089–2111.

282. Kindwall EP. Massive surgical air embolism treated with brief recompression to six atmospheres followed by hyperbaric oxygen. AEMEA 1973; 44:663.

283. Winter PM, Alvis HG, Gage AA. Hyperbaric treatment of cerebral air embolism during cardiopulmonary bypass. JAMA 1971;215:1786.

284. Bove AA, Clark JM, Simon AJ, et al. Successful therapy of cerebral air embolism with hyperbaric oxygen at 2.8 ATA. Undersea Biomed Res 1982; 9:75.

285. Kol S, Ammar R, Melamed Y. Hyperbaric oxygen for arterial air embolism during cardiopulmonary bypass. Ann Thorac Surg 1993;55:401–403.

286. Dahlgren N, Tornebrandt K. Neurological complications after anaesthesia. A follow-up of 18,000 spinal and epidural anaesthetics performed over three years. Acta Anaesthesiol Scand 1995; 39:872–880.

287. Greene NM. Neurological sequelae of spinal anesthesia. Anesthesiology 1961;22:682–698.

288. Moore DC, Bridenbaugh LD. Spinal (subarachnoid) block: a review of 11,574 cases. JAMA 1966;195:907–912.

289. Phillips OC, Ebner H, Nelson AT, et al. Neurologic complications following spinal anesthesia with lidocaine: a prospective review of 10,440 cases. Anesthesiology 1969;30:284–289.

290. Mills GH, Howell SJL, Richmond MN. Spinal cord compression immediately following, but unrelated to, epidural analgesia. Anaesthesia 1994;49:954–956.

291. Vandam LD, Dripps RD. A longterm follow-up of 10,098 spinal anesthetics II. Incidence and analysis of minor sensory neurological defects. Surgery 1955;38:463–469.

292. Liu S, Carpenter RL, Neal JM. Epidural anesthesia and analgesia: their role in postoperative outcome. Anesthesiology 1995;82:1474–1506.

293. Dawkins CJM. An analysis of the complications of extradural and caudal block. Anaesthesia 1969; 24:554–563.

294. Kane RE. Neurologic deficits following epidural or spinal anesthesia. Review article. Anesth Analg 1981;60:150–161.

295. Dripps RD, Vandam LD. Long-term follow-up of patients who received 10,098 spinal anesthetics: failure to discover major neurological sequelae. JAMA 1954;156:1486–1491.

296. Nicholson MJ, Eversole UH. Neurologic complications of spinal anesthesia. JAMA 1946;132:679–685.

297. Kennedy F, Effron AS, Perry G. The grave spinal cord paralysis caused by spinal anesthesia. Surg Gynecol Obstet 1950;91:385–398.

298. Sowter MC, Burgess NA, Woodsford PV, et al. Delayed presentation of an extradural abscess complicating thoracic extradural analgesia. Br J Anaesth 1992;68:103–105.

299. Barsa J, Batra M, Fink BR, et al. A comparative in vivo study of local neurotoxicity of lidocaine, bupivacaine, 2-chloroprocaine and a mixture of 2-chloroprocaine and bupivacaine. Anesth Analg 1982;61:961–967.

300. Moore DC, Spierdijk J, vanKleef JD, et al. Chloroprocaine neurotoxicity: four additional cases. Anesth Analg 1982;61:155–159.

301. Myers RR, Kalichman MW, Reisner LS, et al. Neurotoxicity of local anesthetics: altered perineural permeability, edema, and nerve fiber injury. Anesthesiology 1986;64:29–35.

302. Rigler ML, Drasner K, Krejcie TC, et al. Cauda equina syndrome after continuous spinal anesthesia. Anesth Analg 1991;72:275–281.

303. Lambert LA, Lambert DH, Strichartz GR. Irreversible conduction block in isolated nerve by high concentrations of local anesthetics. Anesthesiology 1994;80:1082–1093.

304. Cheng ACK. Intended epidural anesthesia as possible cause of cauda equina syndrome. Anesth Analg 1994;78:157–159.

305. Beardsley D, Holman S, Gantt R, et al. Transient neurologic deficit after spinal anesthesia: local anesthetic maldistribution with pencil point needles? Anesth Analg 1995;81:314–320.

306. Wang BC, Hillman DE, Spielholz NI, et al. Chronic neurological deficits and Nesacaine-CE – an effect of the anesthetic, 2-chloroprocaine, or the antioxidant, sodium bisulfite? Anesth Analg 1984; 63:445–447.

307. Cope RW. Woolley and Roe versus ministry of health and others. Anaesthesia 1954;9:249–270.

308. Gibbons RB. Chemical meningitis following spinal anesthesia. JAMA 1969;210:900–902.

309. Garfield JM, Andriole GL, Vetto JT, et al. Prolonged diabetes insipidus subsequent to an episode of chemical meningitis. Anesthesiology 1986;64:253–254.

310. Berman RS, Eisele JH. Bacteremia, spinal anesthesia, and the development of meningitis. Anesthesiology 1978;48:376–377.

311. Mamourian AC, Dickman CA, Drayer BP, et al. Spinal epidural abscess: three cases following spinal epidural injection demonstrated with magnetic resonance imaging. Anesthesiology 1993;78:204–207.

312. Green NM. Neurological sequelae of spinal anesthesia. Anesthesiology 1961;22:682–698.

313. Strafford MA, Wilder RT, Berde CB. The risk of infection from epidural analgesia in children: a review of 1620 cases. Anesth Analg 1995;80:234–238.

314. Strong WE. Epidural abscess associated with epidural catheterization: a rare event? Report of two

cases with markedly delayed presentation. Anesthesiology 1991;74:943–946.

315. Baker AS, Ojemann RG, Swartz MN, et al. Spinal epidural abscess. N Engl J Med 1975;293:463–468.

316. Nordstrom O, Sandin R. Delayed presentation of an extradural abscess in a patient with alchol abuse. Br J Anaesth 1993;70:368–369.

317. Jakobsen KB, Christensen MK, Carlsson PS. Extradural anaesthesia for repeated surgical treatment in the presence of infection. Br J Anaesth 1995; 75:536–540.

318. Chestnut DH. Spinal anesthesia in the febrile patient. Anesthesiology 1992;76:667–669.

319. Dripps RD, Vandam LD. Hazards of lumbar puncture. JAMA 1951;147:1118–1121.

320. Reisner LS, Hochman BN, Plumer MH. Persistent neurologic deficit and adhesive arachnoiditis following intrathecal 2-chloroprocaine injection. Anesth Analg 1980;59:452–454.

321. Rigler ML, Drasner K, Krejcie TC, et al. Cauda equina syndrome after continuous spinal anesthesia. Anesth Analg 1991;72;275–281.

322. Owens EL, Kasten GW, Hessel EA. Spinal hematoma after lumbar puncture and heparinization. Anesth Analg 1986;65:1201–1207.

323. Bougher RJ, Ramage D. Spinal subdural haematoma following combined spinal-epidural anaesthesia. Anaesth Intensive Care 1995;23:111–113.

324. Rao TLK, El-Etr AA. Anticoagulation following placement of epidural and subarachnoid catheters: an evaluation of neurological sequelae. Anesthesiology 1981;55:618–620.

325. Odoom JA, Sih IL. Epidural analgesia and anticoagulant therapy: experience with one thousand cases of continuous epidurals. Anaesthesia 1983; 38:254–259.

326. Metzger G, Singbartl G. Spinal epidural hematoma following epidural anesthesia versus spontaneous spinal subdural hematoma. Two case reports. Acta Anaesthesiol Scand 1991;35:105–107.

327. Horlocker TT, Wedel DJ, Offord KP. Does preoperative antiplatelet therapy increase the risk of hemorrhagic complications associated with regional anesthesia? Anesth Analg 1990;70:631–634.

328. Horlocker TT, Wedel DJ, Schlichting JL. Postoperative epidural analgesia and oral anticoagulant therapy. Anesth Analg 1994;79:89–93.

329. Vandermeulen EP, Van Aken H, Vermylen J. Anticoagulants and spinal-epidural anesthesia. Anesth Analg 1994;79:1165–1177.

330. Mayumi T, Dohi S. Spinal subarachnoid hematoma after lumbar puncture in a patient receiving antiplatelet therapy. Anesth Analg 1983;62:777–779.

331. Horlocker TT, Wedel DJ, Schroeder DR, et al. Preoperative antiplatelet therapy does not increase the risk of spinal hematoma associated with regional anesthesia. Anesth Analg 1995;80:303–309.

332. Spurny OM, Rubin S, Wolf JW, et al. Spinal epidural hematoma during anticoagulant therapy. Report of two cases. Arch Intern Med 1964;114:103–107.

333. Onishchuk JL, Carlsson C. Epidural hematoma associated with epidural anesthesia: complications of anticoagulant therapy. Anesthesiology 1992;77: 1221–1223.

334. Owens EL, Kasten GW, Hessel EA. Spinal hematoma after lumbar puncture and heparinization. Anesth Analg 1986;65:1201–1207.

335. Baron HC, LaRaja RD, Rossi G, et al. Continuous epidural analgesia in the heparinized vascular surgical patient: a retrospective review of 912 patients. J Vasc Surg 1987;6:144–146.

336. Bergqvist D, Linblad B, Matzsch T. Low molecular weight heparin for thromboprophylaxis and epidural/spinal anesthesia: is there a risk? Acta Anaesthesiol Scand 1992;36:605–609.

337. Nicholson A. Painless epidural haematoma. Anaesth Intensive Care 1994;22:607–610.

338. Vandam LD, Dripps RD. Exacerbation of pre-existing neurologic disease after spinal anesthesia. N Engl J Med 1956;255:843–848.

339. Shanker KB, Palkar NV, Nishkala R. Paraplegia following epidural potassium chloride. Anaesthesia 1985;40:45–47.

340. McGuinness JP, Cantees KK. Epidural injection of a phenol containing ranitidine preparation. Anesthesiology 1990;73:553–555.

341. Cay DL. Accidental epidural thiopentone. Anaesth Intensive Care 1984;12:61–63.

342. Forestner JE, Raj PP. Inadvertent epidural injection of thiopental: a case report. Anesth Analg 1974; 54:406–407.

343. Liu K, Chia YY. Inadvertent epidural injection of potassium chloride. Report of two cases. Acta Anaesthesiol Scand 1995;39:1134–1137.

344. Bier A. Versuche ueber Cocainisirung des Rueckenmarkes. Deutsche Zeitschrift fuer Deutsch Z Chir 1899;51:361–368.

345. Brownridge P. The management of headache following accidental dural puncture in obstetric patients. Anaesth Intensive Care 1983;11:4–15.

346. Lybecker H, Djernes M, Schmidt JF. Postdural puncture headache (PDPH): Onset, duration, severity, and associated symptoms. Acta Anaesthesiol Scand 1995;39:605–612.

347. Carrie LES. Postdural puncture headache and the extradural blood patch. Br J Anaesth 1993; 71:179–181.

348. Olsen KS. Epidural blood patch in the treatment of post-lumbar puncture headache. Pain 1987; 30:293–301.

349. MacRoberts RJ. The cause of lumbar puncture headache. JAMA 1918;70:1350.

350. Naulty JS, Hertwig L, Hunt CO, et al. Influence of local anesthetic solution on postdural puncture headache. Anesthesiology 1990;72:450–454.

351. Dodd JE, Efird RC, Rauck RL. Cerebral blood flow changes with caffeine therapy for postdural headache. Anesthesiology 1989;71:A679.

352. Camann WR, Murray RS, Mushlin PS, et al. Effects of oral caffeine on postdural puncture headache: a double-blind, placebo-controlled trial. Anesth Analg 1990;70:181–184.

353. Ravindran RS. Epidural autologous blood patch on an outpatient basis. Anesth Analg 1984;63:962.

354. Abouleish E, de la Vega S, Blendinger I, et al. Long-

term follow-up of epidural blood patch. Anesth Analg 1975;54:459–463.

355. Ostheimer GW, Palahniuk RJ, Shnider SM. Epidural bloodpatch for post-lumbar-puncture headache. Anesthesiology 1974;41:307–308.

356. Cohen SE. Epidural blood patch in outpatients: a simpler approach. Anesth Analg 1985;64:458.

357. Ramsay M, Roberts C. Epidural injection does cause an increase in CSF pressure. Anesth Analg 1991;73:676.

358. Beards AC, Jackson A, Griffiths AG, et al. Magnetic resonance imaging of extradural blood patches: appearances from 30 min to 18 hours. Br J Anaesth 1993;71:182–188.

359. Andrews PJD, Ackerman WE, Juneja M, et al. Transient bradycardia associated with extradural blood patch after inadvertent dural puncture in parturients. Br J Anaesth 1992;69:401–403.

360. Edelman JD, Wingard DW. Subdural hematomas after lumbar dural puncture. Anesthesiology 1980;52:166–167.

361. Blake DW, Donnan G, Jensen D. Intracranial subdural hematomas after spinal anesthesia. Anaesth Intensive Care 1987;15:341–342.

362. Jack TM. Post-partum intracranial subdural haematoma: a possible complication of epidural analgesia. Anaesthesia 1979;34:176–180.

363. Wang LP, Fog J, Bove M. Transient hearing loss following spinal anaesthesia. Anaesthesia 1987;42:1258–1263.

364. Sundberg A, Wang LP, Fog J. Influence on hearing of 22 G Whitacre and 22 G Quincke needles. Anaesthesia 1992;47:981–983.

365. Fog J, Wang LP, Sundberg A, et al. Hearing loss after spinal anesthesia is related to needle size. Anesth Analg 1990;70:517–522.

366. Vandam LD, Dripps RD. Long term follow-up of patients who received 10,098 spinal anesthetics: syndrome of decreased intracranial pressure. JAMA 1956;161:586–591.

367. Schneider M, Ettlin T, Kaufmann M, et al. Transient neurologic toxicity after hyperbaric subarachnoid anesthesia with 5% lidocaine. Anesth Analg 1993;76:1154–1157.

368. Hampl KF, Schneider MC, Wolfgang Ummenhofer W, et al. Transient Neurologic symptoms after spinal anesthesia. Anesth Analg 1995;81:1148–1153.

369. Tarkkila P, Huhtala J, Tuominen M. Transient radicular irritation after spinal anaesthesia with hyperbaric 5% lignocaine. Br J Anaesth 1995;74:328–329.

370. Hurley RJ, Lambert DH. Continuous spinal anesthesia with a microcatheter technique: preliminary experience. Anesth Analg 1990;70:97–102.

371. Parks BJ. Postoperative peripheral neuropathies. Surgery 1973;74:348–357.

372. Dhuner KG. Nerve injuries following operations: a survey of cases occurring during a six-year period. Anesthesiology 1950;11:289–293.

373. Martin JT. Postoperative isolated dysfunction of the long thoracic nerve: a rare entity of uncertain etiology. Anesth Analg 1989;69:614–619.

374. Cheney FW, Posner K, Caplan RA, et al. Standard of care and anesthesia liability. JAMA 1989;261:1599–1603.

375. Kroll DA, Caplan RA, Posner K, et al. Nerve injury associated with anesthesia. Anesthesiology 1990;73:202–207.

376. Cooper DE, Jenkins RS, Bready L, et al. The prevention of injuries of the brachial plexus secondary to malposition of the patient during surgery. Clin Orthop 1988;228:33–41.

377. Wood-Smith FG. Postoperative Brachial plexus paralysis. Br Med J 1952;1:115–116.

378. Jackson L, Keats AS. Mechanism of brachial plexus palsy following anesthesia. Anesthesiology 1965;26:190–194.

379. Ewing MR. Postoperative paralysis in the upper extremity: report of five cases. Lancet 1950;1:99–102.

380. Kwaan JHM, Rappaport I. Postoperative brachial plexus palsy: a study of the mechanism. Arch Surg 1970;101:612–615.

381. Lederman RJ, Breuer AC, Hanson MR, et al. Peripheral nervous system complications of coronary artery bypass graft surgery. Ann Neurol 1982;12:297–301.

382. Hanson MR, Bruer AC, Furlan AJ, et al. Mechanism and frequency of brachial plexus injury in open heart surgery: a prospective analysis. Ann Thorac Surg 1983;36:675–679.

383. Paschall RM, Mandel S. Brachial plexus injury from percutaneous cannulation of the internal jugular vein. Ann Emerg Med 1983;12:112–114.

384. Roy RC, Stafford MA, Charlton JE. Nerve injury and musculoskeletal complaints after cardiac surgery: influence of internal mammary artery dissection and left arm position. Anesth Analg 1988;67:277–279.

385. Vander Salm TJ, Cereda JM, Cutler BS. Brachial plexus injury following median sternotomy. J Thorac Cardiovasc Surg 1980;80:447–452.

386. Eggers KA, Asai T. Postoperative brachial plexus neuropathy after total knee replacement under spinal anaesthesia. Br J Anaesth 1995;75:642–644.

387. Anderton JM, Schady W, Markham DE. An unusual cause of postoperative brachial plexus palsy. Br J Anaesth 1994;72:605–607.

388. Dawson DM, Krarup C. Perioperative nerve lesions. Arch Neurol 1989;46:1355–1360.

389. Warner MA, Warner ME, Martin JT. Ulnar neuropathy: incidence, outcome, and risk factors in sedated or anesthetized patients. Anesthesiology 1994;81:1332–1340.

390. Miller RG. The cubital tunnel syndrome: diagnosis and precise localization. Ann Neurol 1979;6:56–59.

391. Miller RG, Camp PE. Postoperative ulnar neuropathy. JAMA 1979;242:1636.

392. Jones HD. Ulnar nerve damage following general anesthesia. Anesthesia 1967;22:471–475.

393. Eisen A. Early diagnosis of ulnar nerve palsy: an electrophysiologic study. Neurology 1974;24:256–262.

394. Williams JR. Postoperative ulnar neuropathy. JAMA 1980;243:1525–1526.

395. Wadsworth TG. The cubital tunnel and the ex-

ternal compression syndrome. Anesth Analg 1974;53:303–208.

396. Stoelting RK. Postoperative ulnar nerve palsy — is it a preventable complication? Anesth Analg 1993;76:7–9.

397. Wadsworth TG, Williams JR. Cubital tunnel external compression syndrome. Br Med J 1973; 1:662–666.

398. Alvine FG, Schurrer ME. Postoperative ulnar nerve palsy: are there predisposing factors. J Bone Joint Surg 1987;69:A255–259.

399. Seyfer AE, Grammer NY, Bogumil GP, et al. Upper extremity neuropathies after cardiac surgery. J Hand Surg 1985;10A:16–19.

400. Caplan RA, Posner KL, Cheney FW. Perioperative ulnar neuropathy: are we ready for shortcuts? Anesthesiology 1994;81:1321–1323.

401. Sy WP. Ulnar nerve palsy possibly related to the use of automatically cycled blood pressure cuff. Anesth Analg 1981;60:687–688.

402. Alexander GD. Mechanism of ulnar nerve injury. Anesthesiology 1990;73:1294–1295.

403. Murphy JP, Devers JC. Prevention of post surgical ulnar neuropathy. JAMA 1974;227:1123–1124.

404. Aita JF. Postoperative ulnar neuropathy. JAMA 1981;245:2295.

405. Mawk JR, Theinprasit P. Postoperative ulnar neuropathy. JAMA 1981;246:2806–2807.

11

HEMATOLOGIC SYSTEM

Charise T. Petrovich

The patient who lies in the postanesthesia recovery room, half awake and half asleep, may be quietly bleeding. There is no sound to alert the physician of the impending danger. The crisis will arise when the patient's vital signs become alarming — the pulse of the patient quickens and the blood pressure falls. Then, the response of the physician must be decisive and astute. Many life-sustaining elements are lost when blood leaves the body: the precious red blood cells that carry oxygen; hemostatic agents, both platelets and clotting factors; and fluid volume, which is necessary to support the beat-to-beat stroke volume of each cardiac cycle. The physician, who arrives on the scene to find the patient's condition deteriorating, must decide which if any of these critical elements must be replaced emergently not only to sustain the life of the patient but also to avoid tissue damage to any vital organs. At this point, resuscitation may be more important than making a definitive diagnosis but, ultimately, the physician must determine whether the patient's bleeding is due to a surgical problem, which requires reoperation, or whether it is secondary to a bleeding disorder, which requires blood component therapy.

The transfusion of hemostatic agents such as platelets and fresh frozen plasma to a patient with surgical defects will only increase the risk of contracting a transfusion-transmitted infection such as acquired immunodeficiency syndrome (AIDS) or hepatitis. Additionally, these blood components cannot seal the large vascular defects created when blood vessels are transected during surgery. Likewise, the rare patient who comes to surgery with an underlying bleeding disorder or who develops a coagulopathy intraoperatively will require blood component therapy. Suture ligaments simply cannot repair a defect in the hemostatic mechanism. However, blood components should neither be transfused in a "shotgun" approach nor according to some predefined recipe. It is more appropriate to correctly diagnose the cause of a bleeding disorder and to transfuse the proper blood component. If a shotgun approach is to be used, then as Glen Gravlee, MD has said, it is best "to fire one barrel at a time."

SURGICAL BLEEDING AND RED BLOOD CELL TRANSFUSIONS

Significant postoperative bleeding is almost always surgical in nature and requires additional sutures to close the anatomic defects. Several mechanisms may serve to decrease blood loss, but eventually, the decision must be made whether to take the patient back to surgery. In response to vascular injury, smooth muscle cells located in the subendothelial layer of the blood vessel wall constrict shunting blood flow away from the site of vascular injury. However, atherosclerotic vessels with stiff calcified walls and vessels that are only partially transected cannot constrict as effectively (1). Also compromised in this regard are large veins, which have relatively thin walls and lack the well-developed smooth muscle layer of their arterial counterparts. In fact, injury to these large veins may result in greater blood loss than arterial injuries despite lower venous blood pressures (1). Eventually, if hemorrhage continues into the surrounding tissues, a tamponade effect will decrease blood loss. Without volume resuscitation or pharmacologic intervention, significant volume loss will inevitably lead to a decline in the patient's systemic blood pressure. This may make the patient's bleeding less evident but more critical.

When faced with a bleeding patient in the recovery room, an attempt should be made to clinically differentiate surgical bleeding from bleeding caused by a hemostatic defect. Bleeding that is surgical in nature is usually localized to the surgical site. In contrast, bleeding that is caused by some hemostatic defect causes generalized oozing from several sites. The presence of blood clots in the surgical field suggests that the patient's hemostatic system is intact. If the cause of a patient's bleeding is unclear, laboratory studies should be ordered, including a platelet count, prothrombin time (PT), an activated partial thromboplastin time (aPTT), a thrombin time (TT), a fibrinogen level, and an assay for the presence of fibrin degradation products (FDPs).

However, when the physician is faced with a bleeding patient, ordering laboratory studies has some disadvantages. Often, the physician is pressed to initiate therapy before the test results are available. Secondly, except for the platelet count, the results of the PT, aPTT, and TT seldom yield information that is precise enough to establish an accurate diagnosis. Despite these drawbacks, the tests should be ordered. If the clotting times are prolonged, the test results will support a clinical impression that the patient's bleeding is due, at least in part, to a hemostatic defect and may justify the use of blood component therapy.

Regardless of the cause, whether surgical or due to a bleeding disorder, volume infusion is critical to the resuscitation of any patient who is actively bleeding. If the patient is bleeding rapidly, transfusion of red blood cells may also be necessary to maintain adequate oxygen delivery to the tissues. For patients with surgical bleeding, however, only the transfusion of red blood cells should be considered. Platelets, fresh frozen plasma, and cryoprecipitate transfusions should be reserved for those patients with bleeding disorders. These blood components can be contaminated with infectious agents such as the human immunodeficiency virus (HIV) virus, the hepatitis B virus, or the non-A, non-B hepatitis virus (2). Because of the possible fatal consequences of transfusion with these hemostatic agents, they should not be given prophylactically to patients who are believed to have a surgical cause of bleeding.

The knowledge that AIDS can be transmitted via red blood cell transfusions has greatly intensified public fear of blood transfusions and it has made physicians reevaluate the criteria they use in deciding when to transfuse a patient with any blood component (3, 4). Before 1985, transfusion decisions were seldom questioned. For decades, anesthesiologists and surgeons used the 10 and 30 rule, i.e., they required patients to have a hemoglobin concentration of 10 g/dL and a hematocrit of 30% before the start of surgery (2, 4, 5). Because of the risks associated with transfusion of blood products, many more factors must be considered.

The primary reason deterring physicians from transfusing red blood cells is the fear of transfusion-transmitted diseases. However, the transfusion of red blood cells has immunomodulatory effects as well (6). In the 1970s, patients who were transfused before renal transplant surgery were observed to have improved subsequent renal graft survival. The transfusion was believed to somehow cause immunosuppression in the recipient. These observations prompted studies on the effect of blood transfusion on tumor recurrence in patients after surgical resection. Retrospective analyses revealed that patients, who had received red blood cell transfusions perioperatively, had an increase in tumor recurrence and a decrease in survival. Although the mechanism is unclear, the evidence for a relationship between perioperative transfusion and tumor recurrence or decreased survival in patients with many types of cancer is convincing (6, 7–9). In addition, it seems that perioperative homologous transfusion may impair host defenses against bacterial infections and increase the risk of postoperative infection (6, 10).

To make rational decisions regarding the administration of red blood cells, the physician must understand the pathophysiology of anemia and be able to evaluate the risks that anemia poses to each patient in the context of their clinical condition. This evaluation requires more than a knowledge of the patient's hemoglobin and hematocrit values. Instead, the risk of transfusion complications must be balanced against the benefit afforded to the patient of increasing the oxygen-carrying capacity of their blood and of avoiding the pathologic affects of severe anemia. This transfusion of red blood cells may be the equivalent of giving the "gift of life" to the patient. However, if fatal infectious agents are also transfused to the patient, it could mean the "kiss of death." The decision to transfuse red blood cells must made carefully and must be based on strong clinical indications.

PHYSIOLOGY OF OXYGEN SUPPLY AND DEMAND AND EXTRACTION RATIOS

The decision to transfuse red blood cells ultimately rests on the clinical judgment that the oxygen-carrying capacity of the patient's blood (oxygen supply) should be increased to avoid impending tissue damage. This implies that the oxygen needs (or oxygen demand) of the tissues may outstrip the oxygen supply. Oxygen delivery to the tissues is dependent on the product of the patient's cardiac output and the arterial oxygen content of their blood (4). The cardiac output for a 70-kg male at rest averages about 5 L/minute (or 70 mL/kg). The arterial content of blood is defined as the number of milliliters of oxygen carried in 100 mL of blood. This can be calculated as follows:

$$CaO_2 = Hb \times 1.34 \times SaO_2 + 0.003 \times PaO_2 \quad \#148$$

In the normal 70-kg male with a hemoglobin of 15 gm/dL (a hematocrit of 45%) and an oxygen saturation of 100%, the arterial oxygen content will be 20 mL/dL. This means that 20 mL of oxygen are contained in each 100 mL of blood. In each liter of blood, there will be 200 mL of oxygen (4). With a cardiac output of 5 L/minute, 1000 mL of oxygen (5 L/m × 200 mL/L) will be delivered to the tissues each minute. The oxygen delivery is primarily dependent on the patient's cardiac output, hemoglobin concentration, and the oxygen saturation of their blood. To improve oxygen supply, it would seem that the body would have to increase cardiac output, hemoglobin concentration, or oxygen saturation of hemoglobin. The body actually has several ways of increasing oxygen delivery to the tissues in response to anemia, but the oxygen consumption or oxygen demand must first be examined to get a handle on the other half of the equation.

Oxygen consumption is equal to the product of the patient's cardiac output and the difference in oxygen content between the arterial and venous blood, as follows:

$$O_2 \text{ consumption} = CO \times (CaO_2 - CvO_2)$$

Under normal circumstances, the difference in the arterial and venous oxygen content is equal to 5 mL/dL or 50 mL/L. With a cardiac output of 5 L/minute, oxygen consumption would normally equal 250 mL/min (5 L/minute × 50 mL/L). In comparing the supply of oxygen to the demand for oxygen, it is obvious that under normal circumstances, 1000 mL of oxygen will be supplied per minute and only 250 mL of oxygen will be consumed. This means that there is a fourfold oxygen reserve under normal circumstances (11).

The problem with this analysis is that is presumes that all tissues of the body receive the identical blood flow and therefore have the same oxygen delivery. It also presumes that all organs consume the same amount of oxygen. This global calculation does not address the fact that blood flow differs to different organs and hence the oxygen reserve is also different. Instead, it is more useful to calculate the extraction ratio of individual organs. The extraction ratio (ER) compares the ratio of oxygen consumed by each tissue to that delivered as follows:

$$ER = \frac{O_2 \text{ consumed}}{O_2 \text{ delivered}}$$

$$ER = \frac{CO \times (CaO_2 - CvO_2)}{CO \times (CaO_2)} = \frac{5 \text{ mL/dL}}{20 \text{ mL/dL}} = 25\%$$

Globally, if the overall extraction ratio is 25%, then mixed venous blood will have a venous oxygen content of 15 mL/dL. This results in a mixed venous oxygen saturation in the range of 75%. Changes in the patient's cardiac output or changes in oxygen consumption as blood passes from the arteries to the veins (the arterial-venous oxygen content difference) will effect the mixed venous oxygen saturation. If cardiac output remains constant, then changes in mixed venous oxygen saturation will indirectly reflect mean tissue oxygen content. The mixed venous oxygen saturation can therefore be used as one method to assess the need for red blood cell transfusions. Factors that increase oxygen extraction may include sepsis, hyperthermia, and any state of increased metabolic activity such as hyperthyroidism (3).

The calculation of extraction ratios implies that one can quantify the "margin of safety" before oxygen demand outstrips oxygen supply. Practically, we cannot monitor blood flow to individual organs or calculate minute-to-minute extraction ratios for these organs. However, the oxygen extraction ratio of various organs has been measured under research conditions. This information is quite valuable because it allows us to compare the extraction ratios of various tissues and to recognize which organs will be at greatest risk under conditions of poor oxygen delivery, such as that which occurs with a decrease in cardiac output, hemoglobin concentration, or oxygen saturation of the blood. These, again, are the determinants of oxygen delivery to the tissues.

The extraction ratio of the heart is about 55 to 70% under basal conditions (4). The extraction ratios of the kidney and skin, which receive a large blood supply relative to low oxygen demands, are closer to 7 to 10%. Obviously, the heart will be much more vulnerable to tissue injury with progressive decreases in oxygen delivery such as occurs with uncompensated anemia.

PHYSIOLOGIC RESPONSES TO ANEMIA

In response to anemia, our bodies have several physiologic mechanisms that allow oxygen delivery to the tissues to be maintained, even in the face of a decreasing hemoglobin concentration. These physiologic responses depend on maintenance of a normal blood volume, however, which becomes critical in the management of patients who have sustained large blood losses. The blood volume must be restored for the body's natural mechanisms to be effective in adapting to anemia.

The first physiologic compensation to acute blood loss involves an increase in cardiac output. In fact, the patient's cardiac output increases in direct proportion to the decrease in hematocrit. The mechanism by which the cardiac output increases — either by an increase in heart rate, by an increase in stroke volume, or both — seems to be different in awake and anesthetized patients (12). In awake patients, increases in heart rate predominate. In anesthetized patients, increases in stroke volume are more common (13–15).

Stroke volume depends on preload, contractility, and afterload or systemic vascular resistance. Decreases in afterload increase stroke volume. The afterload or systemic vascular resistance (SVR) has two components: blood viscosity and vascular tone (12). Decreases in hematocrit result in directly proportional decreases in blood viscosity (4) and, therefore, decreases in SVR. This makes isovolemic hemodilution a self-correcting phenomenon up to a point. As the hematocrit falls, blood viscosity falls, afterload decreases, and stroke volume increases. Consequently, the increase in stroke volume leads to an increase in cardiac output. In this way, decreases in oxygen-carrying capacity of the blood are balanced by decreases in blood viscosity. Although the blood carries less oxygen per 100 mL of blood (decreased arterial oxygen content with isovolemic hemodilution), the increases in cardiac output compensate by delivering a greater volume of blood per minute to the tissues. This means that total oxygen delivery (DO_2) remains constant. At a hematocrit level of about 30% (12), oxygen transport peaks and further decreases in hematocrit do not improve oxygen delivery. At this point, this mechanism to maintain oxygen delivery reaches the limits of compensation.

The cardiac output also can be increased by changes in preload and contractility. The preload may in fact increase as the viscosity of blood decreases because of the improved flow characteristics of blood with a lower hematocrit in the microcirculation. Changes in cardiac contractility, however, play a minor role in the heart's compensation for anemia.

The second physiologic mechanism that helps compensate for decreases in the oxygen-carrying capacity of blood after isovolemic hemodilution is that there is a redistribution of blood flow to different organs of the body. Blood flow increases to organs of the body such as the kidneys, liver, spleen, and the intestines with an increase in cardiac output, but the increase in flow is less than would be expected based solely on increases in cardiac output. In contrast, cerebral and coronary blood flow increases more than can be accounted for by an increase in cardiac output alone (4). Coronary blood flow may increase by 400 to 600%. This redistribution of blood flow is the principal means by which the healthy heart compensates for anemia (12). Because the normal physiologic response to anemia involves increasing cardiac output (and there-

fore cardiac work), and because the heart under normal conditions has such high extraction ratios (50 to 70%), the heart must rely principally on redistribution of blood flow to increase oxygen supply (2). The heart is obviously the organ at greatest risk under conditions of isovolemic hemodilution. When the heart can no longer increase coronary blood flow, the limits of isovolemic hemodilution are reached. Further decreases in oxygen delivery will result in myocardial injury.

Cardiac disease or certain clinical conditions may limit the ability of the heart to increase coronary blood flow and improve oxygen delivery. Coronary artery stenosis, for example, may prevent the redistribution of blood flow in response to oxygen needs (4). Hypertrophy of the left ventricle increases oxygen demand. Tachycardia increases oxygen consumption and also decreases oxygen supply because less time during each cardiac cycle is spent in diastole when coronary perfusion takes place. Finally, any decrease in mean arterial pressure will decrease coronary blood flow and threaten oxygen supply. The heart, indeed, is the organ that is at greatest risk under conditions of isovolemic hemodilution and is most responsible for compensating for anemia.

The third mechanism for adapting to isovolemic hemodilution involves increasing oxygen extraction ratios in the periphery. This mechanism is believed to play an important adaptive role when the normovolemic hematocrit drops below 25% (13, 14). Increases in oxygen extraction will lead to decreases in the oxygen content in the venous blood and will be reflected by decreases in the systemic mixed venous O_2 saturation (SvO_2) (4, 12). As the hematocrit decreases to 15%, whole body oxygen ER increases from 38 to 60% and the SvO_2 decreases from 70 to 50% or less (16). Unfortunately, not all systemic beds can increase oxygen extraction.

The fourth and final mechanism of compensation to anemia is that the binding of oxygen to the hemoglobin molecule changes. The affinity of hemoglobin for oxygen is described by the oxygen-hemoglobin dissociation curve. This curve relates the percentage saturation of the hemoglobin molecule with oxygen to the partial pressure of oxygen in the blood (2). However, the relationship is not linear. As hemoglobin becomes more saturated with oxygen, the affinity of the hemoglobin for the oxygen molecule increases.

The affinity of various hemoglobins for the oxygen molecule can be compared to each other by a number called the P_{50}. The P_{50} is simply the partial pressure of oxygen at which 50% of the hemoglobin molecule is saturated with oxygen at 37°C and a pH of 7.4 (3). The oxygen-hemoglobin dissociation curve is shifted to the left when the hemoglobin has a lower P_{50}. The hemoglobin with a lower P_{50} has a higher affinity for oxygen and is more "stingy;" the hemoglobin with a low P_{50} will only unload oxygen (and become 50% unsaturated) at lower partial pressures of oxygen. This can be damaging to the tissues. In contrast, when the oxygen-hemoglobin dissociation curve is shifted to the right, the hemoglobin has a higher P_{50} and is less "stingy;" the hemoglobin has less affinity for the oxygen molecule. The hemoglobin with the higher P_{50} will release 50% of the oxygen molecules to the tissues at a higher partial pressure of oxygen. This is obviously an advantage at the tissue level. When oxygenation is threatened because of anemia, more oxygen can be delivered to the tissues if the hemoglobin has a lower affinity for oxygen. That hemoglobin will release oxygen at a higher partial pressure of oxygen. In contrast, if the hemoglobin has a low P_{50} and a high affinity for oxygen, the PaO_2 must fall to a lower-than-normal level before oxygen is released from hemoglobin and becomes available to the tissues (3).

Patients with chronic anemias accumulate 2,3-diphosphoglycerate (2,3-DPG) in their red blood cells. The 2,3-DPG alters the affinity of the hemoglobin for oxygen; it shifts the oxygen-hemoglobin dissociation curve to the right and increases the P_{50} for that hemoglobin. This facilitates release of oxygen at higher partial pressures of oxygen and makes the ane-

mia more tolerable. The accumulation of 2,3-DPG in the red cells begins at hemoglobin levels of approximately 9 g/dL and is prominent at levels below 6.5 g/dL (2). The increase in 2,3-DPG levels requires 12 to 36 hours (2).

The affinity of hemoglobin for oxygen is altered by conditions other than the accumulation of 2,3-DPG. Acid-base changes and temperature changes shift the P_{50} of hemoglobin. Acidosis shifts the oxygen-hemoglobin dissociation curve to the right, improving oxygen delivery to the tissues. Hypothermia shifts the curve to the left and should be avoided if possible (10). Storage of red blood cells decreases 2,3-DPG levels and shifts the curve to the left, decreasing the P_{50} of the hemoglobin (3, 4). In fact, Shah et al. have demonstrated that the administration of as little as two units of stored blood may lead to a decreased P_{50} and result in no immediate increase in oxygen delivery despite an increase in oxygen-carrying capacity of the blood (17).

FACTORS TO CONSIDER SYSTEMATICALLY BEFORE TRANSFUSION OF RED BLOOD CELLS

When deciding whether to transfuse a patient with red blood cells, it is important to consider the basic elements that affect oxygen delivery to the tissues (cardiac output and arterial oxygen content) and then evaluate whether the patient's own compensatory mechanisms can be expected to improve oxygen delivery to the tissues in the face of isovolemic hemodilution. The other side of the equation, i.e., oxygen consumption, must also be considered: will the patient's clinical condition increase oxygen demand and require transfusion at a higher level of hemoglobin concentration?

The first factor involved in the formula for oxygen delivery is the patient's *cardiac output*. In this regard, the most important clinical aspect to evaluate is whether the patient has or might have coronary artery disease and whether the patient's heart can respond to isovolemic hemodilution by increasing cardiac output without increasing myocardial oxygen demand. This will depend in large part on the function of the left ventricle, the location of any critical stenoses, and whether left ventricular hypertrophy is present. The heart is the organ that has the highest extraction ratio of oxygen and that depends the most on redistribution of blood flow for adequate oxygen delivery under conditions of isovolemic hemodilution. Critical stenoses in the coronary circulation or other factors that would compromise the myocardial oxygen supply and demand ratio will raise the threshold at which these patients will need to be transfused with red blood cells.

Patients with coronary artery disease undergoing general surgical procedures may tolerate hematocrits as low as 25% if ventricular function is preserved and coronary stenoses are not critical (12). However, ventricular dysfunction may occur with any increases in cardiac output that also increase oxygen consumption. For example, cardiac output may increase with tachycardia, but at higher heart rates, and ventricular dysfunction may occur, decreasing the patient's tolerance to the lower hematocrit. For these reasons, under most circumstances, it is the condition of the patient's heart that will determine the lowest level of hemoglobin that can be tolerated. For the patient with coronary artery disease, the lowest tolerable hematocrit will be influenced by several factors: heart rate, left ventricular function, the presence or absence of left ventricular hypertrophy, the severity of coronary artery stenoses, and the collateral blood flow to areas with critical stenoses (12).

Next to be considered is the *oxygen saturation* of the blood, which impacts the arterial oxygen content of the blood directly (CaO_2 = Hb × 1.34 × SaO_2 + 0.003 × PaO_2) (10). It may be more than obvious that patients who are having difficulty oxygenating their blood — such as those having an asthma attack or a patient who is found to be wheezing in the recovery room following a brief episode of aspiration — will have minimal respiratory reserve and will require higher hemoglobin concentrations to maintain adequate oxygen delivery to their tissues. An arterial blood gas will be helpful in making this clinical judgment.

Because the level of *hemoglobin concentration* is central to this discussion, the patient should be evaluated in terms of whether further blood loss is expected. Also, when evaluating the patient's hematocrit, whether or not the patient's volume status has been repleted should be kept in mind. Although the patient's volume status can best be evaluated with the use of a pulmonary artery (PA) catheter and the measurement of left ventricular filling pressures, such invasive monitoring, is neither present nor indicated for most patients. Observing the contour of an arterial line tracing, following urine output, and serial hematocrits (18) may be useful in establishing the patient's volume status. In the recovery room, a simple tilt test is helpful in this regard.

After the elements of oxygen supply have been evaluated, the patient's ability to use *normal physiologic mechanisms to compensate for anemia* should be assessed. Can the patient increase cardiac output without an increase in oxygen consumption? Does the patient have coronary artery disease, left ventricular dysfunction, or left ventricular hyprertrophy? Is the patient's anemia at least in part chronic in origin, which would result in increased levels of 2,3-DPG in the red blood cells? Has the patient received large quantities of stored blood? Is the patient hypothermic?

Finally, clinical conditions that might affect the other side of the equation, *oxygen consumption*, should be brought to bear on the decision of whether to transfuse the patient with red blood cells. Patients who are cold and shivering have a tremendous increase in oxygen demand. Patients in the recovery room who are in pain are usually tachycardic and also have increases in oxygen consumption. Patients who are febrile or septic obviously have higher tissue oxygen demands and require higher hemoglobin levels.

GENERAL TRANSFUSION GUIDELINES

The National Heart, Lung, and Blood Institutes sponsored consensus conferences to develop recommendations for the transfusion of red blood cells (19), platelets (20), and fresh frozen plasma (21). Their conclusions state that for some patients the transfusion threshold of a hematocrit of 30% was too high and that many patients do not need transfusion until the hemoglobin falls to 7 g/dL (hematocrit 21%) or less. Unfortunately, the report does not address which patients can tolerate which threshold hematocrit.

It is apparent that most patients should be transfused at a hematocrit (Hct) between 18 and 30%. Where each patient falls along this continuum depends on his or her ability to increase oxygen delivery and on his or her rate of oxygen consumption. The patients who could probably tolerate the lower transfusion threshold Hct of approximately 18% would include young healthy patients who have suffered a large blood loss but do not have other perioperative problems (12). Other patients who might tolerate such lower hematocrits are those who have longstanding chronic anemias, such as patients with renal failure who do not have cardiac dysfunction.

Patients who require the middle-of-the-road hematocrit (i.e., about 25%) might be middle-aged patients with well-compensated medical problems but no cardiac disease. This may be the patient with treated hypertension and no left ventricular hypertrophy (12), the patient with diabetes and no signs or symptoms of coronary artery disease, the patient who is somewhat obese but well compensated, or the longtime tobacco smoker who still has normal oxygenation.

Finally, patients who should be transfused to maintain hematocrits of about 30% would be those with coronary artery disease who have not been bypassed recently, cardiac patients with signs or symptoms of left ventricular dysfunction, and those with left ventricular hypertrophy or fast heart rates (4, 12). Patients in whom blood oxygenation is difficult because of longstanding pulmonary disease, bronchospasm, or some other pulmonary complication should also have a higher transfusion threshold. Another class of patients who belong in this category are those with increased oxygen demands, such as those with a systemic infection or those who are critically ill with multisystem problems. Finally, the patient's age should be taken into consideration, because aging decreases cardiac and pulmonary reserves. Older patients should be considered to have higher transfusion thresholds than younger patients with comparable medical problems.

Although the above discussion concerning the decision of when to transfuse a patient may seem a bit belabored, it is for a good reason. Transfusion practices are coming under closer scrutiny because of the significant risks involved. Despite the applicable general guidelines, the decision to transfuse red blood cells must be made on an individual basis and based must be based on solid clinical reasons, which should be clearly stated in the medical record. Such reasons may include that the patient has coronary artery disease, has a low cardiac output or a low arterial pO_2, or that the patient has a fever or is septic. Red blood cells should not be given for volume expansion, wound healing, or to increase well-being but rather only for the express reason to improve oxygen delivery to the tissues (11). Historically, giving blood has meant giving the "gift of life." In fact, the Romans drank the blood of recently slain gladiators to acquire their strength (10). Unfortunately, the infectious complications associated with red blood cell transfusions have changed our attitudes toward blood transfusions and have greatly increased the importance of this clinical decision.

COMPLICATIONS ASSOCIATED WITH RED BLOOD CELL TRANSFUSIONS

Complications that arise with red blood cell transfusions can be classified broadly into those that may occur with any type of volume resuscitation, those that occur with blood component therapy, and those that are specific to red blood cell transfusions. Fluid administration, whether it be colloid, crystalloid, or a blood component, may lead to hypothermia and/or the development of dilutional coagulopathies. Blood component therapy, involving the administration of platelets, fresh frozen plasma, cryoprecipitate or red blood cells, carries the long-term and possibly fatal risks associated with viral infection or bacterial sepsis. Transfusion with red blood cells may lead to some minor biochemical changes (depletion of 2,3-DPG in the stored red blood cells, citrate intoxication, hyperkalemia, and acid-base changes) or may cause an allergic, febrile, or hemolytic transfusion reaction. The more specific complications will be considered first because they are more relevant to the particular subject of red blood cell transfusions.

Minor Complications

Red blood cells can be stored for up to 21 days in an anticoagulant preservative called citrate phosphate dextrose (CPD) (3). The citrate binds calcium and prevents the stored blood from clotting, but this may lead to transient decreases in plasma-ionized calcium levels in the recipient if the red blood cells are transfused at very rapid rates. This "citrate intoxication" or hypocalcemia can produce electrocardiogram changes, but the clinical significance with regard to myocardial performance is debated. If circulatory volume is well maintained, the clinical signs of hypocalcemia — hypotension, narrow pulse pressure, and elevated intraventricular end-diastolic pressure and central venous pressure — do not occur unless the CPD blood is given at rates exceeding 150 mL/70 kg/minute (7). When the red blood cell infusion is terminated, ionized calcium levels rapidly return to normal. In patients with normal cardiac function and normal hepatic perfusion, the citrate is metabolized (3). Therefore, gratuitous routine administration of calcium chloride with red blood cell transfusions is not recommended (7). In fact, that practice could lead to hypercalcemia and serious complications.

Storage of red blood cells leads to increases in plasma potassium concentrations. Serum potassium levels of 3.3 mEq/L on the day of donation increase to 12.3 mEq/L by day 7 of storage and 17.0 mEq/L by day 14 (3). After another week, the potassium levels may be as high as 19 to 30 mEq/L, which makes hyperkalemia theoretically a serious concern. However, there is evidence that transfused potassium must leave the intravascular space rapidly because hyperkalemia is rarely seen except transiently. When it does occur, it is usually under circumstances in which red blood cells are transfused at very rapid rates (greater than 120 mL/minute) and the patient is hypoperfused and acidotic (5, 7).

Hypokalemia is a more common complication caused by the metabolic alkalosis generated by the metabolism of citrate to bicarbonate (5).

CPD solution is acidic in nature and, when added to freshly drawn blood, lowers the pH of the blood to approximately 7.0 to 7.1 (7). During storage, red blood cells metabolize glucose to lactate and they produce pyruvic acid. This acid load generated both from the citrate in the CPD solution and from the products of RBC metabolism would be expected to worsen the lactic acidosis that is often already present in the hypotensive poorly perfused patient in shock. However, the metabolic acid-base consequences of red blood cell transfusions are quite variable and may even produce a metabolic alkalosis (22). This response may be due to several factors: (a) because the citrate from the CPD solution is metabolized to bicarbonate, (b) exogenous bicarbonate is often given, and (c) because these patients are resuscitated with lactated Ringer's solution. Before bicarbonate administration, the patient's blood should be sampled, and only those patients with a severe metabolic acidosis (base excess greater than 7 mEq/L) should receive bicarbonate therapy.

Red blood cells stored at 1 to 6°C lose 2,3-DPG. This increases the affinity of the hemoglobin molecule for oxygen. Theoretically, this can compromise oxygen delivery at the tissue level because the hemoglobin, which now has a higher affinity for oxygen, will not release oxygen to the tissues except at lower partial pressures of oxygen, which can lead to tissue hypoxia. Hypothermia and alkalosis also increase the affinity of hemoglobin for oxygen. Therefore, red blood cells should be warmed before their transfusion and excessive bicarbonate administration should be avoided. Finally, red cells become more fragile with storage and many of them lyse, releasing free hemoglobin into the plasma.

RED BLOOD CELL TRANSFUSION REACTIONS

Red blood cell transfusion reactions can be differentiated into those that are associated with hemolysis and those that are not. It is the intravascular hemolytic reactions that are often associated with a fatal outcome. Of the transfusion-related deaths reported to the U.S. Food and Drug Administration (FDA) since 1975, most were caused by ABO-incompatible transfusions. The fatal mistakes, however, were not due to errors in blood typing in the laboratory. Instead, the patients received the wrong unit of blood because of clerical mistakes made by the person administering the blood on the ward, in the operating room, or in the emergency room. This means that starting a transfusion is a critical step; the person starting the transfusion has the last opportunity to discover a clerical error and the first opportunity to detect a transfusion reaction.

The clinical consequences of an incompatible blood transfusion are variable and depend, in part, on the volume of blood transfused (7). Fever is the most common initial manifestation of immune hemolysis, and this fever is usually accompanied by chills. The patient may complain of a vague uneasiness and chest and back pain. Less commonly, these patients may have generalized flushing, nausea, and lightheadedness. In the setting of the recovery room, most of the signs and symptoms of a hemolytic transfusion reaction may be misleading to the physician because they are common postsurgical signs and symptoms. The patient who has chills and complains of pain on arrival to the recovery room will probably be given warm blankets and be medicated for pain. If the patient is somewhat hypotensive or tachycardic and complains of nausea or lightheadedness, the physician may believe that the patient is hypovolemic. The physician may only suspect that the patient's pain, tachycardia, hypotension, and nausea are related to a blood transfusion when the patient's urine turns red or dark-colored due to hemoglobinuria or when the patient begins to bleed from multiple sites due to the development of dissiminated intravascular coagulation (DIC). When a hemolytic transfusion reaction is suspected, the transfusion should be stopped and supportive care should be started immediately.

When incompatible blood is transfused, antibodies in the recipient plasma react with donor antigens on the surface of the red blood cells. The antibodies activate complement, which leads to lysis of the red blood cells and to the anaphylactic stimulation of mast cells. Histamine and serotonin are released and bronchoconstriction ensues. Throughout the bloodstream, the antigen-antibody complexes activate Hageman factor or factor XII, of the intrinsic coagulation cascade, which leads to DIC. At the same time, the kinin system is activated to produce bradykinin. Bradykinin increases capillary permeability and dilates arterioles, inevitably leading to hypotension. In response, the patient's catecholamine levels rise and vasoconstriction takes place in areas with a high concentration of alpha receptors — in the renal, splenic, pulmonary, and cutaneous capillary beds (23). As a result of this "allergic chemical storm," the patient is tachycardic, wheezing, and hypotensive. Additionally, 30 to 50% of patients will develop DIC (24). As a consequence of these multiple effects, these patients are at great risk for developing renal failure. Renal blood flow is compromised by the systemic hypotension, the renal vasoconstriction, and the fact that intravascular thrombi are deposited throughout all of the capillary beds, including the kidney. The ischemia may progress to acute tubular necrosis and renal failure in less than 48 hours (24).

When a hemolytic transfusion reaction is suspected, the transfusion should be stopped immediately and treatment should be directed at three main goals: (*a*) to support blood pressure, (*b*) to maintain renal blood flow, and (*c*) to prevent DIC. The blood pressure may be maintained with fluid administration and the use of inotropic agents. Urine output should be maintained at a minimum of 75 to 100 mL/hr. If fluid therapy fails to produce adequate urine output, mannitol can be given and furosemide can be added if necessary. Sodium bicarbonate may be administered easily to alkalinize the urine, although the beneficial effects of this are controversial. Initial laboratory studies should include a DIC screen as well as a direct antiglobulin test to confirm whether there are antibodies attached to the transfused donor red blood cells. The patient's blood and urine can also be assayed for hemoglobin concentration. Unused blood should be returned to the blood bank for a recross-match.

Another type of hemolytic transfusion reaction, called a "delayed hemolytic transfusion reaction," also involves recipient antibodies reacting to donor red cell antigens, but red blood cell lysis is delayed and usually occurs extravascularly. These delayed reactions are not as serious as the immediate hemolytic transfusion reactions, because they do not involve the ABO system. Antibodies are manufactured in the Rh or Kidd system only after a previous exposure to these antigens, such as occurs during pregnancy or a previous blood transfusion. Over time, the quantity of antibody decreases. In contrast, patients are born with naturally occurring antibodies to A and/or B antigens and these do not diminish over time. With delayed hemolytic transfusion reactions, their antibody level is too low when they are exposed to the antigen a second time for immediate hemolysis of the red cells to occur. The level of antibody is also too low to be detected with the antibody screen before transfusion. Upon reexposure, new antibody is produced (an anamnestic response) and the delayed hemolytic transfusion reaction is manifest as a gradual decrease in the patient's hematocrit. The patient may have a low-grade fever and complain of fatigue and chills. Diagnosis can be difficult because the symptoms may be mild and the reaction may be delayed for as long as 21 days after a transfusion (24). The primary indication that a delayed hemolytic transfusion reaction has occurred will be the insidious gradual recurrence of anemia in a patient who has received a transfusion.

Transfusion reactions that do not involve red cell hemolysis may be febrile or allergic in nature and, like hemolytic reactions, the patient may present with a fever. Because these nonhemolytic transfusion reactions present with signs and symptoms similar to hemolytic transfusion reactions, it is important to determine which type of reaction is occurring. Febrile reactions are the most common type of transfusion reaction and are believed to be caused by antibodies in recipient plasma reacting against donor white blood cells (lymphocytes, granulocytes, or platelets) (24). The use of leukocyte-poor red blood cells, microaggregate filters, or washed red cells may be helpful in decreasing the incidence of these reactions.

Although relatively benign, febrile reactions present a diagnostic dilemma. The patient with a febrile reaction may complain of chills, headache, nausea, and even chest pain — not unlike the symptoms of a hemolytic transfusion reaction. When in doubt regarding the cause of a patient's symptoms, the transfusion should be stopped until a direct antiglobulin test can be performed. This test will readily differentiate between these two reactions. If the test is negative, the blood transfusion may be continued and the patient's fever can be treated with acetaminophen.

Allergic reactions are believed to be the result of recipient antibodies acting against donor plasma proteins. These reactions are therefore most common after transfusion of fresh frozen plasma, but they can occur with the transfusion of other blood components because some plasma still remains in these other components (24). Patients with an allergic reaction usually complain of urticaria associated with itching. The itching can be alleviated with antihistamines.

In addition to febrile reactions, there is yet another type of transfusion reaction that may occur when antibodies in donor blood react against recipient white blood cells. These leukoagglutinin reactions are usually the result of the donor being multiparous and sensitized to foreign WBCs. Known as graft-versus-host reactions, these serious, life-threatening reactions cause shortness of breath, pulmonary edema, and fever.

INFECTIOUS COMPLICATIONS OF RED BLOOD CELL TRANSFUSIONS

All blood components, except albumin and gamma globulin, can transmit infectious diseases. The more units transfused, the greater the risk of the patient contracting a transfusion-transmitted disease (5). Hepatitis and AIDS are the two most feared diseases, although cytomegalovirus, syphilis, malaria, and several other diseases have also been reported to be transmitted by blood transfusion (7).

The incidence of hepatitis B has been reduced as a result of screening of blood donors for hepatitis B surface antigen (HbsAg). The incidence of non-A, non-B, or hepatitis C has also been reduced by the development of an assay to screen for the antibody against the non-A, non-B, or hepatitis C virus (2, 3). This advancement is an improvement over the previous methods to screen blood for this virus, which relied solely on the presence of abnormal liver enzymes. But screening for the antibody is not as effective as screening for the antigen in controlling the incidence of infected blood, because a person who has recently been infected with the virus but in whom antibodies to the virus have not yet appeared can donate blood. In other words, there is a window of time, before the appearance of antibody in the blood, during which the person may be unknowingly donating contaminated blood. This "latency period" for seroconversion may be up to 60 months or 5 years for the hepatitis C virus. Currently, the incidence of posttransfusion hepatitis due to non-A and non-B is 13 times more prevalent than that due to hepatitis B.

Another problem that makes decreasing the incidence of non-A and non-B hepatitis difficult is that most patients infected with this virus do not become clinically jaundiced and they remain asymptomatic during the acute phase of the disease. Their lack of symptoms, however, does not correlate with the ultimate development of chronic hepatitis or cirrhosis. Forty percent of the anicteric cases progress to chronic hepatitis, and of these, 50% die of fulminate hepatitis (7).

The development of AIDS is the most feared complication of blood transfusion. HIV seroconversion has, in fact, been associated with transfusion of most blood products. This risk has been decreased significantly, like the risk of hepatitis B, by eliminating paid donors and also by discouraging members of high-risk groups from donating blood. Since 1985, all donor blood is tested for the presence of antibodies to the AIDS virus (HIV-1). However, the latency period for seroconversion, or the time before antibodies become detectable in the blood of an infected person, may be several weeks or months after the time of their initial infection. During this time, these blood donors may unknowingly transmit the infection.

The decision to transfuse blood products must balance these risks against the potential benefit to the patient. In the past, many clinicians espoused the concept that any patient who truly needed a blood transfusion should receive a minimum of 2 units of blood. In view of the significant risks involved, perhaps the decision to transfuse blood should be reconsidered with each unit transfused.

NONSURGICAL BLEEDING

Although most patients who show signs of continued bleeding in the recovery room will have a surgical cause for their hemorrhage, at some point in time, the patient's hemostatic mechanism must come into question. The patient may have had a preexisting bleeding disorder that had been overlooked or they may have developed a coagulopathy during the intraoperative period. An obvious surgical cause of bleeding can mask the presence of a bleeding disorder and may lead to a dangerous clinical situation. If the possibility of a bleeding disorder comes to mind, then laboratory tests should be ordered to confirm these clinical suspicions.

Coagulation tests that should be ordered when a bleeding disorder is suspected include a platelet count, a prothrombin time (PT), an activated partial thromboplastin time (aPTT), a thrombin time (TT) if the patient has received heparin, a fibrinogen level, and an assay for fibrinogen degradation products (FSPs). To interpret the results of these coagulation tests, a basic understanding of the hemostatic mechanism and a knowledge of the common causes of bleeding disorders are a prerequisite, because when the coagulation tests are abnormally prolonged, the results are not precise enough to point to a single diagnosis. The prolonged clotting times may confirm your suspicion that the patient has a bleeding disorder but will not define the cause. The laboratory test results must be interpreted in conjunction with this basic knowledge to make the most plausible diagnosis and select the most appropriate course of treatment with the least risk. Otherwise, the clinician may be pressed to transfuse the patient unnecessarily with multiple blood products — red blood cells, fresh frozen plasma, platelets, and/or cryoprecipitate.

THE BASIC HEMOSTATIC MECHANISM

Under normal circumstances, blood flows in a liquid, fluid form throughout the body and clots only at sites of vascular damage. This amazing transformation of liquid blood into a solid clot is controlled by the hemostatic mechanism. The hemostatic mechanism involves three interrelated processes: (a) primary hemostasis, (b) coagulation, and (c) fibrinolysis. All three processes occur almost simultaneously. For ease of understanding, they will be considered sequentially.

In discussing the hemostatic mechanism, some confusion arises because of the use of the word "coagulation" to refer to both the entire hemostatic mechanism that causes blood to "coagulate" or clot and also to the interaction of the clotting factors in the "coagulation" pathways or the second process of the hemostatic mechanism. Therefore, for additional ease of understanding, when the word coagulation refers to the entire hemostatic mechanism (primary hemostasis, coagulation, and fibrinolysis), it will be capitalized, ("Coagulation"). When it refers to the second process of the hemostatic mechanism, it will not be capitalized ("coagulation").

Primary hemostasis involves the blood vessels and platelets. The blood vessels are lined by a single layer of precious endothelial cells. Beneath this endothelial lining is a layer of collagen supporting tissue and smooth muscle cells. When the endothelial lining is denuded after vascular injury, the hemostatic mechanism is set into motion.

Platelets, which are circulating in the blood, come into contact with collagen exposed by the disruption of the endothelial lining (25). The platelets adhere to the collagen via platelet receptors, located on the surface of the platelet. These receptors allow the platelet to stick to a substance circulating in the blood, known as the von Willebrand factor (vWF), which in turn adheres to the collagen layer (1, 26). The von Willebrand factor, which is believed to be released by endothelial cells and by activated platelets, acts as an intercellular glue "sticking" platelets onto collagen (27). This first process in platelet activation is called platelet adherence. It is rapidly followed by a change in the shape of the platelets, a release reaction, and then by their aggregation to one another. The platelets change their shape from that of a disk to a spheroid with the extension of many little pseudopods on their surface (28). During the release reaction, these activated platelets extrude the contents of their cytoplasmic granules, releasing a number of chemical products, including ADP, serotonin, platelet factor 4, β-thromboglobulin, fibronectin, vWF, fibrinogen, factor V, and others (25, 29). The ADP released from the platelet granules is a powerful platelet aggregator and recruits other platelets into the growing platelet mass. With stronger stimuli for platelet activation, prostaglandin synthesis is stimulated in the cytosol of the platelet. A prostaglandin, called thromboxane A_2, is synthesized and released. This prostaglandin has several effects: it causes further release of ADP and, consequently, further platelet aggregation; it is a potent vasoconstrictor and is a powerful platelet agonist (30). The vasoconstriction induced by thromboxane A_2 shunts blood flow away from the site of vascular injury (1). During the process of platelet aggregation induced by thromboxane A_2, fibrinogen receptors are exposed on the surface of the platelet membrane. Aided by calcium, fibrinogen links the platelets together, initiating an irreversible stage of platelet aggregation (25). ADP, epinephrine, and thrombin also expose binding sites on the platelet surface for fibrinogen. The aggregated platelets trap thrombin, one of the clotting factors of the coagulation cascade, and they also trap plasminogen, which is involved in the fibrinolytic system. Together, the aggregated platelets, fibrinogen, trapped thrombin, and plasminogen form the platelet plug, which temporarily arrests bleeding. This process, which involves the blood vessels and platelets, is called primary hemostasis.

In the absence of vascular injury, the intact endothelial lining serves many regulatory functions with regard to the hemostatic mechanism. This endothelial layer prevents platelets from being exposed to collagen. In addition, the endothelial cells synthesize and secrete many substances that aid in regulation of the hemostatic process. One such substance, which is very important to the regulation of primary hemostasis, is a prostaglandin called prostacyclin. Prostacyclin's actions are just the opposite of the thromboxane A_2. Prostacyclin, secreted by the endothelial cells, induces vasodilation, decreases ADP secretion, and inhibits platelet aggregation (30). These actions lead to blood vessels that are dilated and have better blood flow and to blood vessels that are "nonthrombogenic." Because platelets cannot aggregate in the presence of prostacyclin, the smooth flow of liquid blood is promoted.

The balance of these two prostaglandins, thromboxane A_2 and prostacyclin, controls primary hemostasis. At sites of vascular damage where the endothelium is denuded, activated platelets release thromboxane A_2, platelets aggregate, and a platelet plug forms. Beyond the site of vascular damage, endothelial cells secrete prostacyclin and prevent platelet aggregation along the walls of normal endothelium-lined vessels. An imbalance of these two prostaglandins can lead to disorders of primary hemostasis.

Thromboxane A_2 levels can be decreased by the ingestion of aspirin-containing compounds. The aspirin-containing compounds inhibit platelet synthesis of thromboxane A_2 by poisoning the enzymatic machinery of the platelet for its entire life span (29, 30). Nonsteroidal anti-inflammatory drugs inhibit the platelet enzymes for approximately 16 to 24 hours. Prostacyclin levels are decreased when artificial surfaces are placed within the patient's blood stream that are not lined with endothelial cells. This happens with the insertion of vascular grafts and also with the placement of cardiopulmonary bypass tubing before cardiac surgery. Platelets adhere, aggregate, and become activated by contact with a foreign substance that lacks an endothelial lining.

Another type of defect in primary hemostasis is called von Willebrand's disease. It does not involve an imbalance in the synthesis of the prostaglandins, thromboxane A_2 or prostacyclin, which affect platelet aggregation, but instead results from a deficient or defective synthesis of the von Willebrand factor, which affects platelet adherence to collagen. Synthesis of this factor is under genetic control. Von Willebrand's disease, in its various presentations, is the most common hereditary cause of platelet dysfunction.

Several of the clotting factors in the coagulation process can only interact on a phospholipid surface. Such a phospholipid surface is exposed during primary hemostasis. When platelets are activated, not only do they change shape, release the contents of their cytoplasmic granules, and aggregate, but they also expose a phospholipid surface called platelet factor 3 (PF3). PF3 plays a critical role in localizing the Coagulation process because under normal circumstances, platelets are activated and phospholipid (PF3) is exposed, only at sites of vascular injury.

The friable platelet plug, which forms during primary hemostasis, is in danger of being washed away by rapid blood flow if it were not for the second process of the hemostatic mechanism, coagulation. This is discussed below.

COAGULATION

Coagulation involves the interaction of many plasma proteins known as clotting factors. These factors interact with calcium and a phospholipid surface to produce a tough fibrin meshwork that reinforces the friable platelet plug and stops bleeding until tissue repair can occur.

The coagulation process has been made more difficult by the many different names given to the original coagulation factors. In an attempt to standardize the nomenclature, these clotting factors were assigned Roman numerals. However, they were numbered in the order of their discovery, not in the order of the interaction. Most of the clotting factors are referred to by their Roman numeral except for fibrinogen (I), prothrombin (II), calcium (III), and tissue thromboplastin (factor IV). Some of the numbered factors do not exist, such as factor VI. It was found actually to be activated factor V. Also, many new factors have been discovered and have been given multiple names, but no Roman numerals. These new factors are most commonly known as prekallikrein, high molecular weight kininogen, protein C, and protein S. Even though the nomenclature is chaotic and the coagulation reactions are difficult to remember, a few broad principles are helpful in understanding the hemostatic mechanism and the common bleeding disorders that develop.

Most of the clotting factors circulate in an inactive form called a proenzyme. During the process of coagulation, a portion of the molecule is cleaved, forming the active clotting factor. This activated factor, represented by a small letter a next to the Roman numeral, then cleaves the next clotting factor in a chain-reaction–like sequence until fibrin is formed.

Most of the clotting factors are synthesized by the liver, which means that their normal structure and function depend on normal hepatic activity. The one exception may be clotting factor VIII, which is believed to have some extrahepatic synthesis. In addition, this clotting factor is different from the others because it circulates as a huge plasma protein composed of two components with a molecular weight in excess of 1,000,000. The smaller portion of the protein, represented as factor VIII:C, is the coagulant factor VIII portion. The larger component, VIIIR:Ag, is the von Willebrand factor, which plays such an important role in primary hemostasis. Each of these components is under separate genetic control (27). Deficiencies of coagulant factor VIII lead to hemophilia A disease. Because the von Willebrand factor also serves as a carrier protein for the coagulant factor VIII portion, deficiencies of this factor make the patient seem to have both a defect in primary hemostasis and hemophilia A. However, restoration of von Willebrand levels returns the level of coagulant factor VIII to normal.

Four of the clotting factors (factors II, VII, IX, and X) are said to be vitamin-K–dependent clotting factors. This is because the final step in their synthesis requires the presence of vitamin K. In this enzymatic reaction, a carboxyl group (or a carboxy "tail") is added to each of the clotting factors. This carboxyl group enables these vitamin-K–dependent factors to bind via a calcium bridge to phospholipid surfaces. Without vitamin K, or in the presence of coumadin, which competes with vitamin K for binding sites on the hepatocyte, these factors are synthesized and circulate in blood but do not have a carboxyl tail and therefore cannot bind to phospholipid surfaces to participate in the coagulation process. The patient presents with a bleeding disorder that can only be corrected with vitamin K therapy or the transfusion of clotting factors in the form of fresh frozen plasma.

Two of the clotting factors, factors V and VIII, are known as the labile factors. They are said to be labile because their clotting activity does not last long in stored blood. When patients are transfused with whole blood or packed red blood cells that have been stored for more than a few days, the clotting activity of the labile factors, V and VIII, is deficient.

These two clotting factors (V and VIII) are unique in another respect. They do not become active cleavage enzymes but instead serve as cofactors in "reaction complexes." These reactions involve the paired binding of two clotting factors on a phospholipid surface in a particular spatial arrangement such that the two clotting factors can together activate a third clotting factor. The reaction complex requires a vitamin-K–dependent factor that binds with its carboxyl tail via calcium to the phospholipid surface. The other clotting factor, positioned in the reaction complex, is a cofactor (V or VIII). Together, the vitamin-K–dependent factor and its cofactor activate the next clotting factor in the coagulation cascade.

The final broad principle that is helpful in understanding the hemostatic mechanism is that the process of coagulation requires the presence of a phospholipid surface. One phospholipid surface is provided intravascularly by platelets that expose platelet factor 3 (PF3 or platelet phospholipid) when they are activated at the site of vascular injury. The coagulation pathway that occurs on their surface inside the blood vessels is called the intrinsic pathway of coagulation. Another source of phospholipid is liberated from cell membranes of damaged tissues. This phospholipid is variously called tissue thromboplastin or tissue factor. The coagulation pathway that proceeds on the surface of this phospholipid is called the extrinsic pathway of coagulation because a factor that is extrinsic to blood is required for this pathway of coagulation. The intrinsic and extrinsic pathways merge with the activation of factor X and form the common pathway of coagulation. This classical separation of the coagulation cascade into two pathways assists in the interpretation of the standard laboratory tests — the prothrombin time (PT) and the activated partial thromboplastin time (aPTT) — which measure clotting times of the extrinsic and intrinsic pathways, respectively. However, the pathways most likely are not distinct and have many interconnections.

In looking at the classical diagram of the intrinsic and extrinsic pathways, (see Figure 11–1) several useful clinical generalizations can be made. First, it can be noted that the vitamin-K–dependent factors (factors II, VII, IX, and X) are located in both the intrinsic and extrinsic pathways. Therefore, vitamin K deficiency will ultimately affect both pathways. The extrinsic pathway will be affected first, however, because factor VII, which initiates this pathway, has the shortest half-life of all of the clotting factors. For this reason, the extrinsic pathway will also be affected first when coumadin therapy is initiated and this pathway will be most sensitive to liver dysfunction. With increasing vitamin K deficiency, in-

Intrinsic pathway

Extrinsic pathway

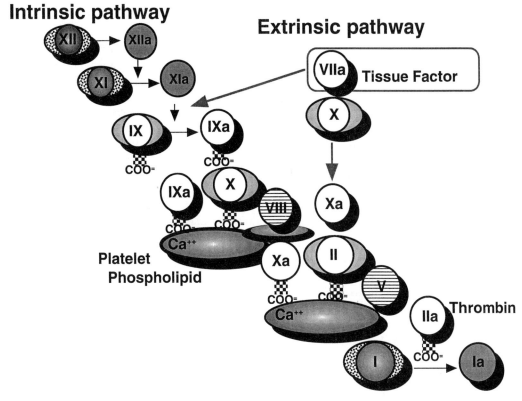

Fig. 11–1. Coagulation proceeds via a series of reactions that require the presence of a phospholipid surface on which clotting factors can interact. The classical extrinsic pathway begins when blood is exposed to tissue factor (also known as tissue thromboplastin), which together with factor VII can activate either factor IX or factor X. The intrinsic pathway provides a source of activated factor IX (IXa) as well. Subsequent reactions take place on the surface of activated platelets, which localizes the coagulation process to the site of vascular injury.

creasing coumadin doses, or increasing liver disease, both pathways will ultimately be affected, prolonging both the PT and the aPTT. This difference in the half-life of the clotting factors may be helpful in interpreting coagulation tests when only the prothrombin time is prolonged. The combination of a prolonged PT with a normal aPTT indicates that the defect is limited to the extrinsic pathway.

Also of note in looking at the pathways is the fact that the labile factors (factors VIII and V) are positioned in the intrinsic and common pathways of coagulation, respectively. A deficiency of factor V, located in the common pathway, will prolong both clotting times, the PT and the aPTT. Massive

transfusion with stored packed red blood cells (deficient in the labile factors) can produce this type of coagulopathy. Although component therapy attempts to separate the red blood cells from plasma, the transfusion of "packed" red blood cells still includes some plasma, and this plasma contains the other clotting factors but is deficient in the labile factors. However, even though a relative deficiency of factors V and VIII may follow massive transfusion with packed red blood cells, dilutional thrombocytopenia is a much greater problem. Factor dilution, or the depletion of factors V and VIII, may contribute to the coagulopathy that follows massive transfusions of red blood cells but rarely is a primary cause. When both the aPTT and PT are prolonged, factor dilution secondary to massive transfusions becomes part of the differential diagnosis.

Just as vitamin K deficiency, liver disease, and coumadin can first affect the extrinsic pathway, heparin therapy when initiated will first affect the intrinsic pathway. Heparin acts via antithrombin III, which is a naturally occurring anticoagulant that circulates in the blood and helps to regulate the normal process of coagulation (31). Just as the name implies, antithrombin III binds to thrombin and prevents it from converting fibrinogen to fibrin (27). Antithrombin III also binds to all of the other active cleavage enzymes in the intrinsic and common coagulation pathway and inhibits their activity. Heparin, man's synthetic anticoagulant, works by making the binding of antithrombin III to thrombin and the other clotting factors 100 to 1000 times more avid. In the presence of heparin, antithrombin III rapidly inactivates these factors and prevents coagulation. Because factor IX, in the intrinsic pathway, is the most sensitive of the clotting factors to the actions of antithrombin III and heparin, the aPTT will be prolonged before the PT is affected. With higher doses of heparin, clotting factors in the common pathway will be inhibited enough to prolong both the aPTT and the PT.

It is tempting to discuss at length the interpretation of coagulation tests when discussing the mechanism of coagulation because the aPTT and the PT test the two principle pathways. However, analysis of these two tests alone will not lead to a specific diagnosis. Instead, the physician must also understand fibrinolysis and have a working knowledge of the common bleeding disorders. Then, the results of all of the tests of the hemostatic mechanism (tests of primary hemostasis, coagulation, and fibrinolysis) can be evaluated together. The pattern of results should suggest the most likely diagnosis. With this in mind, a brief discussion of fibrinolysis follows.

FIBRINOLYSIS

Fibrinolysis is the final process of the hemostatic mechanism. In this process, plasminogen is converted to plasmin, the fibrinolytic enzyme that lyses fibrin clots (32). Plasminogen (not plasmin) circulates in the bloodstream, because antiplasmins, which attack and rapidly neutralize plasmin, circulate in the bloodstream in concentrations 10 times that of plasmin. When plasminogen comes into contact with fibrin, it preferentially binds to the fibrin clot. As the clot evolves, it incorporates the plasminogen and an enzyme called tissue plasminogen activator (TPA). TPA converts the plasminogen to plasmin. This plasmin, produced within the fibrin clot, is "shielded" from antiplasmins in the blood. Bound to the fibrin and protected from antiplasmin attack, the plasmin enzyme literally lyses its way out of the fibrin clot, until it is released again into the bloodstream (27). There, the antiplasmins rapidly neutralize the liberated plasmin and prevent widespread uncontrolled fibrinolysis.

Plasmin, generated by the process of fibrinolysis, is very nonspecific in its actions. Plasmin can lyse fibrinogen, fibrin that is cross-linked, and fibrin that is uncross-linked (33). The resulting family of degradation products are called, collectively, fibrin degradation products (FDPs) or fibrin split products (FSPs). Under normal circumstances, these FDPs have a half-life of 9 hours and are metabolized by the liver, picked up by the reticuloendothelial system, or excreted by the kidney.

COMMON BLEEDING DISORDERS

The patient who is bleeding in the recovery room most likely has a surgical defect (1). However, if no clots are apparent in the shed blood and the patient seems to be oozing generally from many sites, then the presence of a bleeding disorder should also be considered. The patient may have developed a bleeding disorder during surgery or may have come to the operating room with a preexisting bleeding disorder that was overlooked. If the patient develops a coagulopathy intraoperatively, it will most likely be due to the effects of massive transfusions, the administration of heparin, or the development of DIC. The first two causes of intraoperative bleeding are easy to confirm or rule out. If the patient did not receive massive transfusions or heparin before arrival in the recovery room, these two causes can be disregarded. The third cause that leads to the breakdown of the hemostatic mechanism, DIC, is more insidious and causes a pervasive disruption of the hemostatic mechanism. DIC must be included in the differential diagnosis of patients who develop a coagulopathy. In addition to DIC, preexisting bleeding disorders must be considered.

To have a consistent approach to the bleeding patient, the bleeding disorders are classified and discussed according to which component of the hemostatic system is affected: the blood vessels, platelets, coagulation factors, or the fibrinolytic system. Coagulation testing is likewise aimed at diagnosing problems with each component of the hemostatic mechanism. Anesthesiologists most commonly diagnose acquired bleeding defects, not those that are hereditary in origin. The more common hereditary problems, von Willebrand's disease and hemophilia, usually present bleeding complications early in life and the patient seeks the care of a hematologist. Therefore, although it is important for the anesthesiologist to be aware of these hereditary bleeding disorders and keep them in mind when faced with a bleeding patient, the common acquired defects will be the focus of the following discussion.

DEFECTS IN PRIMARY HEMOSTASIS

The formation of the platelet plug during primary hemostasis depends on the interaction of blood vessels and platelets. Primary hemostasis can be defective when vascular integrity is disrupted. This is usually the result of surgical trauma, but the blood vessels can

be compromised by immune or inflammatory processes. Vascular integrity is assessed primarily by inspection of the surgical field, and when this is not helpful, surgical bleeding sometimes becomes a diagnosis of exclusion.

Platelet disorders are characterized as being inherited or acquired, quantitative or qualitative. The most common hereditary defect of primary hemostasis that causes a qualitative platelet defect is that caused by von Willebrand's disease. This deficiency has several variations in its presentation and can cause minor to severe episodes of bleeding. The definitive diagnosis is made by a hematologist and long-term treatment involves the use of desmopressin. The patient with von Willebrand's disease that presents for surgery and has an acute bleeding problem may need treatment with fresh frozen plasma to correct the deficiency of this factor.

Thrombocytopenia, or quantitative platelet deficiencies, result from five general causes: the platelets may be (*a*) inadequately produced, (*b*) sequestered in the spleen, (*c*) consumed with massive tissue damage, (*d*) diluted by massive transfusions, or (*e*) destroyed by immune mechanisms. Inadequate production occurs with conditions that damage the patient's bone marrow such as radiation, chemotherapy, or the invasion of the bone marrow by cancer cells (31). Hypersplenism also leads to thrombocytopenia. Under normal circumstances, the spleen sequesters 30% of the normal platelet pool. With splenomegaly, this proportion increases and thrombocytopenia results.

Massive tissue damage, wherein large areas of endothelium are denuded, exposing collagen and leading to platelet activation, will consume platelets, decreasing their circulating numbers dramatically. This cause of thrombocytopenia, platelet consumption, occurs in burn patients who have large areas of denuded endothelium and with diseases that produce a generalized vasculitis, such as preeclampsia of pregnancy. Platelets are also consumed during the process of DIC. Additionally, the initiation of cardiopulmonary bypass consumes platelets simply because the platelets adhere to the artificial surfaces of the bypass tubing.

A dilutional thrombocytopenia follows massive transfusions with any fluids that do not contain viable platelets. It is obvious that the administration of lactated Ringer's solution and/or normal saline will dilute the patient's platelet count. It may be less obvious, but the massive transfusion of stored whole blood or packed red bloods cells will also lead to a dilutional thrombocytopenia; these blood components do not contain viable platelets. Finally, platelets may be destroyed by immune mechanisms. Particularly troublesome for the anesthesiologist is the syndrome of heparin-induced thrombocytopenia. This coagulopathy has an immune origin and makes anticoagulation for cardiopulmonary bypass problematic.

Like the causes of thrombocytopenia, acquired platelet function disorders are associated with a wide range of disorders and some drugs. Uremia produces a platelet defect (34) that is believed to be caused by the accumulation of certain metabolites that are toxic to the platelets. These substances, such as guanidinosuccinic acid, prolong bleeding time by inhibiting platelet adhesiveness. Dialysis does not totally correct this bleeding disorder but does have some temporary benefit (35). Qualitative platelet defects are also associated with the consumption of large quantities of alcohol over a long period of time. The mechanism of alcohol-related platelet dysfunction is unknown but may relate to the synthesis of prostaglandins. Patients with cirrhosis of the liver predictably display platelet function disorders. Although the above causes of platelet dysfunction are important, the most common cause results from the consumption of aspirin and aspirin-containing medications (1, 36). Aspirin inhibits the synthesis of thromboxane A_2 for the life of the platelet. Many other drugs, such as indomethacin, phenylbutazone, ibuprofen, dipyrimadole, and dextran, inhibit the platelet function to varying degrees. The fourth cause of platelet dysfunction is that caused by the products of fibrinolysis, the fibrin degradation products (FDPs). Patients suffering from DIC will have an active fibrinolytic system that attempts to lyse the many fibrin clots forming throughout the bloodstream. The resulting degradation products (FDPs) may accumulate if they are produced too rapidly for their clearance. The presence of these FDPs inhibits platelet function and may cause the patient to bleed.

COAGULATION FACTOR DISORDERS

As has been stated before, hemophilia A is the most common hereditary defect producing deficiencies of coagulant factor VIII (1). A hematologist should be consulted when these patients are taken to the operating room or when they present with bleeding complications in the recovery room.

Acquired factor deficiencies result from liver disease, vitamin K deficiency, massive transfusions that dilute both the platelet count and the available clotting factors, and conditions that predispose the patient to develop disseminated intravascular coagulation. Because the liver synthesizes most of the clotting factors (except possibly factor VIII), liver disease produces a multifactorial bleeding disorder (1). Because factor VII of the extrinsic pathway has the shortest half-life, the onset of liver dysfunction will initially prolong the prothrombin time. With further hepatic disease, both the PT and the aPTT will be prolonged.

Vitamin K deficiency can result from a variety of causes. Vitamin K is a fat-soluble vitamin that is found in leafy green vegetables (37). With poor diet or after 1 week of intravenous feeding without vitamin supplementation, a person can develop vitamin K deficiency and start producing vitamin-K–dependent factors (II, VII, IX, and X) that are defective. This is because the final step in their enzymatic synthesis involves the addition of a carboxyl group onto the factor and requires the presence of vitamin K. Without this carboxyl group, the factors circulate in the blood but do not bind to phospholipid surfaces (29). Because this fat-soluble vitamin relies on bile secretion for proper absorption, biliary obstruction can also diminish vitamin K stores (1). Malabsorption syndromes or even enema treatments can stop the patient from properly absorbing the vitamin. Finally, the intestinal flora of the gut play an important role in converting the vitamin to its active form. Sterilization of the gut with antibiotic therapy may also contribute to vitamin K deficiency (31). The anticoagulant, coumadin, prolongs bleeding by competing with vitamin K for binding sites in the liver and produces the same bleeding defect as vitamin K deficiency.

The typical scenario in which a patient may develop vitamin K deficiency and, consequently, a bleeding problem is as follows: a patient who has poor nutritional status due to colon cancer is admitted to the hospital for a workup and surgery and is then kept NPO. Preoperative orders include enemas and prophylactic antibiotics to sterilize the gut. Then, although the patient may have been scheduled for surgery, an unpredictable factor causes the surgery to be postponed for 1 or 2 days. By the time the patient is taken to the operating room, the level of vitamin-K–dependent factors is dangerously diminished. Blood loss during surgery and transfusion with crystalloids further dilutes the concentration of the clotting factors. The patient may develop a coagulopathy during surgery or later in the recovery room. This patient presents a dilemma for the physician who evaluates the patient postoperatively because surgical trauma is a more likely cause of the patient's bleeding than the development of a coagulopathy. However, the absence of blood clots and the prolongation of the patient's prothrombin time, considered in the context of this patient's medical condition should suggest the diagnosis. Treatment will depend on the degree of urgency. Vitamin K therapy takes several hours with good hepatic function to replace the deficient factors. Fresh frozen plasma carries the risk of AIDS and hepatitis but corrects the coagulopathy quickly.

Massive transfusions, whether of crystalloid, albumin, or hetastarch, may lead to dilution of the clotting factors. On the other hand, transfusion of packed red blood cells does replace some clotting factors because even "packed cells" contain some plasma. However, the labile factors (V and VIII) become deficient in stored blood so that massive transfusions of stored red blood cells can lead to a bleeding disorder. It must be remembered that dilutional thrombocytopenia is usually the primary cause of a bleeding diathesis developing after massive transfusions; dilution of the labile clotting factors is likely to be only contributory. In reality, the clotting factor levels are almost never low enough to prolong the patient's clotting times. The PT and aPTT require only a minimum of 30% of normal coagulant activity of any of the clotting factors for these tests to be normal. The administration of fresh frozen plasma to replace clotting factors is rarely justified after massive transfusions.

Anticoagulant therapy, coumadin or heparin, predictably creates factor deficiencies. Vascular surgery cases often involve the administration of heparin and although this agent is rapidly metabolized, residual heparin levels can contribute to bleeding disorders. The management of bleeding after cardiac surgery is beyond the scope of this chapter, but the differential diagnosis usually includes surgical problems, platelet dysfunction, thrombocytopenia, and the possibility of residual heparinization and heparin rebound and may even involve factor deficiencies and the presence of excess fibrinolysis.

A review of the patient's medical record will assist in determining whether the likely cause of a patient's bleeding is severe liver disease, vitamin K deficiency, massive transfusions, or anticoagulant therapy. The syndrome of DIC, however, can produce factor deficiencies and may evolve quite insidiously. This bleeding disorder may require the physician to take a closer look at the patient to recognize why that patient's Coagulation system is out of control.

The surgical patient can have or acquire many conditions that predispose to the development of DIC. These conditions include sepsis, tissue injury, liver disease, burns, acidosis, shock, and others. Although these conditions are very different, they may all lead to DIC or "uncontrolled" Coagulation throughout the bloodstream. It is ironic that this syndrome can result in organ dysfunction due to the formation of multiple microthrombi throughout the circulation at one moment and then later produce a patient who is bleeding to death from all orifices. Knowledge of the pathophysiology of DIC and the attempts of the fibrinolytic system to counterbalance the thrombotic events aids in an understanding of why the patient who is first "clotting to death" then "bleeds to death."

Just as primary hemostasis is controlled by the balance of prostaglandins and fibrinolysis is controlled by the presence of antiplasmins in the blood, many mechanisms exist to control and localize Coagulation. Loss of the normal mechanisms that control or limit Coagulation to sites of vascular injury leads to the process of uncontrolled or "disseminated" intravascular coagulation. Normally, the clotting factors circulate in an inactive form. Even when activated, rapid blood flow dilutes the active factors and washes them away from sites where Coagulation should not be activated. In contrast, Coagulation is promoted in patients who have poor perfusion, are hypotensive, or are in shock.

Normal control of Coagulation is promoted by good liver blood flow and by good hepatic function. The liver, as well as the reticuloendothelial system, clears active clotting factors from the circulation. Patients with cirrhosis and portosystemic shunts sometimes develop low-grade DIC because the diseased or partially bypassed liver has a decreased ability to clear activated clotting factors. Additionally, the diseased liver does not clear fibrin degradation products and it releases thromboplastin into the circulation, thereby promoting DIC in these patients.

One more mechanism that serves to localize Coagulation is the fact that several factors involved in the coagulation process require the presence of a phospholipid surface for their proper interaction. This prerequisite for a phospholipid surface, under normal circumstances, limits Coagulation to sites of vascular injury where phospholipid is exposed by activated platelets and to areas of tissue damage where tissue thromboplastin is liberated. However, when phospholipid circulates diffusely throughout the bloodstream, control of Coagulation is lost and the process of DIC begins.

Antithrombin III, the body's natural anticoagulant, helps limit and regulate Coagulation by binding to thrombin and other active cleavage enzymes in the intrinsic pathway. In the process of DIC, the diffuse circulation of phospholipid throughout the bloodstream can produce so much thrombin that the antithrombin III is overwhelmed and consumed. Instead, fibrin clots form throughout the microcirculation, consuming platelets and clotting factors and stimulating fibrinolysis.

Circulating phospholipid may come from two sources: that exposed by platelets when they are activated (PF3) or that released by damaged tissue (tissue thromboplastin). Platelets can be activated throughout the bloodstream by immune complexes or even by bacteria. This is why DIC develops so commonly in septic patients. The activated platelets expose phospholipid, providing a surface for the interaction of clotting factors. When the process overwhelms the ability of antithrombin III to control Coagulation, microthrombi are deposited throughout the circulation. This disseminated intravascular coagulation stimulates fibrinolysis as a defense mechanism to maintain blood flow throughout the body.

Diffuse platelet aggregation and activation may also develop in patients who have large areas of denuded endothelium, such as occurs in burn patients or patients with diffuse vasculitis, such as exists in the preeclamptic patient.

The second type of phospholipid, tissue thromboplastin, may be released into the circulation with massive crush injuries, major strokes, and after some obstetric catastrophes (38). An amniotic fluid embolus, abruptio placenta, and a fetal death in utero are all associated with the release of massive amounts of tissue thromboplastin into the circulation and the development of the all-consuming process of DIC.

As noted above, when Coagulation is rampant and fibrin clots are formed throughout the bloodstream, the fibrinolytic system fires up, lysing the blood clots in an attempt to maintain the fluidity of the blood. Plasmin lyses fibrin that is cross-linked, fibrin that is not cross-linked, and fibrinogen. The action of plasmin produces an entire family of degradation products called fibrin degradation products (FDPs) or fibrin split products (FSPs). These FDPs are normally cleared from the circulation by the liver, by the reticuloendothelial system, and by the kidney. Their normal half-life is about 9 hours. However, if these FDPs are produced at a rate faster than they can be cleared from the circulation, they will begin to accumulate. They become nature's most powerful anticoagulant. The FDPs inhibit platelet aggregation and prevent the normal cross-linking of fibrin, which is necessary to make clots insoluble. With the disruption of primary hemostasis and coagulation, the FDPs cause bleeding where clotting was once occurring throughout the bloodstream.

The patient with DIC bleeds for several reasons. Primarily, they bleed because their platelets are consumed; secondly, they bleed because of the anticoagulant effects of the FDPs; and lastly, they bleed because of the consumption of clotting factors. To treat DIC, the normal mechanisms that control Coagulation must be reinstated. Blood flow, if compromised, should be improved by augmenting cardiac output and correcting any acid-base disturbances that may exist. The source of the circulating phospholipid must be removed from the circulation. If the patient is septic, this means successfully treating the infection. When the stimulus for Coagulation is removed, the fibrinolytic system will be less active and fewer FDPs will be generated. In the interim, platelet transfusions may be necessary and, possibly, fresh frozen plasma (FFP) may be required to replace the platelets and factors that have been consumed. If Coagulation testing reveals that the patient's FDPs are increasing in concentration, a hematologist may be consulted.

COAGULATION TESTING

Tests of Primary Hemostasis

Perioperative bleeding is often very dynamic and may have more than one cause. This makes diagnosis more challenging. If a bleeding disorder is suspected, laboratory tests should include a platelet count, prothrombin time (PT), activated partial thromboplastin time (aPTT), a thrombin time (TT) if the patient has been given heparin, a fibrinogen level, and an assay for the presence of fibrin degradation products (FDPs).

The platelet count is simple, reproducible, and reliable. If the patient's platelet count is below $150,000/mm^3$, by definition, the patient is said to be thrombocytopenic (39). The patient may not develop a clinical coagulopathy, however, until the platelet count drops to $50,000/mm^3$ or less. It is important to make a clinical assessment of the patient's bleeding status and not to just treat the numbers. Instead, the laboratory tests should help to "confirm" clinical suspicions.

The bleeding time (BT) test is used to evaluate platelet function (29). It measures the interaction of platelets with the blood vessel wall and the time it takes to form a platelet plug (35). When this test is prolonged, it may reflect that there is a decrease in the number of platelets, that the platelets do not function normally, or that the platelets cannot interact appropriately with the vessel wall (39). This test is difficult to standardize and is rarely used in the setting of the recovery room. Further, specialized tests of platelet function, such as platelet aggregation studies that use ADP, epinephrine, collagen, and ristocetin are usually only performed in research laboratories and are not readily available at most hospitals (40).

When the patient's platelet count is low, the most likely causes of thrombocytopenia should be evaluated. Either the platelets are inadequately produced, sequestered in the spleen, consumed by massive tissue damage, diluted by massive transfusions, or destroyed by immune mechanisms. When platelet dysfunction is suspected, it is more difficult to confirm because of the paucity of platelet function tests. Instead, this diagnosis is often presumed but not supportable by laboratory evidence. If the patient's clotting tests (PT, PTT) are normal, the platelet count is also normal, and the patient is believed to have a bleeding disorder, the common causes of acquired platelet dysfunction — uremia, liver disease and chronic alcoholism, aspirin ingestion or the ingestion of antiplatelet drugs, and DIC — should be considered.

Tests of the Coagulation Pathways

The intrinsic and extrinsic pathways of coagulation rely on different phospholipid surfaces for the interaction of their clotting factors. Therefore, the two tests of these pathways, the activated partial thromboplastin time (aPTT) and the prothrombin time (PT) differ according to which phospholipid is added to the patient's blood sample (39). The aPTT that measures the intrinsic pathway is initiated by the addition of a platelet phospholipid equivalent called partial thromboplastin (1). The PT is performed by the addition of a tissue factor equivalent and monitors the extrinsic pathway of coagulation.

The usefulness of these tests is diminished by the fact that each pathway involves the interaction of so many clotting factors that even when a test is prolonged, the result does not pinpoint the cause of the delayed clotting. Another drawback to these tests is that they are not very sensitive to deficiencies of the clotting factors. The aPTT and PT clotting

times may be normal even when only 30 to 40% of coagulant activity exists for each of the factors (1, 41). This can be significant clinically because the aPTT can be normal in patients with von Willebrand's disease; factor VIII levels may be decreased and yet the patient has a normal aPTT. Furthermore, neither of these tests, the aPTT or the PT, measure the activity of factor XIII. It should be kept in mind that the aPTT and PT measure coagulation times and do not evaluate primary hemostasis. This means that the patient can be thrombocytopenic and have a normal aPTT because this coagulation test begins with the addition of a platelet phospholipid equivalent to the patient's blood sample.

The aPTT will be prolonged with significant deficiencies of factors XII, XI, IX, and VIII and those factors in the common pathway, X, V, prothrombin (II) and fibrinogen (I) (41). This clotting time will also be affected by circulating anticoagulants, including heparin and fibrin degradation products (41). The aPTT is also prolonged when fibrinogen levels fall below 100 mg/dL. The aPTT will not be affected by deficiencies of factor VII.

The PT will be prolonged with deficiencies of factor VII, and those factors in the common pathway (39). This test also will be prolonged when the fibrinogen concentration is below 100 mg/dL or when heparin or fibrinogen degradation products are present (41).

The sensitivity of the prothrombin time depends, to a large extent, on the particular thromboplastin employed. Because of the tremendous variation in thromboplastins used in North America, an attempt has been made to standardize the sensitivities of the thromboplastins with the use of an international normalized ratio (INR) (39). This ratio compares all thromboplastins used to perform the PT to a standard reference and provides a basis for calibrating the sensitivities of new thromboplastin reagents (39).

The thrombin time (TT) detects abnormalities in the final stage of coagulation, the conversion of fibrinogen to fibrin by thrombin (29). This test is not sensitive to factor deficiencies that precede this step in the coagulation cascade. Thrombin is added to the test plasma and the time that it takes for fibrin to be formed is measured (42). The thrombin time can be prolonged when fibrinogen is depleted or when inhibitors to thrombin, such as heparin or fibrin degradation products, are present (39). The TT is probably the most sensitive indicator of the presence of heparin (40). Because the TT can be prolonged by both heparin and FDPs, the presence of these two in the sample can be differentiated by the use of another test called the reptilase time (39, 42).

Footprints of DIC and Fibrinolysis

To evaluate whether the patient may be developing a hypercoagulable state, it is helpful to measure fibrinogen levels. The patient's fibrinogen concentration is determined by adding large quantities of factor IIa (thrombin) to the patient's sample and comparing the clotting time of the patient to those specimens with known fibrinogen levels (41). Fibrinogen levels are decreased most commonly with hypercoagulable states such as DIC. They may also be decreased with severe liver disease because of the decreased synthesis of this factor (39). Conversely, fibrinogen levels are increased with stress and pregnancy.

FDPs are the byproduct of fibrinolysis and, often, their presence is used as "circumstantial evidence" that DIC is ongoing. Elevated levels of FDPs are also seen with severe liver disease, however (41, 42). Positive tests for fibrin monomers may implicate DIC instead of severe liver disease.

INTERPRETATION OF COAGULATION TESTS

The interpretation of Coagulation tests requires a knowledge of the common bleeding disorders that should be kept in mind as one evaluates these test results. One useful approach to the interpretation of Coagulation tests is to try to decide which combination of test results is consistent with the laboratory picture produced by each bleeding disorder (38). Most clinicians who suspect a bleeding disorder will first order a platelet count, an aPTT, and a PT. Only when a more disruptive process is suspected, such as the presence of circulating anticoagulants (heparin or FDPs), do clinicians order a TT, fibrinogen level, and an assay for the presence of FDPs or fibrin monomers. Therefore, the interpretation of Coagulation tests presented below will follow this sequence.

ONLY PLATELET COUNT IS DECREASED (aPTT AND PT NORMAL)

When only the platelet count is decreased, one of the common causes of thrombocytopenia should be considered: either the platelets are being inadequately produced (bone marrow problem); they are sequestered (splenomegaly), diluted (massive transfusions), or consumed (platelet activation or tissue injury); or they have been destroyed (immune mechanisms).

ONLY PLATELET DYSFUNCTION IS SUSPECTED (PLATELET COUNT, aPTT, PT NORMAL)

Confirmation of platelet dysfunction by laboratory means may be difficult. Although the bleeding time may be useful in evaluating primary hemostasis, it is rarely used in the setting of the operating room or the recovery room. Test results are often questioned, and this test is not as reproducible as other tests of the hemostatic mechanism.

When a patient appears clinically to have a coagulopathy and the Coagulation tests (platelet count, aPTT, PT, and TT) are normal, platelet dysfunction should be considered as a diagnosis of exclusion. Platelet dysfunction occurs with uremia, alcoholic liver disease, in patients taking antiplatelet drugs, and in the presence of DIC. It is also a common cause of bleeding after cardiopulmonary bypass.

ONLY PROLONGED aPTT (PLATELET COUNT AND PT NORMAL)

The bleeding disorders that would produce this combination of test results are limited to those that affect the intrinsic pathway of coagulation. The clotting factors that are unique to the intrinsic pathway include factors XII, XI, IX, and VIII. A deficiency of factor VIII, hemophilia A, will prolong just the aPTT. Because the von Willebrand factor serves as a carrier protein for the coagulant portion of factor VIII, deficiency of this factor may prolong the aPTT. However, von Willebrand's disease will also affect platelet function. Problems with both primary hemostasis and coagulation will be demonstrated (38).

Poor collection techniques when drawing the patient's blood for testing can also prolong just the aPTT. This is because factors V and VIII, the labile factors, may be consumed if the blood is partially clotted before delivery to the laboratory (43).

Heparin therapy is monitored with the aPTT. Initially, only the aPTT is prolonged because of the sensitivity of factor IX to this anticoagulant. With increasing doses, however, both the aPTT and PT will be prolonged because of the effects of heparin on factors in the common pathway of coagulation.

ONLY PROLONGED PT (NORMAL PLATELET COUNT AND aPTT)

Because factor VII has the shortest half-life of the clotting factors, early liver disease, vitamin K deficiency, and coumadin therapy will prolong the extrinsic pathway (PT) before prolonging the intrinsic pathway (29, 38). Eventually, however, these three conditions will prolong both pathways and both tests, the aPTT and the PT.

BOTH PROLONGED aPTT AND PT (NORMAL PLATELET COUNT AND TT)

This combination suggests a defect in both the intrinsic and extrinsic pathways or a defect in the shared factors of the common pathway

(29). Because the TT is normal, the defect must involve factors that precede the conversion of fibrinogen to fibrin by thrombin. This pattern is characteristic of vitamin K deficiency, coumadin therapy, and liver disease wherein the dysfunction has not reduced fibrinogen levels enough to prolong the TT also.

PROLONGED PT, aPTT, TT (NORMAL PLATELET COUNT)

All of these tests will be prolonged when hemorrhage develops secondary to thrombin inhibitors, which block the conversion of fibrinogen to fibrin, as measured by the TT. Such inhibitors include heparin and the presence of fibrin degradation products (FDPs). Hypofibrinogenemia will also prolong these tests. It should be noted that when FDPs are present due to ongoing DIC, the platelet count will usually be decreased.

LOW PLATELET COUNT, PROLONGED aPTT, PT, TT

The patient with a low platelet count and all of their Coagulation tests prolonged, must have a global disruption of their hemostatic mechanism (38). This clinical picture can be produced by DIC, the dilutional effects of massive transfusion, and by excesses of heparin.

LOW FIBRINOGEN AND CIRCULATING FDPs PRESENT

The addition of one more Coagulation test, an assay for FDPs, will be helpful in the differential diagnosis of the patient who has a low platelet count and prolonged aPTT, PT, and TT. The presence of FDPs suggests the diagnosis of DIC.

In summary, interpreting Coagulation tests requires matching the combination of test results with the bleeding disorders that could produce those results. At that point, the patient's clinical condition and medical history must be evaluated to determine which diagnosis is most likely.

TREATMENT OF BLEEDING DISORDERS

Our ability to treat coagulopathies remains rather limited. Individual isolated factors, such as factor VIII, can be transfused for the treatment of genetic defects. But otherwise, component therapy for hemostatic disorders usually involves the transfusion of platelets, fresh frozen plasma, or cryoprecipitate. In deciding to transfuse a patient with hemostatic agents, the clinician should not rely solely on laboratory tests but instead should evaluate whether or not a clinical coagulopathy seems to be present. The results of laboratory tests may not accurately predict the onset of a clinical coagulopathy (3, 4). Often, the Coagulation system demonstrates an amazing tolerance to thrombocytopenia and to clotting factor deficiencies. Even when the clotting times of the PT and aPTT are 1.5 times the control, the patient may not bleed.

Platelets are transfused to correct deficiencies in platelet number or platelet function. Each unit of platelets will increase the platelet count approximately 7,500 to 10,000/mm³. The National Institutes of Health (NIH) sponsored a consensus conference to develop guidelines for the transfusion of platelets. They concluded that indications for pooled platelet concentrates include treatment of thrombocytopenia in association with clinical coagulopathy, which often may not occur until platelet counts reach: (a) 10,000/mm³ in ITP (idiopathic thrombocytopenic purpura), (b) 20,000/mm³ in bone marrow depression, and (c) 40,000/mm³ during massive transfusion. Treatment with platelet concentrates was also recommended with a clinical coagulopathy resulting from platelet dysfunction, even with platelet counts higher than 100,000/mm³ such as occurs: (a) after cardiopulmonary bypass, (b) during surgical procedures in patients taking aspirin or other drugs impairing platelet function, (c) with uremia, and (d) with Glanzmann's thrombasthenia. The NIH consensus further stated that inappropriate uses include prophylaxis in massive transfusion or transfusion prophylactically after cardiopulmonary bypass (44). The July 1989 FDA Drug Bulletin reinforces these guidelines, stating that platelets should not be given: (a) to patients with immune thrombocytopenic purpura (unless there is life-threatening bleeding), (b) for prophylaxis with massive blood transfusion, and (c) for prophylaxis after cardiopulmonary bypass.

In summary, in deciding to transfuse platelets, the clinician should look not only at the platelet count but also for clinical signs of bleeding. In the recovery room, thrombocytopenia that was not present preoperatively will usually be due to massive transfusions, which dilute the patient's platelet count, or due to the presence of DIC, which consumes the patient's platelets. Platelet dysfunction is a presumed diagnosis for patients who have (a) uremia, (b) severe liver disease, (c) a history of antiplatelet drug consumption, or (d) DIC. Platelet dysfunction may also follow cardiopulmonary bypass surgery.

In 1984, the NIH held a multidisciplinary Consensus Development Panel to discuss the indications and risks of transfusion with FFP (45). Indications for FFP administration developed by the consensus conference include: (a) replacement of isolated factor deficiencies (documented by laboratory evidence), (b) reversal of coumadin effect, (c) antithrombin III deficiency, (d) treatment of immunodeficiencies, (e) treatment of thrombotic thrombocytopenic purpura, or (f) massive blood transfusion (rarely an indicated cause for the use of FFP).

The use of FFP in the recovery room will most likely involve treatment of coagulopathies due to the presence of preexisting liver disease or vitamin-K—deficiency, due to the development of a bleeding disorder after massive transfusions, or due to DIC. The decision to give FFP after massive transfusions should only be made after making certain that a clinical coagulopathy is evident, that thrombocytopenia is not the cause of bleeding, and that the aPTT is prolonged (3).

Cryoprecipitate contains significant levels of factor VIII and fibrinogen. It also contains von Willebrand factor. This blood component is used for the treatment of hemophilia, von Willebrand's disease, and fibrinogen deficiencies. In the surgical patient, the consumption of fibrinogen most commonly occurs with the development of DIC.

CONCLUSIONS

The approach to the bleeding patient requires a knowledge of the basic hemostatic mechanism, common bleeding disorders, an ability to interpret Coagulation tests, and an appreciation of the risks involved with blood component therapy. We must rethink the criteria for transfusing patients with red blood cells and be certain that hemostatic agents are appropriately used. None of the blood components should be transfused prophylactically but only when specific recognized indications exist.

REFERENCES

1. Weaver DW. Diferential diagnosis and management of unexplained bleeding. Surg Clin North Am 1993;73:353–361.
2. Welch HG. Prudent strategies for elective red blood cell transfusion. Ann Intern Med 1992;116:393–402.
3. Perez WE. Tranfusion and coagulation: an overview and recent advances in practice modalities Part I: blood banking and tranfusion practices. Nurse Anesth 1990;1.149–161.
4. Crosby ET. Perioperative haemotherapy: I. Indications for blood component transfusion. Can J Anaesth 1992;39:695–707.
5. Kruskall MS. Transfusion therapy in emergency medicine. Ann Emerg 1988;17:327–335.
6. George CD. Immunologic effects of blood transfusion upon renal transplantation, tumor operations, and bacterial infections. Am J Surg 1986; 152:329–337.
7. Miller RD. Transfusion therapy. In: Miller RD, ed. Anesthesia. 3rd ed. New York: Churchill Livingstone, 1990;1467–1499.
8. Burrows L, Tartter P. Effect of blood tranfusions on colonic malignancy recurrence rate. Lancet 1982;2:662.
9. Parrott NR, Lennard TW, Taylor RM, et al. Effect of perioperative blood transfusion on recurrence of colorectal cancer. Br J Surg 1986; 73(12):970–973.
10. Hamilton SM. The use of blood in resuscitation of the trauma patient. (Published erratum appears in Can J Surg 1993;36(2):114.) Can J Surg 1993;36:21–27.
11. Stehling L. Indications for perioperative blood transfusion in 1990. Can Anaesth 1991;38(5):601–604.
12. Robertie PG, Gravlee GP. Safe limits of isovolemic hemodilution and recommendations for erythrocyte tranfusion. Int Anaesthesiol Clin 1990;28:197–204.
13. Von Restorff W, Hofling B, Holtz J, et al. Effect of increased blood fluidity through hemodiliton on general circulation at rest and during exercise in dogs. Pflugers Arch 1975;357:25–34.
14. Tarnow J, Eberlein HJ, Schneider EE. Heodynamic interactions of hemodilution, anaesthesia, propranolol pre-treatment and hypovolaemia. Bas Res Cardiol 1979;74:109–122.
15. Glick G, Plauth WH, Brauwald EE. Role of the autonomic nervous system in the circulatory response to acutley induced anemia in unaesthetized dogs. J Clin Invest 1964;49;2112–2124.
16. Levine E, Rosen A, Sehgal L, et al. Pysiologic effects of acute anaemia: implications for a reduced transfusion trigger. Transfusion 1990;30:11–14.
17. Shah DM, Gottlieb ME, Rahm RLE. Failure of red blood cells transfusion to increase oxygen transport or mixed venous PO, in injured patients. J Trauma 1982;22:746.
18. Ereth MH, Jr. Perioperative interventions to decrease transfusion of allogeneic blood products. Mayo Clin Proc 1964;69:575–586.
19. Office of Medical Applications of Research, National Institute of Health. Perioperative red cell transfusion. JAMA 1988;260:2700.
20. Office of Medical Applications of Research, National Institutes of Health. Platelet transfusion therpay. JAMA 1985;257:1777.
21. Office of Medical Applications of Research, National Institute of Health. Fresh frozen plasma: indications and risks. JAMA 1985;253:551.
22. Miler RD, Tong MJ, Robbins TO. Effects of massive transfusion of blood on acid-base balance. JAMA 1971;216(11):1762–1765.
23. Gloe D. Common reactions to transfusions. Heart and lung 1991;20:506–514.
24. Welborn JL, Hersch J. Blood transfusion reactions: which are life-threatening and which are not? Postgrad med 1991;90:135–138.
25. Shattil SJ, Bennett JS. Platelets and their membtanes in hemostatsis: physiology and pathophysiology. Ann Intern med 1980;94:108–118.
26. Mackey IJ, Pittiolo RM. Vascular integrity and platelet function. Int Anesthesiol Clin 1985;23:3–21.
27. Brandt JT. Current concepts of coagulation. Clin Obstet Gyneocol 1985;28:3–14.
28. Ellison N. Hemostasis and hemotherapy. In: Barash PG, Cullen BF, Stoelting RK, eds. Clinical anesthesia. Philadelphia: J. B. Lippincott Company, 1989;707–710.
29. Triplett DA. Overview of hemostasis. In: Menitove JE, McCarthy LJ, eds. Hemostatic disorders and the blood bank. Arlington: American Association of Blood Banks, 1984;1–23.
30. Pottmeyer E, Vassar MJ, Holcroft JW. Coagulation,

inflammation, and responses to injury. Crit Care Clin 1986;2:683–703.

31. Mansouri A. Acquired hemostatic abnormalities in the elderly. J Am Geriatr Soc 1990;38:809–816.

32. Bone RC. Modulators of coagulation. A critical appraisal of their role in sepsis. Arch Intern med 1992;152:1381–1389.

33. Lewis JH, Spero JA, Hasiba U. Coagulopathies. In: Anonymous disease-a-month. Chicago: Year Book Medical Publishers, 1977.

34. Remuzzi G. Bleeding in renal failure. Lancet 1988;1:1205–1208.

35. Eberst ME. Hemostasis in renal disease: pathophysiology and management. Am J Med 1994;96:168–179.

36. Irving GA. Perioperative blood and blood component therapy. Can J Anaesth 1992;39:1105–1115.

37. Bolan CD. Pharmacologic agents in the management of bleeding disorders. Transfusion 1990;30:541–551.

38. Angelos MG. Coagulation studies: prothrombin time, partial thrombplastin time, bleeding time. Emerg Med Clin North Am 1986;4:95–113.

39. Moir DJ. Investigation of bleeding disorders. Int Anesthe Clin 1985;23:37–47.

40. Ellison N, Silberstein LE. Hemostasis in the Perioperative Period. In: Stoelting RK, Barash PG, Gallagher TJ, eds. Advances in anesthesia. 1st ed. Chicago: Year Book Medical Publishers, 1986;67–101.

41. Bennett JS. Blood coagulation and coagulation tests. Med Clin North Am 1984;68.

42. Freiberger JJ, Lumb PD. How to manage intraoperative bleeding. In: Vaughan RW, ed. perioperative problems/catastrophes. 1st ed. Philadelphia: J B Lippincott Co., 1987;161–172.

43. Colon-Otero G, Cockerill KJ, Bowie EJW. How to diagnose bleeding disorders. Postgraduate Med 1991;90(3):145–150.

44. Consensus Conference Platelet transfusion therapy. JAMA 1987;257:1780.

45. Consensus Conference Fresh frozen plasma: indications and risks. JAMA 1985;253:553.

12

INFECTION CONTROL

Arnold J. Berry

An awareness of the importance of proper infection control procedures in the perioperative period has been augmented during the past two decades as the result of the impact of multiple factors. With the development of new anesthetic techniques and drugs, patients at the extremes of age and with multisystem pathology are undergoing surgical procedures of greater complexity and duration. The development of innovative invasive and noninvasive monitors has enhanced the management of the physiologic alterations associated with both disease processes and surgery. The advent of intensive care units (ICUs) has facilitated continuous preoperative and postoperative vigilance by physicians and nurses. New, more powerful antibiotics have been introduced into practice to be used either prophylactically or to combat the multitude of organisms infecting patients with multiorgan system failure. The global spread of the acquired immunodeficiency syndrome (AIDS) via the human immunodeficiency virus (HIV) has resulted in a population of immunosuppressed individuals at risk for opportunistic infections. With the advent of bone marrow and solid organ transplantation as well as more aggressive chemotherapy for neoplasms, groups of immunosuppressed patients have been created.

The unfortunate consequence of these innovations of medical care has been an increased risk of infection. Invasive monitors and support devices, especially in ICUs, are easily contaminated and provide a portal of entry for pathogenic organisms. The advent of new antibiotics has been countered by the evolution of drug-resistant bacteria. A significant portion of HIV-infected, immunosuppressed persons have been coinfected with tuberculosis, reversing the trend of a decreasing incidence of this respiratory-transmitted disease in the population of the United States. Outbreaks of multidrug-resistant tuberculosis have occurred in healthcare settings affecting both patients and personnel. As physicians have developed more effective drugs and supportive technology, these more aggressive therapeutic modalities often have the undesirable effect of increasing vulnerability to infection.

Concomitant with the advances in anesthesia, surgery, and critical care, there has been an improved surveillance for and understanding of hospital-acquired (nosocomial) infections. Routine surveillance of nosocomial infection and investigation of outbreaks usually has been delegated to hospital epidemiologists and infection control practitioners. Specific recommendations have been derived from data collected through national and local surveys to improve infection control and reduce the risk of infection of hospitalized patients. National organizations such as the Centers for Disease Control and Prevention (CDC) have promulgated guidelines for preventing infections that have been incorporated into hospital policies for patient care. These measures have generally been effective in countering the increasing risk of nosocomial infections associated with the introduction of more complex and invasive clinical procedures.

Anesthesia personnel play a significant role in the treatment of patients in the perioperative period. Because many of the procedures they perform may be associated with significant infectious risk, practitioners must be aware of appropriate infection control techniques. Invasive devices inserted before or during anesthesia may remain in place for a significant interval. An understanding of the mechanisms of and risks for nosocomial infections are primary considerations for their prevention.

SURVEILLANCE OF NOSOCOMIAL INFECTIONS

Infections from microorganisms acquired during hospitalization are called nosocomial infections (1). Although most occur in patients, the term is also applied to personnel and others who develop infection as a result of organisms transmitted from hospitalized patients or the hospital environment. As patients travel around the hospital or are transferred among services or types of care units, surveillance for infection becomes more complex. Economic factors resulting in earlier patient discharge from the hospital have forced a greater reliance on information from referring physicians for detection of hospital-acquired infections.

The diagnosis of infection involves documentation of organisms in tissues of the patient by positive culture or other means along with the clinical findings of associated symptoms or pathology (2). The distinction between infection and colonization of microorganisms in the host may be difficult at times. Obtaining a positive culture by itself is not documentation of infection because colonization or growth of microorganisms in a patient may occur without tissue invasion or resulting pathology. Likewise, contamination of cultures may occur from organisms residing on the skin of the patient, personnel, or surface of equipment.

Nosocomial infections may be classified by the source of the causative organisms: **endogenous**, resulting from flora carried by the patient, or **exogenous**, organisms transmitted from a source outside the patient. Transmission of exogenous organisms may occur via several mechanisms. With contact spread of disease, organisms may be transferred directly by person-to-person contact, indirectly via contamination of a source or object that subsequently contacts the patient, or via droplets produced by sneezing or coughing, which may carry organisms through the air. Another mechanism involves a common vehicle such as a contaminated multidose vial from which aliquots are used on multiple patients. Organisms may be transmitted via airborne particles (droplet nuclei, dust particles, or exfoliated skin cells) that may float in room air for prolonged periods and travel significant distances. Finally, vectors such as mosquitoes may transfer organisms from various sources to patients, although vectorborne spread of nosocomial infections is rare in developed countries.

Successful transmission of an infectious pathogen requires several components. The first consideration is the microorganism which could be either a bacteria, virus, fungus or parasite. The virulence and invasiveness of the organism clearly affect the likelihood of disease. Sufficient numbers of the organism, an infective dose, must be transmitted to cause infection. This quantity will vary for the specific infection. Other factors such as antibiotic resistance will affect the likelihood of an organism's survival. The pathogens responsible for the infection must have a reservoir in which it can replicate and a vehicle for transmission to a vulnerable entrance portal in the host patient. The remaining factors are related to the host. Defense mechanisms such as natural immunity or artificial immunity from vaccination may thwart replication and invasion of organisms that had already been introduced. Other host pathology may also influence the ability of the organism to produce disease. The clinical spectrum of infection will vary as a result of both patient and organism factors.

Surveillance and Infection Control Programs

In the decade after World War II, clinicians recognized an increase in the number of hospitalized patients developing staphylococcal infections resistant to antibiotics. Infection control committees within hospitals attempted to control these infections by educating physicians and personnel on aseptic technique and tracking the incidence of new infections. After this, infection control programs were developed for surveillance and monitoring infections within hospitals. In 1970, the first International Conference on Nosocomial Infections was held by the CDC, and the need for infection control nurses was debated. The CDC instituted training courses for infection control nurses and the Association for Practitioners in Infection Control (APIC) was founded in 1972. Additionally, the National Nosocomial Infections Surveillance System (NNISS), a network of 70 hospitals, was established to gather information on the problem. A landmark study was begun by the CDC in 1974. The Study of the Efficacy of Nosocomial Infection Control (SENIC Project) was designed to determine whether infection surveillance programs had been adopted by United States hospitals and the effectiveness of this approach on reducing nosocomial infections (3–5). The results of the SENIC Project were based on data collected over 10 years (1974–1983). Hospital programs with organized surveillance and control activities (an infection control physician, an infection control nurse for each 250 beds, and a mechanism for informing surgeons of their infection rates) were able to reduce overall infection rates by 32% (3). For hospitals lacking these programs, surveillance from 1970 to 1976 demonstrated an increase in the overall infection rate of 18%.

The findings from surveillance activities permitted the CDC to publish a series of guidelines on infection control practices for hospitals (6–9). These guidelines addressed the major issues in each area of infection control and were used by hospitals to devise local policies. The CDC guidelines were based on both available information and published studies but also included recommendations based on theoretical rationale proposed by panels of experts. Because of their significance in improving the quality of patient care, oversight groups such as the Joint Commission on Accreditation of Healthcare Organizations (JCAHO) incorporated many recommendations from CDC guidelines into their review process.

Hospitals and other healthcare facilities should have an organized surveillance process for infection control. This should include mechanisms for routine monitoring of infection indicators, methods to collect appropriate data for routine surveillance and for identification of outbreaks, a committee for analyzing and interpreting data, and a system to provide information to practitioners for continuous quality improvement or to implement changes to correct deficiencies. The JCAHO standard in 1990 required hospitals to implement surveillance strategies to reduce the risk of nosocomial infections (10). Whereas previous standards had emphasized infection surveillance, the revision equally stressed prevention and control of infections. The JCAHO standards require (a) a hospital-wide program for surveillance, prevention, and control of infection; (b) a multidisciplinary committee to oversee the program; (c) qualified persons responsible for management of the infection control program; (d) written policies and procedures for all patient care areas; and (e) patient care support departments available to assist in prevention and control measures.

To facilitate large-scale disease prevention and control programs, clinicians and/or healthcare facilities are required to report specific infectious diseases to state health authorities (11). The specific diseases to be included vary by state. Additionally, federal legislation in 1970 established the Occupational Safety and Health Administration (OSHA) and the National Institute for Occupational Safety and Health (NIOSH). These agencies are to ensure a safe workplace and to set limits for exposures to hazardous substances (11, 12). Because of the risk of occupational transmission of bloodborne pathogens to healthcare workers who perform certain tasks, OSHA developed a standard to reduce personnel exposures (12).

THE ROLE OF ANESTHESIA PERSONNEL IN INFECTION

The role of the anesthesiologist in the prevention of infection in the perioperative period has been well delineated (13). In 1974, Walter identified multiple areas in which anesthesia personnel could be responsible for disseminating infectious agents and clearly described the occupational infectious hazards of the specialty. Unfortunately, some anesthesiologists have not paid as much attention to sterile technique as they should. An observational study demonstrated that in one hospital, anesthesiologists were more likely than surgical colleagues to violate aseptic techniques in the operating room (14).

Infection control surveillance should identify postsurgical patients who develop infections, but because of the many personnel caring for the patient during the perioperative period, the system may be unable to identify the source responsible for the transmission. Infection rates are usually categorized by the surgeon, and unless there is a large outbreak, the source may not be traced to other personnel.

THE ROLE OF INANIMATE OBJECTS IN INFECTION

The operating room and ICU contain many objects and surfaces that may be contaminated with potentially pathogenic organisms. Although this inanimate environment, including the exterior of the anesthesia machine, can under some circumstances be a source of organisms for transmission to patients or healthcare workers, there are few re-

ported outbreaks. For human pathogens to survive outside an organic environment, adaptations are required that make them less infectious (15). Du Moulin and Hedley-White have suggested that within the anesthesia machine and breathing circuit, changes in relative humidity, oxygen concentration, and exposure to metallic ions and plastics reduce bacteria viability (16). Similarly, operating room walls and floors and surfaces in ICUs have not been shown to serve as a fomite for environmental transmission of microorganisms (15).

In assessing studies linking patient infection to microorganisms found on inanimate objects in the environment, the strength of the conclusion must be judged by the study design. Rhame describes six types of evidence of increasing validity in establishing the role of a fomite in causing disease (15).

1. The weakest evidence is the demonstration that the organism in question can survive on the fomite. Although this is a requirement for transmission, it is only an initial consideration because the infectivity of the organism remains unknown and a mechanism for carrying the organism from the fomite to a portal of entry in the patient must be established.
2. Cultures taken from fomites in the environment yield pathogens. In a similar manner, antigens as markers of virus are sometimes used when an organism cannot be readily cultured. These findings by themselves do not indicate a cause of infection because they could result from contamination of the object from the infected individual.
3. The microbe can grow and remain viable on the fomite. Although this is important in increasing the size of the inoculum and would make infection more likely, the isolated finding does not prove the source of infection.
4. Not all cases of transmission can be assigned to recognized categories of known mechanisms of transmission. Based on this unaccounted portion, some investigators argue that transmission from fomites in the environment have occurred. Proof by exclusion is relatively weak, especially when no mechanism can be demonstrated.
5. Retrospective case-control studies demonstrate a positive relationship between exposure to a contaminated fomite and infection or disease.

The case control method is one of the basic techniques in analytic epidemiology.

6. Prospective or cohort studies demonstrate an association between exposure and infection.

Unfortunately, very few of the studies purported to show causes of infection have used case control or cohort methodology. Although transmission from inanimate objects is rare, airborne transmission does occur for *Mycobacterium tuberculosis*, Varicella-Zoster virus, influenza, and measles.

SURGICAL WOUND INFECTIONS

It has been estimated that nosocomial infections occur in more than 2 million patients annually in the United States with a total cost of more than $4.5 billion in 1992 (17). Surgical wound infection (SWI) is responsible for $1.6 billion of these extra hospital charges annually in the United States (17) (Table 12–1). Patient morbidity and mortality from SWI can be reduced by hospital surveillance, effective reporting, and proper infection control methods. In 1988, the CDC published definitions for diagnosing nosocomial infections that included criteria for SWI (2). Later, the definition of SWI was modified and the name was changed to surgical site infection (SSI) (18). According to the more recent classification, SSI are divided into incisional infections involving superficial (skin and subcutaneous) or deep (fascia and muscle layers) tissues or organ/space that were opened or manipulated during the operative procedure (18).

Because routine surveillance of postoperative patients and reporting the data to surgeons (5) has been effective in reducing rates of infections, hospital accrediting organizations have incorporated these requirements into their reviews (19, 20). To assist in the categorization of surgical procedures for reporting SWI, a classification system based on types of operations has been defined (21). This was later modified to include four classes of operations: clean, clean-contaminated, contaminated, and dirty (Table 12–2).

The incidence of SWI has decreased since 1960 for each of the classes of surgical procedures, but multiple surveys have shown that the rate for comparable patients increases progressively from clean to dirty operations (19, 22) (Table 12–3). Data from the SENIC Project was used to identify four risk factors for SWI, including abdominal surgery, duration of surgery greater than 2 hours, contaminated or dirty operation, and patients with three or more diagnoses at the time of discharge (23). Subsequent data collected from more than 84,600 operations between 1987 and 1990 was used to develop a risk index score that was significantly better for predicting SWI

Table 12–1. Esitmated Average Extra Days and Extra Charges per Infection and Deaths Attributed to Nosocomial Infections Annually in United States Hospitals

Type	Extra Days	Extra Charges[a] Average per Infection	Extra Charges[a] U.S. Total (billion)	Deaths Directly Caused by Infections Total	Deaths Directly Caused by Infections (%)	Deaths to which Infection Contributed Total	Deaths to which Infection Contributed (%)
Surgical wound infection	7.3	$3,152	$1.609	3,251	(0.6)	9,726	(1.9)
Pneumonia	5.9	$5,683	$1.29	7,087	(3.1)	22,983	(10.1)
Bacteremia	7.4	$3,517	$0.36	4,496	(4.4)	8,844	(8.6)
Urinary tract infection	1.0	$ 608	$0.62	947	(0.1)	6,503	(0.7)
Other site	4.8	$1,617	$0.66	3,246	(0.8)	10,036	(2.5)
All sites	4.0	$2,100	$4.53	19,027	(0.9)	58,092	(2.70)

[a] In 1992 dollars

Modified with permission from Martone WJ, Jarvis WR, Culver HR, et al. Incidence and nature of endemic and epidemic nosocomial infections. In: Bennett JV, Brachman PS, eds. Hospital infections. 3rd ed. Boston: Little, Brown & Company, 1992;593.

Table 12–2. Classification of Surgical Wounds

Clean:
Elective operations, not drained and primarily closed.

Clean–Contaminated:
Gastrointestinal or respiratory tract entered without significant spillage, entrance of genitourinary tract in the presence of infected urine, entrance of biliary tract in the presence of infected bile or minor break in technique.

Contaminated:
Major break in operative technique (e.g., surgical entrance of unprepared bowel without gross spillage of bowel contents); acute bacterial inflammation without pus; fresh, traumatic wound from a relatively clean source.

Dirty:
Presence of pus or perforated viscus (before operation), old traumatic wound, or traumatic wound from a dirty source.

Modified with permission from Ehrenkranz NJ, Meakins JL. Surgical infections. In: Bennett JV, Brachman PS, eds. Hospital infections. 3rd ed. Boston; Little, Brown & Company, 1992;689.

Table 12–3. Surgical Wound Infection Rates[a]

Risk Factor	SWI Rate[b]	Percentage of Operations
Wound class		
Clean	2.1	58
Clean-contaminated	3.3	36
Contaminated	6.4	4
Dirty-infected	7.1	2
ASA[c] Physical Status		
1	1.5	26
2	2.1	37
3	3.7	26
4	5.5	11
5	7.1	0.4
Risk Index Category		
0	1.5	47
1	2.9	41
2	6.8	11
3	13.0	1

[a] Data from 84,691 operations.
[b] Number of surgical wound infections (SWI) per 100 operations.
[c] ASA = American Society of Anesthesiologists.
Modified with permission from Culver DH, Horan TC, Gaynes RP, et al. Surgical wound infection rates by wound class, operative procedure, and patient risk index. Am J Med 1991;91(Suppl 3B):152S–157S.

(22). To calculate the risk index score that can range from 0 to 3, one point is assigned for each of the following risks factors: (*a*) American Society of Anesthesiologists Physical Status of 3, 4, or 5; (*b*) a contaminated or dirty operation; and (*c*) an operation lasting longer than the 75th percentile for the same operative procedure performed by all surgeons. The rate of SWI increased directly with higher scores (Table 12–3) and within each wound class relative to the other risk factors. Therefore, simple indicators can be used to predict the likelihood of postoperative SWI.

Factors Affecting Infection Rates

The likelihood of SWI is influenced by patient factors and intraoperative events. Conditions in the host that reduce tissue blood supply may contribute to SWI by decreasing tissue oxygenation and limiting white-cell activity. Examples include diabetes mellitus, obesity, malnutrition, and advanced age.

Some infections result from organisms carried by the patient at sites distant from the surgical incision. Hematogenous spread of bacteria may occur from respiratory or urinary tract infections (24). Bacterial colonization of the skin may be associated with dermatitis and can serve as a source of infection for the operative site. Patients carrying methicillin-resistant *Staphylococcus aureus* in their anterior nares on admission to a surgical intensive care unit were more likely to have a subsequent postoperative infection with this organism (25). Quantitative analysis suggests that an inoculum of at least 10^5 bacteria are usually required to introduce infection at a surgical site (26).

In a prospective study, intraoperative cultures taken from the surgical incision were not predictive of postoperative infection, although positive cultures were associated with an increased rate of infection (27). If patients received perioperative antibiotics and had a postoperative infection, the organism was likely resistant to the antibiotic that had been administered. Therefore, routine intraoperative wound cultures are not useful for identifying patients who will go on to develop SWI. From the NNISS survey, most SWI result from gram-positive cocci or gram-negative bacilli (Table 12–4).

Intraoperative events may also contribute to the likelihood of SWI. Factors within the operative site that may be associated with infection include a fluid collection (seroma or hematoma), choice of suture material, use of foreign bodies (prosthesis or surgical drain), or inadvertent contamination from an unprepared or infected body cavity. Bacteria carried on the skin, scalp, or other body surfaces may be transmitted through the air on desquamated particles to the surgical site (28). Numerous outbreaks of SWI have been traced to attendant personnel and surgeons inadvertently carrying pathogenic organisms. This would suggest that traffic of nonessential personnel in the operating room should be limited and that when specific personnel are identified as sources, antibiotics or treatment of the dermatitis may be indicated. Surgical masks are used to prevent airborne droplet transmission of bacteria from the nasopharynx during speaking, coughing, or sneezing. Hair, including beards, should be routinely covered with appropriate hats or hoods, and masks should be worn in the operating room to prevent dissemination of bacteria from personnel.

Prevention of SWI

In addition to addressing the factors noted above, other strategies can be used to reduce the incidence of surgical infections. Preoperative preparation of the operative site should be performed immediately before surgery rather than the night before as was a common practice. Hair should be removed by clipping rather than shaving to prevent skin cuts, which serve as a nidus for bacterial colonization.

Hand washing remains a primary strategy to prevent nosocomial infections, including SWI (29, 7). Although physicians in ICUs frequently fail to comply with hand-washing protocols, hand washing remains the single most important procedure for preventing nosocomial infections (30). Two populations of organisms reside on the skin: **resident** and **transient** microorganisms. The resident microorganisms routinely survive in the superficial skin layers with a small portion in the deeper epidermis. Hand washing with plain soaps may not remove all resident microorganisms, but they can be inactivated with antimicrobial agents. The resident microorganisms are usually not highly virulent, but they may cause infections in immunocompromised patients or those with prosthetic devices. In contrast, transient microorganisms represent recent contaminates on superficial skin layers that are often found on the hands of hospital personnel. The transient population of organisms are likely pathogens acquired from colonized or infected patients and are associated with nosocomial infections. The transient microbial flora is easily removed with hand washing.

Table 12–4. Microorganisms Responsible for Nosocomial Infections, National Nosocomial Infections Surveillance System, 1986–1989

Pathogen	Pneumonia[a] (%)	SWI[b] (%)	UTI[c] (%)	Bloodstream[d] (%)
Aerobic Bacteria				
Gram-Negative Bacilli	49	36	58	22
Pseudomanas aeruginosa	17	8	12	4
Enterobacter species	11	8	6	5
Klebsiella pneumoniae	7	3	6	4
Escherichia coli	6	10	26	6
Serratia marcescens	4	1	1	1
Proteus mirabilis	3	4	5	1
Citrobacter species	1	2	2	1
Gram-Positive Cocci	21	45	22	55
Staphylococcus aureus	16	17	2	16
Coagulase-negative staphylococci	2	12	4	27
Streptococcus species	1	3	0	4
Enterococcus species	2	13	16	8
Fungi	5	2	9	8
Candida albicans	4	2	7	5
Candida species	1	0	2	3

[a] 11,510 isolates.
[b] SWI, surgical wound infection: 16,727 isolates.
[c] UTI, urinary tract infection: 37,971 isolates.
[d] 10,590 isolates.
Modified with permission from Schaberg DR, Culver DH, Gaynes RP. Major trends in the microbial etiology of nosocomial infection. Am J Med 1991;(Suppl 3B):72S–75S.

Although many antiseptic solutions are effective, the use of chlorhexidine reduced the rate of nosocomial infections more effectively than a protocol using alcohol and soap, probably as a result of better compliance by personnel (31). The CDC has published recommendations on indications for hand washing (Table 12–5). Hand-washing facilities should be conveniently located throughout the hospital, within or near each patient room, and in rooms where diagnostic or invasive procedures are performed (7).

Use of preoperative antibiotic prophylaxis is now an established method for preventing SWI in patients undergoing clean or clean-contaminated operations (32, 33). Because of

Table 12–5. Hand-Washing Indications and Techniques

1. In the absence of a true emergency, personnel should always wash their hands:

   - **Before** performing invasive procedures;
   - **Before** taking care of particularly susceptible patients, such as immunocompromised and newborn patients;
   - **Before and after** touching wounds, whether surgical, traumatic, or associated with an invasive device;
   - **After** regular situations during which microbial contamination of hands is likely to occur, especially those involving contact with mucous membranes, blood or body fluids, secretions, or excretions;
   - **After** touching inanimate objects that are likely to be contaminated with virulent or epidemiologically important microorganisms, including urine, measuring devices, or a secretion-collection apparatus;
   - **After** taking care of an infected patient or one who is likely to be colonized with microorganisms of special clinical or epidemiologic significance, for example, multiple-resistant bacteria;
   - **Between** contacts with different patients in high-risk units.

2. For routine hand washing, a vigorous rubbing together of all surfaces of lathered hands for at least 10 seconds, followed by thorough rinsing under a stream of water, is recommended.

Reproduced from Garner JS, Favero MS. CDC guidelines for the prevention and control of nosocomial infections. Guideline for handwashing and hospital environmental control, 1985. Am J Infect Control 1986;14:114–115.

the significant cost and morbidity associated with postoperative SWI, use of prophylactic antibiotics is extremely cost effective. For most surgical procedures, cefazolin, or vancomycin for penicillin-allergic patients, is the most commonly indicated antibiotic, although references should be consulted for specific procedures and current recommendations (34). The timing of the administration of prophylactic antibiotics is critical. Administration within 2 hours of incision reduces the risk of SWI, whereas effectiveness is reduced when they are given at later times (35). Subsequent doses of antibiotics are sometimes used, especially for patients with contaminated or dirty operations or when prosthetic devices are implanted.

The CDC SENIC study documented the effectiveness of surveillance programs for reduction of nosocomial infections, including SWI. The data collected by hospital infection control programs permit calculation of wound infection rates for reporting confidentially to surgeons. Several groups have recommended that, in addition, SWI rates should be stratified based on measures of patient susceptibility to infection using recognized risk factors (20). When specific surgeons with a greater incidence of SWI are identified, there should be an evaluation of their surgical techniques and judgment, along with other extrinsic factors that may contribute to the problem.

POSTOPERATIVE NOSOCOMIAL PNEUMONIA

Hospital-acquired pneumonia is a significant cause of patient morbidity and mortality (Table 12–1). Surveillance data from the NNISS indicate that pneumonia is responsible for approximately 20% of all nosocomial infections and is the second most common cause of nosocomial infection after the urinary tract (36). This survey reported the incidence of nosocomial pneumonia at 6 per 1000 discharged patients with a greater rate in university-affiliated than in nonteaching hospitals.

Nosocomial pneumonia is a particular risk for postoperative patients. Data from SENIC demonstrated that 75% of cases of nosocomial bacterial pneumonia occurred in postoperative patients (4). Several more recent studies have pointed out specific risk factors for developing nosocomial pneumonias, including endotracheal intubation and/or mechanically assisted ventilation, depressed level of consciousness, prior aspiration of gastric contents, chronic lung disease, age older than 70 years, 24-hour ventilator circuit changes, fall/winter season, stress-ulcer bleeding prophylaxis with cimetidine with or without antacid, administration of antimicrobials, presence of a nasal gastric tube, severe trauma, and recent bronchoscopy (37–39). In a prospective study, 17.5% of 520 patients undergoing elective thoracic, upper abdominal, or lower abdominal surgeries developed pneumonia (40). Factors correlating with postoperative pneumonia included higher American Society of Anesthesiologists (ASA) physical status classification, low serum albumin concentration, history of smoking, longer preoperative hospital stay, longer operative procedure, and thoracic or upper abdominal surgery.

Prolonged mechanical ventilation in critically ill patients is associated with lower respiratory tract infections. The incidence in one study increased from 5% in patients ventilated for 1 day to 69% in patients ventilated for more than 30 days (41). Analysis of this patient population suggested that the greatest risk of infection occurred in the first 8 to 10 days of ventilatory support. The underlying medical condition and patient population seem to be important factors. The incidence of ventilator-associated pneumonia varies from a median rate per 1000 ventilator-days of 4.7 in pediatric intensive care units to 34 in burn units (42).

Analysis of patients requiring mechanical ventilation in a medical, surgical, or cardiothoracic ICU identified four factors associated with pneumonia: failure of three or more organ systems, patient age older than 60 years, prior administration of antibiotics, and supine head position during the first day (43). Pneumonia occurred more frequently in cardiothoracic patients (22%) compared to medical patients (9%) and mortality was greater in patients who had ventilator-associated pneumonia (37% versus 9%).

Nosocomial pneumonia prolongs hospitalization by approximately 6 days; the estimated total cost of the extra hospital stay in the United States amounts to more than $1.2 billion annually (Table 12–1). Assessment of causes of death in 200 consecutive patients at university and community hospitals demonstrated that when a nosocomial infection contributed to the death, nosocomial pneumonia was the most frequent cause occurring in 60% (44). The mortality rate for ventilator-associated pneumonia was 55% in another prospective series (45).

Clinical Features and Diagnosis

The diagnosis of pneumonia involves clinical, radiographic, and laboratory evidence of infection (Table 12–6). In the presence of a positive sputum culture, it is sometimes difficult to differentiate tracheobronchial bacterial colonization from pneumonia. Additionally, noninfectious processes such as atelectasis or pulmonary edema can produce infiltrates on the chest x-rays of postoperative or critically ill patients.

Sputum culture may be unreliable for documentation of causative organisms. Investigators have used more invasive techniques such as transtracheal aspirate, protected specimen brush catheter, or bronchoalveolar lavage to obtain specimens for diagnosis (38, 39). In patients ventilated via an endotracheal tube, sampling via a protected blind brush has been shown to be useful for diagnosing nosocomial pneumonia (46).

The gram-negative bacilli are the most common organisms isolated in nosocomial pneumonia, although concurrent infection with several organisms is not unusual (Table 12–4). Gram-positive organisms are less frequent. Other causes are fungi and occasionally *Legionella pneumophilia*.

Pathogenesis

Although microorganisms may enter the lower respiratory tract by inhalation of contaminated, aerosolized particles or may be spread via the bloodstream from distant sites of infection, the most frequent etiology is from aspiration of organisms colonizing the oropharynx and/or upper gastrointestinal tract (Fig. 12–1). Johanson et al. demonstrated that healthy individuals had a low prevalence of gram-negative bacilli in the oropharyngeal flora, but with severe illness, the prevalence increased markedly (47). The group then demonstrated that only 3% of uncolonized patients developed nosocomial pneumonia and that 85% of patients with pneumonia were colonized with gram-negative rods (48).

Multiple factors are associated with changing of flora in the oropharynx from gram-positive cocci to gram-negative bacilli. Use of antibiotics before surgery may eliminate some types of streptococci that inhibit growth of gram-negative rods. Other medical conditions such as diabetes mellitus or alcoholism are associated with a higher prevalence of gram-negative colonization.

Changes in mucosal surfaces during severe illness create a more favorable environment in which gram-negative bacilli can more easily adhere to oral epithelial cells. When fibronectin, a glycoprotein that is normally present on oral epithelial cells, is intact, gram-positive bacteria more easily adhere to oral epithelial cells. With severe stress, fibronectin is inactivated by elastase, probably from polymorphonuclear leukocytes, which permits gram-negative organisms to bind to epithelial cells and begin colonization (49, 50).

Another major factor contributing to lower respiratory tract infection is the colonization of the stomach when gastric pH is altered. The low, acid pH of the stomach is bactericidal and limits growth of microorganisms. As the acid environment is altered, the concentration of aerobic gram-negative bacilli in the stomach increases proportionately to gastric pH

Table 12–6.   CDC Definition of Nosocomial Pneumonia

Pneumonia must meet one of the following criteria:

1. Rales or dullness to percussion on physical examination of chest **AND** any of the following:
   a. New onset of purulent sputum or change in character of sputum.
   b. Organism isolated from blood culture.
   c. Isolation of pathogen from specimen obtained by transtracheal aspirate, bronchial brushing, or biopsy.

2. Chest radiographic examination shows new or progressive infiltrate, consolidation, cavitation, or pleural effusion **AND** any of the following:
   a. New onset of purulent sputum or change in character of sputum.
   b. Organism isolated from blood culture.
   c. Isolation of pathogen from specimen obtained by transtracheal aspirate, bronchial brushing, or biopsy.
   d. Isolation of virus or detection of viral antigen in respiratory secretions.
   e. Diagnostic single antibody titer (IgM) or fourfold increase in paired serum samples (IgG) for pathogen.
   f. Histopathologic evidence of pneumonia.

3. Patient 12 months of age or younger has two of the following: apnea, tachypnea, bradycardia, wheezing, rhonchi, or cough **AND** any of the following:
   a. Increased production of respiratory secretions.
   b. New onset of purulent sputum or change in character of sputum.
   c. Organism isolated from blood culture.
   d. Isolation of pathogen from specimen obtained by transtracheal aspirate, bronchial brushing, or biopsy.
   e. Isolation of virus or detection of viral antigen in respiratory secretions.
   f. Diagnostic single antibody titer (IgM) or fourfold increase in paired serum samples (IgG) for pathogen.
   g. Histopathologic evidence of pneumonia.

4. Patient 12 months of age or younger has chest radiologic examination that shows new or progressive infiltrate, cavitation, consolidation, or pleural effusion **AND** any of the following:
   a. Increased production of respiratory secretions.
   b. New onset of purulent sputum or change in character of sputum.
   c. Organism isolated from blood culture.
   d. Isolation of pathogen from specimen obtained by transtracheal aspirate, bronchial brushing, or biopsy.
   e. Isolation of virus or detection of viral antigen in respiratory secretions.
   f. Diagnostic single antibody titer (IgM) or fourfold increase in paired serum samples (IgG) for pathogen.
   g. Histopathologic evidence of pneumonia.

Reproduced with permission from Garner JS, Jarvis WR, Emori TG, et al. CDC definitions for nosocomial infections, 1988. Am J Infect Control 1988;16:131.

(51). When H_2 blockers and antacids are used in critically ill patients to prevent stress-ulcer bleeding, gastric colonization is likely and increases the risk of nosocomial pneumonia (52). In a prospective, randomized study of 130 patients requiring mechanical ventilation, the rate of pneumonia was twice as high in patients receiving antacids and H_2 blockers (23%) compared to those receiving sucralfate (12%) (52). Although not quite statistically significant, the mortality rate was 1.6 times higher in the group treated with antacid and H_2 blockers.

Sucralfate forms a viscous gel at low pH in the stomach. The gel seems to prevent gastric ulceration by adhering to cells and absorbing bile acids and pepsin. Use of sucralfate in critically ill patients to prevent gastrointestinal hemorrhage seems to be effective and is less likely to result in gastric colonization (52, 53). Tryba demonstrated that only 10% of patients treated with sucralfate developed nosocomial pneumonia compared to 34% of those treated with antacids (54). Additional work suggests that sucralfate also has antibacterial activity (55).

Short-term use of an H_2-receptor antagonist before cardiac surgery to prevent acid aspiration syndrome significantly increased intraoperative gastric pH (56). Samples of gastric

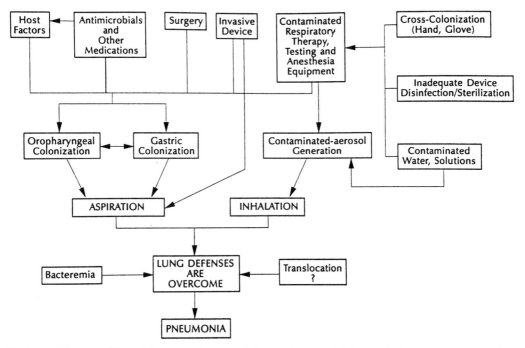

Fig. 12–1. Nosocomial bacterial pneumonia can result from aspiration or inhalation of microorganisms. (Reproduced with permission from Tablan OC, Anderson LJ, Arden NH, et al. Guideline for prevention of nosocomial pneumonia. Part I. Issues on prevention of nosocomial pneumonia — 1994. Am J Infect Control 1994;22:250.)

contents taken during surgery were sterile in 92% of control patients and in only 25% of those receiving H₂ blockers. No control patients developed postoperative pneumonia, but there was a trend toward greater prevalence in those receiving prophylactic H₂ antagonists.

Lower respiratory tract infection may follow aspiration of microorganisms in secretions originating from the colonized oropharynx or upper gastrointestinal tract. Concordance of organisms from the trachea and stomach were demonstrated in a study by duMoulin et al. (51). In sequential cultures, the infecting organism first appeared in the gastric contents before tracheal sampling. Aspiration, the predominate cause of nosocomial pneumonia, is more likely in patients with depressed consciousness, patients with endotracheal or nasogastric tubes, or patients who have recently undergone surgery (Fig. 12–1) (57).

Because of both the underlying illness and the presence of an endotracheal or tracheos-

tomy tube, patients requiring mechanical ventilation have a 6 to 21 times greater risk of nosocomial pneumonia (4, 58, 59). Leakage of bacteria-laden secretions around the cuff of the endotracheal tube permits direct contamination of the lower respiratory tract (60, 61). Hourly aspiration of subglottic secretions via a specially designed endotracheal tube lumen constructed with the distal aperture above the cuff resulted in a lower incidence and prolonged time of onset of nosocomial pneumonia (61). The hourly suctioning required with the device is quite labor intensive, and the cost/benefit associated with the use of the new endotracheal tube design requires further evaluation.

The presence of an endotracheal tube contributes to lower respiratory tract infections via a second mechanism. Bacteria adhering to the tube produce a biofilm or glycocalyx that protects the microorganisms from antibacterial agents and host defenses (62, 63). Translocation of the bacteria-containing matrix during tracheal suctioning or movement of the endotracheal tube may serve to inoculate the lower respiratory tract.

The presence of an orogastric or nasogastric tube increases the colonization of the pharynx by facilitating migration of bacteria from the stomach. The use of enteral feedings via tubes produces an elevated gastric pH, permitting gastric colonization with gram-negative bacilli (64). Increased gastric volumes after feeding may also contribute to gastric reflux. When enteral feeding via nasogastric tube is required, placing the patient in a head-up position, use of small volumes, and frequent assessment for large residual gastric volumes should be considered (65).

Preventive Measures

Certain groups of patients can be identified as having a greater risk for postoperative pneumonia and might benefit from special care. Patients undergoing neurosurgical, ear, nose, and throat (ENT), thoracic, or upper abdominal procedures are prone to impairment of swallowing or inability to cough effectively. Narcotics and sedatives may further impair consciousness and clearance of pulmonary secretions. Use of incentive spirometry may be effective in cooperative patients (66). Improved pain control techniques such as patient-controlled analgesia and regional or epidural analgesia may facilitate coughing, deep breathing, and incentive spirometry to reduce pulmonary complications (67, 68).

SELECTIVE DECONTAMINATION OF THE DIGESTIVE TRACT

In an attempt to reduce the mortality from *Pseudomonas aeruginosa* pneumonia in patients in the respiratory-surgical ICU, investigators aerosolized polymyxin B into the oropharynx and endotracheal tubes (69). Compared to a group of historical controls, there was an increased mortality rate due to nosocomial pneumonia resulting from polymyxin-resistant organisms. Although the results of these interventional studies were disappointing, it led other investigators to consider other prophylactic therapies.

Stoutenbeek believed that selective decontamination of the digestive tract (SDD) would eliminate bacterial colonization of the oropharynx and stomach and thereby prevent nosocomial lower respiratory tract infections (70). A mixture of tobramycin, polymyxin E, and amphotericin B was applied to the oral mucosa as a paste and administered by nasogastric tube to the stomach. Compared to historical controls, the treatment resulted in a reduction in oropharyngeal colonization and a concomitant reduction in the incidence of nosocomial pneumonia.

Multiple studies of various patient populations in the ICU have assessed the efficacy of SDD. Protocols have used a variety of combinations of nonabsorbable antibiotics, including polymyxin, tobramycin, gentamicin, neomycin, norfloxacin, ciprofloxacin, amphotericin B, and nystatin. In most studies, the antibiotic combination was applied to the oropharynx as a paste and administered via nasogastric tube four times per day. For some patients, intravenous antibiotics were also administered. Most of these clinical trials have demonstrated a decrease in the rate of nosocomial pneumonia (71–74), but in some, the overall mortality rate was not different from controls. Kerver used tobramycin, amphotericin B, and polymyxin E along with parenteral antibiotics in a prospective, randomized study (71). There was a decrease in gram-negative rod colonization in the SDD patients, along with a reduction in pneumonia (85% versus 15%). Ulrich et al. used oropharyngeal and gastrointestinal polymyxin E, norfloxacin, and amphotericin B combined with systemic trimethoprim (72). This therapy reduced mortality from nosocomial sepsis (15 to 0%) and overall mortality rate (54 to 31%).

Other investigators have failed to confirm the favorable effects of SDD. A multicenter study of 445 mechanically ventilated patients compared a placebo to topical antibiotics (tobramycin, colistin sulfate, and amphotericin

B) (75). Although pneumonia caused by gram-negative bacilli was less frequent in the patients treated with SDD, survival was not improved and the total charges for antibiotics were 2.2 times greater. The results of a meta-analysis questioned the effect of SDD on mortality and the increased expenses associated with the treatment (76).

With the use of nonabsorbable antibiotics, the risk of resistant organisms must be considered. Gorman et al. have shown that endotracheal tubes used for patients who received SDD had biofilms with a higher prevalence of colonization with yeast and gram-positive bacteria (77). The antibiotics did not inhibit biofilm formation on endotracheal tubes, a possible nidus for infection. Based on the available evidence, the routine use of SDD for all ICU patients cannot be recommended, although further studies may indicate that it is effective for some patients for prevention of nosocomial pneumonia.

Device-Mediated Infection

Contaminated devices used in connection with the respiratory tract can serve as a source of infection (Fig. 12–1). Outbreaks of infection associated with respiratory therapy devices, anesthesia machines, pulmonary function equipment, or endoscopes usually have been related to inadequate disinfection procedures or breaks in sterile technique. The CDC has published recommendations for prevention of nosocomial pneumonia (78).

Multiple reports clearly indicate that the anesthesia machine and respiratory therapy equipment can act as a source of microorganisms that can be transmitted directly to the lower respiratory tract or via the hands of personnel to other patients or equipment. Bacterial typing was used to prove that a contaminated anesthesia machine was responsible for an outbreak of P. aeruginosa in patients undergoing cardiac surgery (79). Outbreaks have occurred with contaminated respiratory monitoring devices (80), bronchoscopes (81), mechanical ventilator circuits (82), resuscitation bags (83), and humidifiers and nebulizers in mechanical ventilator circuits (84). In these outbreaks, implementation of appropriate disinfection and sterilization procedures terminated the problems.

STERILIZATION AND DISINFECTION OF EQUIPMENT

Spaulding proposed a classification system for sterilization or disinfection of medical devices based on the intended use (85). **Critical items** enter tissues, body cavities, or the intravascular space. **Semicritical items** directly or indirectly contact only mucous membranes and do not penetrate body surfaces. **Noncritical items** contact only intact skin or do not come into contact with patients. Based on this classification, critical items (i.e., intravascular catheters, spinal needles, or epidural catheters and needles) are purchased sterile or, if reusable, require sterilization (86–88). Semicritical items (Table 12–7) should be sterile or require high-level disinfection (78). Noncritical devices (i.e., surface of anesthesia machine, blood pressure cuff, electrocardiogram [ECG] cable) can be sanitized with a low-level disinfectant or cleaned with soap and water.

Sterilization is a procedure that kills all microorganisms, including bacterial spores. Several processes can be used to sterilize medical devices, including heat, ethylene oxide, and various liquid germicides (87, 89). To achieve a level of sterilization (the probability of an organism surviving is less than 10^{-6}), a long period of contact with cold liquid germicides is usually needed. The specific modality used for sterilization depends on the recommendation of the manufacturer and the material content of the item.

High-level disinfection kills vegetative bacteria, including the tubercle bacillus, some spores, fungi, and viruses. Chemical germicides are regulated by the U.S. Environmental Protection Agency for efficacy, and the conditions necessary for the desired level of disinfection should be followed. Before any disinfection procedure, the item should be scrubbed to mechanically remove all organic material

Table 12–7.   Semicritical Devices Used on the Respiratory Tract

1. Portions of the anesthesia machine, including:
   Inspiratory and expiratory limbs of the circle system
   Y-piece
   Reservoir bag
   Right angle connector
   Humidifier
2. Endotracheal tubes
3. Bronchoscopes
4. Laryngoscope blades
5. Oral and nasal airways
6. Face masks
7. Monitors that are located in the inspiratory or expiratory limb of the breathing circuit, including CO_2 analyzers, air-pressure monitors, and oxygen analyzers
8. Stylets
9. Suction catheters
10. Temperature probes
11. Esophageal stethoscopes
12. Breathing circuits of mechanical ventilators

From the Centers for Disease Control and Prevention. The Hospital Infection Control Practices Advisory Committee. Guideline for prevention of nosocomial pneumonia. Part II. Recommendations for prevention of nosocomial pneumonia. Am J Infect Control 1994;22:267–292; Favero MS. Principles of sterilization and disinfection. Anesth Clin North Am 1989;7:941–949; and American Society of Anesthesiologists. Prevention of nosocomial infections in patients. In: Recommendations for infection control for the practice of anesthesiology. Park Ridge, IL: Society of Anesthesiologists, 1991;1–16.

to permit the active agents to reach the item's surface.

ANESTHESIA EQUIPMENT

The anesthesia machine and circle breathing system seem to differ from other types of respiratory therapy equipment in that usually they are not reservoirs for pathogens (86, 90). There is no evidence that the internal components of the anesthesia machine, the high-pressure gas source, flow meter, vaporizer, or fresh gas tubing, are sources of infection, and these items do not require disinfection (78, 88). Portions of the breathing system that may become contaminated with microorganisms arising from the patient's oropharynx or lower respiratory tract require high-level disinfection between patients or use of single-use, disposable items with each patient. Although many studies have demonstrated the ability of microorganisms to survive in the inspiratory or expiratory valves and carbon dioxide absorber of circle breathing systems, there is no evidence to suggest that these devices have been associated with patient infections, even with use of low fresh gas flows (91, 92). This may be caused by the bactericidal nature of the changing conditions within the anesthetic circuit (16). Therefore, the carbon dioxide absorber and one-way valves of the circle breathing system require only periodic disinfection (78, 88). Monitoring devices inserted in the inspiratory or expiratory breathing tube, y-piece, or distal connectors should be single-patient-use items or receive high-level disinfection between patients (78, 93). In a prospective, randomized study, use of a sterile anesthesia breathing circuit was not associated with a difference in rate of postoperative pulmonary infection (94).

Because dry anesthetic gases have been found to damage the ciliated tracheobronchial epithelium, recommendations have been made for the use of humidification devices in anesthesia circuits (95). Some clinicians have used heated humidifiers in the inspiratory limb. Sterile, not distilled, water should be used to fill humidifiers. The warming devices should be changed with each patient because contamination can occur when liquid containing microorganisms drains from the patient end of the breathing circuit to the fluid reservoir (78). When condensate forms in the breathing circuit with the use of humidifiers or during long cases with low fresh gas flows, the condensate should be drained away from the patient and emptied from the circuit (78). Personnel performing these procedures should wash their hands as soon as possible to prevent transmission of organisms acquired from the interior of the breathing circuit.

Others have recommended the use of heat-moisture exchangers (HMEs) to provide humidification (96). Many HMEs now include a bacterial filter that can be used to isolate the breathing circuit from the patient when placed directly on the endotracheal tube or at the y-piece (96). Controversy exists regarding the routine use of filters in anesthesia circuits. Although laboratory simulations demonstrate the effectiveness of filters in preventing bacterial spread from simulated patients to the anesthesia circuit (97, 98), other investigators have questioned the need for bacteria filters for reducing patient infection when standard infection control procedures are used (99, 100). In clinical use, bacterial filters placed between the patient and the y-piece effectively reduced bacterial contamination of the circle system during a low-flow technique, but even when no filter was used, there was no growth of organisms in the carbon dioxide absorber, inspiratory tubing, or ventilator circuit (101). A large prospective study of patients undergoing elective thoracic or abdominal surgery demonstrated that use of filters did not affect the rate of postoperative pneumonia (16.7% with use of filters versus 18.3% without) (102). Because there have been no clinical studies demonstrating the need for routine use of bacterial filters in anesthesia circuits, and because complications such as pneumothorax may occur when gas flow is impeded by a filter blocked with secretions (103), the CDC has made no recommendation for their routine use (78). A bacterial filter is recommended for use on the endotracheal tube or expiratory limb of the anesthesia breathing circuit on patients with confirmed or suspected tuberculosis (104).

Between cases, the external horizontal surfaces of the anesthesia machine and equipment contaminated with blood should be cleaned by wiping with a disinfectant (86, 88). Although these surfaces have not been shown to be a source of patient infection, frequently they have found to be contaminated with blood (105).

MECHANICAL VENTILATORS USED IN THE ICU

The role of mechanical ventilators in pulmonary infections has been well studied. There is little evidence to suggest that the internal portions of mechanical ventilators are significant sources of bacterial contamination. Therefore, routine sterilization or high-level disinfection of these components is not required (78). Ventilator circuits are rapidly contaminated by microorganisms from the patient, especially when water from humidifiers condenses in the tubing. Craven demonstrated that within 2 hours after a circuit change, 33% were colonized; at 24 hours, 80% were colonized (82). Based on these findings, they suggested that the condensate be emptied regularly and handled as infectious waste. By serially culturing portions of the ventilator circuit, it was shown that in chronically ventilated patients, contamination occurs initially in the endotracheal tube, followed by the expiratory and then inspiratory breathing tube, again suggesting that the patient is the usual source of contamination (106). Based on a study showing that colonization of mechanical ventilator tubing did not increase between 24 and 48 hours, (107) it was recommended that routine changing of the breathing circuit should occur no more frequently than every 48 hours (78). Breathing circuits and humidifiers should undergo high-level disinfection between uses on patients.

More recent work has shown that the incidence of pneumonia was not increased when the ventilator circuit was used for the entire duration of ventilation for a single patient (108). Another approach assessed the use of an HME bacterial filter between the patient's endotracheal tube and the mechanical ventilator circuit. Cultures taken from the breathing tubing demonstrated that the filter prevented contamination by patient flora and that the circuit could be used for the duration of ventilation for the patient (109). Although there is evidence that alternative methods might permit longer use of mechanical ventilator circuits, current CDC recommendations call for changes no more frequently than every 48 hours (78).

OTHER DEVICES USED ON THE RESPIRATORY TRACT

Because suction catheters are introduced into the lower respiratory tract via endotracheal tubes, these devices should be sterile or receive high-level disinfection (78). Closed, multiuse catheter systems are available, but the limited studies suggest that the rate of patient infection is not reduced with their use (110, 111).

Sterile, not distilled water, should be used for filling humidifiers in respiratory therapy devices (78). *Legionella pneumophila* may be found in water in the hospital environment and is a pathogen associated with hospital-acquired pneumonia (112). Airborne patient-to-patient transmission of *Legionella* has not been documented. Hospital-acquired infections have been traced to contaminated cooling towers or sources of potable water. Hyperchlorination is usually successful in eliminating the organism from water sources (113). When laboratory-confirmed, definite nosocomial Legionnaires" disease is detected, investigations should be undertaken to determine the source of the organism within the hospital's water systems.

Fiberoptic laryngoscopes or bronchoscopes are used to facilitate endotracheal intubation or for diagnostic or therapeutic procedures in critically ill patients. Because endoscopes are constructed with numerous lumens for suctioning or sampling, effective disinfection requires extreme care. High-level disinfection or sterilization is recommended to prevent transmission of bloodborne pathogens, *M. tuberculosis*, or bacteria between patients (78, 114). Sequestered organic material within the working channels poses the greatest risk of cross-contamination, and these lumens must be physically cleaned with brushes and thorough rinsing before disinfection or sterilization. Disinfectants must be compatible with the endoscope material, and some examples that may be appropriate include glutaraldehyde, hydrogen peroxide, and peracetic acid (114). Manufacturers' recommendations should be consulted for compatibility with the individual product and published guidelines for infection control of these devices should be reviewed by personnel caring for these instruments (78, 114). Surveys of healthcare facilities suggest that these procedures are not optimally carried out at some institutions (115).

SINGLE-PATIENT-USE ITEMS

Because of concerns relating to the cost and disposal of single-use devices, some institutions or practices have decided to reuse disposables on more than one patient (116). If an institution decides to reuse devices intended and labeled by the manufacturer to be single-patient-use only (disposable), adequate sterilization or disinfection procedures must be performed between patients and a program should be set up to ensure proper handling (117). Written protocols should be developed to ensure that the devices are safe for reuse, without risk of infection or compromise of the structural integrity of the material. (88) The cost-effectiveness of reusing disposable medical devices requires further study because the cost of the disinfection, handling, and quality assurance programs may not be warranted.

URINARY TRACT INFECTIONS

Urinary tract infections (UTIs) are the most common nosocomial infections, accounting for 40% of hospital-acquired infections (118). The source of most urinary tract infections is microorganisms residing on the patient, but epidemic outbreaks have also been traced to organisms transmitted from contaminated items carried on the hands of personnel (119). Although the proportion of nosocomial infections caused by the urinary tract have remained fairly constant during the past several decades, there may be an increase in UTIs caused by *Candida* species.

The importance of nosocomial UTI as a cause of hospital mortality is pointed out in a study by Platt et al. (120). The investigators prospectively studied 1458 patients with indwelling bladder catheters and noted a three-fold increase in mortality in patients with UTI. The authors noted that the reason for this association was unclear. This study and others (121) suggest that gram-negative rod bacteriuria may be associated with unrecognized bacteremia. Up to 4% of patients having a UTI develop bacteremia, and catheter-associated UTI remains the most likely source of gram-negative bacteremia in hospitalized patients (122).

Most UTIs are produced by gram-negative bacilli (80%), whereas gram-positive cocci, predominately *Enterococcus* and *Staphylococcus*, account for the largest portion of the remainder. Candida infections account for less than 10%.

Mechanisms of Infection

There are several well-known risk factors associated with higher rates of UTI during bladder catheterization (Table 12–8). Microorganisms can enter the urinary tract via two mechanisms in the catheterized patient: through the lumen of the bladder catheter or from the urethra around the catheter. Cultures taken from the urinary tract, catheter, periurethral area, and rectum demonstrated

Table 12–8. Risk Factors Associated with Urinary Tract Infection during Bladder Catheterization

Alterable Factors

  Indications for catheterization
  Length of catheterization
  Catheter care techniques
  Type of drainage system
  Receipt of antimicrobials

Unalterable Factors

  Female gender
  Older age
  Severe underlying illness
  Meatal colonization

Modified with permission from Stamm WE. Nosocomial urinary tract infections. In: Bennett JV, Brachman PS, eds. Hospital infections. 3rd ed. Boston: Little Brown & Company, 1992;598.

that in women, approximately 70% of UTIs are produced by fecal bacteria that enter via the urethra (123, 124). Alternatively, in men, infection of the urinary tract is most commonly caused by catheter or drainage system contamination and infection via the intraluminal route. Contamination of the contents of the urinary drainage bag is likely to result in UTI with the same organism within 48 hours. A small inoculum of bacteria reaching the bladder will quickly proliferate to significant numbers within 24 hours in patients not using antimicrobials.

ROLE OF BIOFILMS

In addition to populations of bacteria that proliferate in the urine, some organisms are capable of growing in a biofilm on the luminal surface of the catheter (125). Species of *Proteus* and *Pseudomonas* most commonly produce a biofilm, which can lead to encrustation on the catheter's inner surface. There are several implications of biofilm formation. The organisms producing the encrustation are more difficult to eradicate with antimicrobial agents, because they may be protected from contact with the urine. This would suggest that indwelling catheters should be changed in the presence of UTI to facilitate treatment. Additionally, urine cultures taken from a catheter may demonstrate organisms that were contained in the biofilm instead of representing bladder bacteriuria.

Prevention

Although local application of antimicrobials to the female periurethral area was not effective in preventing UTIs, other modalities may be more successful. Schaeffer et al. used a silver oxide coating on the urethral catheter and catheter adapter and placed trichloroisocyanuric acid in the urinary drainage bag to reduce the risk of bacteriuria in a prospective, randomized study (126). The incidence of infection was decreased (55% versus 27%), and the median time to bacteriuria was increased

(8 days versus 36 days) in the study group. Although others have not found such widespread improvement in UTI infection rates with antimicrobial impregnated catheters, the approach seems promising.

Because bacteria may spread from the urinary collection bag through the drainage system, disinfection of the bag with antimicrobial agents has been tried. Although addition of disinfectants to the urine collection bag sterilizes its contents, the use of this practice is limited because the other routes for bacterial entry are responsible for most UTIs. In one study, only 7% of patients with bacteriuria were infected with the same organism found in the urinary drainage system (127). For patients on systemic antimicrobials excreted in the urine, addition of germicides to the urinary drainage system is clearly unwarranted. Use of prophylactic systemic antimicrobials decreases the incidence of UTI in catheterized patients, but concern regarding the development of resistant organisms has limited its use (128).

In a prospective study of SDD and systemic trimethoprim, the incidence of gram-negative UTIs was reduced from 27% to 4% (72). Although SDD was originally suggested to prevent pneumonia, the efficacy of SDD for patients at high risk for nosocomial UTI should be investigated.

Breaks in the integrity of the urinary drainage system permit entry of bacteria. Sealed connections between the catheter, drainage tubing, and connection bag reduce the risk of UTI (129). Education of personnel seems to be warranted because disconnections of the urinary drainage system have been identified as a risk factor for UTI.

Chronic Catheterization

The incidence of bacteriuria is approximately 6% per day throughout the period of catheterization, and the likelihood of infection is directly related to the duration (130). After 7 to 10 days of catheterization, approximately 50% of hospitalized patients will have developed UTI. Patients with prolonged urinary catheterization will undoubtedly develop bacteriuria, frequently caused by more than one organism. Studies in patients with chronic catheterization have demonstrated subpopulations of organisms that may be present concurrently. Some of these adhere to uroepithelial cells (*Escherichia coli*), whereas others attach to the catheter via biofilms (131). Prevention of UTI in patients with chronic urinary catheterization has proved difficult.

Routine urinary cultures in asymptomatic patients is not indicated because symptoms usually occur within 24 hours of infection. Antibiotic treatment of asymptomatic bacteriuria is unwarranted.

BACTEREMIA AND INFUSION-RELATED INFECTIONS

Nosocomial bacteremias account for about 8% of hospital-acquired infections in the United States, but they result in significant morbidity and mortality (Table 12–1) (132). The rate of primary bloodstream infections has increased over the last decade and varies between 1.3 (small, nonteaching) and 6.5 (large, teaching) per thousand hospital discharges, depending on hospital size and teaching versus nonteaching facility. Data from NNISS hospitals indicated that the fraction of bloodstream infections caused by gram-negative bacilli has remained relatively stable, but there was an increase in infections produced by coagulase-negative staphylococci, *S. aureus*, *Enterococci*, and *Candida* species (Table 12–4) (132). These organisms, especially *S. aureus* and *Candida* species, frequently colonize the skin and often are responsible for cannula-related septicemia. Catheter-related sepsis may result in shock, distant infection, or endocarditis. These complications are associated with significant mortality, and even if successfully treated, they extend the duration of hospital stay and increase cost. Older reviews have estimated that more than 850,000 device-related infections occur annually in the United States (133).

Although bacteremia may be secondary to other infections, such as pneumonia, wound infection, or UTI, this section will focus on those resulting from intravascular catheters, infusion therapy, and intravenously administered medications.

Sources of Infection

INFUSIONS

Contaminated intravenous products have been a source for bacteremia or septicemia. Epidemics of infusion-related septicemia have resulted from contamination of intravenous fluids during the manufacturing process (134) or from improper technique during preparation or administration (135). A nationwide epidemic of intrinsically contaminated intravenous fluids in 1970–1971 resulted in septicemia in 378 patients in 25 hospitals and contributed to the death of 40 patients (134). In this series of outbreaks, bacteria were isolated from a new design of a liner in the threaded cap of fluid bottles. Organisms were introduced into the intravenous fluid during use.

Pathogens are able to grow in room-temperature solutions of intravenous fluids and medications. With a small number of colonies inoculated into a test solution, *Enterobacter* and *Candida* grow in 5% dextrose in water. *Serratia* species and *P. aeruginosa* can proliferate in distilled water. Many organisms can proliferate in amino acid/25% glucose solutions used for parenteral nutrition and in 10% lipid emulsions. With gram-negative bacilli proliferation, the risk of septicemia and shock secondary to endotoxin is significant.

Extrinsic contamination of solutions or administration sets can happen via multiple mechanisms. Cracks in glass intravenous bottles permit entry of organisms, especially molds. Microorganisms can enter through nonfiltered air intake ports on administration sets used for glass containers. Improper technique may be responsible for contamination during spiking of infusions or addition of agents to carrier fluids. Blood products can be contaminated during processing as well as at the time of collection. Contamination may take place during disconnection or breaks in the administration set or attachment to the intravascular catheter. When intrinsic or extrinsic contamination of infusions is suspected, cultures of the products should be taken to compare with blood cultures from the patient. Procedural errors leading to extrinsic contamination should be corrected through educational programs. If intrinsic contamination of fluids is considered, public health authorities should be notified.

CATHETERS

Intravascular catheters can be colonized via multiple mechanisms (Fig. 12–2). The overwhelming majority of intravascular catheters become colonized from organisms arising from the patient's skin (136). In an animal model, it has been shown that bacteria at the puncture site of percutaneous catheters can rapidly move through the tunnel created in the skin to colonize the intravascular portion of the catheter. For bacteremias related to central venous, arterial, and peripheral intravascular catheters, there is correlation with organisms cultured from the skin around the entry site. Less frequent causes of catheter contamination are related to contaminated infusate, contamination of the catheter hub from the skin or from breaks in aseptic technique by healthcare personnel, or contamination of the device by the manufacturer or during insertion.

Catheter-Related Infections

Maki et al. have developed a semiquantitative culture technique for identifying infection caused by intravascular catheters (137). Based on culture data from the catheter, infusate, and patient, definitions for intravascular device-related infection have been formulated (138, 139).

Local catheter-related infection

Colonization of the catheter documented by a positive semiquantitative culture of the catheter.

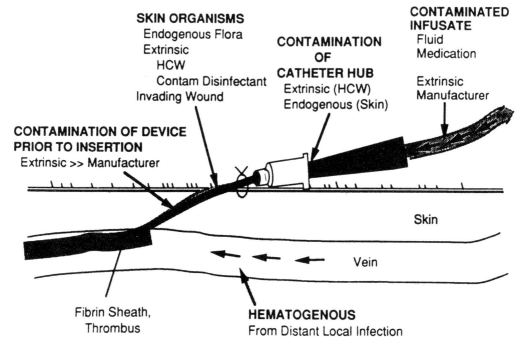

SKIN ORGANISMS
Endogenous Flora
Extrinsic
  HCW
  Contam Disinfectant
Invading Wound

CONTAMINATION OF CATHETER HUB
Extrinsic (HCW)
Endogenous (Skin)

CONTAMINATED INFUSATE
Fluid
Medication

Extrinsic
Manufacturer

CONTAMINATION OF DEVICE PRIOR TO INSERTION
Extrinsic >> Manufacturer

Skin

Vein

Fibrin Sheath,
Thrombus

HEMATOGENOUS
From Distant Local Infection

Fig. 12–2. Possible mechanism of intravascular catheter-related infection. (HCW = healthcare worker). (Reproduced with permission from Maki DG. Infections due to infusion therapy. In: Bennett JV, Brachman PS, eds. Hospital infections. 3rd ed. Boston; Little, Brown, and Co., 1992;861.)

Catheter-related septicemia

Septicemia diagnosed by clinical and microbiologic data without another source and with semiquantitative catheter culture and blood cultures positive for the same organism, with negative culture of infusate.

Septicemia due to a contaminated hub

No other identifiable source for the septicemia with cultures documenting the same species from the catheter hub, from percutaneously drawn blood cultures, and negative culture for the infecting organism from semiquantitative culture of the catheter.

Septicemia due to contaminated infusate

Septicemia without other identifiable source and positive cultures for the same species from infusate and from separate, percutaneously drawn blood cultures and negative

semiquantitative cultures of the catheter for the infecting organism.

The risk of septicemia varies according to the specific intravascular device (Table 12–9). It now seems that infusion-related phlebitis with peripheral venous catheters and thrombosis of central venous catheters are associated with catheter-related infection. Infusion-related phlebitis is believed to be a physicochemical phenomenon resulting in inflammation of the vein with associated erythema, which may proceed to venous thrombosis. In a prospective clinical trial, the risk of phlebitis was greater than 50% by the fourth day after catheterization of a peripheral vein (140). Factors correlating with phlebitis were identified as intravenous antibiotics, female sex, catheterization for longer than 48 hours, and catheter material (polyetherurethane [Vialon] less than tetrafluoroethylene-hexafluoropropylene [Teflon]). (140) Other predictors included phlebitis

Table 12–9. Risks of Septicemia Associated with Various Types of Devices for Intravascular Access

Type of Device	Representative Rate	Range
Short-term temporary access (no. of septicemias per 100 devices)		
Peripheral i.v. cannulas		
Winged steel needles	<0.2	
	0–1	
Peripheral i.v. catheters		
Percutaneously inserted	0.2	
	0–1	
Cutdown	6	—
Arterial catheters	1	0–1
Central venous catheters		
All-purpose, multilumen	3	1–7
Swan-Ganz	1	0–5
Hemodialysis	10	3–18
Long-term indefinite access (no. of septicemias per 100 device-days)		
Peripherally inserted central venous catheters	0.20	—
Cuffed central catheters (e.g., Hickman, Broviac)	0.20	0.10–0.53
Subcutaneous central venous ports (e.g., Infusaport, Port-a-cath)	0.04	0.00–.10

Reproduced with permission from Maki DG. Infections due to infusion therapy. In: Bennett JV, Brachman PS, eds. Hospital infections. 3rd ed. Boston: Little, Brown & Co., 1992;860.

with a previous catheter and anatomic site of placement (forearm > wrist > hand). Additional factors considered important are the experience of the person inserting the catheter and insertion under nonemergent conditions. It is estimated that, at the time of removal, between 5% and 25% of intravascular devices have become colonized by organisms arising from the skin. Although multilumen central venous catheters might be expected to have greater risk of infection, data from ICU patients indicated identical rates of catheter contamination and catheter-related sepsis in patients with single-lumen catheters and those with triple-lumen catheters (141).

DIAGNOSIS

Maki has enumerated clinical findings that might be helpful in identifying infusion or intravascular device-related bacteremia (138). The patient may be otherwise healthy, without local infection or apparent source to cause the sepsis. An intravascular device is being used and may show signs of local inflammation. The septic picture has an abrupt onset and is refractory to antimicrobial therapy until removal of the intravascular device or discontinuation of the infusion. Specific organisms such as staphylococci are more commonly associated with device-related bacteremias.

Bacteremia is diagnosed by positive blood cultures. Optimally, blood cultures are taken from venipuncture of peripheral veins remote from the site of an intravascular catheter. For adults, it is recommended that at least 20 mL of blood be taken with each venipuncture (138). Timing should occur before administration of an antibiotic or, if the patient is taking antimicrobials, immediately before the next dose. In some cases, resins may be used to remove antibiotics from samples to improve the likelihood of obtaining reliable cultures. Although cultures taken through indwelling catheters may correlate with cultures drawn by venipuncture (142), the practice may contribute to further catheter contamination through entry into an otherwise closed administration system. In patients with poor vascular access, obtaining blood cultures through intravascular catheters might be considered.

MECHANISMS FOR CATHETER CONTAMINATION

Microorganisms contaminating intravascular catheters adhere to the surface that becomes coated with proteins such as fibrin and albumin. Clot formation in the vein or on the catheter also seems to contribute to catheter contamination and sepsis (143). Some organisms form a glycocalyx, which enhances adherence. A recent study suggests that hemagglutination of erythrocytes by *S. epidermidis* correlated with adherence of the bacteria to intravenous catheters (144).

PREVENTION OF CATHETER INFECTION

Many studies have assessed the factors relating to the risk of catheter contamination and sepsis. It is recommended that before any invasive procedure, hands should be washed to eliminate transient microorganisms carried by the healthcare personnel (Table 12–5) (7). Maki recommends the use of sterile gloves for insertion of peripheral intravenous cannulas in immunosuppressed patients or those at high risk of infection (138). Sterile gloves are also recommended for all other intravascular devices, including intra-arterial catheters and all central venous catheters (138). A prospective investigation identified a twofold greater risk of infection associated with pulmonary artery catheters inserted in the operating room by anesthesiologists compared with those placed by personnel in the ICU (145). The greater rate of infection occurred even though the ICU catheters remained in place for a longer duration, were more likely placed in infected patients, and were used more frequently for parenteral nutrition. The investigators attributed the lower rate of infection in the ICU-placed catheters to the use of maximal barrier precautions, which included sterile gloves, a long-sleeved sterile surgical gown, a surgical face mask, and a large, sterile sheet drape (not a small fenestrated paper drape)

(146). The rate of catheter-related infection can also be minimized when special personnel or intravenous therapy teams are used for catheter insertion and catheter site care. Cost/benefit analysis suggests that the personnel cost can be offset by reduced expenses for catheter-related complications (145).

Antiseptics

Because of the association between cutaneous flora and catheter contamination, antisepsis of the skin is critical for minimizing catheter infection. A study of central venous and arterial catheters compared the use of 10% povidone-iodine, 70% alcohol, or 2% aqueous chlorhexidine for disinfection of the skin before catheter insertion (147). Chlorhexidine resulted in the lowest incidence in catheter-related bacteremia. In another study assessing skin disinfection during maintenance of implanted central venous catheters, chlorhexidine or tincture of iodine halved the rate of infection compared to the use of 10% povidone-iodine (148). Although iodophors are probably the most commonly used antiseptic for skin preparation, these studies suggest that chlorhexidine may be more effective.

Topical ointments

Application of topical antimicrobial ointment to the catheter insertion site has been suggested to prevent cutaneous flora from gaining access to the intravascular catheter via the tunnel created in the skin. Multiple clinical trials of this therapy have demonstrated little benefit, and use of polyantibiotic ointment resulted in an increase in catheter colonization by *Candida* (149). This suggests that until further data are available, routine use of antibiotic ointment on catheter sites is unwarranted.

Type of dressing

Another factor that seems important to the rate of catheter contamination is the type of dressing used to cover the insertion site. Features required in a dressing include providing an effective barrier to extrinsic microorganisms, removing excess skin moisture, allowing gas exchange, and preventing proliferation of microorganisms on the skin. Transparent plastic films are often used to cover catheters because they permit inspection of the site without removal of the dressing. Because the plastic dressings are more expensive than gauze and tape, they are often left on the catheter site for many days. Because some of these plastics are less permeable to oxygen and water vapor, there is concern that the transparent dressing may increase cutaneous bacterial colonization. In a prospective, randomized clinical trial, sterile gauze, replaced every other day, was compared with gauze or a transparent polyurethane dressing left in place until the peripheral intravenous catheter was removed (150). Cultures taken from under the dressing showed that cutaneous colonization was comparable with all dressings, and the rate of local catheter-related infection did not differ. From this, it was recommended that it was not cost-effective to redress peripheral venous catheters at periodic intervals and that either gauze or the transparent polyurethane dressing could be left on for the duration of the catheterization.

The safety of transparent dressings for central venous catheters has been questioned in several studies. A meta-analysis of multiple studies indicated an increased risk of bacteremia and catheter-related sepsis associated with the use of transparent dressings compared with gauze and tape (151). In one study, the rate of catheter-related septicemia was 16% with catheters dressed with a transparent film compared to 0% with gauze and tape (152). Regardless of the material, dressings on central venous catheters should be routinely changed every other day, especially for patients in the ICU.

Although there are less clinical data available, transparent dressings have not been recommended for arterial catheters (138). Possibly because of the greater likelihood of blood at the arterial puncture site, proliferation of microorganisms can occur readily under the occlusive dressing.

Newer transparent dressings are being developed with a greater vapor transmission rate, which should prevent the buildup of moisture between the dressing and skin. Recommendations on the use of these products must await clinical trials.

Guidewire-assisted catheter changes

In some situations, particularly in patients with difficult vascular access or coagulopathy, an indwelling catheter may be changed over a guidewire. Guidewire catheter exchanges have other advantages, including greater comfort for the patient, decreased incidence of pneumothorax or arterial perforation, and greater likelihood of correct catheter position (153). The decision to change a catheter over a guidewire should be based on the degree of suspicion of catheter-related sepsis and the expected ease of catheter insertion at a new site. For patients with probable catheter-related sepsis and at low risk for percutaneous insertion of a new catheter, the central venous catheter should be removed and cultured and a new catheter should be inserted at another site. Catheter exchange over a guidewire would be permissible if the likelihood of catheter-related sepsis was low or if the patient was at high risk for insertion of a new catheter. After removal, the old catheter should be cultured, and if this is positive, the catheter inserted through the old tract should be removed and a new catheter should be inserted at an alternative site. Catheters replaced for only mechanical malfunctions may be exchanged over a guidewire. Maki has recommended that if a catheter is exchanged over a guidewire, the site and the indwelling catheter should be well cleaned with an antiseptic solution and, after removing the old catheter, the site and guidewire should be reprepped with an antiseptic (138). A second pair of gloves and sterile drapes should be used to place the new catheter because the originals may have been contaminated.

Antimicrobial cuff

New technologies have been developed that seem to be effective in preventing contamination of central venous and pulmonary artery catheters. It has been known that surgically implanted cuffed catheters (Hickman or Broviac) have a low rate of infection because the tunnel through the skin quickly seals, with the growth of scar tissue preventing skin flora from reaching the catheter. An attachable subcutaneous cuff composed of collagen impregnated with silver ions has been developed for placement on catheters placed into the central venous circulation. This device has been shown to significantly reduce catheter colonization and catheter-related bacteremia (139, 149). The cuff comes in several sizes and can be placed on the catheter at the time of insertion. In Maki's study, catheters having the cuff were three times less likely to be colonized and were four times less likely to be associated with bacteremia (139). Although the cost of the cuff is significant, a cost-benefit analysis suggested that its use would be cost effective in an institution with a rate of central venous catheter-related bacteremia in the range of 2 to 3% (139). The beneficial effects of the silver impregnated cuff were limited to its use on catheters at the time of the original placement, and the devices were not effective when used on catheters changed over a guidewire (139). To be cost effective, clinicians might consider using the cuff only for central venous catheters, which will remain in place for longer periods.

Antimicrobial-bonded catheters

Another approach to reducing catheter-related infection has been the development of catheters with either antibiotic (154) or antiseptic (155) bonded to the catheter material. Central venous or arterial catheters bonded with cefazolin reduced catheter contamination from 14% to 2% in a sample of surgical ICU patients (154). *S. epidermidis* was the most common organism cultured from contaminated catheters. The technology of impregnating antimicrobials or antiseptics into the catheter material seems be effective from preliminary studies, but other trials must be conducted and the cost-effectiveness must be evaluated.

Infections From Injectable Medications

PROPOFOL

Postsurgical infections have been reported after extrinsic contamination of propofol, an intravenously administered anesthetic solubilized in a lipid emulsion (156). Investigation of these outbreaks revealed breaks in aseptic technique. In several locations, anesthesia personnel had used a single infusion of propofol on more than one patient. In vitro studies have clearly established that organisms can rapidly proliferate and produce endotoxin in preservative-free propofol (157). Although growth is greater in propofol, bacteria can survive in other preservative-free intravenous anesthetics (158). This suggests that careful aseptic technique should be used in preparing propofol for administration as a bolus or infusion.

Bacteria on the surface of the ampule are carried into its contents on the glass particles created by opening the ampule (159). Therefore, it is recommended that the ampule neck be disinfected with an alcohol swab before opening. Syringes or infusions of propofol should be used for administration to only a single patient, and the drug should be drawn into the syringe as close as possible to the time of use. After propofol is drawn into a syringe, it should be used within 6 hours to prevent any possible contaminating organisms from entering a rapid growth phase. The syringe and any unused propofol should be discarded within 6 hours of the time it was filled.

MEDICATIONS IN MULTIDOSE VIALS

Because of bacteriostatic agents used in multidose vials, the risk of nosocomial infection caused by extrinsic contamination is generally considered to be small. When there are breaks in aseptic techniques, pathogens may be introduced into the contents of multidose vials. In one reported outbreak, six patients died of fulminant hepatic failure as a result of extrinsic contamination of a multidose vial of heparin flush (160). The solution had been contaminated accidentally with blood from a patient carrying the hepatitis B virus. The heparin flush was being used in a hemodialysis unit and apparently a contaminated bloody syringe had been used to enter the vial.

In a study of samples taken from multidose vials used by anesthesiologists, cultures yielded no bacteria, and the investigators concluded that the incidence of extrinsic contamination of multidose vials was low for the drugs studied (161). Highsmith et al. showed that some medications in multidose vials supported bacterial growth, whereas others inactivated organisms slowly, some requiring as long as 48 or 96 hours (162). This suggests that the negative culture found from multidose vials used in the study of an anesthesia practice was possibly due to the study design of sampling weekly. Additionally, endotoxin may be formed by some organisms during the period of growth in contaminated medications. If a multidose vial has been entered without proper aseptic technique or the contents have been grossly contaminated, the vial should be discarded. Multidose vials can be used until the manufacturer's expiration date after opening if appropriate sterile precautions have been used (88). Some practices or institutions have specific policies regarding the permitted duration for use of multidose vials after they have been opened. If some medications in multidose vials are used infrequently, it may be more cost-effective to use single-dose products (163).

USE OF SYRINGES

Plastic syringes should be considered "single-use-only" products and, therefore, should be used to administer medication to only one patient. Although some clinicians reuse syringes after changing the needle, studies have demonstrated that removing the needle from a syringe creates a negative pressure and aspirates the needle contents into the syringe (164, 165). When used for injections into intravenous administration tubing, a syringe may become contaminated even though blood cannot be visually detected (166). In a clinical study, 3% of the injection sites closest to the intravenous catheter were contaminated with blood, even though the administration tubing had a check-valve and the blood pressure cuff was on the contralateral arm.

With multiple cycles of withdrawal and injection of the syringe plunger, the inner portion of the syringe barrel and its contents can be contaminated from microorganisms carried on the back end of the syringe and plunger (167). It is recommended that syringes be used for only one patient and that the contents be discarded after single patient use. Because of the greater risk of proliferation of organisms, syringes of propofol should be discarded within 6 hours after opening the vial.

INFUSIONS

Intravenous infusions may become contaminated in many ways, but the most common are by disconnections of or entry into the infusion system or tubing. Unprotected stopcocks are easily contaminated, especially when filled with blood or when left uncovered (168). Sterile caps or syringes should be used to keep stopcocks covered.

Intravenous administration sets and tubing for hemodynamic monitoring should be replaced every 72 hours (169). Extrinsic contamination of lipid emulsions for intravenous alimentation has been associated with bacteremia (170). Tubing for infusions of lipid emulsions should be changed every 24 hours when a closed system is used. Propofol is being administered more commonly by infusion for sedation of mechanically ventilated patients in the ICU. For propofol administered from a spiked vial, the unused contents of the open vial should be discarded and the tubing changed at 12 hours. Infusions should be used for only one patient.

Hemodynamic pressure transducers and ports used for blood sampling are sources of contamination and have been associated with outbreaks of bacteremia (171). A prospective, randomized study demonstrated that with routine use of disposable transducers in the ICU, the rate of patient bacteremia was not increased when the frequency of transducer replacement was extended from 2 to 4 days (172). The investigators demonstrated that the source of most of the infections were the patients'' own flora. Closed arterial and venous sampling systems are currently available, and their use may reduce extrinsic contamination of tubing and transducers.

INFECTIOUS RISKS TO PERSONNEL

Respiratory Transmitted Infections

TUBERCULOSIS

Recent attention has focused on transmission of *M. tuberculosis* between patients and to staff within hospitals and healthcare facilities (173). Transmission of *M. tuberculosis* has occurred after close contact with infected patients undergoing procedures involving the airway such as bronchoscopy or endotracheal intubation (174, 175). Patients with pulmonary tuberculosis may be unrecognized or incompletely treated and thereby pose an infectious risk to other patients and personnel.

The annual rate of new cases of tuberculosis in the United States had declined until 1985, when the rate began to increase (176). Although 2600 new cases of tuberculosis were reported to the CDC in 1992, data from 1993 suggested a slight decrease and, thus, a reversal of the upward trend. Of particular concern is the emergence of multidrug-resistant organisms. Data from New York City indicated that 33% of new cases of tuberculosis were resistant to isoniazid (177). In outbreaks of multidose-resistant tuberculosis, the orga-

nisms did not seem to be more infectious but resulted in greater mortality (43% to 93%) with a shorter interval between diagnosis and death. The poor outcomes were related to delays in diagnosis, recognition of drug resistance, and initiation of effective therapy (104).

M. tuberculosis is spread via airborne particles, droplet nuclei, generated when patients with pulmonary or laryngeal tuberculosis speak, cough, or sneeze (178). The droplet nuclei (1 to 5 μm in size) can remain suspended in the air for prolonged periods and can travel great distances throughout rooms on air currents. The infectious process begins when the organisms in the droplet are inhaled, reaching the alveoli of a susceptible individual. After the initial infection, the immune response limits the spread of *M. tuberculosis*, but some organisms may remain viable for many years. Approximately 10% of healthy infected individuals progress from latent infection and develop active tuberculosis during their lifetimes. In patients coinfected with HIV, latent tuberculosis infection is more likely to reactivate with a 10% risk per year (179). Other groups with a greater risk of progression from latent infection to active disease include children (younger than 4 years of age), recently infected individuals, and immunosuppressed patients.

Because anesthesiologists frequently instrument their patient's airway, they are at high risk when caring for individuals with pulmonary or laryngeal tuberculosis. The chance of transmission is greater during procedures that induce coughing or acrosolization of *M. tuberculosis*, especially when performed in small spaces with inadequate ventilation. The CDC has published guidelines for preventing transmission of *M. tuberculosis* in healthcare facilities (104, 180). Infection control programs for prevention of tuberculosis involve early identification of infected patients and prompt respiratory isolation of patients suspected of having the disease. Respiratory isolation should be used during the evaluation of the patient and until there has been confirmation that the findings are not caused by tuberculosis. When tuberculosis is diagnosed, the patient should remain in respiratory isolation until there has been documented efficacy of treatment by negative sputum cultures and smears along with improvement of symptoms. Outbreaks of tuberculosis in healthcare facilities have occurred when these precautions have not been taken or when patients were removed from isolation before adequate treatment was ensured.

Care of patients with active tuberculosis

Respiratory isolation. To prevent airborne spread of infectious droplet nuclei to patients and personnel, respiratory isolation should be used for patients suspected of having active pulmonary tuberculosis or other diseases transmitted via the respiratory route (varicella, measles) (104, 181). Respiratory isolation requires a single-patient room with special ventilation maintained at negative pressure relative to the corridor to limit the number of droplet nuclei escaping from the room. The door to the room should be kept closed, except when the patient or healthcare worker needs to enter or exit. To minimize the concentration of droplet nuclei in the room, the ventilation system should provide at least six air exchanges each hour, with the exhaust directed either to the outside or recirculated through a high-efficiency particulate filter (HEPA) and/or an ultraviolet light before reentering the room (104, 182). When it is necessary for the patient to leave the room, he or she should wear a mask to prevent the dissemination of organisms into the air. When healthcare workers enter the isolation room, they should wear a NIOSH approved particulate respirator (classification N-95) (104, 183, 184).

Perioperative care. Elective surgery should not be performed on patients with active pulmonary tuberculosis. If emergency surgical procedures are necessary, a mask should be placed on the patient to prevent exposure of other individuals, and they should be brought directly from their isolation room to the operating room. In the operating room, a positive-pressure environment, personnel should wear particulate respirators with adequate filtration to remove droplet nuclei (104, 183, 184). Respirators with positive-pressure release valves are not appropriate for use in the operating room because microorganisms being exhaled may contaminate the surgical field. A bacterial filter should be used in the expiratory limb of the anesthesia circuit or between the endotracheal tube and y-piece to prevent contamination of the anesthesia machine. After surgery, the patient should recover from anesthesia in the operating room or in a room appropriate for respiratory isolation.

Skin-testing programs should be mandatory for hospital personnel who are at risk for tuberculosis. The frequency of testing should be determined by the prevalence of patients with tuberculosis in the hospital population (104).

RESPIRATORY SYNCYTIAL VIRUS

Respiratory syncytial virus (RSV) causes annual outbreaks of pneumonia during the winter and early spring months and is the single most important respiratory pathogen in infants and children. RSV may also cause disease in adults, especially elderly and immunocompromised patients. The virus is present in respiratory secretions from infected individuals, and transmission to other patients or healthcare personnel is through virus transferred via the hands to the mucous membranes of the eyes or nose. RSV can be found in respiratory secretions for about 7 days in infected patients. The virus may remain viable on environmental surfaces for as long as 6 hours, and transmission of RSV may occur via fomites (185).

Nosocomial transmission of RSV is prevented by isolation of infected patients and use of barriers for healthcare workers. Studies have shown a reduced infection rate in personnel with the use of masks and goggles (186), gloves and gowns (187), and frequent hand washing (188). RSV immune globulin is effective when used prophylactically in infants and children at high risk for RSV infection (189).

Risk of Bloodborne Infections

Anesthesia personnel are frequently exposed to blood and body fluids through cutaneous exposures and needlestick injuries (190–193). Bloodborne pathogens that may be transmitted to susceptible anesthesia personnel include hepatitis B virus (HBV), hepatitis C virus (HCV), and HIV. Although these viruses are spread in the community by homosexual or heterosexual contact, sharing of needles used for injection of drugs, from mother to child in utero or after birth, and from transfusion of contaminated blood or blood products, the prime occupational risk to healthcare workers is through blood or body fluid contact. The CDC warns that occupational transmission of bloodborne pathogens to healthcare workers can take place through exposures to infected patient's blood, blood-tinged fluids, blood products, tissues, or the following body fluids: semen, vaginal secretions, cerebrospinal fluid, synovial fluid, pleural fluid, peritoneal fluid, pericardial fluid, or amniotic fluid (194).

The prevalence of serologic markers for prior HBV infection was 19% in physician-anesthesiologists and certified registered nurse anesthetists (CRNAs) (195) and 13% in anesthesia residents (196) in multicenter studies conducted at university-affiliated hospitals. A similar study conducted at a large inner-city hospital found a seroprevalence rate of 49% for markers of HBV infection (197). These data indicate that anesthesia personnel have a high occupational risk of acquiring HBV. Because HBV serves as a marker for blood exposure, these surveys document that anesthesia personnel should be considered a high-risk group.

The risk of seroconversion for any bloodborne pathogen is a function of the product of three factors: (*a*) the prevalence of patients carrying the virus in the specific population cared for by the worker, (*b*) the number of annual exposures to blood or body fluids, and (*c*) the risk of infection with each exposure to blood carrying the virus (190, 198). Prevention efforts have focused on reducing the frequency of blood exposures because this is the only factor of these three that can be altered.

HEPATITIS B VIRUS

In 1990, the CDC estimated that occupational exposures resulted in 5100 HBV seroconversions in healthcare workers annually (199). Of these infected individuals, 10% become chronic carriers of HBV, and an estimated 170 healthcare workers die annually of long-term complications of HBV infection, cirrhosis, or hepatocellular carcinoma. Surveillance studies in the United States covering the period from 1981 through 1988 have demonstrated a decrease in the fraction of new cases of hepatitis B occurring in healthcare workers (199). This may be attributable to immunization with the hepatitis B vaccine, which became available in 1982, and wider adoption of blood and body fluid precautions recommended by the CDC. For nonimmune individuals, a significant percutaneous injury with a needle contaminated with blood containing HBV carries a 6% to 30% risk of infection (194). Because HBV carriers seropositive for hepatitis B e-antigen have a higher concentration of HBV in the blood, the risk after a percutaneous exposure may be as high as 27% to 43%.

The primary strategy for preventing HBV infection, especially in high-risk healthcare workers such as anesthesia personnel, is use of the hepatitis B vaccine (200). The current vaccines are derived from genetically engineered hepatitis B surface antigen and carry no risk for transmission of HIV. Continued surveillance indicates that the three-dose vaccine regimen produces protective antibodies in 90% to 95% of healthy adults. To ensure adequate immunity, it is recommended that serologic testing for anti-HBs, the protective antibody, be performed approximately 6 weeks after the final dose of vaccine. Inadequate levels of protective antibodies after hepatitis B vaccination is correlated with certain risk factors, including older age, obesity, and smoking (201). Additional doses of vaccine are indicated in individuals with suboptimal antibody titers, because a significant portion of nonresponders will subsequently develop antibodies (202). There is currently no recommendation for routine booster doses of hepatitis B vaccine for healthcare workers with adequate antibody response (200).

When personnel experience a significant HBV-contaminated blood exposure, they should be followed by the Employee Health Service or other designated personnel. Published protocols should be followed for testing the source patient and injured personnel (200). Unimmunized personnel should be offered the hepatitis B vaccine as well as hepatitis B immune globulin to provide passive protection.

HEPATITIS C VIRUS

Infection with HCV is responsible for most cases of sporadic and post-transfusion non-A, non-B hepatitis in the United States (203). The proportion of new cases associated with blood transfusion has declined, whereas that in patients reporting parenteral drug use has increased significantly (204). Approximately 3% of patients with acute non-A, non-B hepatitis are healthcare workers (205).

After either community-acquired or post-transfusion hepatitis C infection, 50% to 60% of patients develop chronic hepatitis (206). The virus persists for several years in most patients, although many do not develop active liver disease. An antibody to HCV (anti-HCV) has been identified and may be useful for diagnosis of HCV infection (207). With early HCV infection, there is usually an initial period of seronegativity for anti-HCV although HCV RNA can be detected as a marker of infection. Anti-HCV does not provide protective immunity or signal resolution of the infection because it may be present in infected patients with persistent hepatitis or a viral carrier state (208). This suggests that an effective vaccine against HCV cannot be based on formation of anti-HCV.

Transmission of non-A, non-B hepatitis has been documented from HCV-infected patients to healthcare workers. In one study, four of 110 workers sustaining an anti-HCV-positive needlestick developed hepatitis (209). Seroprevalence surveys in the United States and Austria identified anti-HCV in 2% of healthcare workers (210, 211). This suggests that the risk of occupational transmission of HCV is significantly lower than for HBV and that the rate of seroconversion after a HCV-contaminated needlestick injury is approximately 3% to 4%.

HUMAN IMMUNODEFICIENCY VIRUS

The CDC estimates that approximately 1 million individuals in the United States are infected with HIV. Since reports of the first cases of AIDS in 1981, more than 496,000 cases were diagnosed through December 1995 in the United States (212). There have been 49 serologic documented occupational HIV infections in the United States (212). Forty-two of these healthcare workers had percutaneous exposures, five had mucocutaneous exposures, one had both percutaneous and mucocutaneous exposures, and one had an unknown route of exposure to HIV-infected material. Forty-four of the exposures were to blood from an HIV-infected person. In a prospective study of healthcare workers exposed to HIV-infected blood or body fluids, there were four seroconversions after 1167 percutaneous exposures (transmission rate of 0.34%), whereas there were none after blood contact with mucous membranes or intact skin (213). From these data, it seems that the greatest risk for occupational transmission of HIV to healthcare workers is via a percutaneous exposure such as needlestick injury (214). Using data published in the literature, Buergler et al. have estimated that the annual risk of HIV infection for anesthesiologists ranges between 0.002 and 0.129%, depending on the prevalence of HIV-infected patients in the population served by the anesthesiologist (198).

Many factors undoubtedly affect the risk of HIV infection after a contaminated needlestick injury. The concentration of virus in the blood is greatest after the initial infection and during the period of immunosuppression (AIDS). The viral dose carried on the sharp device is probably greater when it was contaminated during use on a patient in either of the phases of the disease (215). A hollow-bore needle with a larger lumen is capable of carrying a greater volume of infected blood than a smaller-gauge hollow needle or a solid suture needle (216–218). If the needle traverses a latex glove, a portion of the blood from the outer surface of the needle is removed so that the volume transferred by the injury is reduced (218). Analysis of data from two CDC studies suggests that the greatest risk of HIV infection is related to injuries with large-gauge, hollow-bore, blood-filled needles (219). Other variables possibly affecting the risk of HIV infection include the severity of the exposure, the pathogenicity of the specific virus, host susceptibility, and viral survival in the interval that the virus is exposed to the atmosphere (220).

Some institutions offer postexposure prophylactic zidovudine (AZT) to healthcare workers who have sustained a significant occupational blood exposure, but the CDC suggests that available clinical and laboratory studies in humans are inadequate to prove the effectiveness of this use of the drug (214). Healthcare workers should consider the potential side effects and possible long-term toxicity when choosing to use zidovudine for prophylaxis after occupational blood exposure.

UNIVERSAL PRECAUTIONS

Along with immunization, the primary approach for preventing occupational transmission of bloodborne infections to healthcare workers is the reduction of the potential for exposures to patient's blood and body fluids. Because not all viral carriers can be detected with a routine history, physical examination, and laboratory tests, the CDC has recommended the use of Universal Precautions with all patients (194). Universal Precautions include the use of appropriate barriers when healthcare workers perform tasks that could result in contact with blood or body fluids. The choice of barriers (gowns, eyewear, masks, caps, and gloves) should be based on the specific procedure to be performed and the anticipated degree of exposure. Although the protective barriers should be impervious to fluids, needles and other sharp devices present a risk for penetration. Therefore, the CDC has included specific recommendations to prevent percutaneous injuries caused by sharp objects (194). Disposable syringes with needles and other sharp devices should be directly placed in puncture-resistant containers for disposal immediately after use. The container should be located as close as practical to the use area so that the sharp objects would not require transport over a great distance. Contaminated needles should not be recapped, bent, or broken by hand or removed from syringes before disposable. Reusable needles and sharp devices should be left on the syringe and placed in a puncture-resistant container for transport to the reprocessing area. Sterile needles that have only been used to aspirate sterile medications pose no risk of infection and can be recapped if necessary using a one-hand technique (190). Improperly handled contaminated needles such as those left in a patient's bed or thrown into plastic trash bag pose a threat to personnel, including housekeeping and laundry workers.

Universal Precautions seem to be effective in reducing exposure to blood (221) but often the recommendations are not completely followed (191, 222). A postal survey of a sample of anesthesiologists indicated that most (88%) complied with Universal Precautions when treating a known HIV-infected patient but only 25% adhered to the recommendations when the patient was considered at low risk (191). The same trend was apparent with use of gloves and other barriers. The selective application of Universal Precautions is inappropriate because it has been demonstrated that a significant portion of hospitalized patients, especially trauma victims, may have unrecognized HIV infection (223). Additionally, an observational study of surgical procedures demonstrated that the surgical personnel's knowledge of diagnosed HIV infection or awareness of a patient's high-risk status did not affect the actual rate of exposure (224).

PREVENTION OF NEEDLESTICK INJURIES

Despite recommendations to the contrary, anesthesia personnel continue to recap needles. When the contents of needle disposal containers used by anesthesia personnel were categorized, 41% of all needles had been recapped before disposal (225). In a study of 326 needlestick injuries in a university hospital, one-third were related to recapping of contaminated needles (226). Education has been attempted to reduce needlestick injuries and recapping, but the effectiveness on changing behavior has been limited.

The best method to reduce needlestick injuries is an engineering control approach that would eliminate the use of needles by replacing the standard devices with needleless or protected needle items (226). Multiple safety devices have been designed and are commercially available, but only a few have application to the practice of anesthesiology. Needleless fluid administration systems permit intravenous injection of medications and use secondary infusions without sharp devices (225).

Anesthesia personnel use a large number of intravenous catheters (225). It is desirable for product manufacturers to design safety versions of intravascular catheters that can be used for arterial placement and with the Seldinger approach for placement of central venous catheters. Intravenous catheters have large-bore, hollow-needle stylets, which pose a great risk for transmission of bloodborne pathogens to anesthesia personnel (219, 225). As new safety products become available and are considered for use, cost-effectiveness analysis must be performed because most needleless devices are more expensive than the

standard items they replace (227). Another consideration is the risk of nosocomial infection that may be posed with newer devices (228).

OSHA STANDARD

In 1992, the United States Occupational Safety and Health Administration mandated standards to reduce employee's occupational exposure to bloodborne pathogens (12). The federal standard requires that employers have a written Exposure Control Plan. The standard is based on a hierarchy of preventive measures: engineering controls to remove hazards, work practice controls to change methods of performing tasks, and finally, Universal Precautions to be used when performing procedures not covered by other controls. Changes in work practices (i.e., using an instrument to grasp a needle rather than by hand) should be effective in preventing blood exposures, but institution of this strategy requires analysis of tasks performed by anesthesia personnel and their subsequent modification.

The annual cost of compliance with the OSHA standard was initially estimated to be $813 million; $322 million is required annually by all hospitals in the United States (average cost: $51,950 per hospital) (12). Some analyses are beginning to question the cost effectiveness of Universal Precautions. Data reported from a Canadian 400-bed acute-care teaching hospital indicated that Universal Precautions had an incremental cost increase of $135,000 per year (229). Based on the prevalence of HIV-infected patients in the hospital's population and the annual rate of needlestick injuries at the institution, it was estimated that the cost of Universal Precautions was about $8 million for every case of HIV seroconversion prevented. Because needlestick injuries seem to have a greater risk of transmission of bloodborne pathogens to healthcare workers (212, 213), a more effective strategy for reducing costs might derive from acquiring technology to reduce accidental needlestick injuries.

Isolation Precautions

Because antibiotic-resistant bacterial infections (230, 231) have become more common in acute care hospitals, new modalities to prevent patient-to-patient spread have been proposed (181, 232). Universal precautions have been effective in reducing the exposure of healthcare workers to blood and body fluids, but the emphasis of these recommendations was directed toward protecting the healthcare worker. Pathogenic organisms may be spread to environmental surfaces or from one patient to another when healthcare workers fail to change gloves after they become contaminated (233). Therefore, the CDC has consolidated its isolation recommendations into a single approach to both protect healthcare workers and prevent transmission of organisms from infected patients to other patients or environmental surfaces (181). **Standard Precautions** were proposed to supersede Universal Precautions for use with all patients and apply to situations in which blood, body fluids, nonintact skin, or mucous membranes are contacted. Gloves should be worn by the healthcare workers to prevent exposure to these media. Gloves should be changed between patient contacts and hands should be washed to minimize the possibility of patient-to-patient transmission of microorganisms. In addition, when splashes of blood or body fluids are anticipated, a gown should be worn to protect clothing or body surfaces, and mask and eye protection should be used. Again, these protective barriers should be removed after the patient-care activities and new coverings should be used before contacting another patient.

For patients with specific infections, other control measures may be necessary. These are disease specific and are based on the mode of transmission of the causative agent (181). **Airborne Precautions**, including respiratory isolation (see above), are used to reduce the risk of infectious agents spread via droplet nuclei. **Droplet Precautions** are designed to reduce transmission via large-particle droplets that travel only a few feet through the air to produce infection by entering through the mucous membranes of a susceptible host. Examples of microorganisms transmitted in this way include influenza, rubella, and mycoplasma. Patients infected with microorganisms spread via large droplets should be placed in a private room, and healthcare workers should wear masks when coming within 3 feet of the patient. The patient should wear a mask when being transported from his or her room.

Contact Precautions should be used for patients infected or colonized with microorganisms that can be transmitted by direct contact with the patient or indirect contact with contaminated environmental surfaces (181). Examples include patients with *Clostridium difficile*, skin ulcerations, draining abscesses, wound infections, or RSV. The patient should be placed in a private room because soilage from draining lesions, diarrhea, or secretions can result in widespread contamination. Gloves should be worn by the healthcare workers when they enter the room and should be changed after contacting material that is likely to have high concentrations of infectious organisms. A clean, nonsterile gown should be worn if it is anticipated that the healthcare worker's clothing will have contact with the patient, environmental surfaces, or items in the patient's room. Hands should be washed with an antiseptic soap or waterless antiseptic agent after removing the gloves and gown in the patient's room. When the patient must be transported from the isolation room for surgery or diagnostic tests, personnel in the new location should be informed of the patient's infection and infection control precautions must be continued. In the operating room, the level of barrier protection must be individualized, based on the extent of the expected contamination. When anesthesia personnel are not touching the patient or items that are likely to be contaminated, such as the patient's hospital bed or linen, gloves should be removed to prevent dissemination of organisms to anesthetic equipment or supplies. The extent and nature of the infection and anticipated environmental contamination must be considered when determining whether the patient can go to the recovery room after surgery or must recover from anesthesia in the operating room or isolation room.

LATEX HYPERSENSITIVITY

An unanticipated consequence of the more frequent use of latex gloves by healthcare personnel is an increase in latex sensitivity, both cutaneous and systemic (234–236). When a latex skin prick test was used for testing a group of physicians, including anesthesiologists, 10% of physicians (24% in a subgroup of atopic physicians) demonstrated latex sensitization compared to 3% of controls (235). Anaphylaxis after latex exposure has been reported in healthcare workers with latex sensitivity (234). This suggests that all healthcare workers should limit their exposure to latex by using nonlatex gloves when possible and should limit the use of gloves to tasks that may result in exposure to blood or body fluids. Likewise, all patients should be questioned regarding symptoms of latex sensitivity, and for those at high risk, treatment should involve only use of nonlatex products (237).

REFERENCES

1. Brachman PS. Epidemiology of nosocomial infections. In: Bennett JV, Brachman PS, eds. Hospital infections. 3rd ed. Boston: Little, Brown, and Co., 1992;3–20.
2. Garner JS, Jarvis WR, Emori TG, et al. CDC definitions for nosocomial infections, 1988. Am J Infect Control 1988;16:128–140.
3. Haley RW, Culver DH, White JW, et al. The efficacy of infection surveillance and control programs in preventing nosocomial infection in U.S. hospitals. Am J Epidemiol 1985;121:182–205.
4. Haley RW, Hooton TM, Culver DH, et al. Nosocomial infections by U.S. hospitals, 1975-1976: estimated frequency by selected characteristics of patients. Am J Med 1981;70:947–959.
5. Haley RW, Culver DH, Morgan WM, et al. Increased recognition of infectious diseases in US hospitals through increased use of diagnostic tests, 1970–1976. Am J Epidemiol 1985;121:168–181.
6. Williams WW. CDC guideline for the prevention and control of nosocomial infections: guideline for infection control in hospital personnel. Am J Infection Cont 1984;12:34–57.
7. Garner JS, Favero MS. CDC Guideline for the prevention and control of nosocomial infections: guideline for handwashing and hospital environmental control, 1985: supersedes guideline for hospital environmental control published in 1981. Am J Infection Control 1986;14:110–126.
8. Simmons BP, Hooton TM, Wong ES, et al. Guidelines for prevention of intravascular infections. Infect Control 1981;3:61–72.
9. Simmons BP, Wong ES. CDC guideline for the prevention and control of nosocomial infections: guideline for prevention of nosocomial pneumonia. Am J Infect Cont 1983;11:230–239.
10. Joint Commission on Accreditation of Healthcare Organizations. Standards: infection control. In: JCAHO, accreditation manual for hospitals. Chicago: Joint Commission on Accreditation of Healthcare Organizations, 1990.
11. Centers for Disease Control. Mandatory reporting of infectious diseases by clinicians, and mandatory reporting of occupational diseases by clinicians. MMWR 1990;39(RR-9):1–28.
12. Department of Labor, Occupational Safety and Health Administration. Occupational exposure to bloodborne pathogens; final rule (29 CFR part 1910.1030). Federal Register 1991;56:64004–64182.
13. Walter CW. Cross-infection and the anesthesiologist. Anesth Analg 1974;53:631–644.
14. Crow S, Greene VW. Aseptic transgressions among surgeons and anesthesiologists: a quantitative study. Arch Surg 1982;117:1012–1016.
15. Rhame RS. The inanimate environment. In: Bennett JV, Brachman PS, eds. Hospital infections. 3rd ed. Boston: Little, Brown, and Co., 1992;299–333.
16. du Moulin GC, Hedley-Whyte J. Bacterial interactions between anesthesiologists, their patients, and equipment. Anesthesiology 1982;57:37–41.
17. Martone WJ, Jarvis WR, Culver DH, et al. Incidence and nature of endemic and epidemic nosocomial infections. In: Bennett JV, Brachman PS, eds. Hospital infections. 3rd ed. Boston: Little, Brown, and Co., 1992;577–596.
18. Horan TC, Gaynes RP, Martone WJ, et al. CDC definitions of nosocomial surgical site infections, 1992: a modification of CDC definitions of surgical wound infections. Am J Infect Control 1992;20:271–274.
19. Ehrenkranz NJ, Meakins JL. Surgical infections. In: Bennett JV, Brachman PS, eds. Hospital infections. 3rd ed. Boston: Little, Brown, and Co., 1992;685–710.
20. Society for Hospital Epidemiology of America, Association for Practitioners in Infection Control, Centers for Disease Control, Surgical Infection Society. Consensus paper on the surveillance of surgical wound infection. Am J Infect Control 1992;20:263–270.
21. Ad Hoc Committee on Trauma, Division of Medical Sciences, National Academy of Sciences — National Research Council. Postoperative wound infections: the influence of ultraviolet irradiation of the operating room and of various other factors. Ann Surg 1964;160(Suppl):1–192.
22. Culver DH, Horan TC, Gaynes RP, et al. Surgical wound infection rates by wound class, operative

procedure, and patient risk index. Am J Med 1991;91(Suppl 3B):152S–157S.

23. Haley RW, Culver DH, Morgan WM, et al. Identifying patients at hish risk of surgical would infection. A simple multivariate index of patient susceptibility and wound contamination. Am J Epidemiol 1985;121:206–215.

24. Edwards LD. The epidemiology of 2056 remote site infections and 1966 surgical wound infections occurring in 1865 patients: a four year study of 40,923 operations at Rush-Presbyterian St. Luke's Hospital, Chicago. Ann Surg 1976;184:758.

25. Mest DR, Wong DH, Shimoda KJ, et al. Nasal colonization with methicillin-resistant Staphylococcus aureus on admission to the surgical intensive care unit increases the risk of infection. Anesth Analg 1994;78:644–650.

26. Krizek TJ, Robson MC. Evolution of quantitative bacteriology in wound management. Am J Surg 1975;130:579.

27. Garibaldi RA, Cushing D, Lerer T. Risk factors for postoperative infection. Am J Med 1991;91(Suppl 3B):158S–163S.

28. Mastro TD, Farley TA, Elliott JA, et al. An outbreak of surgical-wound infections due to group A streptococcus carried on the scalp. N Engl J Med 1990;323:968–972.

29. Reybrouck G. Role of the hands in the spread of nosocomial infections. J Hosp Infect 1983;4:103–110.

30. Albert RK, Condie F. Handwashing patterns in medical intensive-care units. N Engl J Med 1981;304:1456–1466.

31. Doebbeling BN, Stanley GL, Sheetz CT, et al. Comparative efficacy of alternative hand-washing agents in reducing nosocomial infections in intensive care units. N Engl J Med 1992;327:88–93.

32. Bernard HR, Cole WR. The prophylaxis of surgical infection: the effect of prophylactic antimicrobial drugs on the incidence of infection following potentially contaminated operations. Surgery 1964;56:151–157.

33. Platt R, Zaleznik DF, Hopkins CC, et al. Preoperative antibiotic prophylaxis for herniorrhaphy and breast surgery. N Engl J Med 1990;322:153–160.

34. Antimicrobial prophylaxis in surgery. The Medical Letter 1992;34:5–8.

35. Classen DC, Evans RS, Pestotnik SL, et al. The timing of prophylactic administration of antibiotics and the risk of surgical-wound infection. N Engl J Med 1992;326:281–286.

36. Horan TC, White JW, Jarvis WR, et al. Nosocomial infection surveillance, 1984. MMWR 1986;35:17SS–29SS.

37. Tablan OC, Anderson LJ, Arden NH, et al. Guideline for prevention of nosocomial pneumonia. Part I. Issues on prevention of nosocomial pneumonia — 1994. Am J Infect Control 1994;22:247–266.

38. Craven DE, Steger KA, Barber TW. Preventing nosocomial pneumonia: state of the art and perspectives for the 1990s. Am J Med 1991;91(Suppl 3B):44S–53S.

39. LaForce FM. Lower respiratory tract infections. In: Bennett JV, Brachman PS, eds. Hospital infections.

3rd ed. Boston: Little, Brown, and Co., 1992;611–639.

40. Garibaldi RA, Britt MR, Coleman ML, et al. Risk factors for postoperative pneumonia. Am J Med 1981;70:677–680.

41. Langer M, Mosconi P, Cigada M, et al. The intensive care unit group of infection control. Long-term respiratory support and risk of pneumonia in critically ill patients. Am Rev Respir Dis 1989; 140:302–305.

42. Jarvis WR, Edwards JR, Culver DH, et al. Nosocomial infection rates in adult and pediatric intensive care units in the United States. Am J Med 1991;91(Suppl 3B):185S–191S.

43. Kollef MH. Ventilator-associated pneumonia: a multivariate analysis. JAMA 1993;270:1965–1970.

44. Gross PA, Neu HC, Aswapokee P, et al. Deaths from nosocomial infections: experience in a university hospital and a community hospital. Am J Med 1980;68:219–225.

45. Craven DE, Kunches LM, Kilinsky V, Lichtenberg DA, Make BJ, McCabe WR. Risk factors for pneumonia and fatality in patients receiving continuous mechanical ventilation. Am Rev Respir Dis 1986;133:792–796.

46. Leal-Noval SR, Alfaro-Rodriguez E, Murillo-Cabeza F, et al. Diagnostic value of the blind brush in mechanically ventilated patients with nosocomial pneumonia. Intensive Care Med 1992;18:410–414.

47. Johanson WG, Pierce AK, Sanford JP. Changing pharyngeal bacterial flora of hospitalized patients. Emergence of gram-negative bacilli. N Engl J Med 1969;281:1137–1140.

48. Johanson WG, Pierce AK, Sanford JP, et al. Nosocomial respiratory infections with gram-negative bacilli: the significance of colonization of the respiratory tract. Ann Intern Med 1972;77:701–706.

49. Woods DE, Straus DC, Johanson WG, et al. Role of fibronectin in the prevention of adherence of Pseudomonas aeruginosa to buccal cells. J Infect Dis 1981;143:784–790.

50. Proctor RA. Fibronectin: a brief overview of its structure, function, and physiology. Rev Infect Dis 1987;9:S317–S21.

51. duMoulin GC, Paterson DG, Hedley-Whyte J, et al. Aspiration of gastric bacteria in antacid-treated patients: a frequent cause of postoperative colonization of the airway. Lancet 1982;1:242–245.

52. Driks MR, Craven DE, Celli BR, et al. Nosocomial pneumonia in intubated patients given sucralfate as compared with antacids or histamine type 2 blockers. N Engl J Med 1987;317:1376–1382.

53. Bresalier RS, Grendell JH, Cello JP, et al. Sucralfate suspension versus titrated antacid for the prevention of acute stress-related gastrointestinal hemorrhage in critically ill patients. Am J Med 1987;83:110–116.

54. Tryba M. Risk of acute stress bleeding and nosocomial pneumonia in ventilated intensive care unit patients: sucralfate versus antacids. Am J Med 1987;83(Suppl 3B):117–124.

55. Tryba M, Mantey-Stiers F. Antibacterial activity of

sucralfate in human gastric juice. Am J Med 1987;83(Suppl 3B):125–127.

56. Lehot JJ, Deleat-Besson R, Bastien O, et al. Should we inhibit gastric acid secretion before cardiac surgery? Anesth Analg 1990;70:185–190.

57. Huxley EJ, Viroslav J, Gray WR, et al. Pharyngeal aspiration in normal adults and patients with depressed consciousness. Am J Med 1973;64:564–568.

58. Craven DE, Kunches LM, Lichtenberg DA, et al. Nosocomial infection and fatality in medical surgical intensive care unit patients. Arch Intern Med 1988;148:1161–1168.

59. Cross AS, Roup B. Role of respiratory assistance device in endemic nosocomial pneumonia. Am J Med 1981;70:681–685.

60. McCrae W, Wallace P. Aspiration around high volume, low pressure endotracheal cuff. Br Med J 1981;2:1220–1221.

61. Mahul P, Auboyer C, Jospe R, et al. Prevention of nosocomial pneumonia in intubated patients: respective role of mechanical subglottic secretions drainage and stress ulcer prophylaxis. Intensive Care Med 1992;18:20–25.

62. Sottile FD, Marrie TJ, Prough DS, et al. Nosocomial pulmonary infection: possible etiologic significance of bacterial adhesion to endotracheal tubes. Crit Care Med 1986;14:265–270.

63. Inglis TJ, Millar MR, Jones JG, et al. Tracheal tube biofilm as a source of bacterial colonisation of the lung. J Clin Microbiol 1989;27:2014–2018.

64. Winterbauer RH, Durning RB, Barron E, et al. Aspirated nasogastric feeding solution detected by glucose strips. Ann Intern Med 1981;95:67–68.

65. Jacobs S, Chang RWS, Lee B, et al. Continuous enteral feeding: a major cause of pneumonia among ventilated intensive care unit patients. J Parent Enter Nutr 1990;14:353–356.

66. Stock MC, Downs JB, Gauer PK, et al. Prevention of postoperative pulmonary complications with CPAP, incentive spirometry, and conservative therapy. Chest 1985;87:151–157.

67. Wasylak TJC, Abbott FV, English MJM, et al. Reduction of postoperative morbidity following patient-controlled morphine. Can J Anaesth 1990;37:726–731.

68. Cushieri RJ, Morran CG, Howie JC, et al. Postoperative pain and pulmonary complications: comparison of three analgesic regimens. Br J Surg 1985;72:495–498.

69. Feeley TW, duMoulin GC, Hedley-Whyte J, et al. Aerosol polymyxin and pneumonia in seriously ill patients. N Engl J Med 1975;293:471–475.

70. Stoutenbeek CP, Van Saene HKF, Miranda DR, et al. The effect of selective decontamination of the digestive tract on colonisation and infection rate in multiple trauma patients. Intensive Care Med 1984;10:185–192.

71. Kerver AJH, Rommes JH, Mevissen-Verhage EAE, et al. Prevention of colonization and infection in critically ill patients: a prospective randomized study. Crit Care Med 1988;16:1087–1093.

72. Ulrich C, Harinck-de Weerd HJEH, Bakker NC, et al. Selective decontamination of the digestive

tract with norfloxacin in the prevention of ICU-acquired infections: a prospective randomized study. Intensive Care Med 1989;15:424–431.

73. Pugin J, Auckenthaler R, Lew DP, et al. Oropharyngeal decontamination decreases incidence of ventilator-associated pneumonia: a randomized, placebo-controlled, double-blind clinical trial. JAMA 1991;265:2704–2710.

74. Cockerill FR, Muller SR, Anhalt JP, et al. Prevention of infection in critically ill patients by selective decontamination of the digestive tract. Ann Intern Med 1992;117:545–553.

75. Gastinne H, Wolff M, Delatour F, et al. A controlled trial in intensive care units of selective decontamination of the digestive tract with nonabsorbable antibiotics. N Engl J Med 1992;326:594–599.

76. Selective Decontamination of the Digestive Tract Trialists Collaborative Group. Meta-analysis of randomised controlled trials of selective decontamination of the digestive tract. Br Med J 1993;307:525–532.

77. Gorman S, Adair C, O'Neill F, et al. Influence of selective decontamination of the digestive tract on microbial biofilm formation of endotracheal tubes from artificially ventilated patients. Eur J Clin Microbiol Infect Dis 1993;12:9–17.

78. Centers for Disease Control and Prevention. The Hospital Infection Control Practices Advisory Committee. Guideline for prevention of nosocomial pneumonia. Part II. Recommendations for prevention of nosocomial pneumonia. Am J Infect Control 1994;22:267–292.

79. Olds JW, Kisch AL, Eberle BJ, et al. Pseudomonas aeruginosa respiratory tract infection acquired from a contaminated anesthesia machine. Am Rev Respir Dis 1972;105:628–632.

80. Ahmed J, Brutus A, D'Amato RF, et al. Acinetobacter calcoaceticus anitratus outbreak in the intensive care unit traced to a peak flow meter. Am J Infect Control 1994;22:319–321.

81. Centers for Disease Control and Prevention. Nosocomial infection and pseudoinfection from contaminated endoscopes and bronchoscopes — Wisconsin and Missouri. MMWR 1991;40:675–678.

82. Craven DE, Goularte TA, Make BJ. Contaminated condensate in mechanical ventilator circuits: a risk factor for nosocomial pneumonia? Am Rev Respir Dis 1984;129:625–628.

83. Hartstein AI, Rashad AL, Liebler JM, et al. Multiple intensive care unit outbreak of Acinetobacter calcoaceticus subspecies anitratus respiratory infection and colonization associated with contaminated, reusable ventilator circuits and resuscitation bags. Am J Med 1988;85:624–631.

84. Craven DE, Lichtenberg DA, Goularte TA, et al. Contaminated nebulizers in mechanical ventilator circuits. Am J Med 1984;77:834–838.

85. Spaulding EH. Chemical sterilization of surgical instruments. Surg Gynecol Obstet 1939;69:738–744.

86. Favero MS. Principles of sterilization and disinfection. Anesth Clin North Am 1989;7:941–949.

87. Favero MS, Bond WW. Clinical disinfection of medical and surgical materials. In: Block S, ed. Disinfec-

tion, sterilization, and preservation. 4th ed. Philadelphia: Lea & Febiger, 1991;617–641.

88. American Society of Anesthesiologists. Prevention of nosocomial infections in patients. In: Recommendations for infection control for the practice of anesthesiology. Park Ridge, IL: Society of Anesthesiologists, 1991;1–16.

89. Rutala WA. APIC guidelines for selection and use of disinfectants. Am J Infect Control 1990; 18:99–117.

90. duMoulin GC, Saubermann AJ. The anesthesia machine and circle system are not likely to be sources of bacterial contamination. Anesthesiology 1977; 47:353–358.

91. Bengtson JP, Brandberg Å, Brinkhoff B, et al. Low-flow anaesthesia does not increase the risk of microbial contamination through the circle absorber system. Acta Anaesthesiol Scand 1989;33:89–92.

92. Murphy PM, Fitzgeorge RB, Barrett RF. Viability and distribution of bacteria after passage through a circle anaesthetic system. Br J Anaesth 1991; 66:300–304.

93. Klick JM, duMoulin GC. An oxygen analyzer as a source of Pseudomonas. Anesthesiology 1978; 49:293–294.

94. Feeley TW, Hamilton WK, Xavier B, et al. Sterile anesthesia breathing circuits do not prevent postoperative pulmonary infection. Anesthesiology 1981; 54:369–372.

95. Chalon J, Chandrakant P, Ali M, et al. Humidity and the anesthetized patient. Anesthesiology 1979; 50:195–198.

96. Mebius C. Heat and moisture exchangers with bacterial filters: a laboratory evaluation. Acta Anaesthesiol Scand 1992;36:572–576.

97. Berry AJ, Nolte FS. An alternative strategy for infection control of anesthesia breathing circuits: a laboratory assessment of the Pall HME filter. Anesth Analg 1991;72:651–655.

98. Leijten DTM, Rejger VS, Mouton RP. Bacterial contamination and the effect of filters in anaesthetic circuits in a simulated patient model. J Hosp Infect 1992;21:51–60.

99. Ping FC, Oulton JL, Smith JA, et al. Bacterial filters — are they necessary on anaesthetic machines? Canad Anesth Soc J 1979;26:415–419.

100. Shiotani GM, Nicholes P, Ballinger CM, Shaw L. Prevention of contamination of the circle system and ventilators with a new disposable filter. Anesth Analg 1971;50:844–855.

101. Luttropp HH, Berntman L. Bacterial filters protect anaesthetic equipment in a low-flow system. Anaesthesia 1993;48:520–523.

102. Garibaldi RA, Britt MR, Webster C, et al. Failure of bacterial filters to reduce the incidence of pneumonia after inhalation anesthesia. Anesthesiology 1981;54:364–368.

103. McEwan AI, Dowell L, Karis JH. Bilateral tension pneumothorax caused by a blocked bacterial filter in an anesthesia breathing circuit. Anesth Analg 1993;76:440–442.

104. Centers for Disease Control and Prevention. Guidelines for preventing the transmission of Mycobacterium tuberculosis in health-care facilities, 1994. MMWR 1994;43(RR-13);1–132.

105. Hall JR. Blood contamination of anesthesia equipment and monitoring equipment. Anesth Analg 1994;78:1136–1139.

106. Comhaire A, Lamy M. Contamination rate of sterilized ventilators in an ICU. Crit Care Med 1981; 9:546–548.

107. Craven DE, Connolly MG, Lichtenberg DA, et al. Contamination of mechanical ventilators with tubing changes every 24 or 48 hours. N Engl J Med 1982;306:1505–1509.

108. Dreyfuss D, Djedaini K, Weber P, et al. Prospective study of nosocomial pneumonia and of patient and circuit colonization during mechanical ventilation with circuit changes every 48 hours vs. no change. Am Rev Respir Dis 1991;143:738–743.

109. Gallagher J, Strangeways JEM, Allt-Graham J. Contamination control in long-term ventilation: a clinical study using a heat- and moisture-exchanging filter. Anaesthesia 1987;42:476–481.

110. Deppe SA, Kelly JW, Thoi LL, et al. Incidence of colonization, nosocomial pneumonia, and mortality in critically ill patients using Trach Care closed-suction system versus open-suction system: prospective, randomized study. Crit Care Med 1990; 18:1389–1393.

111. Ritz R, Scott LR, Coyle Mb, et al. Contamination of a multiple-use suction catheter in a closed-circuit system compared to contamination of a disposable, single-use suction catheter. Respir Care 1986; 31:1087–1091.

112. Alary MA, Joly JR. Factors contributing to the contamination of hospital water distribution systems by Legionellae. J Infect Dis 1992;165:565–569.

113. Hoge CW, Breiman RF. Advances in the epidemiology and control of Legionella infections. Epidemiol Rev 1991;13:329–340.

114. Martin MA, Reichelderfer M, Association for Professionals in Infection Control and Epidemiology. APIC guideline for infection prevention and control in flexible endoscopy. Am J Infect Control 1994;22:19–38.

115. Kaczmarek RF, Moore RM, McCrohan J, et al. Multi-state investigation of the actual disinfection/ sterilization of endoscopes in health care facilities. Am J Med 1992;92:257–261.

116. Campbell BA, Wells GA, Palmer WN, et al. Reuse of disposable medical devices in Canadian hospitals. Am J Infect Control 1987;15:196–200.

117. Greene VW. Reuse of disposable medical devices: historical and current aspects. Infect Control 1986;7:508–513.

118. Haley R, Culver D, White J, et al. The nationwide nosocomial infection rate: a new need for vital statistics. Am J Epidemiol 1985;121:159–167.

119. Rutala WA, Kennedy VA, Loflin HB, et al. Serratia marcescens nosocomial infections of the urinary tract associated with urine measuring containers and urinometers. Am J Med 1981;70:659–663.

120. Platt R, Polk BF, Murdock B, et al. Mortality associated with nosocomial urinary-tract infection. N Engl J Med 1982;307:637–642.

121. van Deventer SJH, de Vries I, van Eps LWS, et al. Endotoxemia, bacteria, and urosepsis. In: Bacterial endotoxins: pathophysiological effects, clinical significance, and pharmacological control. London: Alan R. Liss, 1988;213–224.

122. Kreger BE, Craven DE, Carling PC, et al. Gram-negative bacteria. III. Reassessment of etiology, epidemiology and ecology in 612 patients. Am J Med 1980;68:332–355.

123. Daifuku R, Stamm W. Association of rectal and urethral colonization with urinary tract infection in patients with indwelling catheters. JAMA 1984; 252:2028–2030.

124. Stamm WE, Hooton TM, Johnson RJ, et al. Urinary tract infections: from pathogenesis to treatment. J Infect Dis 1989;159:400–406.

125. Cox AJ, Hukins DWL, Sutton TM. Infection of catheterized patients: bacterial colonization of encrusted Foley catheters shown by scanning electron microscopy. Urol Res 1989;17:349–352.

126. Schaeffer AJ, Story KO, Johnson SM. Effect of silver oxide/trichloroisocyanuric acid antimicrobial urinary drainage system on catheter-associated bacteriuria. J Urol 1988;139:69–73.

127. Thompson RL, Haley CE, Searcy MA, et al. Catheter-associated bacteriuria: failure to reduce attack rates using periodic instillations of a disinfectant into urinary drainage systems. JAMA 1984; 251:747–751.

128. Britt MR, Garibaldi RA, Miller WA, et al. Antimicrobial prophylaxis for catheter-associated bacteriuria. Antimicrob Agents Chemother 1977;11:240–243.

129. Platt R, Murdock B, Polk BF, et al. Reduction of mortality associated with nosocomial urinary tract infection. Lancet 1983;1:1893–1897.

130. Garibaldi RA, Burke JP, Britt MR, et al. Meatal colonization and catheter-associated bacteriuria. N Engl J Med 1980;303:316–318.

131. Mobley HLT, Chippendale GR, Tenney JH, et al. MR/K hemagglutination of providencia stuartii correlates with catheter adherence and with persistence in catheter-associated bacteriuria. J Infect Dis 1988;157:264–271.

132. Banerjee SN, Emori TG, Culver DH, et al. Secular trends in nosocomial primary bloodstream infections in the United States, 1980-1989. Am J Med 1991;91(Suppl 3B):86S–89S.

133. Stamm WE. Infections related to medical devices. Ann Intern Med 1978;89:764–769.

134. Maki DG, Rhame FS, Mackel DC, et al. Nationwide epidemic of septicemia caused by contaminated intravenous products. I. Epidemiologic and clinical features. Am J Med 1976;60:471–485.

135. Maki DG, Anderson RL, Shulman JA. In-use contamination of intravenous infusion fluid. Appl Microbiol 1974;28:778–784.

136. Cooper Gl, Schiller AL, Hopkins CC. Possible role of capillary action in pathogenesis of experimental catheter-associated dermal tunnel infections. J Clin Microbiol 1988;26:8–12.

137. Maki DG, Weise CE, Sasafin HW. A semiquantitative culture method for identifying intravenous-catheter-related infection. N Engl J Med 1977; 296:1305–1309.

138. Maki DG. Infections due to infusion therapy. In: Bennett JV, Brachman PS, eds. Hospital infections. 3rd ed. Boston: Little, Brown, and Co., 1992; 849–898.

139. Maki DG, Cobb L, Garman JK, et al. An attachable silver-impregnated cuff for prevention of infection with central venous catheters: a prospective randomized multicenter trial. Am J Med 1988; 85:307–314.

140. Maki DG, Ringer M. Risk factors for infusion-related phlebitis with small peripheral venous catheters: a randomized controlled trial. Ann Intern Med 1991;114:845–854.

141. Farkas JC, Liu N, Bleriot JP, et al. Single- versus triple-lumen central catheter-related sepsis: a prospective randomized study in a critically ill population. Am J Med 1992;93:277–282.

142. Wormser GP, Onorato IM, Preminger TJ, et al. Sensitivity and specificity of blood cultures obtained through intravascular catheters. Crit Care Med 1990;18:152–156.

143. Raad II, Luna M, Khalil SAM, et al. The relationship between the thrombotic and infectious complications of central venous catheters. JAMA 1994; 271:1014–1016.

144. Rupp ME, Archer GL. Hemagglutination and adherence to plastic by Staphyloccus epidermidis. Infect Immunity 1992;60:4322–4327.

145. Tomford JW, Hershey CO. The IV therapy team. Impact on patient care and costs of hospitalization. NITA 1985;8:387.

146. Mermel LA, McCormick RD, Springman SR, et al. The pathogenesis and epidemiology of catheter-related infection with pulmonary artery Swan-Ganz catheters: a prospective study utilizing molecular subtyping. Am J Med 1991;91(Suppl B):197S–205S.

147. Maki DG, Alvarado CJ, Ringer M. A prospective, randomized trial of povidone-iodine, alcohol and chlorhexidine for prevention of infection with central venous and arterial catheters. Lancet 1991; 338:339.

148. Rannem R, et al. Catheter-related sepsis in long-term parenteral nutrition with Broviac catheters. An evaluation of different disinfectants. Clin Nutr 1990;9:131.

149. Flowers RH, Schwenzer KJ, Kopel RF, et al. Efficacy of an attachable subcutaneous cuff for the prevention of intravascular catheter-related infection: a randomized, controlled trial. JAMA 1989; 261:878–883.

150. Maki DG, Ringer M. Evaluation of dressing regimens for prevention of infection with peripheral intravenous catheters: gauze, a transparent polyurethane dressing, and an iodophor-transparent dressing. JAMA 1987;258:2396–2403.

151. Hoffmann KK, Weber DJ, Samsa GP, et al. Transparent polyurethane film as an intravenous catheter dressing: a meta-analysis of the infection risks. JAMA 1992;267:2072–2076.

152. Conly JM, Grieves K, Peters B. A prospective, randomized study comparing transparent and dry

gauze dressings for central venous catheters. J Infect Dis 1989;159:310–319.

153. Galloway JR, Hooks MA, Millikan WJ. Catheter-related sepsis. Anesth Clin N Am 1989;7:827–844.

154. Kamal GD, Pfaller MA, Rempe LE, et al. Reduced intravascular catheter infection by antibiotic bonding: a prospective, randomized, controlled trial. JAMA 1991;265:2364–2368.

155. Bach A, Böhrer H, Motsch J, et al. Prevention of catheter-related infections by antiseptic bonding. J Surg Res 1993;55:640–646.

156. Centers for Disease Control. Postsurgical infections associated with an extrinsically contaminated intravenous anesthetic agent — California, Illinois, Maine, and Michigan, 1990. MMWR 1990; 39:426–433.

157. Arduino MJ, Bland LA, McAllister SK, et al. Microbial growth and endotoxin production in the intravenous anesthetic propofol. Infect Control Hosp Epidemiol 1991;12:535–539.

158. Sosis MB, Braverman B. Growth of Staphylococcus aureus in four intravenous anesthetics. Anesth Analg 1993;77:766–768.

159. Zacher AN, Zornow MH, Evans G. Drug contamination from opening glass ampules. Anesthesiology 1991;75:893–895.

160. Oren I, Hershow RC, Ben-Porath E, et al. A common-source outbreak of fulminant hepatitis B in a hospital. Ann Intern Med 1989;110:691–698.

161. Schubert A, Hyams KC, Longfield RN. Sterility of anesthetic multiple-dose vials after opening. Anesthesiology 1985;62:634–636.

162. Highsmith AK, Greenhood GP, Allen JR. Growth of nosocomial pathogens in multiple-dose parenteral medication vials. J Clin Microbiol 1982; 15:1024–1028.

163. Sheth NK, Post GT, Wisniewski TR, Uttech BV. Multidose vials versus single-dose vials: a study in sterility and cost-effectiveness. J Clin Microbiol 1983;17:377–379.

164. Plott RT, Waggner RF, Trying SK. Iatrogenic contamination of multidose vials in simulated use: a reassessment of current patient injection technique. Arch Dermatol 1990;126:1441–1444.

165. Koepke JW, Reller B, Masters HA, et al. Viral contamination of intradermal skin test syringes. Ann Allergy 1985;55:776–778.

166. Trépanier CA, Lessard MR, Brochu JG, et al. Risk of cross-infection related to the multiple use of disposable syringes. Can J Anaesth 1990;37:156–159.

167. Huey WY, Newton DW, Augustine SC, et al. Microbial contamination potential of sterile disposable plastic syringes. Am J Hosp Pharm 1985;42:102–105.

168. Dryden GE, Brickler J. Stopcock contamination. Anesth Analg 1979;58:141–142.

169. Maki DG, Botticelli JT, LeRoy ML, et al. Prospective study of replacing administration sets for intravenous therapy at 48- vs. 72-hour intervals: 72 hours is safe and cost-effective. JAMA 1987; 258:1777–1781.

170. Freeman J, Goldmann DA, Smith NE, et al. Association of intravenous lipid emulsion and coagulase-negative staphylococcal bacteremia in neonatal intensive care units. N Engl J Med 1990;323:301–308.

171. Weinstein RA, Emori TG, Anderson RW, et al. Pressure transducers as a source of bacteremia after open heart surgery: report of an outbreak and guidelines for prevention. Chest 1976;69:338–344.

172. Luskin RL, Weinstein RA, Nathan C, et al. Extended use of disposable pressure transducers: a bacteriologic evaluation. JAMA 1986;255:916–920.

173. Beck-Sague O, Dooley SW, Hutton MD, et al. Outbreak of multidrug-resistant Mycobacterium tuberculosis infections in a hospital: transmission to patients with HIV infection and staff. JAMA 1992;268:1280–1286.

174. Catanzaro A. Nosocomial tuberculosis. Am Rev Respir Dis 1982;125:559–562.

175. Ehrenkranz NJ, Kicklighter JL. Tuberculosis outbreak in a general hospital: evidence of airborne spread of infection. Ann Intern Med 1972; 77:377–382.

176. Centers for Disease Control. Tuberculosis morbidity — United States, 1992. MMWR 1993;42:696.

177. Goble M, Iseman MD, Madsen LA, et al. Treatment of 171 patients with pulmonary tuberculosis resistant to isoniazid and rifampin. N Engl J Med 1993;328:527–532.

178. American Thoracic Society/Centers for Disease Control. Diagnostic standards and classification of tuberculosis. Am Rev Respir Dis 1990;142:725–735.

179. Selwyn PA, Hartel D, Lewis VA, et al. A prospective study of the risk of tuberculosis among intravenous drug users with human immunodeficiency virus infection. N Engl J Med 1989;320:545–550.

180. Centers for Disease Control. Guidelines for preventing the transmission of tuberculosis in healthcare settings, with special focus on HIV-related issues. MMWR 1990;39(RR-17):1–29.

181. Centers for Disease Control and Prevention. Draft guideline for isolation precautions in hospitals. Federal Register 1994;59:55552–55570.

182. Nardell EA. Fans, filters, or rays? Pros and cons of the current environmental tuberculosis control technologies. Infect Control Hosp Epidemiol 1993;14:681–685.

183. Rosenstock L. 42 CFR Part 84: Respiratory protective devices: implications for tuberculosis protection. Infect Control Hosp Epidemiol 1995; 16:529–531.

184. National Institute for Occupational Safety and Health. Centers for Disease Control and Prevention. Respiratory protective devices (42 CFR Part 84). Federal Register 1995;60:30336–30398.

185. Hall CB, Douglas RG, Geiman JM. Possible transmission by fomites of respiratory syncytial virus. J Infect Dis 1980;141:98–102.

186. Agah R, Cherry JD, Garakian AJ, et al. Respiratory syncytial virus (RSV) infection rate in personnel caring for children with RSV infections: routine isolation procedure vs routine procedure supplemented by use of masks and goggles. Am J Dis Child 1987;141:695–697.

187. Leclair JM, Freeman J, Sullivan BF, et al. Prevention of nosocomial respiratory syncytial virus infections through compliance with glove and gown isolation precautions. N Engl J Med 1987;317:329–334.

188. Isaacs D, Dickson H, O'Callaghan C, et al. Hand-washing and cohorting in prevention of hospital acquired infections with respiratory syncytial virus. Arch Dis Child 1991;66:227–231.

189. Groothuis JR, Simoes EAF, Levin MJ, et al. Prophylactic administration of respiratory syncytial virus immune globulin to high-risk infants and young children. N Engl J Med 1993;329:1524–1530.

190. Berry AJ, Greene ES. The risk of needlestick injuries and needlestick-transmitted diseases in the practice of anesthesiology. Anesthesiology 1992;77:1007–1021.

191. Tait AR, Tuttle BD. Prevention of occupational transmission of human immunodeficiency virus and hepatitis B virus among anesthesiologists: a survey of anesthesiology practice. Anesth Analg 1994; 79:623–638.

192. Maz DA, Lyons G. Needlestick injuries in anaesthetists. Anaesthesia 1990;45:677–678.

193. Kristensen MS, Sloth E, Jensen TK. Relationship between anesthetic procedure and contact of anesthesia personnel with patient body fluids. Anesthesiology 1990;73:619–624.

194. Centers for Disease Control. Guidelines for prevention of transmission of human immunodeficiency virus and hepatitis B virus to health-care and public safety workers. MMWR 1989;38(S-6):3–37.

195. Berry AJ, Isaacson IJ, Kane MA, et al. A multicenter study of the prevalence of hepatitis B viral serologic markers in anesthesia personnel. Anesth Analg 1984;63:738–742.

196. Berry AJ, Isaacson IJ, Kane MA, et al. A multicenter study of the epidemiology of hepatitis B in anesthesia residents. Anesth Analg 1985;64:672–676.

197. Fyman PN, Hartung J, Weinberg S, et al. Prevalence of hepatitis B markers in the anesthesia staff of a large inner-city hospital. Anesth Analg 1984; 63:433–436.

198. Buergler JM, Kim R, Thisted RA, et al. Risk of human immunodeficiency virus in surgeons, anesthesiologists, and medical students. Anesth Analg 1992;75:118–124.

199. Alter MJ, Hadler SC, Margolis HS, et al. The changing epidemiology of hepatitis B in the United States, need for alternative vaccination strategies. JAMA 1990;263:1218–1222.

200. Centers for Disease Control. Protection against viral hepatitis: recommendations of the Immunization Practices Advisory Committee (ACIP). MMWR 1990;39(RR-2):1–26.

201. Wood RC, MacDonald KL, White KE, et al. Risk factors for lack of detectable antibody following hepatitis B vaccination of Minnesota health care workers. JAMA 1993;270:2935–2939.

202. Strickler AC, Pavone ED. Hepatitis B immunization: effect of 4th and 5th injections following suboptimal seroconversion in health care workers. Can J Pub Health 1987;78:315–317.

203. Alter MJ. Hepatitis C: a sleeping giant? Am J Med 1991;91(Suppl 3B):112S–115S.

204. Donahue JG, Muñoz A, Ness PM, et al. The declining risk of post-transfusion hepatitis C virus infection. N Engl J Med 1992;327:369–373.

205. Alter MJ, Hadler SC, Judson FN, et al. Risk factors for acute non-A, non-B hepatitis in the United States and association with hepatitis C virus infection. JAMA 1990;264:2231–2235.

206. Alter MJ, Margolis HS, Krawczynski K, et al. The natural history of community-acquired hepatitis C in the United States. N Engl J Med 1992; 327:1899–1905.

207. Farci P, Alter HJ, Wong D, et al. A long-term study of hepatitis C virus replication in non-A, non-B hepatitis. N Engl J Med 1991;325:98–104.

208. Farci P, Alter HJ, Govindarajan S, et al. Lack of protective immunity against reinfection with hepatitis C virus. Science 1992;258:135–140.

209. Kiyosawa K, Sodeyama T, Tanaka E, et al. Hepatitis C in hospital employees with needlestick injuries. Ann Intern Med 1991;115:367–369.

210. Cooper BW, Drusell A, Tilton RC, et al. Seroprevalence of antibodies to hepatitis C virus in high-risk hospital personnel. Infect Control Hosp Epidemiol 1992;13:82–85.

211. Hofmann H, Kunz C. Low risk of health care workers for infection with hepatitis C virus. Infection 1991;18:286–288.

212. Centers for Disease Control and Prevention. HIV/AIDS surveillance report. 1995;7:1–27.

213. Marcus R, and the CDC Cooperative Needlestick Surveillance Group. Surveillance on health care workers exposed to blood from patients infected with the human immunodeficiency virus. N Engl J Med 1988;319:1118–1123.

214. Centers for Disease Control. Public Health Service statement on management of occupational exposure to human immunodeficiency virus including consideration regarding zidovudine postexposure use. MMWR 1990;39(RR-1):1–14.

215. Daar EX, Moudgh T, Meyer RD, et al. Transient high levels of viremia in patients with primary human immunodeficiency virus type 1 infection. N Engl J Med 1991;324:961–964.

216. Shirazian D, Herzlich BC, Mokhtarian F, et al. Needlestick injury: blood, mononuclear cells, and acquired immunodeficiency syndrome. Am J Infect Control 1992;20:133–137.

217. Bennett NT, Howard RT. Quantity of blood inoculated in a needlestick injury from suture needles. J Am Coll Surg 1994;178:107–110.

218. Mast ST, Woolwine JD, Gerberding JL. Efficacy of gloves in reducing blood volumes transferred during simulated needlestick injury. J Infect Dis 1993;168:1589–1592.

219. Berry AJ. Are some types of needles more likely to transmit HIV to health care workers? (letter). Am J Infect Control 1993;21:216–217.

220. Henderson DK, Fahey BJ, Willy M, et al. Risk for occupational transmission of human immunodeficiency virus type 1 (HIV-1) associated with clinical exposures. Ann Intern Med 1990;113:740–746.

221. Wong ES, Stotka JL, Chinchilli VM, et al. Are universal precautions effective in reducing the number of occupational exposures among health care work-

ers? A prospective study of physicians on a medical service. JAMA 1991;265:1123–1128.

222. Becker MH, Janz NK, Band J, et al. Noncompliance with universal precautions policy: why do physicians and nurses recap needles? Am J Infect Control 1990;18:232–239.

223. Kelen GB, Fritz S Qaqish B, et al. Unrecognized human immunodeficiency virus infection in emergency department patients. N Engl J Med 1988;318:1645–1650.

224. Gerberding JL, Littell C, Tarkington A, et al. Risk of exposure of surgical personnel to patients blood during surgery at San Francisco General Hospital. N Engl J Med 1990;322:1788–1793.

225. Berry AJ. The use of needles in the practice of anesthesiology and the effect of a needleless intravenous administration system. Anesth Analg 1993;76:1114–1119.

226. Jagger J, Hunt EH, Brand-Elnaggar J, et al. Rates of needle-stick injury caused by various devices in a university hospital. N Engl J Med 1988; 319:284–288.

227. Laufer FN, Chiarello LA. Application of cost-effectiveness methodology to the consideration of needlestick-prevention technology. Am J Infect Control 1994;22:75–82.

228. Larson EL, Cheng G, Choo JTE, et al. In vitro survival of skin flora in heparin locks and needleless valve infusion devices. Heart & Lung 1993; 22:459–462.

229. Stock SR, Gafni A, Bloch RF. Universal precautions to prevent HIV transmission to health care workers: an economic analysis. Can Med Assoc J 1990; 142:937–946.

230. Brumfit W, Hamilton-Miller J. Methicillin-resistant Staphlococcus aureus. N Engl J Med 1989; 320:1188–1196.

231. Tomasz A. Multiple-antibiotic-resistant pathogenic bacteria. A report on the Rockefeller University Workshop. N Engl J Med 1994;330:1247–1251.

232. Centers for Disease Control and Prevention. Recommendations for preventing the spread of vancomycin resistance. Hospital Infection Control Practices Committee (HICPAC). Infect Control Hosp Epidemiol 1995;16:105–113.

233. Hall JR. Blood contamination of anesthesia equipment and monitoring equipment. Anesth Analg 1994;78:11346–11349.

234. Sussman GL, Tarlo S, Dolovich J. The spectrum of IgE-mediated responses to latex. JAMA 1991;265:2844–2847.

235. Arellano R, Bradley J, Sussman G. Prevalence of latex sensitization among hospital physicians occupationally exposed to latex gloves. Anesthesiology 1992;77:905–908.

236. Hirshman CA. Latex anaphylaxis (editorial). Anesthesiology 1992;77:223–225.

237. Gerber AC, Jörg W, Zbinden S, et al. Severe intraoperative anaphylaxis to surgical gloves: latex allergy, an unfamiliar condition. Anesthesiology 1989;71:800–802.

13

THERMOREGULATION IN THE POSTOPERATIVE PATIENT

Gary Okum, Henry Rosenberg

This chapter focuses on the regulation of body temperature in the postoperative patient and the mechanisms leading to altered heat generation and dissipation in the anesthetized patient. The adverse consequences of altered body temperature will be enumerated to demonstrate the importance of meticulous attention to thermal conservation. The physiologic thermoregulatory responses will also be discussed, in addition to techniques of augmenting heat conservation or dissipation.

NORMAL THERMOREGULATION

Core temperature is normally maintained within a very narrow range +/–0.2°C of the individual's baseline temperature. The maintenance of temperature is an extraordinarily complex neuroregulatory response consisting of afferent input, central modulation, and efferent responses.

Afferent thermal input is provided principally by A delta fibers, which are responsible for cold sensation, and C fibers, which are responsible for heat sensation. As with pain and other sensory pathways, the afferent impulses for temperature travel primarily through the spinothalamic tract. Although the integumentary system provides most of the environmental contact, the central tissues such as the thorax, abdomen, and neuraxis provide the most input.

Satinoff postulated a caudal-to-rostral hierarchy in which lower centers such as the spinal cord are modulated by more sophisticated rostral centers (1). This is likely because the thermoregulatory response incorporates neural pathways also used for other vital homeostatic functions, including modulation of vascular tone in response to blood pressure fluctuation and muscular control of posture. In man, the most precise central control of temperature originates in the preoptic region of the hypothalamus. This region, in turn, receives input from other areas of the brain, as well as the aforementioned peripheral input. Although much remains unknown about the exact mechanism of temperature regulation, it is apparent that over a narrow range of core temperatures (approximately 0.2°C either side of baseline) there is no activation of heat-conserving or heat-wasting mechanisms.

As temperature deviates further from the setpoint, different compensatory responses initiate in sequence. As the perturbation becomes more extreme, additional mechanisms are recruited and the ongoing mechanisms become more intense. The thermoregulatory window may be defined by the range in temperature separating the initial response to hypothermia (vasoconstriction) from the initial response to hyperthermia (sweating, vasodilation). The degree of temperature control required by homeotherms mandates that the thermoregulatory window be narrow and that responses to thermal perturbations be prompt and effective. Whereas the responses to temperature alteration occur in a defined and predictable sequence, and there seems to be roughly a 0.2°C "thermoregulatory window," the exact temperature range in which this regulation occurs varies by gender, diurnally, and even over the course of the menstrual cycle. The diurnal effect is such that core temperature increases approximately 0.1°C from the time of awakening until approximately 3 pm, at which point the process reverses. The menstrual effect is superimposed upon this so that temperatures average 0.5°C lower from the onset of menses until ovulation. Despite the variability in setpoint, the response cascade remains the same for all humans. The degree of responsiveness to a given change in temperature from the setpoint is less in extremes of age, thus rendering the very young and the elderly more susceptible to environmentally induced temperature changes. Goldberg and Roe showed that the degree of difficulty in maintaining core temperature during anesthesia is age related (2).

There are several mechanisms employed by the human body to maintain temperature. Initial responses are primarily behavioral and, of course, may not be seen in patients emerging from general anesthesia. The second tier response involves nonshivering thermogenesis and vasoconstriction in the case of hypothermia and sweating and vasodilatation in hyperthermia. Finally, shivering is seen in response to profound hypothermia.

Behavioral responses to altered temperature need no discussion here other than to emphasize that they exceed the combined capabilities of the autonomic responses. This should heighten the awareness of the practitioner whose patient is rendered incapable of the behavioral response for whatever reason.

In the case of central hypothermia, the first response seen is constriction of arteriovenous shunts. A reduction of core temperature by as little as 0.1 to 0.2°C at constant skin temperature will trigger constriction of these shunts, which are found mainly in fingers and toes. Despite their small diameter (approximately 100 microns), their large number ensures that even slight reduction of blood flow will result

in tremendous heat sparing effect. This response is largely mediated by peripheral α-adrenergic fibers, but the degree of alpha response is largely centrally mediated. Only at extreme peripheral temperatures is this response primarily locally mediated (e.g., frostbite in a patient whose central temperature is maintained while proper extremity protection is not used). Although reduction in blood flow via arteriovenous shunts is more important, reduction in capillary flow can be an important contributor to heat conservation. Sessler et al. induced hypothermia in volunteers previously vasodilated in a hot environment and demonstrated that the hands and feet contributed disproportionately to the total heat loss compared to arms, legs, trunk, and head (3) (Figures 13–1 and 13–2).

Nonshivering thermogenesis is not an important mechanism for heat production in adult humans although it is significant in infants, in whom the use of brown fat allows for a doubling of metabolic heat production. The minimal nonshivering thermogenesis seen in adult humans is mainly believed to occur in skeletal muscle.

Shivering is the primary nonbehaviorally induced mechanism for heat production in adults. Heat production may increase sixfold in the presence of adequate muscle mass, although a twofold to threefold increase is more typical. The temperature threshold for shivering is roughly a full degree Celsius below that for vasoconstriction assuming constant skin temperature. If skin temperature decreases, however, shivering will occur at a higher core temperature than if skin temperature were held constant.

Akin to vasoconstriction, sweating is very precisely regulated. A core temperature increase of 0.1 to 0.2°C in the presence of a constant skin temperature will reliably trigger sweating. Sweating is a function of postganglionic sympathetic neurons that, unlike all other postganglionic sympathetic fibers, are mediated by cholinergic pathways. The response is severely inhibited by atropine and enhanced by anticholinesterases. A typical patient may

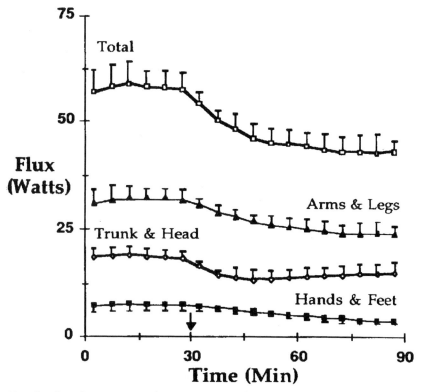

Fig. 13–1. Heat flux from the ten measured sites were grouped to incorporate losses from the head trunk (head, back, chest, and abdomen); legs and arms (upper arm, lower arm, thigh, and calf); and hands and feet. Total heat flux from the arms and legs decreased ~25% after infusion of cold fluid (arrow). Heat loss from the trunk and head decreased only 17%; in contrast, loss from the hands and feet decreased 60%. All values obtained for epochs > 35 min differed significantly from control. Heat losses indicated in the lower three curves (arms and legs; trunk and head; hands and feet) comprise the total loss indicated at the top of the figure.

sweat up to 1 L/hour, whereas an athlete may sweat twice as much. However, sweating does not dissipate heat; instead, it is the evaporation of sweat. Thus, the nearer the relative humidity to 100%, the less efficient the sweating mechanism becomes, as anyone who has been exposed to summer in the eastern United States will attest. Assuming that the operating room environment is dry, as it usually is, the evaporative process is extremely efficient. Each gram of water evaporated from the skin will remove 0.58 kcal of heat (the latent heat of vaporization of water). Thus, in a dry environment, up to 10 times basal heat production may be dissipated.

Active vasodilation of the precapillary beds may tremendously increase skin blood flow to values approximating a normal resting cardiac output. This enlarges the interface between core blood and the periphery, thus promoting additional heat loss via sweating and conduction. The vasodilatory response to hyperthermia seems to be mediated by a nonadrenergic factor.

THERMOREGULATION DURING GENERAL ANESTHESIA

All anesthetics decrease the threshold for vasoconstriction. For isoflurane, this decrease is 3°C/percent isoflurane (4). Typical doses of other inhalational agents and nitrous-oxide/fentanyl will lower the threshold to approxi-

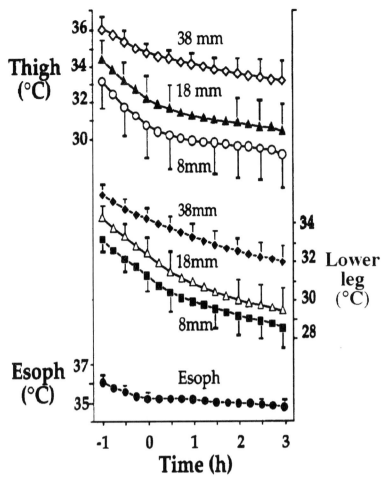

Fig. 13–2. Thigh and lower leg tissue temperatures continued to decrease after the core temperature reached a plateau indicating that body heat content also continued to decrease. In contrast, esophageal temperature remained nearly constant after constriction. Elapsed time of zero indicates calf minus toe, skin-temperature gradient of 0° C. Alternate error bars were omitted for clarity. All muscle temperatures differed significantly from values at the time of vasoconstriction at elapsed time before −0.25 h and after +0.5 h. In contrast core temperatures (Esoph) differed signficantly from values at the time of vasoconstriction before −15 h and after +1.75 h.

mately 34.5°C. A propofol/nitrous-oxide anesthetic seems to lower the threshold even more (5). When the vasoconstrictor response is triggered, it seems to proceed with the same intensity as in a nonanesthetized patient.

In adults, the shivering threshold is substantially lower than the vasoconstriction threshold. Shivering is almost never seen in surgical planes of anesthesia, regardless of the degree of hypothermia. However, if the anesthetic effect dissipates before the restoration of normothermia, shivering will occur. The implications and treatment of this common problem will be detailed later.

The sweat response is inhibited by anesthetics, but not nearly as much as the vasoconstrictive response. One MAC of isoflurane will increase the sweating threshold to 38.2°C while it decreases the vasoconstriction threshold to 33°C. This helps to explain the lower incidence of intraoperative hyperthermia versus hypothermia. Of course, there are several well-documented disease states (e.g., thyroid storm, malignant hyperthermia) that may be life threatening and may be manifested by hyperthermia intraoperatively and during the early postoperative stage. When the sweating threshold is reached in the anesthetized patient, the response is no different in intensity than in the awake patient. Because sweating does not occur in anesthetized infants, they are particularly at risk for intraoperative overheating.

The vasodilatory response to hyperthermia begins at a higher temperature in the anesthetized patient, but as with the other responses to temperature disturbance, the response seems to be fully intact after it is triggered.

HEAT BALANCE DURING GENERAL ANESTHESIA

Whereas core temperature is nearly constant in the unanesthetized patient, the same cannot be said for peripheral temperatures. The peripheral tissues act as a first-line thermal buffer. There can be as much as a 5°C gradient between core and peripheral tissues owing to vasoconstriction. Roughly 150 kcal of heat can be lost from the periphery or gained into the periphery before core temperature is affected. The patient under general anesthesia loses the ability to guard against heat gain from or loss to the environment due to anesthetic-induced alterations in the central nervous system (CNS) and peripheral vasculature.

HEAT TRANSFER

Heat is gained or lost through four processes: evaporation, conduction, convection, and radiation. Although heat may be gained or lost through any of these mechanisms, the transfer of heat must follow any existing gradient. Because the operating room environment is always cooler than the patient, the general heat budget will favor loss to the environment.

Heat loss via radiation is proportional to the fourth power of the temperature gradient. However, because in a thermodynamic sense (i.e., degrees Kelvin), the difference between skin and room temperature is minimal, matters are simplified by considering radiated heat loss proportional to temperature gradient from skin to surroundings.

Heat loss via conduction is proportional to temperature gradient as well, but another factor must be considered — the conductivity of the substance adjacent to the skin. Air is a relatively poor conductor of heat, whereas water and metal can conduct tremendous amounts of heat from the patient.

Whereas still air is a relatively poor conductor of heat from the patient, convective heat loss refers to the transfer of heat from the patient via *moving* air. The heat loss is proportional to the square root of the air speed. It should be apparent that the high air flow used in a typical operating room will promote convective heat loss and the very-high-flow laminar flow units used in some settings, such as the orthopedic operating room will promote even greater losses.

Evaporative heat loss normally results in about 10% of total body heat loss. This tends to increase in the surgical patient from three sources: the evaporation of surgical preparation solutions, the unheated gases used to ventilate most patients, and the added surface area exposed by exteriorizing such large surface area regions as the peritoneum and pleura. Still, evaporative heat loss is not a large factor in perioperative hypothermia.

The *major* etiologic factor in intraoperative hypothermia is the anesthesia-induced alteration of vasomotor tone resulting in the loss of the ability of the peripheral tissues to buffer the central core from the combined effects of the environment. This is evidenced by the fact that during the first hour under a general anesthetic, core temperature decreases 0.5 to 1.5°C followed by a much slower decrease over the next 2 to 3 hours. Because this is the primary etiologic factor in anesthesia-induced heat loss, it stands to reason that hypothermia will be a potential problem in any patient undergoing general anesthesia, whether the procedure is brief or prolonged and whether the procedure involves a surgical preparation, unless the patient has been "preheated."

In cases lasting longer than 1 hour, there is a slow, linear decrease in core temperature that results from the inability of metabolic heat production to match environmental losses. Although there is a decline in metabolic heat production in the patient undergoing general anesthesia, the loss to the environment is a more important etiologic factor. Factors such as low room temperature, high air flow, evaporation from the wound, and cold intravenous solutions primarily account for this slow, steady heat loss.

The limit to this temperature decline for most patients seems to be at approximately 34.5°C, which is the temperature at which vasoconstriction will initially occur. The vasoconstriction ensures that relatively little blood reaches the skin for loss to the environment and also permits the limited metabolic heat produced to remain confined to the smaller area represented by the core tissues. However, the clinician must not be misled by this new thermal plateau, as the peripheral temperatures continue to decline, reestablishing the normal core to periphery temperature gradient with lower temperatures. The ability of small children to initiate nonshivering thermogenesis may allow significant warming to occur without external assistance.

Although discussion so far has centered general anesthesia, patients undergoing major conduction anesthesia are far from immune to the problem of perioperative hypothermia. Core temperature may decrease as much as 2.5°C in the patient undergoing regional anesthesia. The hypothermia will usually resolve as the block dissipates. Unfortunately, this degree in hypothermia may go unrecognized because of the invasiveness of most intraoperative temperature-measuring devices and resulting unsuitability for the awake patient. Although hypothermia may be more difficult to detect in the patient undergoing regional anesthesia, it is no less harmful. Reflex vasoconstriction is seen above the level of the block, and shivering may contribute to increased oxygen extraction, decreased arterial saturation, and substantially increased myocardial oxygen consumption as seen in the patient emerging from general anesthesia (6). Although this heat loss was once believed to be caused solely by vasodilation in the anesthetized areas, Hynson et al. showed in volunteers given epidural anesthesia that skin temperature increased, core temperature decreased, and heat loss to the environment increased minimally. Heat production actually increased because of shivering. The fall in core temperature despite increased heat production and minimal heat loss is explained by heat redistribution within the body. The unanesthetized patient will constrict cutaneous blood flow, restricting metabolic heat to the central core to prevent environmental heat loss. As the ability to constrict cutaneous blood vessels is lost in the region of the block, heat redistributes to the skin and core temperature falls despite minimal change in total body heat (7).

Although it would be expected that the awake patient could complain if rendered cold by regional anesthesia, it has been shown that there is no clear relationship between core temperature and thermal sensation. Perception of temperature is mainly a function of input from the skin, although details of the mechanism remain unknown (8). Epidural opioids also have been associated with perioperative hypothermia (9).

TEMPERATURE MEASUREMENT IN THE PERIOPERATIVE PATIENT

Body temperature is routinely measured via oral, axillary, rectal, esophageal, nasopharyngeal, urinary, intravascular (e.g., Swan-Ganz), or tympanic membrane probes. Each method has its drawbacks. The oral and axillary approaches are influenced by the temperature of surrounding air. The lower extreme of typical oral probes is 34°C, so that the severity of hypothermia may not be evident. Rectal temperatures tend to be slow in reacting to rapid temperature fluxes and may be insulated by feces. Distal esophageal probes are quite accurate but impractical in the awake patient and nasopharyngeal probes carry the minimal risk of epistaxis. Foley catheter probes are reliable but are only useful if the patient requires catheterization. Tympanic membrane temperatures are highly reflective of brain temperature, but otic trauma is possible with repeated measurements. Less invasive aural temperature-measurement devices are now available. Pulmonary artery probes may be influenced by the temperature of inspired gases.

NONANESTHETIC-RELATED FACTORS PREDISPOSING HYPOTHERMIA

Many causes exist for hypothermia in the postoperative patient. Burns are a significant predisposing factor because, despite increased metabolic heat production, patients whose burns exceed 20% of body surface area will often lose sufficient heat via the disrupted integumentary system, causing clinically significant hypothermia. Patients with impaired myocardial function are at special risk because the usual compensatory responses to hypothermia require increased cardiac output, which may not be possible. These patients also may be unusually susceptible to ventricular irritability and myocardial ischemia. Patients with CNS lesions may be at added risk if the lesion influences the hypothalamic regulatory centers.

The intoxicated patient may suffer from hypothermia because alcohol causes vasodilation and suppresses shivering and hepatic gluconeogenesis. Therefore, increased heat loss and decreased heat production from shivering and gluconeogenesis will occur. Similarly, malnourished patients are also at risk.

Patients with endocrine disorders affecting metabolic heat production are at added risk for hypothermia, as are septic patients. In sepsis, impairment of gluconeogenesis will decrease metabolic heat production, and endotoxin-induced vasodilation will enhance heat loss. The presence of hypothermia in the septic patient is an ominous sign (10).

Hypothermia in trauma patients is a serious problem. This is evidenced by increased attention in the Advanced Trauma Life Support Manual of the American College of Surgeons (11).

Patients at extremes of age are more likely than other patients to suffer from perioperative hypothermia. Pediatric patients are at added risk because of their disproportionately high ratio of body surface area to body mass, which increases susceptibility to convective and radiational heat loss. This is especially true of neonatal patients. The neonatal patient is unique, however, in its ability to increase heat production up to 100% through sympathetic stimulation of brown fat for nonshivering thermogenesis. The vasoconstrictive threshold differs little between pediatric and adult patients (12). Elderly patients are at increased risk of hypothermia for several reasons. The basal rate of metabolic heat production under anesthesia decreases with age, such that the 80-year-old patient produces 10% less heat under general anesthesia than the 40-year-old patient (13). Muscle mass decreases with age, thereby reducing the contribution of shivering to thermogenesis. In addition, the use of neuromuscular blockers in the postoperative patient requiring ventilation will decrease the metabolic heat production from muscle. Poor nutritional status, often seen in elderly patients, results in hypoproteinemia and lack of energy producing substrates (14). In the cachectic patient, the loss of body mass leads to an increased ratio of surface area to body mass as in the infant, with the same consequences. Concomitant disease states reducing heat production include hypothyroidism, hypoadrenalism, diabetes mellitus, congestive heart failure, and severe hepatic dysfunction. In peripheral vascular disease, the already cool extremities are rendered even cooler during anesthesia, leading to even greater heat transfer from the body core (13). In addition, the type of anesthesia may affect the risk of hypothermia in elderly patients (15).

HYPOTHERMIA IN THE POSTSURGICAL PATIENT

Now that the normal physiologic mechanisms governing temperature regulation in the awake and anesthetized patient have been reviewed, along with potential concomitant factors, attention will turn to the patient recovering from anesthesia. In these patients, the ability to autoregulate temperature may be fully or partially intact. An understanding of the consequences of hypothermia will emphasize to the clinician the need to return the patient to a thermally neutral state. Hypothermia is defined as a core temperature of less than 36°C.

CONSEQUENCES OF HYPOTHERMIA

The consequences of hypothermia depend on the degree of heat loss, duration of hypothermia, and underlying conditions. The initial effects on the cardiovascular system include elevation of plasma catecholamine levels, increased heart rate, peripheral vasoconstriction, increased central blood volume, and a resultant increase in cardiac output, systemic vascular resistance and mean arterial blood pressure. As hypothermia becomes more severe, bradycardia and decreased myocardial contractility are seen. At 32 to 33°C, Osborn or "J" waves are seen, which are pathognomonic of hypothermia (16). Ventricular irritability is common in the hypothermic patient; ventricular fibrillation is common by 30°C. The threshold for dysrhythmias is decreased in the presence of underlying cardiac pathology. The effect of resuscitative drugs is unpredictable. Bradycardia may not respond to atropine. Pacing and cardioversion may be ineffective.

Blood loss in the hypothermic surgical patient is increased owing to impairment of the intrinsic and extrinsic coagulation pathways as well as platelet sequestration in the liver and spleen (17). Blood viscosity increases because of water losses from cold diuresis and extravas-

cular fluid redistribution. Cold diuresis is the result of increased central blood volume owing to peripheral vasoconstriction. As hypothermia becomes more profound, renal blood flow decreases, with resulting oliguria and azotemia.

Basal metabolic rate declines about 7% per degree Celsius. The resulting lower oxygen consumption is partially negated by the leftward shift of the oxyhemoglobin dissociation curve. For each 1°C decrease in temperature, pH increases by 0.015 U and PCO_2 decreases by about 7% (19). Serum sodium decreases while potassium increases because of disruption of the sodium-potassium pump. Hyperglycemia is the result of stress-induced gluconeogenesis, depressed insulin release, and impaired insulin uptake at the receptor site.

Progressive hypothermia results in decreased mental acuity leading to narcosis at 28 to 30°C. Moderate hypothermia has a sparing effect on brain tissue, because metabolic demand decreases more than cerebral blood flow.

Compensatory shivering accompanies hypothermia until temperatures fall below about 32°C. Below 30°C, muscle tone is rigid and neuromuscular transmission is impaired. Resistance to nondepolarizing agents may be seen because of reduced acetylcholine mobilization (20).

A centrally mediated hyperventilation is seen at first in the hypothermic patient, but as the severity increases, decreased respiratory rate and tidal volume are seen until 24°C, when respiratory effort ceases (21).

Hypothermia may profoundly influence anesthetic action and duration. MAC for inhalational agents decreases with temperature. For halothane, MAC decreases 5% per degree Celsius (22). Neuromuscular blocking agents may have prolonged action and may be difficult to reverse (23). Decreases in hepatic and renal blood flow and metabolism may prolong the effect of all drugs.

In summary, hypothermia affects all major organ systems through a combination of slowed enzymatic activity, increased blood viscosity, decreased oxygen availability, and microcirculatory changes (24).

STRATEGIES FOR MAINTENANCE OF BODY TEMPERATURE IN THE PATIENT RECOVERING FROM ANESTHESIA

The treatment of postoperative hypothermia of necessity begins in the operating room. However, despite the most meticulous efforts of clinicians, hypothermia, defined as temperature below 36°C, is present in as many as 85% of adult patients admitted to the recovery room (25). The previous discussion has emphasized the protean effects of hypothermia on all major organ systems. The organ systems of most immediate concern to the anesthesiologist, of course, are the cardiovascular and respiratory systems. In the operating room, the use of general anesthetics that lessen cerebral metabolic demand and neuromuscular blocking agents, which lessen muscle metabolic needs, combined with controlled ventilation can easily circumvent the physiologic perturbations seen in hypothermia. Thus, it is easy for the clinician to subjugate temperature management to a role subordinate to control of heart rate, blood pressure, end-tidal carbon dioxide, and other homeostatic parameters.

However, after the patient arrives in the postanesthesia care unit (PACU), all of the derangements caused by hypothermia will be manifest. Although severe hypothermia may lead to ventricular fibrillation or standstill resistant to therapy, the moderate hypothermia more commonly seen in the recovery room leads to vasoconstriction and shivering. Although shivering is certainly a commonly observed behavior in the postoperative patient, it is probably less commonly seen today because of the increased intraoperative usage of opioids. Two patterns of muscular activity are seen in postanesthetic shivering: a tonic pattern resembling normal shivering, and a phasic pattern resembling pathologic clonus (26). Both patterns are thermoregulatory, but the clonic pattern is not present in normal thermoregulatory shivering and is unique to recovery from volatile anesthetics (27). Although the precise cause of the clonic pattern is unknown, a disinhibition of normal descending attenuation of spinal reflexes seems likely. When it does occur, the metabolic cost of shivering is very high. Oxygen consumption may increase by 300 to 800%, although more typically, the increase is in the range of 40 to 100% (28, 29). As a result, CO_2 production must increase by nearly as much. Even a healthy, unanesthetized patient may not be able to increase minute ventilation sufficiently to eliminate all of the CO_2. Residual anesthetic drugs attenuate the ventilatory response to CO_2 so that respiratory acidosis may be expected. Even trace quantities of residual anesthetics have been shown to blunt or eliminate the hypoxic respiratory drive. Thus, the arterial hypoxemia that can result from increased oxygen demand and venous admixture may not stimulate respiration. In addition, the inability of the heart to increase its output sufficiently will lead to a metabolic acidosis. Because many postoperative patients have preexisting derangements of the cardiovascular system, any additional insults may prove overwhelming. Perhaps this explains the increased postoperative mortality in these patients (30).

Skin surface warming, especially to the chest, inhibits postanesthetic tremor (31). Thus, skin surface warming may be beneficial for the patient recovering from anesthesia independent of the ability to increase core temperature by attenuating tremor and the resulting metabolic consequences. Maintenance of normothermia will prevent most cases of postanesthetic shivering, but temperature must remain at or above the individual patient's baseline temperature; there is no "magic" temperature above which shivering is not observed.

Postanesthetic shivering may also be treated with meperidine or clonidine. Meperidine is more effective in treating shivering than equipotent doses of other opioids (32). The effect of meperidine is preserved in the presence of moderate doses of naloxone but obliterated by large doses, suggesting a role for non-μ receptors (33).

As discussed earlier, the four main sources of heat transfer are radiation, conduction, evaporation, and convection. Less than 10% of metabolic heat production is lost via the respiratory tract. Therefore, even active airway heating and humidification offers little benefit to the hypothermic patient. The reported clinical efficacy is probably an artifact of heating of the temperature probe, which is usually in proximity to the heated gases (34). Passive humidification using hygroscopic condenser humidifiers may benefit the patient for several reasons; however, they are of little benefit in temperature conservation. The intraoperative or postoperative administration of cold intravenous fluids may further contribute to the perioperative heat deficit. The extent of heat loss is proportional to the temperature of the fluid, its specific heat, and the infusion rate. The rapid infusion of 2 units of blood at refrigerator temperature (4°C) may decrease temperature by 0.5°C (35). This may be of serious concern when one considers all of the other factors provocative of hypothermia in the perioperative period. However, it is apparent that only in massive resuscitations involving cold fluid will hypothermia develop solely because of the temperature of intravenous fluids. Still, warming of fluids, in combination with other modalities, may be of benefit for hypothermic postsurgical patients. Blood warmers using a metal plate, as commonly seen in operating rooms, may be used in the postanesthesia care unit as well. If these are not available, warmed intravenous solutions may substitute.

Morris showed that if operating room temperature is maintained above 21°C, adults will remain normothermic (36). Heat transfer by radiation is a function of the temperature gradient, and thermodynamically speaking, the difference between operating room temperature of 21°C (294°K) and body temperature of 37°C (310°K) is minimal. Thus, little is gained by heating the operating room or recovery room to temperatures unbearable to those who must work there. However, because redistribution of core heat is such an important factor in intraoperative hypothermia, prewarming the patient to increase core temperature before the induction of anesthesia is an effective strategy. Warming blankets present the risk of burns for unconscious or semiconscious patients. The limited surface area exposed to the warmer and peripheral vasoconstriction may also explain the relative inefficiency of warming blankets (37).

The easiest method of decreasing cutaneous heat loss is to apply passive insulation to the skin surface. Cotton blankets, surgical drapes, and plastic and reflective blankets are equally effective (38). The primary insulating effect is provided by air trapping beneath the blanket and, therefore, the type of blanket is unimportant. Furthermore, little is gained from additional blankets. It is not true that a large fraction of metabolic heat is lost from the head in the adult patient. Cutaneous heat loss is proportional to the surface area exposed and, thus, the amount of skin covered is more important than the location (39). To reiterate, passive skin warming is effective in attenuating postanesthetic shivering but is relatively ineffective in raising the core temperature of the hypothermic patient. However, the initial redistribution hypothermia could be prevented by prewarming the patient for up to 1 hour before inducing anesthesia. Although this has minimal effect on the core temperature, the lack of a core to periphery temperature gradient will prevent thermal redistribution (40). Alternatively, a patient may be vasodilated before anesthetic induction. This allows normal heat-conserving mechanisms to preserve core temperature as the periphery is warmed. Redistribution of central heat is thus prevented (41).

Because preoperative warming is usually not feasible and vasodilation may have significant side effects, only cutaneous warming represents an effective and practical method to transfer heat to the patient. The two commonly used methods to transfer heat are circulating water and forced air. Of these, forced air is far superior. Relatively little heat is lost from the back into the foam insulation of most operating tables. Also, the combination of heat and decreased local perfusion caused by compression of the capillaries increases the likelihood for burns even if the temperature of the blanket is held under 40°C (42). For this reason, circulating water is more safe and effective if placed over, and not underneath, the patient.

The most effective perianesthetic warming system is forced air. The best forced-air systems transfer at least 50 watts across the skin surface to rapidly increase body temperature (43). Forced air maintains normothermia even during the most major surgeries (44, 45). Forced air is far superior to circulating water (46). Of the warmers commercially available, the Bair Hugger type remains superior, based on current studies (47). The effectiveness of the Bair Hugger depends on the ability to transfer heat from the periphery to the core. Thus, the device is more effective intraoperatively, when the patient is vasodilated, than postoperatively, when patients are vasoconstricted.

To summarize, although mild intraoperative hypothermia protects against tissue ischemia and hypoxia, the consequences of postoperative hypothermia are deleterious. These consequences include myocardial ischemia, prolongation of drug action, coagulopathy, and discomfort. Airway heating and humidification are of little benefit. Although it is difficult to warm a patient with intravenous fluids, heat may be conserved by warming intravenous solutions, especially if more than 2 L/hour is administered. Forced-air warmers are by far the most effective and can maintain body temperature even during major surgery.

HYPERTHERMIA DURING ANESTHESIA

Although hypothermia is a frequent occurrence in perioperative patients, hyperthermia is a rare but worrisome phenomenon. Of course, whereas the malignant hyperthermia

syndrome is well described and is solely seen in the perioperative patient, there are numerous other entities in the differential diagnosis of postoperative hyperthermia.

NEUROLEPTIC MALIGNANT SYNDROME

Although neuroleptic malignant syndrome (NMS) is seen primarily in patients undergoing treatment for severe mental disorders, the use of phenothiazines and butyrophenones in anesthesia for sedation and antiemesis mandates a discussion here. The NMS may be indistinguishable from malignant hyperthermia. The syndrome is most commonly seen in young to middle-aged adults receiving large doses of neuroleptics but may be seen in any patient receiving these drugs. For some patients, a prodromal phase characterized by altered mental status, catatonia, tachycardia, tachpnea, hypertension, diaphoresis, incontinence, low-grade fever, rigidity, clonus, or tremor may herald the arrival of the fulminant syndrome. The full-blown syndrome is characterized by hyperthermia, often exceeding 40°C, rigidity including cogwheeling, other extrapyramidal signs, rhabdomyolysis-clouded consciousness, and verbal unresponsiveness. Serum creatine phosphokinase (CPK) is nearly always elevated. Treatment is supportive and is usually successful, assuming prompt recognition, discontinuance of the offending agent, and care to avoid end-organ damage. Dantrolene is effective in the NMS patient and should be given if the diagnosis of malignant hyperthermia cannot be ruled out. Unlike malignant hyperthermia (MH), NMS may respond to muscle relaxants and central dopamine agonists.

BACTEREMIA AND SEPSIS

Although hyperthermia is rare in the postanesthetic patient who is usually hypothermic, it will recur in the septic patient and is often accompanied by severe vasoconstriction and rigors. Blood products may be contaminated by bacteria. Platelets are most susceptible, because they may be stored at room temperature for as long as 5 days. Other blood products, even refrigerated red blood cells, are not immune, however. Obviously, the transfusion should be discontinued immediately, and both the specimen and the patient should be cultured. Broad-spectrum antibiotics should be started. Intravenous solutions may become contaminated, and propofol, in particular, has been implicated when not handled appropriately (48). In addition, in the critical care patient, invasive lines must always be considered a source of potential septic complications.

THYROID STORM AND THYROTOXICOSIS

Thyroid storm is an exaggerated form of hyperthyroidism characterized by hyperthermia, tachycardia, heart failure, blood pressure lability, dehydration, and shock. There is always a precipitating event, which may be an infection, surgical stress, or iodine contamination as in contrast dye in the known hyperthyroid patient. The diagnosis of thyroid storm is confirmed by the laboratory, but clinically, it resembles MH. However, in thyroid storm, muscle rigidity is not seen and acidosis is rare. Treatment of thyroid storm includes cooling by any appropriate means, sodium iodide to block thyroid secretion, beta blockers to blunt the cardiac effects, and oral propylthiouracil or intravenous methimazole to decrease the synthesis of new thyroid hormone. Glucocorticoids are useful to block the peripheral conversion of T_4 to T_3.

PHEOCHROMOCYTOMA

Previously undiagnosed pheochromocytoma may present as a hypermetabolic state in the patient under or recovering from anesthesia. It may be extremely difficult to distinguish pheochromocytoma from MH, but muscular rigidity is rarely seen in the former.

Although serum CPK may be elevated in pheochromocytoma, the elevation is usually not as massive as that seen in MH. Rhabdomyolysis and myoglobinuria are rarely seen in pheochromocytoma. Unfortunately, dantrolene, when administered to a patient whose hypermetabolic state results from pheochromocytoma, has been reported to cause cardiac arrest (49, 50). However, rapid improvement of the patient after dantrolene, supports the diagnosis of malignant hyperthermia.

CENTRAL NERVOUS SYSTEM DYSFUNCTION

Perioperative hyperthermia may occur in patients suffering from any of numerous CNS pathologies. In status epilepticus, the intense muscle activity may induce fever, which could even be interpreted as MH. Major CNS catastrophies such as intraventricular hemorrhage and anoxic encephalopathy may lead to loss of thermoregulatory function. Again, muscular rigidity may lead the clinician to entertain the diagnosis of MH.

TRANSFUSION REACTIONS

Hemolytic transfusions are infrequent but may be fatal. Most are caused by human errors, leading to administration of ABO-incompatible blood, but incompatibility of other antibodies can occasionally cause a fatal hemolytic reaction. The classic signs of transfusion reaction, such as chills, fever, chest, and flank pain and nausea, are easily missed or confused with other etiologies in patients under or recovering from anesthesia. If a hemolytic reaction to blood is suspected, the unit must be stopped, the blood bank must be notified, and verifying tests such as urine and plasma hemoglobin levels, Coombs test, bilirubin, and haptoglobin should be ordered. Treatment is directed at maintaining urine output using intravenous fluids, diuretics, and perhaps dopamine. Febrile nonhemolytic reactions to blood products are common and are usually self-limited. They do not require discontinuance of the blood product, except that a hemolytic reaction must be ruled out as described above. When hemolysis is ruled out, the transfusion may resume. Microaggregate filters may be helpful in removing leukocytes, which frequently precipitate the reaction. In addition, prophylactic antipyretics may be useful for subsequent transfusions.

GENETIC ABNORMALITIES MANIFESTING AS HYPERTHERMIA

Several well-described genetic syndromes are associated with perianesthetic fever. Osteogenesis imperfecta (OI) patients present with limitations to neck and jaw mobility, kyphoscoliosis, propensity to skeletal fractures, and intraoperative hyperthermia. Although MH has been reported in a patient with osteogenesis imperfecta (51), the potent inhalational agents are generally considered safe in OI patients. Riley-Day syndrome includes postural hypotension, dysphagia, indifference to pain, and deranged temperature control. Perioperative fever is usually infectious or atelectatic in origin and is treated as such. Arthrogryposis refers to many different entities involving congenital contractures. Some of these are associated with hypermetabolic states different from MH.

IATROGENIC FEVER

Postoperative fever not attributable to the etiologies outlined above may result from intraoperative measures taken to avoid hypothermia, such as warming blankets or airway humidifiers, particularly if the area exposed for surgery is small (52). Prolonged use of a tourniquet may cause a slow rise in body temperature in pediatric patients, probably because of catecholamine release and constraint of body heat to the central compartment (53).

In summary, perturbations in thermoregulation are a hallmark of the perioperative state. These disturbances may have iatrogenic etiologies or may be symptoms of other more profound disease states. Whether one observes hypothermia or hyperthermia in the patient recovering from anesthesia, failure to promptly recognize and treat the condition may lead to an adverse preventable outcome.

HYPERTHERMIA IN THE PACU

The differential diagnosis of postoperative fever is large and varied (Table 13–1). It is obviously important to distinguish the etiology of the hyperthermia, because the treatment is quite different for many of the syndromes. For example, antipyretics and antibiotics are the agents of choice in treating sepsis from bacteremia, whereas dantrolene is specific for MH and NMS and anticonvulsants are used in the treatment of seizures.

Although it is not possible to discuss each of these entities in detail, an overview of these causes of hyperthermia will be presented, along with recommended steps in the treatment.

MALIGNANT HYPERTHERMIA

Currently, MH is a well-known disorder described in many standard references (54). MH is an inherited disorder affecting patients when they are exposed to potent volatile anesthetic agents and succinylcholine. For susceptible patients, these drugs induce a rise in intracellular calcium ion in skeletal muscle. This leads to muscle contraction and increase in tone (not always recognized) and activation of enzymes and biochemical intermediates that seek to control intracellular calcium ion concentration. The ensuing hypermetabolic state leads to tachycardia, tachypnea, and sometime muscle rigidity. The biochemical changes include respiratory and metabolic acidosis, elevation of arterial CO_2, hyperkalemia, and hypercalcemia, which result from muscle cell membrane damage. Arrhythmias are believed to be a result of the elevated CO_2 and potassium levels. Fever is a late sign of MH and

Table 13–1.   Causes of Temperature Elevation in the PACU

Sepsis
    Bacteremia from surgical manipulation of infected lesions
    Atelectasis and pulmonary infection
    Aspiration pneumonia
Central nervous system (CNS) causes
    Neuroleptic malignant syndrome (NMS)
    Hypothalamic damage (e.g., hypoxia)
    Seizures, especially continuous
Endocrine
    Thyrotoxicosis
    Pheochromocytoma
Pharmacologic
    Neuroleptic malignant syndrome
    Malignant hyperthermia
    Central anticholinergic syndrome
    Radiologic contrast agents in CNS
    Cocaine, amphetamine overdose
    Interaction of meperidine with monoamine oxidase inhibitors
Iatrogenic
    Transfusion reaction
    Overaggressive heating
Genetic/inherited
    Riley-Day syndrome (familial dysautonomia)
    Malignant hyperthermia
    Osteogenesis imperfecta
Miscellaneous
    Postbypass temperature overshoot
    Faulty temperatures-monitoring device

may not be prominent, particularly if the patient was hypothermic before the onset of MH.

Treatment with dantrolene, beginning with 2.5 mg/kg, is essential, along with cooling the patient, if the temperature is above about 38.5°C. Dantrolene treatment should be available immediately whenever general anesthesia is given in adequate quantities (at least 36 vials each containing 20 mg of dantrolene). Prompt response to dantrolene is a feature of clinical MH.

To prevent problems related to MH, a treatment plan should be available (Figure 13–3, as well as dantrolene and a source of ice for surface and internal cooling.

MH usually presents upon induction of anesthesia or during maintenance of anesthesia. The presentation of MH in the PACU is rather unusual(perhaps less than 10% of cases). Nevertheless, muscle biopsy studies reveal that up to 18% of cases presenting with high fever in the PACU may represent the initial onset of MH (55).

When a patient experiences an episode of MH during anesthesia and is initially treated with dantrolene, recrudescence of the syndrome in the early postoperative period may occur in up to 25% of cases. It is for that reason that after initial control of an MH episode continued dantrolene treatment in an approximate dose range of 1 mg/kg every 4 hours should be continued for at least 36 hours. Of course, the dose of dantrolene should be titrated to clinical signs of MH.

The diagnosis of MH in the PACU may be difficult because many of the signs of MH are not specific to this disorder. For example, tachycardia, tachypnea, and acidosis may result from respiratory or cardiovascular abnor-

LOOK FOR • *tachycardia* • *muscle stiffness* • *hypercarbia* • *tachypnea* • *cardiac dysrhythmias*
• *respiratory & metabolic acidosis* • *fever* • *unstable/rising blood pressure* • *cyanosis/mottling* • *myoglobinuria*

Emergency Therapy for

Malignant Hyperthermia

· * Revised 1993 *

ACUTE PHASE TREATMENT

1. Immediately discontinue all volatile inhalation anesthetics and succinylcholine. Hyperventilate with 100% oxygen at high gas flows; at least 10 L/min. The circle system and CO_2 absorbent need not be changed.
2. Administer dantrolene sodium 2-3 mg/kg initial bolus rapidly with increments up to 10 mg/kg total. Continue to administer dantrolene until signs of MH (e.g. tachycardia, rigidity, increased end-tidal CO_2 and temperature elevation) are controlled. Occasionally, a total dose greater than 10 mg/kg may be needed. Each vial of dantrolene contains 20 mg of dantrolene and 3 grams mannitol. Each vial should be mixed with 60 mL of sterile water for injection USP without a bacteriostatic agent.
3. Administer bicarbonate to correct metabolic acidosis as guided by blood gas analysis. In the absence of blood gas analysis, 1-2 mEq/kg should be administered.
4. Simultaneous with the above, actively cool the hyperthermic patient. Use IV iced saline (not Ringer's lactate) 15 mL/kg q 15 min X 3.
   a. Lavage stomach, bladder, rectum and open cavities with iced saline as appropriate.
   b. Surface cool with ice and hypothermia blanket.
   c. Monitor closely since overvigorous treatment may lead to hypothermia.
5. Dysrhythmias will usually respond to treatment of acidosis and hyperkalemia. If they persist or are life threatening, standard anti-arrhythmic agents may be used, with the exception of calcium channel blockers (may cause hyperkalemia and CV collapse).
6. Determine and monitor end-tidal CO_2, arterial, central or femoral venous blood gases, serum potassium, calcium, clotting studies and urine output.
7. Hyperkalemia is common and should be treated with hyperventilation, bicarbonate, intravenous glucose and insulin (10 units regular insulin in 50 mL 50% glucose titrated to potassium level). Life threatening hyperkalemia may also be treated with calcium administration (e.g. 2-5 mg/kg of $CaCl_2$).
8. Ensure urine output of greater than 2 mL/kg/hr. Consider central venous or PA monitoring because of fluid shifts and hemodynamic instability that may occur.
9. Boys less than 9 years of age who experience sudden cardiac arrest after succinylcholine in the absence of hypoxemia should be treated for acute hyperkalemia first. In this situation calcium chloride should be administered along with other means to reduce serum potassium. They should be presumed to have subclinical muscular dystrophy.

POST ACUTE PHASE

A. Observe the patient in an ICU setting for at least 24 hours since recrudescence of MH may occur, particularly following a fulminant case resistant to treatment.
B. Administer dantrolene 1 mg/kg IV q 6 hours for 24-48 hours post episode. After that, oral dantrolene 1 mg/kg q 6 hours may be used for 24 hours as necessary.
C. Follow ABG, CK, potassium, calcium, urine and serum myoglobin, clotting studies and core body temperature until such time as they return to normal values (e.g. q 6 hours). Central temperature (e.g. rectal, esophageal) should be continuously monitored until stable.
D. Counsel the patient and family regarding MH and further precautions. Refer the patient to MHAUS. Fill out an Adverse Metabolic Reaction to Anesthesia (AMRA) report available through the North American Malignant Hyperthermia Registry (717) 531-6936.

**CAUTION: This protocol may not apply to every patient and must of necessity
be altered according to specific patient needs.**

*Names of on-call physicians available
to consult in MH emergencies may be
obtained 24 hours a day through:*

**MEDIC ALERT
FOUNDATION INTERNATIONAL
(209) 634-4917
Ask for: INDEX ZERO**

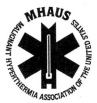

For Non-Emergency
or Patient Referral Calls:
MHAUS
(203) 847-0407
P.O. Box 191
Westport, CT 06881-0191

3/93/12K

Fig. 13–3. Emergency Therapy for Malignant Hyperthermia.

malities. Shivering and increased muscle tone upon emergence from anesthesia is not uncommon, particularly in hypothermic patients and may be mistaken for MH.

If a suspicion of MH exists and the patient is extubated, arterial and femoral venous blood gases should be drawn. Elevated venous PCO_2 above about 70 in the patient who has no respiratory compromise is strongly suggestive of MH. Defervescence in response to antibiotics and antipyretics strongly suggests that the cause of fever is not MH. The response of signs to dantrolene is suggestive but not diagnostic of MH. Dantrolene may produce a resolution of fever in a nonspecific manner.

Other helpful clues may be the presence of myoglobinuria and elevation of potassium or creatine kinase (CK). Blood and urine samples for myoglobin, as well as determination of CK levels every 12 hours, should be obtained when the diagnosis of MH is entertained. For additional help, the Malignant Hyperthermia Association of the United States (MHAUS) hotline should be contacted (209-634-7917, index zero).

Unfortunately, the only way to determine with accuracy whether the patient actually experienced an episode of MH is muscle biopsy. Fourteen muscle biopsy centers are located in the United States and Canada. Further information is available through the MHAUS (800-98-MHAUS).

MH Variants

Recently, information concerning sudden unexpected cardiac arrest in apparently healthy children, usually males, has surfaced. Children who have a genetic predisposition to developing muscular dystrophy, but who display few or no signs or symptoms, are at risk of developing hyperkalemic cardiac arrest when administered succinylcholine or even volatile anesthetics without succinylcholine. The incidence of Duchenne Muscular Dystrophy is about 1:3500 live male births. Because of the low incidence of surgery in children, and the appearance of signs of myopathy at about 4 years of age in most cases, the occurrence of cardiac arrest is very low. Nevertheless, a few cases of cardiac arrest in the PACU after a brief anesthetic in patients with an underlying myopathy have been described (56). During the arrest, elevation of body temperature is sometimes noted and, hence, the cause of the arrest is believed to be MH. In fact, the cause is hyperkalemia. Therefore, hyperkalemia and rhabdomyolysis should be sought actively in young patients who experience an unexpected cardiac arrest (57).

Reaction to Radiologic Contrast Agents

Another uncommon cause of fever in the PACU is the instillation of certain radiologic contrast agents in the CSF. The scenario usually involves a patient who, during anesthesia or without anesthesia, receives an ionic contrast agent injection during a myelogram. When such agents ascend into the cerebral ventricles, a syndrome of ascending tonic/clonic seizure activity occurs, along with fever, rhabdomyolysis, coma, and acidosis. This syndrome does not occur (or occurs very rarely) when nonionic agents are used. The progression of the syndrome is quite typical and dramatic. The signs of muscle "jerking" movements appear within a few hours of the myelogram and progress to coma over a brief interval. Therapy involves management of the respiratory failure and control of seizures in a standard fashion. Dantrolene has been used as an adjunctive treatment on an empiric basis. The mortality from the syndrome is approximately 50% if untreated. Recent case reports show no mortality with aggressive critical care management (58, 59).

Postbypass Hyperthermia

When cardiac surgery is conducted with hypothermic cardiopulmonary bypass, patients are rewarmed before separation from bypass. However, because of the extreme degrees of hypothermia, rewarming of the entire body takes longer than merely rewarming blood. As a result, there is usually an afterdrop of body temperature, followed by a period of rewarming. Of course, during this period, patients are usually mechanically ventilated and passively warmed. Several studies have documented overshoot of body temperature at 4 to 6 hours after admission to the intensive care unit (60, 61). Sometimes, elevated PCO_2 is documented. The cause of this overshoot is not always apparent but is probably a result of a resetting of the hypothalamic thermostat in conjunction with aggressive heating measures and active hypermetabolism of skeletal muscle due to increase in tone, but not sufficient to manifest as shivering. The reason for the hypercarbia is often the failure to readjust the ventilator to higher minute ventilation after the patient has become warmer. Shivering often will occur at this time also, further accentuating the temperature rise. This hypermetabolic state, together with hypermetabolism, may be mistaken for MH.

Included in the differential diagnosis is hypothalamic damage and failure of the central temperature regulating system as a consequence of hypoxemia. Treatment with cooling blankets is effective.

Miscellaneous Causes of Hyperthermia

Many drugs, particularly those with sympathetic stimulating properties, may induce hyperthermia. Among those are cocaine and amphetamines (usually secondary to agitation and muscle hyperactivity), as well as ketamine.

The central anticholinergic syndrome may result from agitation secondary to the use of scopolamine and similar compounds. The cause of the temperature elevation is either muscle hyperactivity secondary to agitation or failure of sweating to dissipate heating.

The combination of meperidine and monoamine oxidase (MAO) inhibitors also may produce marked and dramatic hyperthermia (62).

Several inherited disorders are characterized by fluctuating elevations in body temperature. Two of the more unusual ones are the Riley-Day syndrome (familial dysautonomia), which is marked by mental retardation, failure to produce tears and decreased pain sensation, and osteogenesis imperfecta. The cause(s) of the temperature elevation in these cases is unclear.

Treatment of Hyperthermia

The treatment of increased body temperature depends on the etiology of the hyperthermia. Clearly, dantrolene is most effective in treating MH or the NMS, whereas antibiotics and antipyretics are effective in sepsis. As stated above, dantrolene may, through its ability to reduce muscle tone, produce a nonspecific lowering of body temperature (63).

When body temperature, for whatever reason, begins to exceed approximately 39°C, active cooling measures should be considered. In most cases, simply uncovering the patient and placing bags of ice over the axillae and groin and neck area are sufficient. Infusion of cold solutions and nasogastric lavage with iced saline or water are also effective and more aggressive techniques. A particularly effective technique, used often in the treatment of heat stroke, is the spraying of the patient with tepid water (to avoid vasoconstriction) while directing a current of air from a fan over the patient. Shivering, which may raise body temperature, can be prevented by administering 25- to 50-mg increments of meperidine (for adults).

REFERENCES

1. Satinoff E. Neural organization and evolution of thermal regulation in mammals. Science 1978;201:16–22.
2. Goldberg MJ, Roe F. Temperature changes during anesthesia and operations. Arch Surg 1966;93:365.
3. Sessler DI, Moayeri A, Stoen R, et al. Thermoregulatory vasoconstriction decreases cutaneous heat loss. Anesthesiology 1990;73:656.
4. Stoen R, Sessler DI. The thermoregulatory threshold is inversely proportional to isoflurane concentration. Anesthesiology 1990;72:822.
5. Hynson JM, Sessler DI, Belani K, et al. Thermoregulatory vasoconstriction during propofol/nitrous oxide anesthesia in humans: threshold and S_pO_2. Anesth Analg 1991;75:947.
6. Glosten B. Thermoregulation and regional anesthesia. (In: Lopez M, Sessler DI, Walter K, et al. Rate

and gender dependence of the sweating, vasoconstriction, and shivering thresholds in humans. Anesthesiology 1994;80:780–788.) Anaesthesia 1994;8(1):99–107.

7. Hynson JM, Sessler DI, Glosten B, et al. Thermal balance and tremor patterns during epidural anesthesia. Anesthesiology 1991;74:680.

8. Glosten B, Sessler DI, Faure EAM, et al. Central temperature changes are poorly perceived during epidural anesthesia. Anesthesiology 1992;77:10.

9. Liu WHD, Luxton MC. The effect of prophylactic fentanyl on shivering in elective caesarean section under epidural analgesia. Anaesthesia 1991;46:344.

10. Clemmer TP, Fisher CJ Jr, Bone RC, et al. Hypothermia in the sepsis syndrome and clinical outcome. Crit Care Med 1992;20:1395.

11. Ramenofsky ML, Ali J, Brown R, et al. Advanced trauma life support (ATLS) manual. 5th ed. Chicago: American College of Surgeons, 1993;89.

12. Bissonnette B. Temperature monitoring in pediatric anesthesia. Int Anesthesiol Clin 1992;30:63.

13. Morrison RC. Hypothermia in the elderly. Int Anesthesiol Clin 1988;26:124.

14. Morley-Foster PK. Unintentional hypothermia in the operating room. Can Anaesth Soc J 1986;33:516.

15. Frank SM, Beattie C, Christopherson R, et al. Epidural v. general anesthesia, ambient operating room temperature, and patient age as predictors of inadvertent hypothermia. Anesthesiology 1992;77:252.

16. Osborn JJ. Experimental hypothermia; respiratory and blood pH changes in relationship to cardiac function. Am J Physiol 1953;75:389.

17. Rohrer MF, Natale AM. Effect of hypothermia on the coagulation cascade. Crit Care Med 20:1402, 1992.

18. Hessell EA, Schner G, Dillard DH. Platelet kinetics during deep hypothermia. J Surg Res 1980;28:23.

19. Ream AK, Reitz BA, Silverberg G. Temperature correction of PCO_2 and pH in estimating acid-base status. Anesthesiology 1982;56:41.

20. Miller RD, Roderick LL. Pancuronium-induced neuromuscular blockade and its antagonism by neostigmine at 29, 37 and 41 degrees C. Anesthesiology 1977;46:333.

21. Nunn JF. Applied respiratory physiology. 2nd ed. London: Butterworths, 1977;220.

22. Eger EI, Saidman LJ, Brandstater B. Temperature dependence of halothane and cyclopropane anesthesia: correlation with some theories of anesthetic action. Anesthesiology 1965;26:764.

23. Miller RD, Roderick LL. Pancuronium induced neuromuscular blockade and its antagonism by neostigmine at 29, 37 and 41°C. Anesthesiology 1977;46:333.

24. Elder PT. Accidental hypothermia. In: Shoemaker WC, Ayres S, Grevnik A, et al., eds. Textbook of critical care. 2nd ed. Philadelphia: WB Saunders, 1989;101.

25. Stewart SMB, Lujan E, Ruff CL. Innovations and excellence: the incidence of adult hypothermia in the postanesthesia care unit. Periop Nurs Q 1987;3:57–62.

26. Sessler DI, Lee KA, McGuire J. Isoflurane anesthesia and circadian temperature cycles. Anesthesiology 1991;75:985–989.

27. Sessler DI, Rubinstein EH, Moayeri A. Physiological responses to mild perianesthetic hypothermia in humans. Anesthesiology 1991;75:594–610.

28. Horvath SM, Spurr GB, Hutt BK, et al. Metabolic cost of shivering. J Appl Physiol 1956;8:595–602.

29. Benzinger TH. Heat regulation: homeostasis of central temperature in man. Physiol Rev 1969;49: 671–759.

30. Slotman GJ, Jed EH, Burchard KW. Adverse effects of hypothermia in postoperative patients. Am J Surg 1985;149:495–501.

31. Sharkey A, Lipton JM, Murphy MT, et al. Inhibition of postanesthetic shivering with radiant heat. Anesthesiology 1987;66:249–252.

32. Pauca AL, Savage RT, Simpson S, et al. Effect of pethidine, fentanyl, and morphine on post-operative shivering in man. Acta Anaesthesiol Scand 1984;28:138–143.

33. Kurz M, Belani K, Sessler DI, et al. Naloxone, meperidine and shivering. Anesthesiology 1993;79: 1193–1201.

34. Kaufman RD. Relationship between esophageal temperature gradient and heart and lung sounds heard by esophageal stethoscope. Anesth Analg 1987;66:1046–1048.

35. Morley-Foster PK. Unintentional hypothermia in the operating room. Can Anaesth Soc J 1986;33:516.

36. Morris RH. Operating room temperature and the anesthetized, paralyzed patient. Arch Surg 1971;102;95.

37. Morris RH, Kumar A. The effect of warming blankets on maintenance of body temperature of the anesthetized, paralyzed adult patient. Anesthesiology 1972;36:408.

38. Sessler DI, McGuire J, Sessler AM. Perioperative thermal insulation. Anesthesiology 1991;74:875–879.

39. Sessler DI, Moayeri A, Stoen R, et al. Thermoregulatory vasoconstriction decreases cutaneous heat loss. Anesthesiology 1990;73:656–660.

40. Hynson JM, Sessler DI, Moayeri A, et al. The effects of pre-induction warming on temperature and blood pressure during propofol/nitrous oxide anesthesia. Anesthesiology 1993;79:219–228.

41. Vassilieff N, Rosencher N Sessler DI, et al. Nifedipine and intraoperative core body temperature in humans. Anesthesiology 1994;80:123–128.

42. Gendron F. "Burns" occurring during lengthy surgical procedures. J Clin Engineering 1980;5:20–26.

43. Hynson J, Sessler DI. Intraoperative warming therapies: a comparison of three devices. J Clin Anesth 1992;4:194–199.

44. Camus Y, Delva E, Just B, et al. Thermal balance using a forced air warmer (Bair Hugger) during abdominal surgery. Anesthesiology 1991;75:A491.

45. Kelley SD, Prager MC, Sessler DI, et al. Forced air warming minimizes hypothermia during orthotopic liver transplantation. Anesthesiology 1990;73:A433.

46. Kurz A, Kurz M, Poeschl B, et al. Forced-air warming maintains intraoperative normothermia better than circulating-water mattresses. Anesth Analg 1993;77:89–95.

47. Giesbrecht GG, Ducharme MB, McGuire JP. Comparison of forced-air patient warming systems for

perioperative use. Anesthesiology 1994;80:671–679.

48. Arduino MJ, Bland LA, McAllister SK, et al. Microbial growth and endotoxin production in the intravenous anesthetic agent propofol. Infect Control Hosp Epidemiol 1991;12:535.

49. Crowley KJ, Cunningham AJ, Conroy R, et al. Phaeochromocytoma — a presentation mimicking malignant hyperthermia. Anaesthesia 1988;43:1031.

50. Wajon P. Phaeochromocytoma in a malignant hyperthermia patient under anaesthesia. Anaesthesia Intens Care 1990;18:570.

51. Rampton AJ, Kelley DA, Shannahan EC, et al. Occurrence of malignant hyperthermia in a patient with osteogenesis imperfecta. Br J Anaesth 1984;56:1443.

52. Clark RE, Orkin LR. Body temperature studies in anesthetized man. JAMA 1954;154:311.

53. Rosenberg H, Horrow JC. Causes and consequences of hypothermia and hyperthermia. In: Benumof JL, Saidman LJ, eds. Anesthesia and perioperative complications. St. Louis: Mosby-Year Book, 1992;337.

54. Gronert GA, Antongnini JF. Malignant hyperthermia. In: Miller R, ed. Anesthesia. 4th ed. New York: Churchill Livingstone, 1994;1075–1093.

55. Allen GC, Larach MG. Does postoperative fever predict susceptibility to malignant hyperthermia? Anesthesiology 1993;79:A1078.

56. Kelfer HM, Singer WD, Reynolds RN. Malignant hyperthermia in a child with Duchenne muscular dystrophy. Pediatrics 1983;71:118–119.

57. Larach MG, Rosenberg H, Gronert GA, et al. Pediatric perianesthetic cardiopulmonary resuscitation: epidemiology and prediction of survival. Anesth Analg 1995;80:S265.

58. Ong RO, Rosenberg H. Malignant hyperthermia-like syndrome associated with metrizamide myelography. Anesth Analg 1989;68:795–797.

59. Karl HW, Talbott GA, Roberts TS. Intraoperative administration of radiologic contrast agents: potential neurotoxicity. Anesthesiology 1994;81:1068–1071.

60. Sladen RN. Temperature and ventilation after hypothermic cardiopulmonary bypass. Anesth Analg 1985;64:816–820.

61. Chiara O, Giomarelli PP, Bagioli B, et al. Hypermetabolic response after hypothermic cardiopulmonary bypass. Crit Care Med 1987;15:995–1000.

62. Baldessarini RJ. Drugs and the treatment of psychiatric disorders. In: Goodman-Gilman A, Goodman L, Rall T, et al., eds. The pharmacologic basis of therapeutics. 7th ed. New York: Macmillan Publishing Co., 1985;426.

63. Hotchkiss RS, Karl JE. Dantrolene ameliorates the metabolic hallmarks of sepsis in rats and improves survival in a mouse model of endotoxemia. Proc Natl Acad Sci U S A 1994;91:3039–3043.

14

NAUSEA AND VOMITING

Roger S. Mecca, Stephen V. Sharnick

Nausea and vomiting are among the most common complications that occur during the immediate postanesthesia interval (1). These problems can affect both the real and the perceived course of a surgical procedure and often generate significant patient and family dissatisfaction with an otherwise flawless anesthetic. In an era of evolving competition between facilities for surgical patients and of random litigation related to outcome, maintaining patient confidence and satisfaction with the "quality" of anesthetic care is important.

MEDICAL RISKS

Postoperative vomiting poses genuine medical risks to a patient. Sedation from residual anesthesia or postoperative analgesic medications often diminishes the effectiveness of airway reflexes during early recovery, as does marginal reversal of neuromuscular relaxation. If the ability to protect the upper airway is compromised, vomiting increases the risk of aspirating gastric contents with subsequent serious airway obstruction or aspiration pneumonitis. Surgical procedures that interfere with swallowing or require oral fixation can also interfere with a sedated patient's ability to expel vomitus, increasing the risk of aspiration. During emergence from general anesthesia, vomiting can precipitate serious laryngospasm with consequent hypoxemia. Forceful retching or vomiting increases intraabdominal pressure, which in turn jeopardizes abdominal or inguinal suture lines. Muscle strains, rib fractures, and esophageal tears or

rupture all can occur. Elevation of central venous pressure increases risk of surgical complications after tympanic, ocular, or intracranial operations. Uncontrolled movement during vomiting may dislodge indwelling catheters, disrupt dressings, or cause incidental injury such as contusion from contact with side rails or corneal abrasion from displaced oxygen apparatus.

Vomiting also elicits a significant sympathetic nervous system response, which generates tachycardia and systemic hypertension. These hemodynamic changes increase risk of myocardial ischemia in patients with coronary artery disease and can precipitate dysrhythmias in patients with a history of paroxysmal or multifocal atrial tachycardia, atrial fibrillation, or sympathetically induced premature ventricular contractions. Forceful muscular contraction during vomiting worsens postoperative pain, accentuating the sympathetic response. Increased pain may act as an additional stimulus for nausea and may prolong the vomiting. Gagging or retching can also elicit a parasympathetic response, leading to bradycardia and hypotension. Protracted postoperative emesis can generate dehydration and a hypokalemic, hypochloremic metabolic alkalemia.

PSYCHOLOGICAL IMPACT

Postoperative nausea is a particularly unpleasant sensation for the sufferer and is often the outstanding negative factor that a patient recalls about recovery from anesthesia. Unhappiness and discomfort caused by nausea intensifies other unpleasant elements of recovery, such as pain, boredom, frustration, or fear. Emesis is messy and personally embarrassing for the patient and enhances perceptions of helplessness and loss of control. Nausea after surgery and anesthesia might also generate an acquired physical or psychological aversion to future anesthetics, similar to the aversion a patient might acquire to a food that triggered nausea in the past.

Postoperative nausea and vomiting also have a negative impact on staff and/or family after surgery. Caring for a patient with intractable nausea and vomiting is an unpleasant, physically demanding component of postanesthesia care unit (PACU) and postsurgical nursing roles that usually is not greeted with enthusiasm. Dealing with vomiting patients might also marginally increase the risk to medical personnel from bloodborne and secretion-borne pathogens such as hepatitis and immunodeficiency viruses. Family members are often ill equipped, inexperienced, and displeased to deal with this problem in a home setting after discharge from an ambulatory facility. Staff or family can inadvertently communicate their displeasure to the patient, further increasing his or her discomfort.

ADMINISTRATIVE IMPACT

Postoperative nausea and vomiting can increase the cost of completing a surgical procedure, which in turn negatively affects the overall "cost-effectiveness" of surgical care in a facility. Vomiting frequently extends the time a patient spends in the PACU, requiring additional investment of expensive personnel and capacity. Use of antiemetic medications increases overall pharmacy expenditures, especially if newer, expensive agents are chosen. Nausea and vomiting can delay discharge of ambulatory patients or necessitate unanticipated overnight admission, increasing both direct care costs for personnel or supplies and allocation of indirect facility costs. Frequent, unanticipated admissions of ambulatory patients for postoperative vomiting will raise

concern during use, review, or analysis of cost-effectiveness. In a traditional payment environment, these additional expenses make the overall procedure less attractive to third-party payors or managed care entities and can interfere with subsequent referrals or contracts. In a capitated reimbursement environment, additional costs related to nausea and vomiting reduce operating margins for the surgical procedure, turning a potential profit into a loss. Unfortunately, in the current health care environment, these considerations are achieving an importance that rivals clinical outcome.

Many patients believe that nausea and vomiting should be avoidable or that its emergence somehow represents a shortcoming in the anesthetic care. This perception is reinforced by thoughtless comments from physicians, staff, or lay people about newer anesthetic medications that "avoid" postoperative nausea or about favored anesthetic practitioners whose patients "never" experience postoperative nausea. Misinformation about the relationship between anesthetic quality and postoperative nausea is not restricted to patients. Physician referrals to individual practitioners, practices, and even surgical facilities can be affected if a perception exists that the incidence of postoperative vomiting is unnecessarily high or somehow related to suboptimal anesthetic technique.

Every effort should be made to minimize the negative impact of postoperative nausea and vomiting on patients and staff. The potential for nausea and vomiting should be frankly and objectively addressed with the patient and the family during the preoperative evaluation and informed consent, especially when patients are at unusually high risk. If nausea occurs, adequate preoperative information improves patient acceptance while reducing fear and anxiety in the PACU. It is equally important to educate surgeons, referring physicians, PACU staff, and others caring for postoperative patients about the causes and implications of postoperative nausea. This will not only eliminate misconceptions about the relationship of nausea to the quality of anesthesia care but will also help these professionals intelligently inform and reassure patients and families about postoperative nausea.

PHYSIOLOGY OF NAUSEA AND VOMITING

To discuss potential causes of postoperative emesis, it is important to understand the basic physiologic mechanisms governing nausea and vomiting and how various anesthetic and surgical factors might interact with these mechanisms. Nausea and vomiting are components of a broad defensive gastrointestinal response that protects against ingestion and absorption of toxic matter in the upper gastrointestinal system (2). Nausea is an unpleasant pharyngeal and epigastric sensation that is often phasic in intensity and associated with a feeling that vomiting is about to occur. Gastric relaxation and intestinal retroperistalsis impede distal passage of gastric contents into the intestine and promote return of previously passed contents to the stomach for expulsion. Nausea frequently leads to vomiting but can occur with varying intensity in the absence of retching or vomiting. It is often accompanied by parasympathetically mediated salivation and by sympathetically mediated sweating and pupillary dilation.

Vomiting is often preceded by retching, which involves synchronized contractions of the diaphragms, abdominal obliques, and intercostal muscles, leading to a marked increase in intra-abdominal pressure. Vomiting involves relaxation of the hiatal portion of the diaphragm, which allows intrathoracic pressure to increase as well. A series of forceful contractions of striated muscles then occurs in the abdomen and thorax in conjunction with contractions of appropriate portions of the intestines and stomach. Increased intraabdominal and intrathoracic pressure leads to forceful, high-velocity expulsion of gastric and upper duodenal contents through a relaxed gastroesophageal sphincter into the pharynx and out of the mouth. This complex series of events is regulated by the "emetic center,"

which is probably located in the lateral reticular formation of the brain stem, near the tractus nucleus solitarius.

Many different stimuli trigger this broad gastrointestinal response. Receptors in the stomach or intestine can directly detect a noxious substance after ingestion and initiate nausea and vomiting. In humans, chemoreceptors in the mucosa of the upper gut can initiate afferent stimuli to the emetic center in response to mechanical stimulus, irritants, pH changes, and osmotic or temperature gradients. These responses may be linked to release of 5-hydroxy-tryptamine (5-HT) from damaged or irritated enterochromaffin cells in the gastric mucosa. 5-HT, in turn, might activate $5\text{-}HT_3$ receptors on vagal afferents in the mucosa, creating an afferent stimulus for nausea. Vomiting can also be initiated by afferent signals from mechanoreceptors in the gastric antrum and proximal duodenum, which respond to distention or smooth muscle contraction. Central receptors in the "chemoreceptor trigger zone," which monitor the blood for absorbed components of a noxious substance, can also trigger afferent input to the emetic center and cause nausea and vomiting. In humans, this central mechanism probably exists in the nucleus tractus solitarius and in the area postrema of the caudal fourth ventricle. The nucleus tractus solitarius contains receptors for histamine and muscarinic mediators, whereas the area postrema contains a high concentration of receptors for $5\text{-}HT_3$, opioids, and dopamine. The structure of the blood-brain barrier at the chemoreceptor trigger zone allows sampling of both the cerebrospinal fluid and the blood, yielding access to circulating substances that might not diffuse into the central nervous system. Finally, the emetic center receives afferent input from higher central nervous system centers, which modulate nausea and vomiting. Central nervous system responses to pain, anxiety, or fear can therefore elicit nausea and vomiting, as can tympanic membrane stimulation, initiation of the gag reflex during pharyngeal stimulation, or vestibular labyrinthine activation secondary to motion or irritation. Cortical input probably accounts for "learned" aversion to substances from previous exposures.

INCIDENCE AND RISK

Incidence of postoperative nausea and vomiting reported in studies of postanesthetic outcomes varies so widely that discussion of an overall incidence for this problem loses real significance (3–12). Wide variation is in large part caused by inconsistencies in the approach used in the study of this problem (13). Lack of universal agreement about what degree of symptomatology constitutes clinically significant nausea leads to lack of comparability among studies. In addition, a large number of poorly defined factors correlate with an increased incidence of postoperative emesis, including age, gender, body habitus, individual sensitivities, type of surgical procedure, anesthetic technique and duration, and type of antiemetic regimen employed (14, 15). Incidence also varies across individual practitioners (16). Given this large number of variables, construction of reproducible, controlled studies with comparable patient groups and conditions are difficult. For the practicing clinician, it is more effective to assess each patient in view of predisposing factors and then to qualitatively estimate the patient's individual risk of developing postoperative nausea and vomiting.

PREDISPOSING FACTORS

The incidence of postoperative nausea and vomiting seems to vary with several individual characteristics, although clear relationships among different characteristics is lacking. Age seems to bear a relationship to risk of developing nausea. Incidence seems lowest (approximately 5%) for infants less than 1 year of age, increases to approximately 20% through 5 years of age and peaks between 34 and 51% between 6 and 16 years of age (17). Incidence seems lower and more constant throughout adulthood into the geriatric age group. Correlation of incidence with age may be related to variation in the types of surgical procedures performed among age groups, levels of pain and anxiety, premedication or anesthetic regimens, frequency of intubation during general anesthesia, or sensitivity to triggers of nausea and vomiting between children and adults.

Gender apparently influences the risk of developing postoperative nausea (14). A perceived higher risk of nausea in women may be skewed by a relatively high incidence after gynecologic procedures, which are only performed on women (18). However, an increased incidence noted in women after surgical procedures that are performed on both sexes is probably related to hormonal differences. It seems that the risk of developing postoperative nausea and vomiting is highest during the luteal phase of the menstrual cycle (e.g., the third and fourth week of the cycle) (9, 18–20), perhaps related to an increase in circulating E2 estrogen levels (10). The potential role of hormonal differences between males and females is supported by evidence that risk is independent of gender in prepubertal children or in the extreme geriatric population.

Patients who have a history of motion sickness are at higher risk of developing postoperative nausea, as are patients who have a low threshold for nausea. Certainly, individuals who have suffered postoperative nausea and vomiting after previous anesthetics are at increased risk. This relationship might reflect individual hypersensitivity to labyrinthine stimulation and other triggers of nausea or an acquired aversion to previously encountered stimuli (21, 22).

Presence of food in the stomach before induction of anesthesia increases the risk of postoperative vomiting as well as the risk of vomiting during induction (2). This correlation is possibly caused by vagally mediated mechanoreceptor and/or chemoreceptor stimulus from the food in the stomach. Increased secretion of gut hormones and 5-HT might stimulate and "sensitize" the area postrema or increase the sensitivity of gastrointestinal afferent receptors. However, decreased gastric emptying secondary to pain or anxiety coupled with increased intragastric volume may also play a role. Other conditions that delay gastric emptying or increase gastric volume (e.g., intestinal or gastric outlet obstruction, cholecystitis, diabetes, neuropathies, uremia, neuromuscular conditions) also increase the risk of postoperative nausea, most likely in a similar fashion (15). Conditions that affect the integrity of the gastroesophageal junction, such as pregnancy or hiatal hernia, also increase the likelihood of emesis in the PACU. It is interesting that starvation can also increase the likelihood of postoperative nausea (6), especially for patients whose surgery is performed late in the day after an all-night fast. The net effect of shorter NPO intervals on the incidence of postoperative nausea and vomiting still remains to be elucidated.

Obese patients seem to exhibit an increased incidence of postoperative nausea and vomiting (6). This correlation may result from physiologic aberrations inherent in obesity, such as increased intragastric pressure, increased gastric acidity, decreased gastric emptying, and incompetence of the gastroesophageal junction. Obese patients may suffer proportionally greater insufflation of air into the stomach during difficult face mask ventilation, increasing risk of postoperative vomiting. Also, in longer cases, adipose tissue might act as a reservoir for both inhaled and intravenous agents, causing more prolonged exposure to offending agents during subsequent gradual washout.

Preoperative anxiety, fear, and agitation seem to increase the risk of nausea (6, 15). Worry about death, pain, separation, surgical outcome, and the economic or personal impact that a procedure might have all increase preoperative anxiety. The intensity of preoperative emotional responses is difficult to quantify, given individual variations in expression and methods of coping. Surgical procedures that cause an unusually high degree of emotional stress (e.g., breast biopsy, mastectomy,

testicular procedures, curettage for fetal demise) may entail a higher risk of postoperative nausea and vomiting. Autonomic and endocrine components of fear and anxiety probably play a role. Release of endogenous catecholamines resulting in α-adrenergic stimulation has been implicated as a likely cause (23). Given the relationship between emotional state and incidence of nausea and vomiting, control of preoperative anxiety should help avoid postoperative nausea. When necessary, administration of midazolam in small doses yields very effective relief of anxiety. Midazolam can be administered orally to pediatric patients (0.25 to 0.75 mg/kg mixed in 5 mL of Caro or maple syrup) 30 minutes before induction. Benzodiazepines such as lorazepam may also exert a direct antiemetic effect (24).

TYPE OF SURGERY

Certain surgical procedures carry a higher risk of postoperative nausea and vomiting. A widely appreciated correlation exists between surgery on extraocular muscles and postoperative emesis in pediatric patients (25–28). Increased risk of nausea after laparoscopy and other gynecologic procedures (16, 18, 29) may be related to hormonal factors or to stimulation of vagal afferents from peritoneal irritation. Increased risk of nausea after surgical procedures involving middle ear manipulation is most likely secondary to stimulation of labyrinthine afferents (5, 30). Nausea and vomiting after surgery in the upper airway are probably secondary to direct stimulation of the gag reflex by the surgical manipulations, although accumulation of blood in the stomach may act as a noxious substance during emergence (31–33). Procedures that involve peritoneal or intestinal irritation may increase risk of emesis because of afferent vagal activity or liberation of active polypeptides from gastric and bowel manipulation. Nausea during or after testicular traction is most likely secondary to increased vagal input (34). Procedures that generate significant postoperative pain seem to precipitate more nausea and vomiting.

PREMEDICATION

The reduction in frequency and intensity of premedication use in ambulatory and same-day-admission surgery programs have made the impact of premedications on postoperative nausea and vomiting somewhat less important. Using opioids such as morphine (35–37) or transmucosal fentanyl (38) for premedication increases the risk of postoperative emesis when compared with no premedication at all. Most likely, administration of benzodiazepines for preoperative sedation does not increase the risk of nausea (39). Administration of anticholinergics as premedications has appropriately fallen into disfavor. Unfortunately, some anticholinergics exhibit a significant antiemetic effect when used for premedication, so their exclusion from anesthetic regimens may have inadvertently increased incidence of postoperative nausea. Antiemetic effects of atropine and scopolamine have been repeatedly demonstrated (35, 40, 41). These antiemetic properties are believed to result from a central rather than a peripheral anticholinergic effect, because glycopyrrolate (a polarized molecule that does not cross the blood-brain barrier) is much less effective as an antiemetic (42).

ANESTHESIA

General Factors

Without question, exposure to anesthetic medications increases the risk of postoperative nausea and vomiting. Whether this is due to direct effects of anesthetics on chemotactic centers, autonomic nervous system imbalance, interference with central inhibitory mechanisms, or secondary effects on end organs is unclear.

Incidence of nausea and vomiting varies among individual anesthesiology practitioners, even when all other factors are held constant (16). This difference probably reflects individual variations in technique, timing of interventions, skills at airway management, and a host of other elements that will never be fully elucidated. It seems that the experience of the practitioner correlates inversely with the incidence of postoperative nausea and vomiting (43). It is tempting to attribute this correlation to simple factors. Inexperience with airway management could lead to more gastric distention in patients treated by inexperienced anesthesiologists, whereas lack of confidence may lead to maintenance of deeper levels of anesthesia with correspondingly higher incidence of drug side effects. Quality of training may also play a role, although this has not been examined. Regardless, this variation among practitioners confounds attempts to scientifically determine how various medications or anesthetic influences affect the incidence of nausea and vomiting.

Induction Agents

The choice of induction agent for general anesthesia has a definite impact on the risk of postoperative nausea, although firm comparison among agents is difficult. Use of short-acting barbiturates such as thiopental seems less offensive than etomidate, which has been related to a high incidence of postoperative nausea (44). Ketamine is suspected of causing an increased incidence of nausea (45), which may be related to release of catecholamines. Induction with propofol probably offers the lowest incidence (46–48). Propofol may actually act as an antiemetic when administered in small doses postoperatively (47, 49–51), although its efficacy has not been clearly established. Whether these salutary effects on reducing incidence of postoperative nausea outweigh the cost differential of propofol over other induction agents is a decision that each facility must consider.

Maintenance Agents

Some investigators have reported a decrease in postoperative vomiting when nitrous oxide is excluded (52–55), although these findings are still controversial (22, 32, 56–59). Nevertheless, general consensus is that use nitrous oxide increases the incidence of postoperative nausea in some patients. Several possible mechanisms could explain this relationship. Nitrous oxide may exert a central action that induces nausea and vomiting. Nausea could also be triggered by afferent input caused by diffusion of nitrous oxide into trapped gas in the stomach, intestine, or middle ear. When nitrous oxide is employed as part of a general anesthetic, it is prudent to minimize accumulation of trapped gastric air. This could decrease both the risk of nausea and the risk of regurgitation related to increased intragastric pressure.

Incidence of nausea does not seem to differ significantly whether halothane, enflurane, isoflurane, desflurane, or sevoflurane is used for inhalation anesthesia (60–62). Use of propofol by continuous infusion for maintenance of anesthesia seems to offer an improvement in postoperative nausea and vomiting, although cost is still a significant issue (26, 48–50, 63, 64). When opioids such as fentanyl or morphine are added to an inhalation or propofol infusion anesthetic regimen, the incidence of postoperative nausea increases (62, 65–70). This implies that for ambulatory patients, employment of a "pure" inhalation or propofol infusion technique probably entails a lower risk of postoperative nausea than employment of a "balanced" narcotic anesthetic technique using opioids and nitrous oxide. Meperidine seems to generate a higher incidence of postoperative nausea than morphine. Although newer opioids are touted as causing less nausea, both alfentanil (71) and sufentanil (72) have been implicated as causing postoperative nausea when used as the main agent for general anesthesia. Using small doses of the shorter-acting narcotics (e.g., fentanyl 1 to 1.5 $\mu g/kg$, alfentanil 6 to 8 $\mu g/kg$) in ambulatory patients may partially circumvent this problem. The impact of agonist-antagonist agents on postoperative nausea and vomiting is inconsistent (15). Supplementation of analgesia

with nonnarcotic analgesics such as ketorolac may also help decrease the incidence of nausea (73, 74).

Neuromuscular Relaxation/Reversal

There is little evidence that neuromuscular paralysis or any specific neuromuscular relaxant specific relaxant has a significant impact on postoperative nausea. However, administration of neostigmine for reversal of neuromuscular relaxants does increase the incidence of postoperative nausea, even when atropine is administered at the same time (75). A similar increase in nausea occurs when intravenous physostigmine is employed to counteract sedation (76).

Airway Management

Gastric insufflation and distention during face mask ventilation seems to increase the incidence of postoperative nausea (22). Postoperative vomiting may occur secondary to increased intragastric pressure or secondary to stimulation of vagally mediated mechanoreceptors. Gastric irritation from anesthetic vapors or gases may also play a role (43). Risk of nausea might be lower when tracheal intubation is used, because the amount of gastric insufflation is less than during face mask ventilation. However, pharyngeal or laryngeal stimulation secondary to minor trauma during laryngoscopy or to irritation during extubation may increase incidence. Postoperative nausea can also be triggered by pharyngeal stimulation from an indwelling nasogastric tube (77).

Regional Anesthesia

Use of subarachnoid anesthesia probably generates a lower incidence of postoperative vomiting than general, although this difference becomes less significant if pain is perceived during surgery (78) or if parenteral narcotics are administered for intraoperative sedation and supplementation. Blockade above a T5 sensory level increases the incidence of nausea and vomiting during and after subarachnoid block, perhaps related to complete blockade of sympathetic outflow leading to unbalanced parasympathetic influence (78, 79). The appearance of systemic hypotension during surgery also increases the incidence of postoperative nausea, whereas administration of ephedrine to avoid hypotension during subarachnoid block offsets this increase (80). Most likely, this effect of ephedrine indicates that maintenance of appropriate perfusion pressure reduces the stimulus for nausea, although a direct antiemetic effect of ephedrine administration has also been postulated (81, 82). Epidural anesthesia may offer a slightly lower incidence of nausea in selected patient groups (83), but this correlation is not consistent. Use of intrathecal sympathomimetics such as phenylephrine or epinephrine also increases the risk of nausea after subarachnoid anesthesia, as does administration of epidural or intrathecal opioids (84, 85). Administration of opioids for postoperative pain relief after the regional block has resolved also increases incidence of nausea.

For appropriate procedures, peripheral regional technique or a local infiltration technique is associated with an incidence of nausea and vomiting, which is lower than either general anesthesia or subarachnoid block (86, 87). Again, addition of opioid supplements during or after surgery attenuates this advantage.

PROPHYLAXIS AND TREATMENT

Conservative Measures

Protracted nausea and vomiting are leading causes of unplanned admissions after ambulatory surgery and highly undesirable outcomes from the patient's point of view. A problem of this magnitude has almost as many solutions as there are anesthesiologists to treat it. Treatment regimens are highly individualized, based on the experience of the practitioner, the anesthetic regimen used, the particular

clinical circumstances surrounding the patient, and whatever limitations are present within the facility. When assessing a patient, it is important to rule out other serious causes of nausea and vomiting, such as hypotension, hypovolemia, hypoxemia, hypoglycemia, cerebral ischemia or increased intracranial pressure, gastric bleeding, or bowel obstruction before instituting treatment.

Basic conservative interventions during the postoperative course can affect both the incidence of nausea and the success of antiemetic therapy. Clearly, significant postoperative pain can either trigger or exacerbate nausea caused by other factors (6, 88). Obviously, providing adequate analgesia during the PACU interval is one of the anesthesiologist's primary responsibilities. Reliance on parenteral opioids for postoperative analgesia is a two-edged sword, because opioids themselves undoubtedly trigger postoperative nausea when administered to some patients in the PACU. Striking an appropriate balance can only be performed with careful consideration of each individual patient. Certainly, innovative use of analgesic supplements such as preoperative oral ibuprofen, intramuscular ketorolac, incisional infiltration with local anesthetic, or regional analgesic blocks reduces the amount of parenteral opioids necessary for adequate pain control, thereby reducing the stimulus for nausea. Careful titration of opioids to a measured endpoint using small incremental intravenous doses will also minimize doses necessary to achieve adequate analgesia, as well as unwanted side effects. It is probably more effective to ensure a baseline level of analgesia before emergence to avoid a period of intense discomfort that may initiate nausea. This can be achieved by administration of parenteral narcotics and/or nonnarcotic supplements near the end of surgery, timed to exert their peak effect early in the PACU course when discomfort can be most intense. Similarly, administration of postoperative analgesic blocks at the end of surgery or very early in the PACU course can minimize the amount of discomfort a patient experiences and the secondary stimulus for nausea. It is also important to differentiate agitation or anxiety from pain in the PACU. Opioids are relatively poor sedatives, so large doses are often required to resolve psychological components of discomfiture. Judicious use of sedation to treat undue agitation or anxiety, in conjunction with analgesics to treat pain, will often minimize doses of opioids and the risk of triggering nausea.

Stimulation of the gag reflex in the PACU can be a strong trigger for postoperative nausea. Offending foreign bodies in the upper airway, such as artificial airways, should be removed as soon as possible. Suctioning of the pharynx in emerging patients should be minimized and should only be performed for strict indications. Insertion of nasogastric tubes should be accomplished in the operating room under anesthesia whenever possible, and movement of indwelling nasogastric tubes in the PACU should be minimized. Although gargling with viscous lidocaine or spraying the airway with topical local anesthetics can reduce stimulation from an indwelling nasogastric tube, it is unclear whether these interventions affect the incidence of postoperative nausea. One should also consider whether attenuating airway protective reflexes will increase risk of aspiration should regurgitation or vomiting occur.

Inappropriate positioning can sometimes precipitate postoperative nausea. Obese patients or those suffering from symptomatic hiatal hernia should be recovered in a semisitting position as soon as feasible to avoid gastroesophageal reflux, as should patients who undergo emergency surgery with a "full stomach." Motion often seems to trigger postoperative nausea, most probably secondary to stimulation of the labyrinthine apparatus (21, 22). During recovery, brisk head motions and frequent axial rolling should be avoided as much as possible. Stretchers should be wheeled gently without sudden motions, especially when turning corners. Movements from stretcher to bed should be slow and gentle. Avoiding tight packing of the external auditory meatus and concha can decrease postoperative nausea

after ear surgery (30). For nauseated "one-day" patients awaiting discharge, postoperative ambulation should not be overemphasized. Waiving a requirement to demonstrate the ability to walk before discharge can often make the difference between a relatively smooth transition to bed at home and an admission for protracted nausea. Certainly, nauseated patients should be sent with an emesis basin to avoid unpleasant circumstances during the ride home.

A relationship exists between postoperative oral intake and postoperative emesis, although its exact nature needs elucidation. In some instances, taking small amounts of clear liquids or ice chips soon after surgery seems to calm postoperative nausea and avoid vomiting. However, in other patients, being forced to drink or eat seems to trigger emesis. This is especially evident in children who have undergone upper airway procedures such as tonsillectomy (89, 90). Probably the most prudent approach is to allow each patient who is a candidate for postoperative fluid or food intake to act as his or her own barometer. As experience with ambulatory procedures has grown, the requirement that ambulatory patients drink without vomiting before discharge has become less rigid. In selected instances, discharge without drinking is appropriate, as long as clear instructions are given to a responsible companion to contact the facility if inability to tolerate oral fluids persists.

There is obviously a strong psychogenic component to postoperative nausea. Patients who experience nausea should be aggressively reassured that nausea is not a serious complication, that it can be easily dealt with, and that it will probably pass quickly. Focusing a patient's attention away from the nausea by having them concentrate on deep breathing, conversation, or some other distraction can often preclude progression to vomiting. Some evidence exists that delivery of positive suggestions during surgery will decrease the incidence of vomiting (91). The "contagious" nature of nausea and vomiting should not be discounted in the postoperative period. Patients should be isolated as much as possible from those suffering from protracted nausea and vomiting, to avoid triggering the same response.

Elimination of postoperative anxiety should help avoid postoperative nausea. Administration of small doses of midazolam yields effective relief of anxiety without prolonging recovery time. Benzodiazepines such as lorazepam may also exert a direct antiemetic effect (24), although their effects on arousal and psychomotor performance make them poor substitutes for more potent antiemetics.

Evacuation of stomach contents with an orogastric tube during surgery may decrease the incidence of postoperative emesis (77, 92–94), although this benefit is not evident in all patient groups (95). Routine passage of a gastric tube for gastric decompression is probably not advisable, especially during face mask general anesthesia. However, if serious insufflation of the stomach has occurred during mask anesthesia, intubation and decompression may be appropriate to decrease the risk of regurgitation and to reduce the incidence of postoperative nausea. Maintenance of adequate hydration may decrease the incidence of postoperative vomiting in adults (96), although the impact of hydration seems to be less in children (97).

Obviously, any suspicion that postoperative nausea and vomiting are caused by hypoxemia, acidemia, or hypotension should be clarified immediately. Appearance of central symptoms from these conditions indicates a degree of severity that is threatening end-organ viability and constitutes a medical emergency that should be rectified immediately.

Antiemetic Medications

Several medications can be used successfully to prophylactically decrease the incidence of postoperative nausea and vomiting or to treat nausea once it emerges during the postoperative period. The controversy concerning whether every patient undergoing general anesthesia should receive prophylactic antiemetic medications is unresolved. Some anesthesiologists believe that antiemetic medications are an integral part of a general anesthetic regimen. Others do not administer prophylactic antiemetics but prefer to treat nausea and vomiting if they emerge in the PACU. As a general guideline, patients who are at increased risk for postoperative nausea based on previous history, surgical procedure, etc. probably benefit from prophylactic treatment with antiemetics.

Although less controversial, some difference of opinion also exists concerning what degree of nausea and/or emesis constitutes an appropriate indication for administration of an antiemetic medication in the PACU. Some anesthesiologists treat any complaint of nausea or any sign of vomiting or retching with an antiemetic regimen. Others believe that a percentage of nauseated patients suffer only transient, benign nausea, which does not justify potential risks and side effects of antiemetics. As a general guideline, very mild postoperative queasiness can often be observed for a short time to see if the sensation resolves as emergence progresses. During this period of observation, conservative measures should be implemented in an attempt to resolve the problem. In the authors' opinion, nausea that causes a patient significant discomfort or persists for more than 10 minutes should be treated with an antiemetic regimen. Similarly, one might choose to observe a patient who suffers only transient retching or one short episode of vomiting that resolves nausea. However, if retching or vomiting persists for more than one brief episode, an antiemetic regimen should be initiated.

Although volumes have been written, the optimal antiemetic regimen for all circumstances has yet to emerge in the literature. This lack of definition is caused partly by the difficulty in achieving tight control over studies of efficacy between regimens. Also, a wide variety of physiologic influences and systems affect the emergence of postoperative nausea and vomiting, most likely through several different mediator pathways. Finally, the incidence of nausea and vomiting is highly dependent on each patient's individual characteristics, the surgical procedure, and the anesthesia practitioner. The likelihood that one particular drug or combination of drugs will be optimally effective in each of these different circumstances is small. Each practitioner should determine which antiemetic approach yields the best results for his or her individual anesthetic techniques in various types of patients and proceed accordingly.

The prophylactic antiemetic effect of intravenous droperidol has been extensively evaluated (25, 26, 33, 98–105). Droperidol is a butyrophenone that exhibits an antiemetic effect that is probably mediated by antagonism of dopaminergic receptors. Most studies show that perioperative administration of intravenous droperidol decreases incidence and severity of postoperative nausea. Efficacy varies widely among different procedures and among individual patients. General consensus is that droperidol is one of the more effective antiemetic agents for postoperative vomiting, although a universally valid comparison against other antiemetic medications may never be clearly defined. Some studies indicate that prophylactic droperidol may be more effective if given before induction or initiation of a nauseating stimulus, such as eye muscle manipulation (26, 104). Side effects of droperidol include sedation, extrapyramidal symptoms, and anxiety or restlessness. Intravenous droperidol is also effective to treat breakthrough nausea in the PACU. If total dosage is kept below 20 μg/kg (approximately 1.25 mg total for adults), the use of droperidol should not prolong recovery time or cause excessive sedation. Appearance of extrapyramidal symptoms or postoperative agitation is rare in these dosage ranges (106). Increasing total dosage to 50 to 75 μg/kg (approximately 1.25 mg total for adults) yields more profound antiemetic effects but can prolong recovery time to ambulation and discharge and can increase the possibility of undesirable central side effects (107). Droperidol also exhibits α-adrenergic-blocking properties and can conceivably cause hypotension in hypovolemic patients or in those with high levels of peripheral sympathetic tone. However, with commonly used dosages, reduction of systemic blood pressure is seldom problematic. Akathisia, dysphasia, and acute dystonia have been reported after even small doses of droperidol, but such reactions are idiosyncratic. Haloperidol (another butyrophenone) and domperidone (a structurally similar benzimidazole) possess antiemetic properties but have achieved less acceptance than droperidol for treatment of postoperative nausea.

Metoclopramide, a benzamide, exhibits a central antiemetic effect that is probably secondary to blockade of both dopaminergic and 5-HT$_3$ receptors. Metoclopramide also exerts a peripheral antiemetic effect in that it increases the tone of the gastroesophageal sphincter, relaxes the pylorus, and increases gastric and small bowel motility. These changes promote gastric emptying. This medication has been widely assessed for prophylaxis and treatment of postoperative nausea (29, 93, 100, 108–112). Administration of intravenous metoclopramide 0.1 to 0.2 mg/kg (up to 10 to 20 mg for adults) before induction can reduce the incidence of nausea and vomiting without causing excessive sedation or prolonged recovery time. In awake patients, intravenous administration should be performed over 5 minutes to avoid abdominal cramping. Because metoclopramide has a relatively short half-life compared with other antiemetics, it may be more efficacious for prophylaxis when administered toward the end of a surgical procedure. Metoclopramide is also effective for treating nausea and vomiting in the PACU. Its relative effectiveness with respect to other antiemetics has not been established clearly, but it clearly is among the more effective agents. Sedation after administration of lower doses (0.1 to 0.2 mg/kg; 10 to 20 mg for adults) does not usually prolong recovery or delay discharge with the same frequency as droperidol (29, 100). Metoclopramide has also been implicated in causing dysphoria

(111, 112) and dystonic reactions. Frequency of such side effects in these dosage ranges is somewhat lower than droperidol. However, these dosages can elicit extrapyramidal symptoms, especially in children. The antiemetic potency of metoclopramide in these dosage ranges seems somewhat less than offered by droperidol in patients with severe nausea. Increasing dosage of metoclopramide to enhance antiemetic potency increases the incidence of undesirable side effects.

Medications that exert an antiemetic effect by blocking serotonin receptors have achieved prominence in antiemetic therapy for nausea after chemotherapy. Ondansetron is a selective 5-HT$_3$ receptor blocker that seems to exhibit potent antiemetic properties when used to treat postoperative nausea (113–123). Although side effects such as mild sedation, headache, and dizziness can occasionally occur, the degree of impairment of psychomotor performance seems inconsequential (124). Use of ondansetron does not seem to prolong recovery time or delay discharge of ambulatory patients (125–127). Ondansetron does not elicit bothersome extrapyramidal symptoms or dystonias that occur with metoclopramide or droperidol. Intravenous ondansetron does not potentiate respiratory depression from potent opioids (128) or cause direct cardiovascular changes (129). The major disadvantage of ondansetron is its extremely high cost. An antiemetic dose of ondansetron can cost 20 to 40 times as much as an equipotent dose of droperidol. Routine use of this drug must be subjected to cost-benefit analysis for individual institutions. In institutions in which cost control is important, use of prophylactic ondansetron might be reserved for patients with a history of severe postoperative emesis. Similarly, ondansetron might be reserved for PACU use in patients whose nausea is refractory to more inexpensive medications or when fear of unacceptable side effects requiring admission makes the expenditure worthwhile.

Ganisetron, another 5-HT$_3$ receptor blocker, has received less attention as a post-operative antiemetic, although its properties are probably similar to those of ondansetron. Other, more potent 5-HT$_3$ receptor blockers are in development (130).

Prochlorperazine (Compazine) is a phenothiazine that has been in wide clinical use since 1950. Phenothiazines probably exert a central antiemetic action through inhibition of dopaminergic receptors. Prochlorperazine can be used to effectively suppress postoperative nausea (25 mg rectally, 5 to 10 mg intramuscularly, 2.5 to 5 mg intravenously). However, the incidence of side effects is inordinately high (6, 131). Prochlorperazine can cause blurred vision, drowsiness, and acute dystonias, which can significantly prolong recovery or delay discharge. Hypotension, acute dystonia, decrease in the seizure threshold, and neuroleptic malignant syndrome have also been reported. Children with acute illness such as measles, chickenpox, or gastroenteritis are more susceptible to acute dystonias than are adults. Compazine is not recommended for use in children less than 2 years of age or less than 20 pounds. Other phenothiazines such a perphenazine or dyxrazine exhibit antiemetic properties but are not particularly advantageous for postoperative nausea.

Use of low dose propofol (10 mg intravenously in an adult) as a postoperative antiemetic has been described (47, 49, 51), although effectiveness of this treatment should be clarified. It may be that propofol has a direct central antiemetic effect or that it merely exerts sedative or analgesic effects that reduce a stimulus for nausea from anxiety or pain, respectively.

Ephedrine (0.5 mg/kg intramuscularly or 10 mg intravenously) has been used to treat postoperative nausea (81, 82), although its efficacy has been questioned (101). Ephedrine may be most effective when nausea is related to ambulation or motion. Efficacy for nausea related to vasovagal reactions or hypotension is probably secondary to its sympathomimetic effects on α- and β-adrenergic receptors.

Administration of "H2" histamine receptor blocking agents such as oral or intravenous cimetidine or ranitidine can attenuate gastric acid secretion. These medications effectively increase the gastric fluid pH, which may decrease the stimulus for nausea and decrease the risk of aspiration pneumonitis if vomiting and aspiration occur. However, H_2 blockers do not reliably decrease gastric fluid volume or gastric emptying time and have limited application as antiemetics. Other antihistamines, such as diphenhydramine, dimenhydrinate, and hydroxyzine, are useful in treating motion sickness, probably by a direct central effect on vestibular pathways and on the vomiting center. These medications may be useful for control of nausea after surgical procedures on the middle ear.

Anticholinergics exhibit weak antiemetic properties but are not usually included in postoperative antiemetic regimens because of their side effects. Use of atropine is limited by tachycardia, dry mouth, and blurred vision. Intravenous scopolamine causes unacceptable psychogenic reactions during recovery when used as an antiemetic. Although transdermal scopolamine has some benefit as a prophylactic agent, its low efficacy and tendency to cause anticholinergic side effects such as visual disturbances, dry mouth, and urinary retention make it a poor substitute for other agents, especially in an ambulatory setting (132–138). Transdermal scopolamine is contraindicated for patients at risk for glaucoma or urinary retention and in pregnant or elderly patients.

Various combinations of antiemetics can be used to minimize side effects of any one agent while optimizing antiemetic potency. Experienced practitioners know that addition of a second antiemetic will often improve control of nausea. The idea that each drug in a combination might eliminate a specific type of triggering influence or block a different central receptor is appealing but unsubstantiated. A combination of 10 mg of metoclopramide and 0.625 mg of droperidol intravenously seems to be as effective as using a higher dose of droperidol (2.5 mg) but to cause less sedation (109). As with multidose, single-drug therapy, the risk of precipitating side effects by

adding a second drug must be balanced against benefit of suppressing nausea.

Effectiveness of hypnosis, transcutaneous electrical stimulation, acupuncture, or acupressure stimulation as prophylaxis for postoperative nausea is controversial and inconsistent. However, these modalities may reduce the incidence of postoperative vomiting in selected patients (139–142).

REFERENCES

1. Hines HR, Barash PG, Watrous G, et al. Complications occurring in the postanesthesia care unit: a survey. Anesth Analg 1992;74:503–509.
2. Andrews PLR. Physiology of nausea and vomiting. Br J Anaesth 1992;69(S1):2S–19S.
3. Dawson B, Reed WA. Anaesthesia for day care surgery: a symposium III. Anaesthesia for surgical outpatients. Can Anaesth Soc J 1980;27(4):409–411.
4. Ahlgren EW, Bennett EJ, Stephen CR. Outpatient pediatric anesthesiology: a case series. Anesth Analg 1971;50(3):402–406.
5. Patel RI, Hannallah RS. Anesthetic complications following pediatric ambulatory surgery. A three year study. Anesthesiology 1988;69:1009–1012.
6. Palazzo MG, Strunin L. Anesthesia and emesis I: etiology. Can Anaesth Soc J 1984;31(2):178–187.
7. Palazzo MG, Strunin L. Anesthesia and emesis II: prevention and management. Can Anaesth Soc J 1984;31(4):407–415.
8. Hines RL, Barash PG, Dubow H, et al. Ambulatory surgical complications in the postoperative period: we can't just walk away. Anesth Analg 1989;86:S122.
9. Lindblad T, Beattie WS, Buckley DN, et al. Increased incidence of postoperative nausea and vomiting in menstruating women. Can J Anaesth 1989;36:S78–S79.
10. Beattie WS, Lindblad T, Buckley DN, et al. The incidence of postoperative nausea and vomiting in women undergoing laparoscopy is influenced by the day of menstrual cycle. Can J Anaesth 1991;38:298–302.
11. Cohen MM, Duncan PG, Pope WDB, et al. The Canadian four center study of anaesthetic outcomes: II. Can outcome be used to assess the quality of anaesthesia care? Can J Anaesth 1992;39:430–439.
12. Clarke RSJ. Nausea and vomiting. Br J Anaesth 1984;56:19–27.
13. Kortilla K. The study of postoperative nausea and vomiting. Br J Anaesth 1992;69(Suppl 1):20S–24S.
14. Lerman J. Surgical and patient factors involved in postoperative nausea and vomiting. Br J Anaesth 1992;69(S1):24S–32S.
15. Watcha MF, White PF. Postoperative nausea and vomiting. Anesthesiology 1992;77:162–184.
16. Cohen MM, Duncan PG, DeBoer DP, et al. The postoperative interview: assessing risk factors for nausea and vomiting. Anesth Analg 1994;78(1):7–16.

17. Cohen MM, Cameron CB, Duncan PG. Pediatric anesthesia morbidity and mortality in the perioperative period. Anesth Analg 1990;70:160–167.

18. Haigh CG, Kaplan LA, Durham FM, et al. Nausea and vomiting after gynaecological surgery; a meta-analysis of factors affecting their incidence. Br J Anaesth 1993;71(4):517–522.

19. Beattie WS, Lindblad T, Buckley DN, et al. Menstruation increases the risk of nausea and vomiting after laparoscopy: a prospective randomized study. Anesthesiology 1993;78(2):272–276.

20. Honkavaara P, Lehtinen A, Hovorka J, et al. Nausea and vomiting after gynecological laparoscopy depends upon the phase of the menstrual cycle. Can J Anaesth 1991;38:876–879.

21. Kamath B, Curran J, Hawkley C, et al. Anaesthesia, movement, and emesis. Br J Anaesth 1990;64:728–730.

22. Muir JJ, Warner MA, Offord KP, et al. Role of nitrous oxide and other factors in postoperative nausea and vomiting: a randomized and blinded prospective study. Anesthesiology 1987;66:513–518.

23. Jenkins JC, Lahay D. Central mechanisms of vomiting related to catecholamine response: anesthetic implications. Can Anaesth Soc J 1971;18:434–441.

24. Leigh TJ, Link CGG, Fell GL. Effects of granisetron and lorazepam, alone and in combination, on psychometric performance. Br J Clin Pharmacol 1991;31:333–336.

25. Abramowitz MD, Oh TH, Epstein BS, et al. The antiemetic effect of droperidol following outpatient strabismus surgery in children. Anesthesiology 1983;59(6):579–583.

26. Lerman J, Eustis S, Smith DR. Effect of droperidol pretreatment on postanesthetic vomiting in children undergoing strabismus surgery. Anesthesiology 1986;65:322–325.

27. Hardy JF, Charest J, Girouard G, et al. Nausea and vomiting after strabismus surgery in preschool children. Can Anaesth Soc J 1986;33:57–62.

28. Weir PM, Munro HM, Reynolds PI, et al. Propofol infusion and the incidence of emesis in pediatric outpatient strabismus surgery. Anesth Analg 1993;76(4):760–765.

29. Madej TH, Simpson KH. Comparison of the use of domperidone, droperidol, and metoclopramide in the prevention of nausea and vomiting following major gynaecological surgery. Br J Anaesth 1986;58:884–887.

30. Ridings P, Gault D, Khan L. Reduction in postoperative vomiting after surgical correction of prominent ears. Br J Anaesth 1994;72(5):592–593.

31. Smith BL, Manford MLM. Postoperative vomiting after paediatric adenotonsillectomy. Br J Anaesth 1974;46:373–378.

32. Pandit U, Pryn S, Randel G, et al. Nitrous oxide does not increase postoperative nausea/vomiting in pediatric outpatients undergoing tonsillectomy-adenoidectomy. Anesthesiology 1990;73:A1245.

33. Grunwald Z, Scheiner MS, Pamess J, et al. Droperidol decreases vomiting after tonsillectomy and adenoidectomy in children. Anesth Analg 1990;70:S138.

34. Caldamone AA, Rabinowitz R. Outpatient orchiopexy. J Urol 1982;127:286–288.

35. Riding JE. Post-operative vomiting. Proc R Soc Med 1960;53:671–677.

36. Clark RSJ, Dundee JW. Clinical studies of induction agents XII: the influence of some premedicants on the course and sequelae of propanidid anaesthesia. Br J Anaesth 1965;37:511–556.

37. Dundess JW, Loan WB, Clarke RSJ. Studies of drugs given before anaesthesia XI: diamorphine (heroin) and morphine. Br J Anaesth 1966;38:610–619.

38. Friesen RH, Lockhart CH. Oral transmucosal fentanyl citrate for preanesthetic medication of pediatric day surgery patients with and without droperidol as a prophylactic anti-emetic. Anesthesiology 1992;76:46–51.

39. Forrest JB, Beattie WS, Goldsmith CH. Risk factors for nausea and vomiting after general anesthesia. Can J Anaesth 1990;37:S90.

40. Clarke RSJ, Dundee JW, Love WJ. Studies of drugs given before anaesthesia VIII: morphine 10 mg alone and with atropine or hyoscine. Br J Anaesth 1962;34:523–526.

41. Salmenpera M, Kuoppamaki R, Salmenpera A. Do anti-cholinergic agents affect the occurrence of postanaesthetic nausea? Acta Anaesthesiol Scand 1992;36:445–448.

42. Mirakhur RK, Dundes JW. Lack of anti-emetic action of glycopyrrolate. Anaesthesia 1981;36:819–820.

43. Hovorka J, Korttila K, Erkola O. The experience of the person ventilating the lungs does influence postoperative nausea and vomiting. Acta Anaesthesiol Scand 1990;34:203–205.

44. Hoorigan RW, Moyers JR, Johnson BH, et al. Etomidate versus thiopental with and without fentanyl: a comparative study of awakening in man. Anesthesiology 1980;52:362–364.

45. White PR, Dworsky WA, Horai Y, et al. Comparison of continuous infusion fentanyl or ketamine versus thiopental: determining the mean effective serum concentrations for outpatient surgery. Anesthesiology 1983;59:564–569.

46. Marais ML, Maher MW, Wetchler BV, et al. Reduced demands on recovery room resources with propofol (Diprivan) compared to thiopental — isoflurane. Anes Rev 1989;16:29–40.

47. McCollum JSC, Milligan KR, Dundess JW. The antiemetic action of propofol. Anaesthesia 1988;43:239–240.

48. Watcha MF, Simeon RM, White PF, et al. Effect of propofol on the incidence of postoperative vomiting after strabismus surgery in pediatric outpatients. Anesthesiology 1991;75:204–209.

49. Smith I, White PF, Nathanson M, et al. Propofol: an update on its clinical use. Anesthesiology 1994;81(4):1005–1043.

50. Borgeat A, Wilder-Smith OHG, Suter PM. The non-hypnotic therapeutic applications of propofol. Anesthesiology 1994;80(3):642–656.

51. Borgeat A, Wilder Smith OHG, Saiah M, et al, Subhypnotic doses of propofol possess direct antiemetic properties. Anesth Analg 1992;74:539–541.

52. Alexander GD, Skupski JN, Brown EM. The role of nitrous oxide in postoperative nausea and vomiting. Anesth Analg 1984;63:A175.

53. Lonie DS, Harper NJN. Nitrous oxide anaesthesia and vomiting. Anaesthesia 1986;41:703–707.

54. Melnick BM, Johnson LS. Effects of eliminating nitrous oxide in outpatient anesthesia. Anesthesiology 1987;67:982–984.

55. Felts JA, Poler M, Spitznaggel EL. Nitrous oxide, nausea, and vomiting after outpatient gynecologic surgery. J Clin Anesth 1990;2:168–171.

56. Sengupta P, Plantevin OM. Nitrous oxide and day-case laparoscopy: effects on nausea, vomiting and return to normal activity. Br J Anaesth 1988;60:570–573.

57. Hovorka J, Korttila K, Erkola O. Nitrous oxide does not increase nausea and vomiting following gynaecological laparoscopy. Can J Anaesth 1989;36:145–148.

58. Korttila K, Hovorka J, Erkola O. Nitrous oxide does not increase the incidence of nausea and vomiting after isoflurane anesthesia. Anesth Analg 1987;66:761–765.

59. Ranta P, Nuutinen L, Laitinen J. The role of nitrous oxide in postoperative nausea and recovery in patients undergoing upper abdominal surgery. Acta Anaesthesiol Scand 1991;35:339–341.

60. Carter JA, Dye AM, Cooper GM. Recovery after day-case anaesthesia. The effect of different inhalational anaesthetic agents. Anaesthesia 1985;40:545–548.

61. Jones RM. Desflurane and sevoflurane: Inhalation anesthetic for this decade? Br J Anaesth 1990;65:527–536.

62. Forrest JB, Cahalan MK, Rehder K, et al. Multicenter study of general anesthesia II. Results. Anesthesiology 1990;72:262–268.

63. Sebel PS, Lowdon JD. Propofol: a new intravenous anesthetic. Anesthesiology 1989;71:260–277.

64. Millar JM, Jewcks CF. Recovery and morbidity after day case surgery: a comparison of propofol with thiopentone-enflurane with and without alfentanil. Anaesthesia 1988;43:738–743.

65. Epstein BS, Levy ML, Thein MH, et al. Evaluation of fentanyl as an adjunct to thiopental-nitrous oxide-oxygen anesthesia for short surgical procedures. Anesthesiol Rev 1975;2(3):24–28.

66. Hunt TM, Plantevin OM, Gilbert JR. Morbidity in gynaecological day-case surgery: a comparison of two anaesthetic techniques. Br J Anaesth 1979;5l:785–787.

67. Sanders RS, Sinclair ME, Sear JW. Alfentanil in short procedures: a comparison with halothane using etomidate or methohexitone for induction of anesthesia. Anaesthesia 1984;39(12):1202–1206.

68. White PF, Chang T. Effect of narcotic premedication on the intravenous anesthetic requirement. Anesthesiology 1984;61:A389.

69. Weinstein MS, Nicolson SC, Schreiner MS. A single dose of morphine sulfate increases the incidence of vomiting after outpatient inguinal surgery in children. Anesthesiology 1994;81(3):572–577.

70. Haley S, Edelist G, Urbach G. Comparison of alfentanil, fentanyl, and enflurane as supplement to general anesthesia for outpatient gynecologic surgery. Can J Anaesth 1986;35:570–575.

71. White PF, Coe V, Shafer A, et al. Comparison of alfentanil with fentanyl for outpatient anesthesia. Anesthesiology 1986;64:99–106.

72. White PF, Sung M-L, Doze VA. Use of sufentanil in outpatient anesthesia — determining an optimal preinduction dose. Anesthesiology 1985;63:A202.

73. Ding Y, Terkonda P, White PF. Use of ketorolac and dezocine as alternatives to fentanyl during outpatient anesthesia. Anesth Analg 1992;74:S67.

74. Watcha MF, Jones MB, Lagueruela R, et al. A comparison of ketorolac and morphine when used during pediatric anesthesia. Anesthesiology 1991;75:A942.

75. King MJ, Milazkiewicz R, Carli F, et al. Influence of neostigmine on postoperative vomiting. Br J Anaesth 1988;61:403.

76. Toro-matos A, Rendon-Platas AM, Avil-Valez E, et al. Physostigmine antagonizes ketamine. Anesth Analg 1980;59:644.

77. Burtles R, Peckett BW. Postoperative vomiting: some factors affecting its incidence. Br J Anaesth 1957;29:114–123.

78. Carpenter RL, Caplan RA, Brown DL, et al. Incidence and risk factors for side effects of spinal anesthesia. Anesthesiology 1992;76:906–916.

79. Crocker JS, Vandam LD. Concerning nausea and vomiting during spinal anesthesia. Anesthesiology 1959;20:587–592.

80. Datta S, Alper MH, Ostheimer GW, et al. Method of ephedrine administration and nausea and hypotension during spinal anesthesia for cesarean section. Anesthesiology 1982;56:68–70.

81. Rothenberg DM, Parnass SM, Newman L, et al. Ephedrine minimizes postoperative nausea and vomiting in outpatients. Anesthesiology 1989;71:A322.

82. Rothenberg DM, Parnass SM, Litwack K, et al. Efficacy of ephedrine in the prevention of postoperative nausea and vomiting. Anesth Analg 1991;72:58–62.

83. Bridenbaugh LD. Regional anaesthesia for outpatient surgery: a summary of 12 years experience. Can Anaesth Soc J 1983;30:548–552.

84. Chadwick RS, Ready LB. Intrathecal and epidural morphine sulfate for post-cesarean analgesia. A clinical comparison. Anesthesiology 1988;68:925–929.

85. Bromage PR, Camporesi EM, Durant PAC, et al. Non-respiratory side effects of epidural morphine. Anesth Analg 1982;61:490–495.

86. Dent S, Ramachandra V, Stephen CR. Postoperative vomiting; incidence, analysis and therapeutic measures in 3000 patients. Anesthesiology 1995;16:564–572.

87. Bonica JJ, Crepps W, Monk B, et al. Postanesthetic nausea, retching and vomiting. Anesthesiology 1958;19:532–540.

88. Anderson R, Crohg K. Pain as a major cause of postoperative nausea. Can Anaesth Soc J 1976;23(4):366–369.

89. Berry FA. Postoperative vomiting: causes and treatment. Curr Rev Clin Anesth 1991;11:91–95.

90. Vandenberg AA, Lambourne A, Yazji NS, et al. Vomiting after ophthalmic surgery: effects of intraoperative antiemetics and postoperative oral fluid restriction. Anaesthesia 1987;42:270–276.

91. Williams AR, Sweeney BP. Incidence and severity of postoperative nausea and vomiting in patients exposed to positive intraoperative suggestions. Br J Anaesth 1992;69:216P–217P.

92. McCarroll SM, Mori S, Bras PJ, et al. The effect of gastric intubation and removal of gastric contents on the incidence of postoperative nausea and vomiting. Anesth Analg 1990;70:S262.

93. Kraynack BJ, Bates MF, Gintautas J, et al. Antiemetic efficacy of ranitidine, metoclopramide, and gastric suctioning in outpatient laparoscopy. Anesth Analg 1990;70:S218.

94. Smessaert A, Schehr CA, Artusio JF. Nausea and vomiting in the immediate postanesthetic period. JAMA 1959;170:2072–2076.

95. Hovorka J, Korttila K, Erkola O. Gastric aspiration at the end of anaesthesia does not decrease postoperative nausea and vomiting. Anaesth Intensive Car 1990;18:58–61.

96. Keane PW, Murray PF. Intravenous fluid in minor surgery: their effect on recovery from anaesthesia. Anaesthesia 1986;41:635–637.

97. Blackstock D, DaSilva CA, Demars PD, et al. Intravenous fluid administration does not reduce nausea and vomiting in children. Can J Anaesth 1989;36:S126.

98. Eustis S, Lerman J, Smith D. Droperidol pretreatment in children undergoing strabismus repair: the minimal effective dose. Can Anaesth Soc J 1986;33:S115.

99. Wetchler BV, Collins IS, Jacob L. Antiemetic effects of droperidol on the ambulatory surgery patient. Anes Rev 1982;9:23–26.

100. Pandit SK, Kothary SP, Pandit UA, et al. Dose-response study of droperidol and metoclopramide as antiemetics for outpatient anesthesia. Anesth Analg 1989;68:798–802.

101. Poler SM, White PF. Does ephedrine decrease nausea and vomiting after outpatient anesthesia? Anesthesiology 1989;71:A995.

102. Brustowicz RM, Nelson DA, Betts EK, et al. Efficacy of oral premedication for pediatric outpatient surgery. Anesthesiology 1984;60:475–477.

103. Williams JJ, Goldberg ME, Boerner TF, et al. A comparison of three methods to reduce nausea and vomiting after alfentanil anesthesia in outpatients. Anesth Analg 1989;68:S311.

104. Jorgensen NH, Coyle JP. Effect of intravenous droperidol upon nausea and vomiting using alfentanil anesthesia. Anesth Analg 1989;68:S139.

105. Grunwald Z, Torjman M, Schieren H, et al. The pharmacokinetics of droperidol in anesthetized children. Anesth Analg 1993;76(6):1238–1242.

106. Melnick BM. Extrapyramidal reactions to low-dose droperidol. Anesthesiology 1988;69:424–426.

107. Melnick B, Sawyer R, Karambelkar D, et al. Delayed side effects of droperidol after ambulatory general anesthesia. Anesth Analg 1989;69:748–751.

108. Cohen SE, Woods WA, Wyner J. Antiemetic efficacy of droperidol and metoclopramide. Anesthesiology 1984;60(1):67–69.

109. Doze VA, Shafer A, White PF. Nausea and vomiting after outpatient anesthesia: effectiveness of droperidol alone and in combination with metoclopramide. Anesth Analg 1987;66:S41.

110. Broadman LM, Ceruzzi W, Patane PS. Metoclopramide reduces the incidence of vomiting following strabismus surgery in children. Anesthesiology 1990;72:245–248.

111. Horton BF, Chadwick D. Metoclopramide may cause dysphoria. Anesthesiology 1990;73:A38.

112. Caldwell C, Raions G, McKiterick K. An unusual reaction to preoperative metoclopramide. Anesthesiology 1987;60:67–69.

113. Bodner M, Poler SM, White PF. Initial evaluation of ondansetron — a novel antiemetic. Anesthesiology 1990;73(3A):A328.

114. Wetchler BV, Sung YF, Duncalf D, et al. Ondansetron decreases emetic symptoms following outpatient laparoscopy. Anesthesiology 1991;73:A36.

115. Furst SR, Rodarte A. Prophylactic antiemetic treatment with ondansetron in children undergoing tonsillectomy. Anesthesiology 1994;81(4):799–803.

116. Ummenhofer W, Frei FJ, Urwyler A, et al. Effects of ondansetron in the prevention of postoperative nausea and vomiting in children. Anesthesiology 1994;81(4):804–810.

117. Scuderi P, Wetchler B, Sung Y-F, et al. Treatment of postoperative nausea and vomiting after outpatient surgery with the 5-HT$_3$ antagonist ondansetron. Anesthesiology 1993;78(1):15–20.

118. McKenzie R, Kovac A, O'Connor T, et al. Comparison of ondansetron versus placebo to prevent postoperative nausea and vomiting in women undergoing ambulatory gynecologic surgery. Anesthesiology 1993;78(1):21–28.

119. Khalil SN, Kataria B, Pearson K, et al. Ondansetron prevents postoperative nausea and vomiting in women outpatients. Anesth Analg 1994;79(5):845–851.

120. McKenzie R, Tantisira B, Karambelkar DJ, et al. Comparison of ondansetron with ondansetron plus dexamethasone in the prevention of postoperative nausea and vomiting. Anesth Analg 1994;79(5):961–964.

121. Rosenblum F, Azad SS, Bartkowski RR, et al. Ondansetron: a new effective antiemetic prevents postoperative nausea and vomiting. Anesth Analg 1991;72(Suppl):S230.

122. Larijani GE, Gratz I, Afshar M, et al. Treatment of postoperative nausea and vomiting with ondansetron: a randomized double blind comparison with placebo. Anesth Analg 1991;73:246–249.

123. Lesser J, Lip H. Prevention of postoperative nausea and vomiting using ondansetron, a new, selective, 5-HT$_3$ receptor antagonist. Anesth Analg 1991;72:751–755.

124. Hall ST, Ceuppens PR. A study to evaluate the effect of ondansetron on psychomotor performance after repeated oral dosing in healthy subjects. Psychopharmacology 1991;104:86–90.

125. Lessin J, Azad SS, Rosenblum F, et al. Does anti-

emetic prophylaxis with ondansetron prolong recovery time? Anesth Analg 1991;72:S162.

126. Kovac A, Steer P, Hutchinson M, et al. Effect of ondansetron on recovery time, sedation level, and discharge from ambulatory surgery. Anesthesiology 1991;75:A7.

127. Pearson KS, From RP, Ostman LP, et al. Psychomotor effects of IV ondansetron in female outpatients. Anesthesiology 1991;75:A8.

128. Dershwitz M, Di Biase PM, Roscow CE, et al. Ondansetron does not affect alfentanil induced ventilatory depression. Anesthesiology 1991;75:A321.

129. Conahan TJ, Young ML, Levy WJ, et al. Cardiovascular stability with rapid intravenous infusion of ondansetron. Anesth Analg 1992;74:S52.

130. Russell D, Kenny GNC. 5-HT$_3$ antagonists in postoperative nausea and vomiting. Br J Anaesth 1992;69(Suppl):63S-68S.

131. Loesser EA, Bennet G, Stanley TH, et al. Comparison of droperidol, haloperidol, and prochlorperazine as postoperative antiemetics. Can Anaesth Soc J 1979;26:125-127.

132. Bailey PL, Streisand JB, Pace NL, et al. Transdermal scopolamine reduces nausea and vomiting after outpatient laparoscopy. Anesthesiology 1990;72:977-980.

133. Reinhart DJ, Klein KW, Schroff E. Transdermal scopolamine for the reduction of postoperative nausea in outpatient ear surgery: a double-blind, randomized study. Anesth Analg 1994;79(2):281-284.

134. Gibbons PA, Nicolson SC, Betts EK, et al. Sco-polamine does not prevent postoperative emesis after pediatric eye surgery. Anesthesiology 1984;61:A435.

135. Uppington J, Dunnet J, Blogg CE. Transdermal hyoscine and postoperative nausea and vomiting. Anaesthesia 1986;41:16-20.

136. Loper KA, Ready LB, Dorman BH. Prophylactic transdermal scopolamine reduces nausea in postoperative patients receiving epidural morphine. Anesth Analg 1989;68:144-146.

137. Tigerstedt I, Salmela L, Aromaa U. Double-blind comparison of transdermal scopolamine, droperidol and placebo against postoperative nausea and vomiting. Acta Anaesth Scand 1988;32:454-457.

138. Bailey PL, Bubbers SJM, East KA, et al. Transdermal scopolamine reduces postoperative nausea and vomiting. Anesthesiology 1988;69:A641.

139. Lewis IH, Pryn SJ, Reynolds PI, et al. Effect of P6 acupressure on postoperative vomiting in children undergoing strabismus correction. Br J Anaesth 1991;67:73-78.

140. Dundee JW, Ghaly RG, McKinney MS. P6 acupuncture antiemesis comparison of invasive and noninvasive techniques. Anesthesiology 1989;71:A130.

141. Sacco JJ, Grant WD, Luthringer DD, et al. The reduction of postsurgical nausea and vomiting in patients receiving N$_2$O. Anesthesiology 1990;73:A15.

142. Fassoulaki A, Papilas K, Sarantopoulos C, et al. Transcutaneous electrical nerve stimulation reduces the incidence of vomiting after hysterectomy. Anesth Analg 1993;76(5):1012-1015.

15

CARE OF THE CRITICALLY ILL PATIENT IN THE PACU

Athos J. Rassias, Andrew Gettinger

Critically ill patients may be cared for in the postanesthesia care unit (PACU) under many circumstances. For example, a patient may have undergone an elective surgical procedure that resulted in an unexpectedly complicated recovery course, necessitating prolonged intensive care. Alternatively, a patient may undergo a surgical procedure on an elective or emergent basis, with the expectation that he or she will require a high degree of care postoperatively but not to the extent to require the services of the intensive care unit (ICU). Not uncommonly, this sort of patient has a complicated and prolonged recovery course. Other patients actually may be transferred to the PACU for intensive care from other locations in the hospital. In some institutions, the PACU serves as a source of critical care beds when other critical care units are unable to accept additional patients. For example, patients may be transferred to the PACU in lieu of going to the ICU, coronary care unit, or pediatric intensive care unit. This practice, of course, is particularly institution-dependent and is a function of the resources available locally.

The types of patients described above may be cared for completely in the PACU or they may be transferred to the ICU as their courses are prolonged. The policy of transfer to the appropriate geographical location is also dependent on the resources available within the institution.

The critically ill patient will present healthcare providers with a complex set of is-sues, frequently in addition to the issues of the usual postoperative patient. It is of paramount importance that the physicians, nurses, respiratory therapists, and all other personnel caring for the patient are cognizant of each patient's long-term issues. For example, critically ill patients frequently require nutritional support and have multiple infectious disease issues, which are concerns that are not usually addressed during the typical short-term care provided in the PACU.

An additional problem is that these patients present more of a diagnostic challenge than the usual PACU patient and, thus, may require trips out of the PACU unit. For example, a patient may require a computed tomography scan in the radiology department, which presents caregivers with the task of continuously providing intensive care in a changing and unfamiliar environment. Indeed, it is estimated that at least one-third of intrahospital transports of critically ill patients suffer from a mishap in patient care (1). These mishaps vary in severity, but it is clear that transporting a critically ill patient places the patient at an increased risk of incurring iatrogenic problems.

Critically ill patients optimally should be cared for by physicians who are willing and capable of providing longitudinal medical care. The usual model for the PACU is collaborative coverage by both the primary surgical service and the anesthesia service. In contrast, the typical model for the care of patients in the ICU is a collaborative effort on the part of the primary surgical service and a critical care service. The PACU model of medical care serves the recovery of the typical postoperative patient well; however, the prolonged care required for the typical critically ill patient may be better served by the ICU model of medical care. Of course, the distinction between when a patient is best served by a typical PACU model and when they are best served by an ICU model is not easily made.

A final issue is that the family visitation policy of most PACUs is more strict than that of the typical ICU, and consequently, this may create problems of a social nature. It seems obvious that a family member should be able to visit a relative who requires prolonged care, but many PACUs are not structured to accommodate this easily. Limitations to access are created by various problems, often including a physical structure that separates the PACU from family waiting areas. Furthermore, unit policies on patient visitation are typically more restrictive in the PACU than in the ICU, again reflecting the usual short-term stay of most patients. However, it is perhaps true that the visitation policies of PACUs are evolving toward a less restrictive policy, although this is certainly not a universal occurrence. In addition, the typical PACU has a physical structure resembling an open ward, which does not provide a private space for family members to visit. It is, therefore, of paramount importance that these issues be addressed whenever a patient will be cared for over a prolonged period of time.

PULMONARY

Many patients who are critically ill will require mechanical ventilation, either for intrinsic cardiopulmonary disease, or for protection of the airway in patients with central nervous system disorders or who have sustained head and neck trauma. In addition, the critically ill postoperative patient may require mechanical ventilation to allow for emergence from a long-acting anesthetic. This section will discuss the various methods of mechanical ventilation and will then address the question of prolonged weaning from mechanical ventilation.

Ventilator Modes

CONTROL MODE VENTILATION (CMV)

In this mode, a predetermined volume is delivered at a specified rate. The patient is not able to trigger the ventilator and, thus, cannot breathe spontaneously. Hence, weaning must be performed with trials of T-piece ventilation. In addition, patients frequently require sedation to tolerate this mode, because they may feel uncomfortable being unable to take a spontaneous breath. This mode of ventilation is rarely used for a conscious patient.

INTERMITTENT MANDATORY VENTILATION (IMV)

This mode also delivers a predetermined volume and rate but allows the patient to breath spontaneously between ventilator breaths. In synchronized IMV (SIMV), the patient is allowed to trigger the mechanical ventilator-assisted breaths. Weaning from the ventilator is achieved by decreasing the IMV rate, thus allowing the patient to assume increasing amounts of respiratory work (see below).

The advantages of IMV over CMV include increased patient comfort (hence, minimization of sedation), respiratory muscle training, and technically easier weaning from the ventilator. Any parameter that can be performed by CMV mode can also be performed by IMV mode, and it is the provision for the patient to initiate spontaneous breaths that has led to IMV supplanting CMV.

ASSIST CONTROL VENTILATION (A/C)

All breaths initiated by the patient, while being ventilated in this mode, trigger the ventilator to deliver a predetermined volume. A baseline frequency is also specified, and the ventilator delivers breaths if the patient's rate does not meet this requirement.

Each patient breath of sufficient magnitude to trigger the ventilator will ensure the delivery of a full tidal volume. Thus, any cause of tachypnea by the patient can result in hyperventilation and respiratory alkalosis. In addition, weaning the patient from the ventilator is difficult, because decreasing the preset respiratory rate will change very little the amount of respiratory work done by the patient.

PRESSURE CONTROL VENTILATION (PC)

This mode differs from IMV, CMV, and A/C in that it is the airway pressure, and not the volume to be delivered, which is preset. When a preset pressure is delivered to the airway, the tidal volume that is achieved is dependent upon the pressure, as well as the compliance and resistance of the respiratory system. In addition, it depends on the level of PEEP, as it is the difference between the peak pressure and the PEEP that is the driving pressure for achieving a volume change. Other parameters that must be preset are the respiratory rate and the inspiratory time (or the inspiratory:expiratory ratio.)

The capacity to control the peak airway pressure is one way in which PC ventilation differs from volume ventilation. This capability allows greater control over the airway pressures achieved, which may be important in the development of barotrauma (2, 3).

PRESSURE-SUPPORT VENTILATION (PSV)

PSV was developed to overcome the resistive properties of the endotracheal tube and ventilatory circuit. PSV functions by delivering a specified pressure when triggered by the patient's spontaneous breaths. The pressure applied to the airway is terminated and, hence, inspiration ceases when flow reaches 25% of the original flow required to trigger the ventilator.

As with PC ventilation, the tidal volume that is achieved is dependent upon the pressure delivered, as well as the patient's respira-

tory compliance and resistance. It has been found that many patients can be ventilated and weaned successfully using PSV as the only form of ventilation (4). PSV can be used to provide total ventilatory support, to provide partial support, or as an adjunct to another mode (most commonly IMV).

Weaning from Mechanical Ventilation

Most patients who are recovering from anesthesia do not need a prolonged trial of weaning from mechanical ventilation. As the patient emerges from the anesthetic, the clinician must ascertain whether the patient has adequate strength to maintain respirations, has adequate respiratory drive to maintain gas exchange, and is neurologically intact to protect his or her airway. When these parameters are met, most patients' tracheas may be extubated successfully, although a period of close observation is mandatory. The critically ill patient, however, may not meet these criteria. Typically, a prolonged course of mechanical ventilation has occurred, to allow the patient to recover from the acute illness, which leaves the patient in a debilitated state. Thus, special attention must be paid to weaning these patients from mechanical ventilation.

As discussed in a review by Tobin and Yang (5), the main factors that determine weaning failure are hypoxemic respiratory failure, ventilatory pump failure, and psychological problems.

Hypoxemic respiratory failure is related to either insufficient ventilation, inadequate gas exchange, or a decreased venous oxygen content (5). Ventilatory pump failure is a common problem for critically ill patients, and it is most frequently because of decreased respiratory muscle strength, from muscle atrophy and generalized malnutrition. Other causes of ventilatory pump failure include a decreased central respiratory center output, phrenic nerve dysfunction, and an increased load on the respiratory system, such as with increased ventilatory requirements or increased dead space ventilation. Finally, patients occasionally become anxious or even develop fear with attempts at weaning from mechanical ventilation (5), and this can pose a serious impediment to weaning.

As Civetta discussed in a recent editorial (6), by the initiation of mechanical ventilation, we may have created a subset of patients with "iatrogenic ventilator dependency." The increased work of breathing imposed on patients by the breathing apparatus encourages respiratory muscle atrophy. Civetta conceptualizes the work of breathing for the patient as three components: the first is the normal work of breathing; the second is the imposed work of breathing caused by the breathing apparatus; and the third is the work imposed on the patient because of the disease process. As a goal for respiratory support, he states that we should, "Never make the patient supply more than the normal physiologic work of breathing nor supply so much ventilatory assistance that the patient's contribution is eliminated" (6).

Predicting Outcome from Weaning

Various methods have been advocated to allow clinicians to predict which patients will be weaned successfully from mechanical ventilation. The use of such an index would be that one could select which patients will need further therapy of aggressive pulmonary and respiratory muscle rehabilitation and which patients will tolerate cessation of mechanical ventilation.

Yang and Tobin (7) performed a prospective trial (in medical ICU patients) of various indices used to predict outcome in weaning. They used standard indices, such as minute ventilation, the negative inspiratory force, and tidal volume. In addition, they also evaluated the ratio of frequency to tidal volume (in breaths per minute per liter), as well as an index that combined elements of pulmonary compliance, rate, oxygenation, and pressure; therefore, it was termed the "CROP" index. The threshold values chosen by the authors are listed in Table 15–1. The accuracy of the

Table 15–1. Threshold Values of Indexes Used to Predict Weaning Outcome

Index	Value[a]
Minute ventilation (L/min)	≤15
Respiratory frequency (breaths/min)	≤38
Tidal volume (mL)	≥325
Tidal volume (mL)/patient's weight (kg)	≥4
Maximal inspiratory pressure (cm H_2O)[b]	≤−15
Dynamic compliance (mL/cm H_2O)	≥22
Static compliance (mL/cm H_2O)	≥33
PaO_2/P_AO_2 ratio	≥0.35
Frequency/tidal volume ratio (breaths/min/L)	≤105
CROP[c] index (mL/breath/min)	≥13

[a] Threshold values were those that discriminated best in the training data set between the patients who were successfully weaned and those in whom a weaning trial failed; ≥ and ≤ indicate whether the values above the threshold value or those below it are those that predicted a successful weaning outcome.
[b] To convert value to kilopascals, multiply by 0.09807.
[c] CROP = compliance, rate, oxygenation, pressure.

indexes tested are shown in Table 15–2. The authors concluded that rapid shallow breathing, as reflected by the ratio of frequency to tidal volume, was the most accurate predictor of failure to wean. Furthermore, the authors felt that if rapid shallow breathing was not present, then this was the most accurate predictor of success.

Techniques of Weaning from Mechanical Ventilation

T-PIECE OR CPAP TRIAL

Some patients who have undergone brief episodes of tracheal intubation, such as those emerging from anesthesia, will do well with an abrupt cessation of mechanical ventilation. This provides the opportunity to observe the patient's respiratory status before tracheal extubation. A trial of T-piece ventilation, however, should not be prolonged, as an endotracheal tube and the respiratory circuit can add a significant amount of resistance to breathing (5), especially if the patient is breathing through the ventilator (e.g., with CPAP through the ventilator circuit).

Failure of patients to do well with this type of weaning is manifest by discoordination be-

Table 15–2. Accuracy of the Indexes Used to Predict Weaning Outcome[a]

Index	Sensitivity	Specificity	Positive Predictive Value	Negative Predictive Value
Minute ventilation	0.78	0.18	0.55	0.38
Respiratory frequency	0.92	0.36	0.65	0.77
Tidal volume	0.97	0.54	0.73	0.94
Tidal volume/patient's weight	0.94	0.39	0.67	0.85
Maximal inspiratory pressure	1.00	0.11	0.59	1.00
Dynamic compliance	0.72	0.50	0.65	0.58
Static compliance	0.75	0.36	0.60	0.53
PaO_2/P_AO_2 ratio	0.81	0.29	0.59	0.53
Frequency/tidal volume ratio	0.97	0.64	0.78	0.95
CROP[b] index	0.81	0.57	0.71	0.70

[a] Values shown were derived from the complete prospective-validation data set, comprising 36 successfully weaned patients and 28 patients in whom weaning failed.
[b] CROP = compliance, rate, oxygenation, pressure.
From Yang KL, Tobin MJ. A prospective study of indexes predicting the outcome of trial of weaning from mechanical ventilation. N Engl J Med 1991; 324:1445–1450.

tween the motion of the rib cage and the abdomen and the worsening of ventilation-perfusion mismatch (5).

An established method of weaning patients is a gradual T-piece wean. This method consists of increasing duration of spontaneous ventilation with a T-piece setup, interspersed with periods of mechanical ventilation. When the duration has increased to about 30 minutes, and this has been tolerated over several trials, and provided that the clinical condition is satisfactory, then the patient's trachea may be extubated. Some experts say that the duration of T-piece ventilation may be extended for as long as 2 hours (5).

INTERMITTENT MANDATORY VENTILATION WEAN

The typical IMV wean consists of gradually decreasing the IMV rate, which necessitates that the patient increases the amount of respiratory work that he or she performs. Monitoring of tolerance of weaning is performed by: (*a*) observing the clinical status, watching for evidence of respiratory discoordination, tachypnea, or fatigue; (*b*) maintenance of an adequate pH, usually recommended to be above 7.35 (8); and (*c*) maintenance of adequate oxygenation. If these criteria are met, when the IMV rate has reached zero or is close to zero, then the patient's trachea is extubated.

Although IMV weaning is straightforward and well tolerated by most patients, there are some disadvantages to this technique. Importantly, to initiate a spontaneous breath, the patient must first open a demand valve that allows the flow of fresh gas for a spontaneous inspiration. In many ventilator systems, the work of breathing is increased significantly by the effort needed to open the demand valve (9). It is important to reduce the sensitivity of the demand valve to a low level, to reduce the work of breathing imposed on patients.

Despite the popularity of the technique, there is little evidence to show that IMV weaning is a great improvement in long-term ventilator-dependent patients who are difficult to wean (5).

PRESSURE SUPPORT WEANING

The technique of weaning with pressure support involves gradually decreasing the amount of pressure employed. Thus, a patient may be weaned from a level of pressure support that is essentially full ventilatory support to a level of minimal ventilatory support by decrements of 2 to 6 cm H_2O, depending on the clinical situation.

Several studies have attempted to demonstrate a benefit to PSV weaning. Jounieaux et al. (10) in a group of chronic obstructive pulmonary disease (COPD) patients compared weaning using IMV with or without PSV. They decreased the IMV rate concurrent with a decrease in the pressure support and found that there was only a marginal decrease in weaning time when PSV was added to IMV.

It should be noted that there is a large variation in the level of pressure support that is required to overcome the resistance of the endotracheal tube and the breathing apparatus. Banner et al. (11) evaluated the work imposed by the breathing apparatus with the goal of reducing this to zero, by increasing the pressure support level. They found that the mean level of PSV needed to overcome imposed work was 13.5 cm H_2O. However, they also found that the range was from 5 to 22 cm H_2O. This indicates that there is a lot of variation in the amount of work imposed by the breathing apparatus for a given setup and patient.

ADULT RESPIRATORY DISTRESS SYNDROME

Since the adult respiratory distress syndrome (ARDS) was first described by Ashbaugh in 1967 (12), the mortality rate has remained 40 to 60% (13–15). This has remained true, despite intensive investigation into the pathophysiology and treatment of ARDS. It has become clear that ARDS is a complex response. Indeed, the pulmonary process is believed to be one aspect of a systemic response (16), which may or may not involve multiple organs. The following will include only a discussion specific to ARDS; related issues will be discussed in the section on sepsis.

The main pathophysiologic process involved in ARDS is the alteration of the alveolar-capillary membrane (17). This leads to the characteristic alveolar edema, causing a reduction in pulmonary compliance, diffuse patchy infiltrates on chest roentgenogram, and hypoxemia associated with normal left ventricular filling pressures. Currently, there are many postulated mechanisms that lead to

the pathophysiology found in ARDS, including activated neutrophils or macrophages or activated circulating mediators, such as complement factors, cytokines, prostaglandins, or oxygen-derived radicals (17, 18). ARDS has been associated with many disease states, including systemic sepsis, pulmonary contusion, aspiration, fat emboli from long bone fractures, pneumonia, and pancreatitis (18).

The clinical picture of hypoxemia and tachypnea, seen so frequently in ARDS, can be related to the increased extravascular lung water causing intrapulmonary shunting, as well as to the reduction in functional residual capacity (FRC) and lung compliance (18). The loss of FRC means that a patient's closing capacity will be in the range of the tidal volume, leading to atelectasis and worsened ventilation/perfusion mismatching.

The goals of therapy for patients with ARDS should be twofold: initially, the patient requires stabilization and support; just as importantly, there must be an ongoing search for an etiology of the ARDS, leading to definitive therapy. The latter topic will be covered in sections below.

Stabilization of the patient with ARDS is first centered on ensuring the patency of the airway and the adequacy of ventilation. Any hemodynamic instability must then be corrected. The impairment of oxygenation is variable. In patients with early or mild ARDS, supplemental oxygen therapy may be adequate. However, refractory hypoxemia or worsening tachypnea will necessitate tracheal intubation and mechanical ventilation. The mainstay of respiratory support is positive end-expiratory pressure (PEEP). PEEP, by its ability to recruit collapsed airways, can increase the functional residual capacity, and therefore improve oxygenation and compliance (18, 19).

There are major detrimental aspects to PEEP, including impeded venous return, which can lead to decreased cardiac output and worsened ventilation/perfusion mismatching. The other main side effect of PEEP is barotrauma. Therefore, this modality of therapy must be carefully titrated against its effects. Basically, the goals of therapy are to achieve an acceptable PaO_2 (usually > 60 mm Hg), at a minimum FiO_2 (usually < 0.6), with the least cardiovascular compromise possible (19). It should be noted that PEEP therapy should be reevaluated frequently.

In ARDS, there is a heterogeneous distribution to lung damage, as has been demonstrated by both computed tomography of the lungs and gas exchange analysis (3). Thus, whereas some lung units are not undergoing gas exchange, because of either edema or atelectasis, there remain other units of lung that are relatively normal. Hence, to achieve a normal tidal volume, high ventilatory pressures must be used, and this places the preserved normal units of lung at increased risk for barotrauma (3).

It is now believed that volume changes leading to lung overdistention are at least as important, and perhaps more important, than high ventilatory pressures, in the pathogenesis of barotrauma (2, 3, 20). An animal study compared the microvascular permeability of pressure-cycled mechanically ventilated animals who had either a whole body cast in place versus animals who were not casted (21). The restriction to chest expansion by the body cast led to a lower tidal volume for a given airway pressure. At high levels of airway pressure, the uncasted animals had changes in microvascular permeability associated with areas of hemorrhage and atelectasis, whereas the animals whose thoraces were restricted by a cast had completely normal lungs. This work, and other studies, suggests that overdistention of the small remaining normal areas of lung, by ventilating with too large a tidal volume, will lead to barotrauma (2). Hence, it is advisable to use either smaller tidal volumes or to initiate ventilation with pressure control mode and maintain low peak alveolar pressures (3), which is related to peak airway pressure; see the review by Marcy and Marini (3), to avoid overdistention. Unfortunately, other than these broad guidelines, there are no reliable recommendations on avoidance of overdistention in a particular patient, because of the absence of randomized prospective studies of these issues.

Inverse Ratio Ventilation

In an attempt to both improve oxygenation and minimize ventilator-associated lung damage, the technique of inverse ratio ventilation (IRV) was proposed. The basic principle behind this method of ventilation is that one can achieve increased alveolar recruitment at lower airway inflating pressures. One of the goals of this technique is to increase the mean pressure at the alveolar level, averaged over the entire respiratory cycle. This has been correlated with alveolar recruitment, oxygenation, and shunt reduction (3). Because this pressure cannot be measured directly, the mean airway pressure is used as an estimation of the pressure at the alveoli (3). This is accomplished by increasing the inspiratory time (and decreasing the expiratory time), so that the I:E ratio is increased from the normal 1:2 to 1:1 or more (3, 19). There are two ways to achieve this, either with volume-cycled ventilation and reducing the flow rate markedly or by using pressure control mode and altering the inspiratory and expiratory times. In this way, the mean airway pressure can be maintained at a lower level of PEEP, as long as end-expiratory trapping of air is not excessive.

The advantage to IRV is that more non-aerated alveoli will be recruited with a sustained increase in airway pressure. Improvements in oxygenation may be seen only after a few hours of initiation of IRV. If, however, air trapping is excessive, then the real end-expiratory pressure will exceed the applied PEEP. This will lead to increased peak pressure in volume-cycled ventilation or to decreased tidal volume in pressure-cycled ventilation. Furthermore, if no improvement in oxygenation is seen, then raising the mean airway pressure farther probably will not lead to increased alveolar recruitment. Indeed, ventilation/perfusion mismatch may worsen if the cardiac output is decreased significantly.

If high levels of airway pressure are obtained, then a significant impact on the hemodynamic status should be expected. On the other hand, one recent study (22) demonstrated an actual improvement in cardiac output, when measured by transesophageal echocardiography, in patients with ARDS who were switched from volume ventilation to pressure-controlled IRV at a 2:1 I:E ratio. Certainly, this is not to be expected in all patients, and those who demonstrate a tenuous hemodynamic status after initiation of IRV should be considered candidates for invasive hemodynamic monitoring or cessation of IRV therapy.

It should be noted that IRV requires a patient who is not initiating respiratory efforts independently. Most frequently, profound sedation is required, perhaps in addition to neuromuscular blockers, which carries the inherent risk of the inability of the patient to breath spontaneously if a ventilator disconnection occurs. The other problems with neuromuscular blocking agents is that atrophy of the respiratory muscles is promoted, by preventing any respiratory effort whatsoever, and the extended use of these agents may induce a syndrome of prolonged paralysis.

Despite the theoretical advantages of IRV, no studies have been able to demonstrate an improvement in patient outcome. Indeed, a recent study by Lessard et al. (23) compared pressure-controlled IRV with conventional volume-controlled ventilation. In a group of patients with moderate to severe ARDS, tidal volume, respiratory rate, FiO_2, and total-PEEP remained constant in each of the two modes. No improvement in ventilatory parameters could be demonstrated by using 2:1 I:E ratio, in comparison to volume-controlled ventilation. However, this was a short-term study, and it may be that the lower peak airway pressures obtainable with IRV would lead to less ventilator-induced airway damage. Clearly, this issue must be studied further, and the role of IRV is as yet undetermined.

Nitric Oxide

A promising therapy is the use of inhaled nitric oxide, a potent pulmonary vasodilator that is metabolized before reaching the systemic circulation. One trial of the use of this agent for patients with severe ARDS demonstrated improvement in oxygenation and an associated reduction in the pulmonary-artery pressures (24). However, a prospective randomized controlled trial will be needed to ascertain whether an improvement in outcome for patients with ARDS can be attained.

Permissive Hypercapnia

To avoid lung overdistention in patients with ARDS, the technique of permissive hypercapnia has been suggested. The basic premise of this technique is to decrease minute ventilation by decreasing peak inspiratory pressure (PIP) and tidal volume. This, in theory, causes a lessened degree of lung distention and less ventilator-associated lung damage (25). By decreasing minute ventilation, the PCO_2 is allowed to rise; in one study, it rose to a mean of 62 mm Hg (26). If the associated respiratory acidosis becomes problematic, it may be treated with the judicious use of sodium bicarbonate. Unfortunately, no prospective controlled trials of this technique exist, so it is difficult to ascertain whether outcome is improved.

Hypercapnia may be deleterious, however, by its ability to increase the pulmonary vascular resistance. This may lead to worsened ventilation/perfusion mismatch. Recently, it was demonstrated that inhaled nitric oxide completely reversed the permissive hypercapnia-induced elevation in pulmonary vascular resistance in patients with ARDS (27). In addition, this led to a significant improvement in arterial oxygenation. A technique of using nitric oxide to lessen the potentially deleterious effects of permissive hypercapnia may lead to a reduction in the impact of mechanical ventilation on lung parenchyma. Prospective clinical trials to confirm the safety and efficacy of this therapy must be performed.

Extracorporeal Carbon Dioxide Removal

A related technique was developed by Gattinoni et al., which incorporates low frequency and low tidal volume ventilation with the removal of carbon dioxide by an extra-corporeal circuit and membrane gas exchanger (28). This technique, termed "extra-corporeal carbon dioxide removal," would not be feasible to apply to all patients with severe ARDS because of lack of equipment; however, it does, perhaps, support the concept of attempting to minimize ventilator-associated lung damage.

CIRCULATORY SHOCK

The patient in circulatory shock has inadequate oxygen delivery (DO_2) to meet the needs of the body to maintain adequate adenosine triphosphate (ATP) production. Thus, shock leads to states of oxygen debt, anaerobic metabolism, and tissue acidosis (29). Shock may result from various causes, such as hemorrhage, cardiac failure, anaphylaxis, or sepsis. The clinical picture is one of hypotension, tachycardia, and evidence of poor organ perfusion, such as neurological changes and oliguria. A patient may be in a state of compensated shock, such that the blood pressure and oxygen transport values are normal, but nonetheless, evidence of poor tissue perfusion remains (29, 30). The cardiac output may be redistributed away from certain organs, such as the kidneys and splanchnic organs (31). In the splanchnic vascular bed, for example, inadequacy of regional tissue oxygenation may lead to increased gastrointestinal mucosal permeability (29). In some studies, this has been shown to lead to translocation of toxins from enteric bacterial flora to body fluids (32) and may even lead to the translocation of bacteria (32, 33).

Goals

The traditional goals of resuscitation should be considered of paramount impor-

tance. Namely, initial attention should be directed at determining that the "ABC" mnemonic of airway, breathing, and circulation is fulfilled. That is, establishing an adequate airway must be the initial step in any resuscitative effort. The breathing aspect of resuscitation refers to determining that adequate gas exchange is occurring. This can be monitored by following the arterial blood gases.

Traditionally, resuscitation of the circulatory system has referred to determining that hypovolemia has been corrected and then directing attention toward the optimization of cardiac function. Algorithms have been constructed to aid in the administration of intravenous fluids (IVF), inotropes, and vasopressors, with sequential escalation in circulatory monitoring. For example, a typical algorithm would suggest that if a patient is hypotensive and has a low urine output and is suspected of having intravascular volume depletion, then IVF should be administered. If this therapy leads to no improvement, or equivocal results, then the central venous pressure (CVP) probably should be monitored. If the CVP rises with IVF administration, but other signs of circulation are unsatisfactory, such as the blood pressure or urine output, then a pulmonary artery catheter is inserted. The measurement of the pulmonary artery occlusion pressure (PAOP) is used to optimize IVF administration. After the PAOP has been brought to a reasonable range, then inotropes and vasopressors are initiated, using the guidance of the cardiac output (CO) measurement and systemic vascular resistance (SVR) calculation.

Although fulfillment of the above circulatory goals are essential, much work has been performed recently to demonstrate that a perfusion-based approach to circulatory resuscitation may lead to improved outcome (30, 34, 35). Various endpoints have been proposed to guide perfusion-based therapy, and these include the mixed venous oxygen saturation, measures of oxygen extraction, lactate concentrations, metabolic acidosis, and more recently, tissue oxygenation or gastric mucosal pH (36). The basic premise to all of these endpoints has been that they are a better indicator of the adequacy of perfusion than the traditional parameters.

Much of the initial work in this area was performed by Shoemaker et al., who observed that high-risk surgical patients who were treated to "supranormal" goals had improved survival when compared to a control group that was treated to normal goals (34). The "supranormal" goals consisted of an oxygen delivery of >600 mL/min/m², oxygen consumption of >170 mL/min/m², and a cardiac output >4.5 L/min/m². An association between oxygen consumption and oxygen delivery was noted. That is, oxygen consumption was dependent upon the amount of oxygen delivered, until a certain level of delivered oxygen was reached, and then a plateau of the amount of oxygen consumed was found (37). In theory, if, in an individual patient, this plateau can be found, then one can ensure an adequate oxygen delivery for the perfusion of all organ systems. Although this work focused attention on oxygen delivery and use, these issues have remained controversial.

More recently, Boyd et al. (35) performed a prospective, randomized controlled trial involving high-risk surgical patients. After ensuring adequate hemoglobin concentration and oxygen saturation, they used dopexamine, which increases cardiac output while causing peripheral vasodilatation, to increase oxygen delivery to a goal of 600 mL/min/m². A 75% reduction in mortality was observed, when compared to a control group that was treated to goals of normal hemodynamic values.

Another recent study (38) also prospectively randomized critically ill patients to either a treatment group, which had a goal of oxygen delivery of >600 mL/min/m², or to a control group, which received treatment to normal parameters. They did not find a statistically significant difference in the control versus treatment groups. However, they did find that patients had increased survival if they actually achieved the supranormal goals, whether they were in the treatment group or the control group, but had generated the supranormal values independent of the goals of treatment. The authors concluded that maximization of oxygen delivery, whether by treatment intent or through self-generation, leads to improved survival in critically ill patients.

The three studies cited above all relied on a mathematical calculation of oxygen delivery and oxygen consumption that uses a common set of measured variables, namely cardiac output and arterial oxygen content. It has been suggested that this coupling of variables may lead to error when calculating the oxygen extraction ratio. To investigate this theory, Ronco et al. (39) increased oxygen delivery in a group of patients with severe adult respiratory distress syndrome by giving a blood transfusion. They found that oxygen consumption remained constant as measured by the analysis of respiratory gases. Furthermore, Hanique et al. (40) recently performed a study in which they compared calculated oxygen consumption with the actual oxygen uptake. They found that by increasing oxygen delivery with a colloid infusion, there was an increase in the calculated but not the measured oxygen consumption. This highlights that further studies into the question of oxygen delivery and consumption should rely on actual measurements of oxygen consumption.

An important issue is that the goals discussed above are measures of global body perfusion. Thus, the effectiveness of the use of oxygen at the end-organ level is not being assessed directly. This, of course, subjects the measure to discrepancies introduced by heterogeneity of the different tissue beds and their differing degrees of microvascular flow reserve, as well as their different metabolic needs (36). Efforts has been concentrated recently into developing monitors that are useful in the clinical arena to guide therapy in the perfusion-based resuscitation of circulatory shock. One method that is promising, although not yet substantiated, is the monitoring of interstitial pH of the gastrointestinal tract using balloon tonometry via a specially adapted nasogastric tube. It has been proposed that the measurement of intramucosal pH in the stomach changes in parallel with the intramucosal pH in the small and large intestines in shock and resuscitation (29, 41). Thus, this may be a convenient measure of the adequacy of oxygenation in one tissue bed, although more work is needed to determine whether this can function as a guide to the resuscitation of shock.

It should be noted that developments of the future may lead to significant changes in the therapy of shock states. For example, reperfusion injury can cause local tissue damage through the generation of oxygen-free radicals. If it is possible to significantly alter the course of reperfusion injury, then this may avoid some consequences of shock, such as the multiple organ dysfunction syndrome (42, 43).

ACUTE RENAL FAILURE

Acute renal failure (ARF) is a common problem, having a prevalence rate of about 5% in hospitalized patients (44), and this is increased in the ICU. During the last few decades, the mortality rate for ARF of 40 to 50% has changed little, despite advances in the diagnosis, treatment, and supportive therapy of renal failure. In addition to a high mortality rate, ARF is associated with increased length of stay in the hospital and increased morbidity (45).

ARF is usually defined as a decrease in renal function, manifested by the failure of the kidney to regulate fluid and electrolyte balance and to excrete nitrogenous waste products. ARF may be associated with oliguria (usually defined as a urine output of less than 400 mL/day); however, nonoliguric renal failure is common.

The etiology for ARF is typically divided into three groups: prerenal, renal, and postrenal (see Table 15–3). Prerenal causes of ARF are consequences of hypoperfusion of the kidney caused by either decreased intravascular volume or decreased cardiac function. In addi-

Table 15–3. Causes of Acute Renal Failure

Prerenal causes of ARF
  Intravascular hypovolemia
  Decreased cardiac output
  Renal vascular disease
Intrinsic renal causes of ARF
  Glomerular diseases
  Tubulointerstitial diseases
  Vascular diseases
Postrenal causes of ARF
  Ureteral obstruction
  Bladder obstruction
  Urethral obstruction

tion, renal vascular disease may be categorized as prerenal. ARF caused by intrinsic renal disease can be related to abnormalities of the glomerulus, tubules, interstitium, or vessels and is due to a large variety of causes. Postrenal ARF is caused by one of the various etiologies of urinary obstruction.

Various theories have been proposed regarding the pathogenesis of ARF from ischemic and nephrotoxic causes; however, a unifying theory is lacking. Factors that have been believed to be important include intratubular obstruction by cellular debris, backleak of filtrate through damaged tubular epithelia, decrease in renal blood flow, and a defect in glomerular permeability (44). It is likely that the pathogenesis of ARF involves factors from each of these theories.

Diagnosis

The etiology for ARF should be diagnosed expediently, to allow specific therapy to be instituted. The first step should be to differentiate between prerenal, renal, and postrenal causes. This will then allow therapy to be targeted toward the specific etiology.

A careful history of the patient's recent course can provide invaluable information regarding the etiology of ARF. The patient's concurrent diseases, cardiac status, exposure to nephrotoxins, and any recent events such as angiography or hypotension may be important clues. The physical examination is usually most helpful in providing information about the patient's state of hydration — both intravascular and total body water.

The urinalysis can be helpful in providing information about ARF. For example, the presence of protein is suggestive of intrinsic renal disease with glomerular injury (44). A microscopic examination of the sediment from a centrifuged sample of a patient with ischemic acute tubular necrosis (ATN) may have coarse pigmented granular casts, tubule epithelial cells and casts, and cellular debris (44). In addition, the presence of white cells and bacteria suggests infection.

The urinary sodium excretion may, in some instances, differentiate between certain etiologies of ARF. In states of renal hypoperfusion, with maintained tubule function, the kidney will retain sodium.

An ultrasound examination of the kidney can be a helpful diagnostic technique in the patient with ARF. It can detect obstruction with a high degree of sensitivity (44) and determines renal size. The latter may help in determining the chronicity of the renal disease, because chronic renal disease frequently results in the loss of nephrons and, hence, a reduction in size.

Other radiological procedures, such as intravenous urography, computed tomography, angiography, and radionucleotide scans, may be helpful in certain groups of patients. Renal biopsy can also be helpful in providing information in select patients with ARF.

Treatment

The basic principle for management of a patient with established ARF is that control is maintained over the metabolic processes normally regulated by the kidney. As such, this would include control of the balance of water and electrolytes. In addition, the maintenance of adequate cardiovascular and hematologic parameters is of paramount importance.

POTASSIUM

The combination of decreased renal excretion of potassium and systemic acidosis, which increases release of intracellular potassium, can lead to life-threatening hyperkalemia in patients with ARF. Hyperkalemia is most toxic in its effects on the heart, and it can precipitate peaking of the T-waves, widening of the QRS complex, and eventually, ventricular fibrillation.

Measures that can decrease the potassium concentration in the short term are the administration of insulin with glucose intravenously and the administration of sodium bicarbonate. If the patient is mechanically ventilated, forced respiratory alkalosis can also acutely decrease the hydrogen ion concentration and, thus, the potassium concentration. In addition, the administration of intravenous calcium may stabilize the cardiac membranes against the effects of hyperkalemia (46).

Steps to decrease the total body potassium concentration include administering a cation-exchange resin (as an enema or orally) or performing the more definitive therapy: dialysis. Although peritoneal dialysis will lower the potassium level, hemodialysis will perform the desired effect far more quickly.

ACIDOSIS

The inability of the kidney to excrete the normal acid load will lead to a metabolic acidosis. Most experts (47) do not advocate the administration of sodium bicarbonate unless the acidosis is severe (e.g., bicarbonate level less than 15 mEq/L), as such therapy presents a large salt and water load. However, one may estimate the bicarbonate deficit: $[(0.5) \cdot (\text{body weight in kg}) \cdot (24\text{-plasma } [HCO_3])]$. Approximately one-half of the deficit may be replaced during the initial 12 hours of therapy.

Hemodialysis, of course, is indicated in cases of life-threatening acidosis and is the definitive method for controlling acidosis.

SODIUM/WATER

The basis for management of fluids in patients with ARF is the assessment of fluid status. This is done by the physical examination and perhaps in association with hemodynamic monitoring. If the patient is euvolemic, fluids may be administered by matching input and output, taking insensible losses into account. The daily weight of the patient should be followed.

Hyponatremia may occur secondary to a defect in the ability to excrete free water gained from the intake of free water.

Dialysis

Indications for dialysis include hyperkalemia, severe acidosis, volume overload, or worsening signs of uremia (e.g., changing mental status or lethargy). The decision to initiate dialysis is based on these indications and the overall clinical condition. In addition, the question frequently arises regarding whether early and intensive dialysis will have an improved outcome over postponing dialysis until a more specific indication occurs. This subject remains controversial; most studies show no improvement in survival with early and intensive dialysis (47).

HEMODIALYSIS

The major advantage of hemodialysis is that it can be used to rapidly correct metabolic disturbances and volume overload. Access is usually obtained for temporary needs via a catheter placed in a centrally located vein. The major disadvantage of this technique is that it may induce hemodynamic instability, especially in critically ill patients. In addition, removing a large amount of excess total body water by an intermittent technique may be problematic. A continuous technique may be better suited to this purpose (see below).

PERITONEAL DIALYSIS

Peritoneal dialysis cannot rapidly correct states of volume or metabolic abnormalities. However, the gradual correction of such abnormalities may provide the advantage of being less of a hemodynamic and metabolic stress. Catheters may be placed either percutaneously or surgically. The main complication is peritonitis, and this usually can be treated without having to remove the catheter, unless the infection is due to *Candida*, which may require catheter removal (47).

CONTINUOUS VENO-VENOUS AND ARTERIOVENOUS HEMOFILTRATION

Continuous arteriovenous hemofiltration (CAVH) and continuous veno-venous hemofiltration (CVVH) are techniques that are well suited for use in critically ill patients with renal failure, especially those with volume overload (48, 49). Ultrafiltration can be performed for 24 hours/day and can be continued for as long as is necessary. The ultrafiltrate is driven by either the arteriovenous pressure difference with CAVH or by a small roller pump with CVVH. This technique is especially good for the removal of excess volume, although a certain amount of solutes are also removed (50).

The major advantage of a continuous technique is that it is usually very well tolerated from a hemodynamic standpoint, often even by patients who do not tolerate hemodialysis (49, 51). The disadvantages of this technique are that it usually requires anticoagulation, it is nursing intensive, and unanticipated clearance of crucial drugs, such as antibiotics, may occur.

SEPSIS

It has been realized recently that what has been termed "sepsis" is actually part of a spectrum of a systemic reaction. In an attempt to clarify the description of this complex reaction, the term *systemic inflammatory response syndrome* (SIRS) was introduced to replace the term *sepsis syndrome* (15, 52). Briefly, SIRS would include clinical signs of a systemic response to endothelial inflammation in the setting (or strong suspicion) of a known cause of endothelial inflammation. This response can occur with or without the presence of a documented infection and is manifest by two or more of the following: (*a*) temperature >38° or <36°, (*b*) heart rate > 90 beats/minute, (*c*) respiratory rate > 20 or $PaCO_2$ < 32 mm Hg, (*d*) white blood cell (WBC) count > 12,000 or < 4,000 or >10% immature forms present (53). For the sake of simplicity, however, the remainder of this discussion will use the term "sepsis" in the general sense.

Sepsis involves a series of characteristic clinical derangements, which is usually induced by infection and frequently precipitates the multiple organ dysfunction syndrome (MODS) (15, 30, 53, 54). Despite prodigious work on the pathogenesis and therapy of sepsis, the mortality rate remains in the range of 10 to 50% (15, 30). Indeed, much of the variation in mortality has been said to be caused by differences in criteria for describing sepsis (16).

Current evidence consistently explains the pathophysiologic processes involved in the induction of the septic response as the result of a cascade of endogenous mediators expressed by an individual, in the face of a precipitating event. Such events are most frequently an infection, although noninfectious causes also exist (53, 54). Much of the initial investigations were performed on the model of sepsis from Gram-negative bacterial endotoxin; however, Gram-positive bacteria, pathogenic viruses, fungi, and rickettsia may also produce a similar syndrome. In addition, noninfectious causes such as severe trauma or pancreatitis may induce the same systemic reaction (53, 54).

As an example of the cascade sequence, examine the result of the reaction to Gram-negative bacterial endotoxin (Fig. 15–1). Endotoxin causes the release of other factors, including tumor necrosis factor (TNF). These factors induce the release of arachidonic acid metabolites, the activation of the coagulation cascade and the complement system, and the release of various interleukins. These all effect the vascular endothelium, and probably the myocardium, to produce the characteristic picture of increased endothelial permeability and septic shock (53, 54). This is truly a sys-temic process, and virtually all organs become involved to one degree or another. The characteristic picture of myocardial dysfunction, increased vascular permeability, neurological dysfunction, respiratory failure, and renal insufficiency is all too common.

In a subgroup of patients with SIRS, the systemic response leads to a progressive deterioration in individual organ systems, leading to MODS. Although it is still possible for a patient to recover, as more and more organs become involved, the likelihood of survival diminishes (55).

Currently, therapy consists of supporting the pulmonary and cardiovascular systems, the provision of nutritional support, and the elimination of the inciting event — whether it is infectious or otherwise. As discussed above, many etiologies can cause sepsis, and the systemic reaction may continue after resolution of the inciting event. However, the resolution of a persisting etiology is of utmost importance. This may involve, for example, the drainage of an abscess and the administration of appropriate antibiotics.

Efforts are being made to alter the high mortality rate of sepsis by directing research into areas that include: (*a*) improving the delivery of oxygen to tissues and (*b*) interrupting the cascade of mediators of systemic inflammation. The treatment of septic shock and the concept of oxygen use are discussed in the *Circulatory Shock* section.

It is becoming apparent that there is a very important difference between the laboratory model of sepsis and the clinical picture. Namely, in the laboratory model, one provides an insult to produce a septic subject in a very controlled fashion. In contrast, in the common clinical scenario, a patient may have suffered an insult before entering the medical system and thus, when he or she is first seen, the cascade of mediators is firmly established. Therefore, an intervention designed to prevent the elaboration of these mediators may be too late, and the challenge is both to identify patients at risk of developing sepsis and to

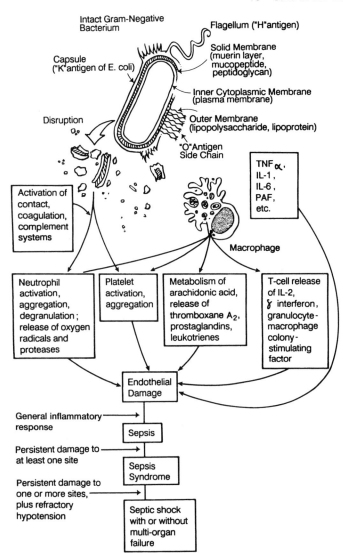

Labels in figure:
Intact Gram-Negative Bacterium
Flagellum ("H"antigen)
Capsule ("K"antigen of E. coli)
Solid Membrane (muerin layer, mucopeptide, peptidoglycan)
Inner Cytoplasmic Membrane (plasma membrane)
Disruption
Outer Membrane (lipopolysaccharide, lipoprotein)
"O"Antigen Side Chain
$TNF\alpha$, IL-1, IL-6, PAF, etc.
Activation of contact, coagulation, complement systems
Macrophage
Neutrophil activation, aggregation, degranulation; release of oxygen radicals and proteases
Platelet activation, aggregation
Metabolism of arachidonic acid, release of thromboxane A_2, prostaglandins, leukotrienes
T-cell release of IL-2, γ interferon, granulocyte-macrophage colony-stimulating factor
Endothelial Damage
General inflammatory response
Sepsis
Persistent damage to at least one site
Sepsis Syndrome
Persistent damage to one or more sites, plus refractory hypotension
Septic shock with or without multi-organ failure

Fig. 15–1. Schematic of sepsis. Note that although the schematic illustration somewhat oversimplifies the pathophysiologic process, it does provide a framework for understanding a complex chain of events. The pathways are not distinct, and the effects of any one mediator may vary with physiologic conditions. Massive endothelial damage does not ordinarily occur because there are many points at which feedback loops downregulate mediator release. If the body cannot restore homeostasis, however, the generalized inflammatory response will produce clinical evidence of sepsis. Persistent endothelial damage to at least one site will produce signs of organ failure (the sepsis syndrome); if hypotension develops and proves refractory to treatment, the patient will meet the criteria for septic shock. (From Bone RC. The pathogenesis of sepsis. Ann Intern Med 1991;115:457–469.)

design an intervention that is efficacious in the clinical arena.

Work to interrupt the cascade of mediators has concentrated on several different approaches. In Figure 15–2, the regulation of TNF biosynthesis, which leads to the secretion of the mediator proteins, in macrophages is schematized. The steps include (*a*) transcription (messenger ribonucleic acid [mRNA] is synthesized from the deoxyribonucleic acid [DNA] template), (*b*) the processing of mRNA, (*c*) mRNA translation into protein, and (*d*) modification and secretion of proteins.

Theoretically, the secretion of proteins from the stimulation of the lipopolysaccharide (LPS)-binding protein (LPS-LBP) may be interrupted at any regulated point. As noted in the figure, agents that increase cyclic adenosine monophosphate (cAMP) production will inhibit mRNA transcription. The agents that have been studied in this regard include pentoxifylline, amrinone, and dobutamine, and preliminary studies in animal models and hu-

Fig. 15–2. Regulation of tumor necrosis factor (TNF) biosynthesis in macrophages. After binding of lipopolysaccharide (LPS)-binding protein (LPS-LBP) to the CD14 molecule, the synthesis of TNF is begun by translation of preformed tumor necrosis factor messenger ribonucleic acid (TNF mRNA) and accelerated transcription of the TNF gene. After translation of mRNA into preprotein monomers, posttranslational modification and trimer formation are required to generate the mature secreted form of TNF. Transcriptional activation is inhibited by agents that increase the intracellular cyclic adenosine monophosphate (cAMP) concentration. Translation of TNF mRNA is inhibited by corticosteroids. After secretion of TNF, toxicity may be inhibited by monoclonal antibodies directed against TNF of by artificial protein inhibitors of TNF. UTR = untranslated region. (From Giroir BP. Mediators of septic shock: new approaches for interrupting the endogenous inflammatory cascade. Crit Care Med 1993;21:780–789.)

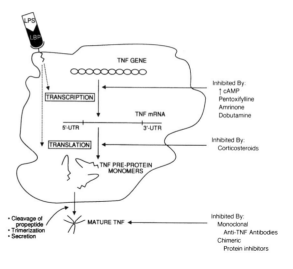

man volunteers demonstrate a reduction in TNF synthesis (54). However, this has not been rigorously tested in a population of human patients with sepsis.

Corticosteroids are inhibitors of the translation of mRNA and have been promising in animal models of septic shock (54, 56). However, two large randomized human trials did not show any benefit to the use of corticosteroids in sepsis (57, 58). This subject remains somewhat controversial, because it may be that corticosteroids would be beneficial if administered before antibiotics, in low doses, or if given to a small subset of patients.

Intense research has been focused on the use of monoclonal antibodies directed against various steps in the synthesis of TNF and the elucidation of the cascade phase of sepsis. The latter aspect refers to the secretion of other mediators, such as various interleukins, prostaglandins, and leukotrienes, as well as the activation of neutrophils. In animal models, monoclonal antibodies against TNF have provided significant protection from the toxic effects of the infusion of endotoxemia (54).

Other targets for the use of monoclonal antibodies have been endotoxin (59, 60) and interleukin-1 (IL-1) (61). Two monoclonal antibodies against endotoxin have been tested in large clinical trials in patients with evidence of Gram-negative sepsis (59, 60). The E5 murine monoclonal antibody resulted in improved survival only in the subgroup of patients who were not in shock at study entry (60). The HA-1A human monoclonal IgM antibody improved survival in the subgroup of patients who eventually had Gram-negative bacteremia proven by blood culture, but survival was unchanged in the study population as a whole (59). Because these results were inconclusive, a second study was initiated, but this was suspended after excess mortality was noted in patients treated with HA-1A (62). In addition, the safety of HA-1A has been called into question in animal models of sepsis (63). Because of these questions of efficacy and safety, neither antibody against endotoxin is currently available in the United States, although HA-1A is available in Europe (62).

Antibodies against IL-1 have proven promising in animal models (54), and human trials are in progress. These studies must be awaited for further recommendations.

NOSOCOMIAL PNEUMONIA

Diagnosis and Treatment

Pneumonia has been shown to be the most common nosocomial infection in patients who are mechanically ventilated. Furthermore, hospital-acquired pneumonia is the leading cause of mortality from nosocomial infection in the United States (64, 65). In a multivariate analysis of the risk factors for developing nosocomial pneumonia, patients at increased risk included those who undergo mechanical ventilation, have a depressed level of consciousness, have underlying chronic lung disease, or are elderly, have undergone thoracic or upper abdominal surgery, or have had a large volume aspiration (64). Mortality rates of 20 to 70% have been reported for nosocomial pneumonia (64, 65).

The diagnosis of pneumonia in a critically ill patient can be problematic. The familiar clinical signs of a roentgenographic infiltrate, fever, leukocytosis, and a pathogenic organism obtained from sputum are not always reliable in the critically ill patient. All too frequently, these patients have pulmonary pathology that makes the roentgenographic diagnosis of an infiltrate very difficult. Likewise, there may be many reasons for these patients to be febrile or have a leukocytosis, or the patients may be too debilitated to mount such a response. In addition, a blind tracheal aspirate has been shown in numerous studies to have a low specificity but a somewhat higher sensitivity (66–68). This probably is due to the colonization

of the tracheobronchial system with multiple organisms. Thus, inappropriate antimicrobial therapy may be instituted, which may alter a particular patient's flora and can lead to the selection of resistant pathogens.

It is, therefore, often a difficult task to diagnose and empirically treat a patient who is suspected of having a nosocomial pneumonia. Fagon et al. prospectively provided a team of ICU physicians with complete clinical data for a series of 84 patients who were suspected to have nosocomial pneumonia (69). All patients had a new pulmonary infiltrate and purulent tracheal secretions. With this information, the physicians created a diagnosis and a treatment plan. The group of patients then underwent quantitative culture of protected specimen brush (PSB) samples of the affected lobe, a technique with high specificity (67, 68, 70). They found that patients were diagnosed correctly as having pneumonia only 62% of the time. In addition, 16% of the time, patients were unnecessarily subjected to antibiotics.

Techniques have been devised in attempts to improve the diagnostic capability of detecting nosocomial pneumonia. These include bronchoalveolar lavage (BAL) and protected specimen brush (PSB). Both of these techniques are performed with fiberoptic bronchoscopy. For bronchoalveolar lavage, sterile saline is irrigated into the lobe in question by wedging the bronchoscope in a medium-sized bronchus. The saline is then aspirated and sent for Gram's stain and semiquantitative culture. To obtain a PSB culture, the bronchoscope is introduced into the lobe of interest. A brush with a sterile protective covering is advanced several centimeters through the suction port. The brush is then advanced out of its protective covering into the airway. It is then withdrawn into its covering and sent for semiquantitative culture. Both BAL and PSB have been shown to have improved specificity over tracheal aspirate cultures. If a cutoff of 10^3 colony-forming units per mL (CFU/mL) is chosen for PSB, then various series have shown a specificity of between 85 and 100% (66). For a cutoff of 10^5 CFU/mL with BAL, various series have shown a specificity of between 70 and 100% specificity (66). However, these procedures are invasive and require specialized training and, therefore, may not be applicable to all clinical situations.

Considering the difficulties in diagnosing nosocomial pneumonia and the risks both of treating and not treating patients who are not infected, what are specific recommendations that can be applied to most clinical situations? Certainly, an acute change in any of the clinical parameters, such as newly purulent tracheal secretions and a new infiltrate, together with a rising white blood cell (WBC) count or fever, are signs that most clinicians would associate with nosocomial pneumonia. The difficulty in this situation may lie in determining the proper empiric antibiotics to use. A tracheal aspirate has been shown to be poorly specific but probably will be sensitive enough to include most of the organisms causing the pneumonia (66). Therefore, following the Gram's stain and culture data and the response to therapy will provide a basis for treatment.

The more perplexing situation, when the clinical parameters may be conflicting (e.g., the Gram's stain of the tracheal aspirate is nonspecific), may be a situation in which one of the more invasive techniques may be helpful in diagnosis and therapy decisions.

Prophylaxis Against Nosocomial Pneumonia

GASTRIC pH AND NOSOCOMIAL PNEUMONIA

Considering the high rate of nosocomial pneumonia in mechanically ventilated ICU patients, various prophylactic techniques have been attempted. In addition to the use of standard precautions against the transmission of nosocomial infections, much research has centered on gastrointestinal microbes colonizing and infecting the upper and lower airways of patients. Two methods that have received widespread attention are the management of gastric pH and selective gut decontamination.

Stress ulcers occur frequently in ICU patients and can induce significant morbidity. However, with the use of stress ulcer prophylaxis, this can be reduced by a large degree. The main methods are the use of H_2-receptor antagonists, sucralfate, or antacids, all of which have been shown to be efficacious in reducing stress ulcers (71–73). However, it is controversial whether agents that raise the pH of the stomach, and thereby change the gastric flora to more pathogenic organisms, predispose patients to developing pneumonia. Two recent meta-analyses have reached somewhat disparate conclusions. Tryba found that pneumonia occurred more frequently in patients undergoing long-term mechanical ventilation receiving either H_2 antagonists or antacids than in patients receiving sucralfate (72). He concluded that sucralfate is effective prophylaxis against stress bleeding and minimizes the risk of nosocomial pneumonia.

Cook et al., in a meta-analysis comparing patients who received either stress prophylaxis or placebo, found that drugs that raised the gastric pH did not increase the incidence of pneumonia (74). In contrast, sucralfate was associated with a lower incidence of pneumonia when compared to agents that raised gastric pH. However, they noted that methodological deficiencies and small sample sizes in many of the studies may make these conclusions suspect.

In a recent prospective randomized trial of 85 patients comparing sucralfate versus ranitidine in stress ulcer prophylaxis, there was found to be no difference in pneumonia rate in mechanically ventilated patients with trauma (71). Clearly, the issue remains controversial. However, it can be concluded that stress ulcer prophylaxis is efficacious in reducing bleeding. In addition, a large prospective randomized trial is necessary to determine whether there is a reduction in pneumonia rates with sucralfate.

SELECTIVE GUT DECONTAMINATION

As Gram-negative bacteria from the digestive tract have been implicated in nosocomial infections, particularly those of the lower respiratory tract (75), attempts have been made to lower this infection rate by preventing bacterial colonization. This is accomplished by the administration of nonabsorbable antibiotics to the digestive tract. Typical regimens have included such antimicrobials as polymyxin E, amphotericin B, and norfloxacin (76), which are typically administered via the oropharynx, via the nasogastric tube, and as an enema.

Results of gut decontamination have been conflicting. A study by Tetteroo et al. (76) demonstrated increased survival and decreased ICU time in a subgroup of prospectively treated postoperative patients who were decontaminated successfully. They did not find much improvement in survival in those patients who were not decontaminated successfully. However, there was no comparison control group in this study. Instead, patients' expected mortality rate was calculated from group data.

Hammond et al. (77) performed a double-blind placebo controlled trial of selective gut decontamination in critically ill patients. They did not find any difference in incidence of secondary infection, ICU length of stay, or mortality rate between the treatment and placebo groups. Furthermore, a meta-analysis into this subject revealed equivocal results (78).

HEAD TRAUMA

Patients who sustain multiple trauma may develop a closed head injury. The initial event causes a destructive injury to the brain that cannot be repaired and has an associated high morbidity and mortality. Intensive efforts have been directed toward minimizing what has been described as secondary injuries due to cerebral hypoxia, ischemia, and compression (79–81). The brain lacks metabolic reserves and, hence, is very susceptible to alterations in cerebral blood flow (CBF). In addition, because the intracranial pressure (ICP) increases in a hyperbolic fashion with increases

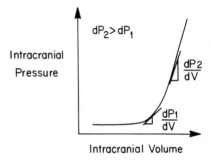

Fig. 15–3. Cerebral compliance curve. Intracranial pressure (ICP) increases in a hyperbolic fashion with increasing intracranial volume. At lower intracranial volumes, ICP does not change with changing intracranial volume. At dP1/dV, increasing intracranial volume is reflected in an increase in ICP. At dP2/dV, small increases in intracranial volume are associated with large changes in pressure. (From Borel C, Hanley D, Diringer MN, et al. Intensive management of severe head injury. Chest 1990;98:180–189; modified from Davis RJ, et al. Head and spinal cord injury. In: Rogers MC, ed. Textbook of pediatric intensive care. Baltimore: Williams & Wilkins, 1986;655.)

in intracranial volume (Fig. 15–3), the brain is particularly vulnerable to changes in the intracranial contents, from either edema or bleeding. Therefore, efforts to reduce the secondary injuries in head trauma have been directed toward preventing cerebral hypoxia and compression, through the management of ICP and CBF.

Clearly, the most important initial efforts are to ensure a patent airway and adequate ventilatory and circulatory systems. Any surgical problems, such as a subdural hematoma, must be detected and treated. In addition, other injuries suffered by the patient must be stabilized.

The level of consciousness of the patient at initial assessment is indicative of the seriousness of the primary injury. In evaluating consciousness, the Glasgow Coma Scale (GCS) is frequently used in patients with head trauma (see Table 15–4). Severe depression of consciousness is generally accepted to correlate with a GCS of 8 or lower. The GCS is influenced by any modifiers of consciousness, such as drugs, alcohol, hypoxia, or hypotension. In addition to evaluating consciousness,

Table 15–4. Glasgow Coma Scale

	Points
Eye opening	
No response	1
Response to pain	2
Response to voice	3
Spontaneously	4
Verbal response	
No response	1
Incomprehensible sounds	2
Inappropriate words	3
Oriented and appropriate	4
Motor response	
No response	1
Extensor posturing	2
Flexor posturing	2
Withdrawal	4
Localizes pain	5
Obeys command	6

a complete neurological examination must be performed and any associated injuries must be evaluated.

Attention may then be directed toward attempting to lessen the secondary injury from traumatic head injury. Most of the research has been directed toward the monitoring and treatment of elevated intracranial pressure (ICP), ensuring an adequate CBF, and trials of agents to "protect" the brain from a decreased CBF.

Becker et al. (79) proposed aggressive ICP monitoring in patients with severe head trauma. They used hyperventilation, cerebral spinal fluid (CSF) drainage, and mannitol as techniques to treat elevated ICP. When compared with series of head trauma patients at other centers, Becker et al. demonstrated improved outcome. ICP monitoring and treatment became widely used, due in large part to this study's favorable results. In centers that manage ICP aggressively, it is generally accepted to maintain an ICP of 20 mm Hg or less (82).

Many medical techniques have been proposed as methods of controlling ICP, including barbiturate coma, osmotic agents, hypothermia, hyperventilation, and steroids. The mainstay of therapy for control of ICP is dehydration, which attenuates cerebral swelling. The osmotic diuretic mannitol is often used initially, and loop diuretics may be used to promote cerebral dehydration. Hyperventilation is a very effective method of reducing ICP. However, the effects of a decreased PCO_2 on cerebral vasoconstriction are of a short duration, because the CSF bicarbonate level will adjust to the altered CSF pH and counteract the effects on the vasculature. Other methods of managing ICP include avoidance of excessive coughing and maintaining the head of the patient's bed in an upright position. Many other techniques, such as barbiturate coma, have been used; the reader is referred to a neurosurgical textbook for additional sources.

Several years after the initial favorable work on ICP management, Stuart et al. (80) presented a series of patients in whom ICP monitoring was not performed, although the patients received standard medical and surgical therapy. Importantly, any hematomas were surgically removed. Their results compared favorably to those of other groups using ICP monitoring. This subject has remained controversial.

More recently, Rosner and Daughton presented a protocol that questions much of what has become standard care for severe head trauma (81). This group attempted to maintain the cerebral perfusion pressure (CPP) at 70 to 80 mm Hg. (CPP is the mean arterial pressure [MAP] minus the ICP, or the central venous pressure, depending on which is greater). Maintaining an elevated blood pressure traditionally has been believed to be potentially deleterious, because it is felt that damaged areas of brain will have an abnormal autoregulation of blood flow. The authors of this study, however, did not demonstrate any deleterious effects of an elevated MAP and CPP and, in fact, presented data that support the converse, namely that increasing the CPP resulted in a decrease in the ICP. Their patient outcome was favorable. It must be noted that this subject remains quite controversial.

SEDATION

One of the most important issues facing caregivers of hospitalized patients is the assessment/alleviation of stress and anxiety. This concept is magnified for critically ill patients, who are in very threatening and often painful situations. The feeling of helplessness can be pervasive and can lead to much distress. In addition to wreaking psychological havoc, these reactions can lead to activation of the stress response, causing activation of the sympathetic system, among other mechanisms (83, 84). For the critically ill patient with a poor physiological reserve, this may lead to cardiopulmonary decompensation, such as myocardial ischemia. Thus, for both humane and physiological reasons, it is imperative to alleviate stress and pain in critically ill patients. Because pain control is reviewed in other chapters, the discussion that follows will center on anxiety. Clearly, however, many critically ill patients experience pain, and the alleviation of such symptoms is a mandatory part of the treatment of stress and anxiety.

Diagnosis

Anxiety is, unfortunately, a very common problem among critically ill patients, and it frequently can escalate to maladaptive levels (83, 84). Therefore, one must suspect anxiety in most hospitalized patients, and certainly in most of those who are critically ill. Anxiety and its manifestations must be differentiated from delirium, which is also common in critically ill patients. Delirium, of course, is usually the result of the underlying disease process causing neurological impairment. This frequently results from metabolic or infectious problems. Furthermore, the most important aspect of treating anxiety is to reverse any processes causing metabolic derangements, such as hypotension, hypoxemia, or acidosis. It should be noted that there is a large spectrum of what actually comprises anxiety, ranging from heightened awareness, through inability

Table 15–5. Physical Signs and Symptoms of Anxiety

Anorexia	Muscle tension
"Butterflies" in stomach	Nausea
Chest pain or tightness	Pallor
Diaphoresis	Palpitations
Diarrhea	Paresthesias
Dizziness	Sexual dysfunction
Dry mouth	Shortness of breath
Dyspnea	Stomach pain
Faintness	Tachycardia
Flushing	Tremulousness
Headache	Urinary frequency
Hyperventilation	Vomiting
Lightheadedness	

From Pollack MH, Stern TA. Recognition and treatment of anxiety in the ICU patient. In: Rippe JM, Irwin RS, Alpert JS, et al., eds. Intensive care medicine. Boston: Little, Brown and Co., 1991;1875–1887.

to concentrate, to distortion of perception (see Table 15–5).

Treatment

NONPHARMACOLOGIC

The first line of therapy to alleviate anxiety is the use of techniques that do not involve pharmacologic agents. As reviewed by Pollack and Stern (84), this would involve a combination of the techniques outlined in Table 15–6.

PHARMACOLOGIC

In addition to use of the nonpharmacologic methods to alleviate stress, many patients re-

Table 15–6. Nonpharmacologic Interventions

Nonpharmacologic interventions
  Education
  Support
  Behavioral techniques
    Hypnosis
    Relaxation techniques
    Imagery
  Cognitive therapy
  Family therapy

Modified from Pollack MH, Stern TA. Recognition and treatment of anxiety in the ICU patient. In: Rippe JM, Irwin RS, Alpert JS, et al., eds. Intensive care medicine. Boston: Little Brown and Co., 1991;1875–1887.

quire additional methods, such as the use of pharmacologic techniques. Many approaches can be used successfully in the pharmacologic control of anxiety in the critically ill patient. The exact goals of therapy must be determined before choosing a technique. Specific endpoints will help guide therapy, and these might include analgesia, anxiolysis, amnesia, chemical control of agitation or delirium, maximization of favorable oxygen balance and/or ventilatory parameters, and terminal comfort. Thus, a patient who is experiencing anxiety probably would respond well to an anxiolytic, such as a benzodiazepine, whereas the patient who is delusional and psychotic probably would respond better to an antipsychotic, such as haloperidol. In addition, if the patient is experiencing pain, then administration of an opioid would be beneficial.

It is equally important to determine what level of sedation is desired. This can range from mild to very profound sedation, depending on the clinical situation. Clearly, the patient who cannot maintain oxygenation unless he or she is in a state of deep sedation requires different therapy than the patient who merely requires an oral sedative to maintain a calm, controlled state. Unfortunately, no assessment tools to measure anxiety in critically ill patients have been tested adequately. A scale, derived by investigators at Duke University Medical Center, that has been used at our institution is as follows:

1. No response to painful stimuli
2. Responds to painful stimuli only (not verbal stimuli)
3. Eyes closed, calm, responds to loud verbal command or physical stimuli
4. Eyes closed, calm, responds appropriately to verbal command
5. Eyes open, awake, calm
6. Eyes open, awake, agitated

It is recommended that this scale be used as any medication is titrated to produce sedation. In general, there is no indication for further doses of medication as long as the patient is in levels 1 through 5.

A final goal would be to define the predicted time course involved. For example, a patient needing sedation and analgesia for a brief bedside procedure will require a different technique than the patient requiring long-term sedation for the purpose of coordinating synchrony with the ventilator.

After the goals of therapy have been delineated, a pharmacologic agent best suited to achieve these goals may be chosen. The choice between different agents would best be made by considering the differing potencies, half-lives, and rates of efficacy of the drugs (83, 84). Another guiding principle would be the ease of administration via different techniques. For example, whether a particular drug lends itself to administration via a bolus or by a constant infusion would be an important factor.

It should be noted that neuromuscular blockers play almost no role in the patient who is difficult to control because of anxiety or confusion. Except in the rare case in which the patient presents an immediate danger to himself or herself, and he or she is mechanically ventilated, would it be appropriate to administer a short-acting neuromuscular blocking agent. In general, the risks of iatrogenic respiratory insufficiency and the risk of having a paralyzed but not sedated patient would be too great to assume. It should be expected that almost all patients could be controlled with sedative/hypnotic agents.

The following discussion of sedative agents and the accompanying Table 15–7 are intended to be of a general nature. Each patient warrants individualized titration of sedation.

Benzodiazepines

Oral and parenteral benzodiazepines seem to be most useful in patients with mild to moderate anxiety, those experiencing alcohol withdrawal with a concomitant illness, and in patients for whom sedative and amnestic effects are desired. In these situations, several drugs have been used with great success. Close titration is always necessary. Problems en-

Table 15–7. Commonly Used Sedative Agents

Drug	Route	Initial dose (mg)	Dosing interval (hr)	Onset of action (min)	Duration of action (hr)	Elimination (beta) T1/2
Diazepam	p.o.	2–10	6–12	15–45	—	30–56
	i.v.	2–10	3–4	1–5	0.25–1	30–56
Midazolam	i.v.	1–2	4–6	1–3	—	1.2–12.3
Lorazepam	p.o.	2–3	8–12	—	—	12–18
	i.v.	1–2	—	15–20	6–8	—
Morphine	i.v.	2–10	3–6	2–3	4–5	—
Meperidine	i.v.	50–100	3–4	30–60	4–6	13–47
Fentanyl	i.v.	0.05–0.1	1–2	1–2	0.5–1	3.6
Haloperidol	p.o.	0.5–2	8–12	—	—	11.5–24
	i.m.	0.5–2	1–8	<30–45	—	—
	i.v.	0.5–2	1–8	10–19	10–20	—

countered may include delay in onset of effect, short-acting agents that require frequent boluses or a continuous infusion, long-acting agents that may persist after sedation is no longer needed, respiratory depression, and paradoxical agitation.

Opioids

Opioids are most useful for patients who have underlying pain, which may contribute to agitation. These agents may be used alone or in conjunction with a drug from another class (e.g., a benzodiazepine). Strictly speaking, they are not anxiolytic agents, but they have a secondary anxiolytic effect if pain is partially responsible for causing agitation. In addition, they will cause sedation and hypnosis if given in larger doses.

Neuroleptics

Neuroleptics are most useful for patients with severe agitation and delirium. They may be especially useful for patients who do not respond to benzodiazepines or who become paradoxically agitated with benzodiazepines. The most commonly used agent is haloperidol, a butyrophenone. It should be noted that haloperidol has not been approved for intravenous use by the U.S. Food and Drug Administration, although there is a large amount of literature to support this route (85).

Propofol

Propofol recently has been approved by the FDA for sedation in the ICU. The advantage of this agent is its titratability, which allows patients to recover quickly from profound sedation. An example of when this would be of importance is when it is crucial to follow a patient's neurological examination, but sedation is still required for recovery of function. This short-acting agent may have limited application for long-term sedation because of cost concerns.

NUTRITION

Critically ill patients are usually dependent on physicians to meet their nutritional needs. In addition, these patients are frequently chronically malnourished or have increased metabolic demands. Not providing adequate caloric substrates can lead to malnutrition, which is associated with decreased muscle function and can lead to ventilator dependency. In addition, critically ill patients who are metabolically stressed may require larger increases in nutrients than nonstressed patients. On the other hand, providing more calories than needed can lead to increased carbon dioxide production, necessitating increased minute ventilation for patients who may have a decreased ventilatory reserve. Thus, it is imperative that critically ill patients be assessed from a nutritional standpoint and that their needs are addressed soon after their risk for malnutrition and inability to meet requirements independently are determined.

Many institutions have a multidisciplinary team consisting of physicians and nutritionists that addresses the nutritional needs of patients. By applying a standardized approach to the assessment of nutritional status, the creation of a therapeutic plan, and the continual reassessment of the effectiveness of therapy, critically ill patients can be better served.

Assessment

The nutritional status of critically ill patients can be assessed by history, physical examination, and laboratory techniques. Patients may have a history of weight loss or decreased food intake before the development of illness. On physical examination, they may demonstrate signs such as muscle wasting. The degree of wasting can be quantitated by anthropometric measurements, for example, triceps skinfold thickness. Laboratory measurements, such as electrolytes, blood urea nitrogen (BUN), and creatinine will provide information as to water and metabolite status. An estimate of visceral protein mass can be obtained by a serum albumin measurement, although this is fraught with inaccuracies because albumin has a long half-life and can be redistributed during states of diffuse capillary leak. Larger proteins, such as prealbumin, transferrin, or retinal binding protein have been proposed as an improvement in estimating protein balance (86).

Caloric requirements can be estimated by the use of equations, such as the familiar Harris-Benedict equation: Resting Energy Expenditure (REE) (males) = 66.473 + (13.7516 · Weight [kg]) + (5.0033 · Height [cm]) – (6.755 · Age [years]); REE (females) = 655.0955 + (9.5634 · Weight) + (1.8496 · Height) – (4.6756 · Age). Inaccuracies that may arise for the prediction of caloric needs for the critically ill patient are usually compensated for by factors that take into account the degree that the patient is considered to be stressed. Although such equations are easily used, they have been shown to be inaccurate in critically ill patients. Makk et al. (87) compared the use of the Harris-Benedict equation versus the measurement of caloric requirements via a metabolic cart, which analyzes respiratory gases. In their study of hospitalized patients, they demonstrated that 41% of patients were underfed and 27% were overfed. This study highlights the importance of using a metabolic cart, especially for patients who are critically ill and who can have large variations in caloric needs (86).

The protein requirements of critically ill patients may be estimated from the measurement of a 24-hour urine urea nitrogen, as well as the volume of the urine. One must allow for insensible losses of nitrogen, from sources such as stool and skin, of approximately 4 g/day (86). In this way, a positive nitrogen balance of approximately 1 to 2 g/day can be a goal.

Nutritional Supplementation

Nutrition can be provided to critically ill patients either enterally or parenterally. Enteral feeding is generally preferred, if it is tolerated by the patient. Using the gastrointestinal tract has the advantages of reduced cost, probable reduced morbidity, possible preservation of the gut mucosal barrier, and favorable modulation of the immune system by certain supplements (88). However, providing enteral nutrition requires a functioning gastrointestinal tract, which may not be present in many critically ill patients.

Enteral feedings may range from either protein-calorie supplementation to complete forced feedings, usually via either a flexible nasoenteric tube or a gastroenterostomy. Many different types of feeding preparations that provide all of the essential nutrients are available. A typical polymeric formula contains 30% fat and 70% carbohydrates and has an osmolality of about 350 mOsm/L. Such formulas contain 1 kCal/mL. Other formulas exist for special needs, such as elemental preparations that might be better absorbed in the immediate postoperative period.

Complications of enteral nutrition may be related to the delivery device or to the feeding itself. Flexible nasoenteric tubes have a notoriously high rate of tracheal passage; therefore, a roentgenogram should be obtained, at least for all patients with a compromised neurological status. Once in place, these small bore tubes are generally well tolerated and do not have high rates of causing sinusitis or other physical complications. With feeding tubes that remain in the stomach (and do not enter the duodenum), patients may be at increased risk of pulmonary aspiration, especially if the feedings are not well tolerated. Complications that pertain to the feeding itself can be large gastric residuals or severe diarrhea (89).

Total parenteral nutrition (TPN) is required when enteral feedings are not able to meet complete nutritional requirements. To administer TPN, a central venous catheter is needed, because the solutions can induce sclerosis of peripheral veins. A typical standard formulation of TPN contains a 3.5% amino acid solution, 25% dextrose, and approximately 850 nonprotein kCal/L. Intralipids can be added, which also increases the nonprotein kCal/L (a 10% solution of intralipids has 1.1 kCal/mL). Vitamins, trace minerals, and electrolytes must be added to the formulation to prevent deficiencies.

The response to supplemental nutrition must be monitored on a continual basis. Measurements of electrolytes, renal function, liver function, divalent ions, and glucose are usually sufficient to monitor for complications (86). Glucose intolerance is common, especially when commencing TPN, and is usually easily treated with insulin.

REFERENCES

1. Smith I, Fleming S, Cernaianu A. Mishaps during transport from the intensive care unit. Crit Care Med 1990;18:278–281.
2. Manning HL. Peak airway pressure: why the fuss? Chest 1994;105:242–247.
3. Marcy TW, Marini JJ. Inverse ratio ventilation in ARDS. Rationale and implementation. Chest 1991;100:494–504.
4. Hershey MD. Ventilatory support of patients with respiratory failure. Int Anesthesiol Clin 1993;31:149–168.
5. Tobin MJ, Yang K. Weaning from mechanical ventilation. Crit Care Clin 1990;6:725–747.
6. Civetta JM. Nosocomial respiratory failure or iatrogenic ventilator dependency. Crit Care Med 1993;21:171–173.
7. Yang KL, Tobin MJ. A prospective study of indexes predicting the outcome of trial of weaning from mechanical ventilation. N Engl J Med 1991;324:1445–1450.
8. Milbern SM, Downs JB, Jumper LC, et al. Evaluation of criteria for discontinuing mechanical ventilation support. Arch Surg 1978;113:1441–1443.
9. Sassoon CSH, Giron AE, Ely EA, et al. Inspiratory work of breathing on flow-by and demand-flow continuous positive airway pressure. Crit Care Med 1989;17:1108–1114.
10. Jounieaux V, Duran A, Levi-Valensi P. Synchronized intermittent mandatory ventilation with and without pressure support ventilation in weaning patients with COPD from mechanical ventilation. Chest 1994;105:1204–1210.
11. Banner MJ, Kirby RR, Blanch PB, et al. Decreasing imposed work of the breathing apparatus to zero using pressure-support ventilation. Crit Care Med 1993;21:1333–1338.
12. Ashbaugh DG, Bigelow DB, Petty TL, et al. Acute respiratory distress in adults. Lancet 1967;2:319–323.
13. Villar J, Slutsky AS. The incidence of the adult respiratory distress syndrome. Am Rev Respir Dis 1989;140:814–816.
14. Suchyta MR, Clemmer TP, Orme JF Jr, et al. Increased survival of ARDS patients with severe hypoxemia (ECMO criteria). Chest 1991;99:951–955.
15. Bone RC. Toward an epidemiology and natural history of SIRS (systemic inflammatory response syndrome). JAMA 1992;268:3452–3455.
16. Bone RC, Balk R, Slotman G, et al. Adult respiratory distress syndrome. Sequence and importance of development of multiple organ failure. Chest 1992;101:320–326.
17. Cunningham AJ. Acute respiratory distress syndrome — two decades later. Yale J Biol Med 1991;64:387–402.
18. Taylor RW, Norwood S. The adult respiratory distress syndrome. In: Civetta JM, Taylor RT, Kirby RR, eds. Critical care. Philadelphia: JB Lippincott Co., 1992;1237–1248.
19. Stoller JK, Kacmarek RM. Ventilatory strategies in the management of the adult respiratory distress syndrome. Clin Chest Med 1990;11:755–772.

20. Rouby JJ, Lherm T, Martin de Lassale E, et al. Histologic aspects of pulmonary barotrauma in critically ill patients with acute respiratory failure. Intensive Care Med 1993;19:383–389.

21. Hernandez LA, Peevy KJ, Moise AA, et al. Chest wall restriction limits high airway pressure-induced lung injury in young rabbits. J Appl Physiol 1989;66:2364–2368.

22. Poelaert JI, Visser CA, Everaert JA, et al. Acute hemodynamic changes of pressure-controlled inverse ratio ventilation in the adult respiratory distress syndrome. Chest 1993;104:214–219.

23. Lessard MR, Guerot E, Lorino H, et al. Effects of pressure-controlled with different I:E ratios versus volume-controlled ventilation on respiratory mechanics, gas exchange, and hemodynamics in patients with adult respiratory distress syndrome. Anesthesiology 1994;80:983–991.

24. Rossaint R, Falke KJ, Lopez F, et al. Inhaled nitric oxide for the adult respiratory distress syndrome. N Engl J Med 1993;328:399–405.

25. Bidani A, Tzouanakis AE, Cardenas VJ, et al. Permissive hypercapnia in acute respiratory failure. JAMA 1994;272:957–962.

26. Hickling KG, Henderson SJ, Jackson R. Low mortality associated with low volume pressure limited ventilation with permissive hypercapnia in severe adult respiratory distress syndrome. Intensive Care Med 1990;16:372–377.

27. Puybasset L, Stewart T, Rouby JJ, et al. Inhaled nitric oxide reverses the increase in pulmonary vascular resistance induced by permissive hypercapnia in patients with acute respiratory distress syndrome. Anesthesiology 1994;80:1254–1267.

28. Gattinoni L, Pesenti A, Mascheroni D, et al. Low frequency positive ventilation with extracorporeal CO_2 removal in severe acute respiratory failure: clinical results. JAMA 1986;256:881.

29. Fiddian-Green RG, Haglund U, Gutierrez G, et al. Goals for the resuscitation of shock. Crit Care Med 1993;21:S25–S31.

30. Shoemaker WC, Appel PL, Kram HB. Hemodynamic and oxygen transport responses in survivors and nonsurvivors of high-risk surgery. Crit Care Med 1993;21:977–990.

31. Gutierrez G, Bismar H. Distribution of blood flow in the critically ill patient. In: Wendt M, Lawin P, eds. Oxygen transport in the critically ill patient: anaesthesiology and intensive care medicine. Berlin: Springer-Verlag, 1990;127–135.

32. Van Leeuwen PA, Boermeester MA, Houdijk AP, et al. Clinical significance of translocation. Gut 1994;35:S28–S34.

33. Sori AJ, Rush BF, Lysz TW, et al. The gut as a source of sepsis after hemorrhagic shock. Am J Surg 1988;155:185–192.

34. Shoemaker WC, Appel PL, Kram HB, et al. Prospective trial of supranormal values of survivors as therapeutic goals in high-risk surgical patients. Chest 1988;94:1176–1186.

35. Boyd O, Grounds M, Bennett ED. A randomized clinical trial of the effect of deliberate perioperative increase of oxygen delivery on mortality in high-risk surgical patients. JAMA 1993;270:2699–2707.

36. Dantzker DR: Adequacy of tissue oxygenation. Crit Care Med 1993;21:S40–S43.

37. Shibutani K, Komatsu T, Hubal K, et al. Critical level of oxygen delivery in anesthetized man. Crit Care Med 1983;11:640.

38. Yu M, Levy MM, Smith P, et al. Effect of maximizing oxygen delivery on morbidity and mortality rates in critically ill patients: a prospective, randomized, controlled study. Crit Care Med 1993;21:830–838.

39. Ronco JJ, Phang PT, Walley KR, et al. Oxygen consumption is independent of changes in oxygen delivery in severe adult respiratory distress syndrome. Am Rev Respir Dis 1991;143:1267–1273.

40. Hanique G, Dugernier T, Laterre PF, et al. Significance of pathologic oxygen supply dependency in critically ill patients: comparison between measured and calculated methods. Intens Care Med 1994;20:12–18.

41. Montgomery A, Hartmann M, Jonsson K, et al. Intramucosal pH measurement with tonometers for detecting gastrointestinal ischemia in porcine hemorrhagic shock. Circ Shock 1989;29:319–327.

42. Schiller HJ, Reilly PM, Bulkley GB. Tissue perfusion in critical illnesses. Antioxidant therapy. Crit Care Med 1993;21:S92–S102.

43. Strieter RM, Kunkel SL, Bone RC. Role of tumor necrosis factor-alpha in disease states and inflammation. Crit Care Med 1993;21:S447–S463.

44. Corwin HL, Bonventre JV. Acute renal failure in the intensive care unit. Part 1. Intens Care Med 1988:14:10–16.

45. Corwin HL, Bonventre JV. Factors influencing survival in acute renal failure. Semin Dialysis 1989;2:220–225.

46. Bisogno JL, Langley A, Von Dreele MM. Effect of calcium to reverse the electrocardiographic effects of hyperkalemia in the isolated rat heart: a prospective, dose-response study. Crit Care Med 1994;22:697–704.

47. Corwin HL, Bonventre JV. Acute renal failure in the intensive care unit. Part 2. Intens Care Med 1988;14:86–96.

48. Vesconi S, Sicignano A, De Pietri P, et al. Continuous veno-venous hemofiltration in critically ill patients with multiple organ failure. Int J Artif Organs 1993;16:592–598.

49. Tominaga GT, Ingegno MD, Scannell G, et al. Continuous arteriovenous hemodiafiltration in postoperative and traumatic renal failure. Am J Surg 1993;166:612–615.

50. Bickley SK. Drug dosing during continuous arteriovenous hemofiltration. Clin Pharmacol 1988;7:198–206.

51. Bellomo R, Boyce N. Continuous venovenous hemodiafiltration compared with conventional dialysis in critically ill patients with acute renal failure. ASAIO J 1993;39:M794–M797.

52. Bone RC, Balk RA, Cerra FB, et al. Definitions for sepsis and organ failure and guidelines for the use of innovative therapies in sepsis. Chest 1992;101:1644–1655.

53. Bone RC. The pathogenesis of sepsis. Ann Intern Med 1991;115:457–469.

54. Giroir BP. Mediators of septic shock: new approaches for interrupting the endogenous inflammatory cascade. Crit Care Med 1993;21:780–789.
55. Beal AL, Cerra FB. Multiple organ failure syndrome in the 1990s. JAMA 1994;271:226–233.
56. Jansen NJG, Van Oeveren W, Hoiting BH, et al. Methylprednisolone prophylaxis protects against endotoxin-induced death in rabbits. Inflammation 1991;15:91–101.
57. Bone RC, Fisher CJ Jr, Clemmer TP, et al. A controlled clinical trial of high-dose methylprednisolone in the treatment of severe sepsis and septic shock. N Engl J Med 1987;317:653–658.
58. The Veterans Administration Systemic Sepsis Cooperative Study Group. Effect of high-dose glucocorticoid therapy on mortality in patients with clinical signs of systemic sepsis. N Engl J Med 1987;317:659–665.
59. Ziegler EJ, Fisher CJ Jr, Sprung CL, et al. Treatment of gram-negative bacteremia and septic shock with HA-1A human monoclonal antibody against endotoxin. A randomized, double-blind, placebo-controlled trial. N Engl J Med 1991;324:429–436.
60. Greenman RL, Schein RM, Martin MA, et al. A controlled clinical trial of E5 murine monoclonal IgM antibody to endotoxin in the treatment of gram-negative sepsis. JAMA 1991;266:1097–1102.
61. McNamara MJ, Norton JA, Nauta RJ, et al. Interleukin-1 receptor antibody (IL-1 rab) protection and treatment against lethal endotoxemia in mice. J Surg Res 1993;54:316–321.
62. Luce JM. Introduction of new technology into critical care practice: a history of HA-1A human monoclonal antibody against endotoxin. Crit Care Med 1993;21:1233–1241.
63. Quezado ZM, Natanson C, Alling DW, et al. A controlled trial of HA-1A in a canine model of gram-negative septic shock. JAMA 1993;269:2221–2227.
64. Celis R, Torres A, Gatell JM, et al. Nosocomial pneumonia. A multivariate analysis of risk and prognosis. Chest 1988;93:318–324.
65. Rodriguez JL, Gibbons KJ, Bitzer LG, et al. Pneumonia: incidence, risk factors, and outcome in injured patients. J Trauma 1991;31:907–912.
66. Baselski V. Microbiologic diagnosis of ventilator-associated pneumonia. Infect Dis Clin North Am 1993;7:331–357.
67. Sauaia A, Moore FA, Moore EE, et al. Diagnosing pneumonia in mechanically ventilated trauma patients: endotracheal aspirate versus bronchoalveolar lavage. J Trauma 1993;35:512–517.
68. Chastre J, Fagon JY, Lamer C. Procedures for the diagnosis of pneumonia in ICU patients. Intensive Care Med 1992;18:S10–S17.
69. Fagon JY, Chastre J, Hance AJ, et al. Evaluation of clinical judgment in the identification and treatment of nosocomial pneumonia in ventilated patients. Chest 1993;103:547–553.
70. Middleton R, Broughton WA, Kirkpatrick MB. Comparison of four methods for assessing airway bacteriology in intubated, mechanically ventilated patients. Am J Med Sci 1992;304:239–245.
71. Pickworth KK, Falcone RE, Hoogeboom JE, et al. Occurrence of nosocomial pneumonia in mechanically ventilated trauma patients: a comparison of sucralfate and ranitidine. Crit Care Med 1993;21:1856–1862.
72. Tryba M. Sucralfate versus antacids or H2-antagonists for stress ulcer prophylaxis: a meta-analysis on efficacy and pneumonia rate. Crit Care Med 1991;19:942–949.
73. Lacroix J, Infante-Rivard C, Jenick M, et al. Prophylaxis of upper gastrointestinal bleeding in intensive care units: a meta analysis. Crit Care Med 1989;17:862–868.
74. Cook DJ, Laine LA, Guyatt GH, et al. Nosocomial pneumonia and the role of gastric pH: a meta analysis. Chest 1991;100:7–13.
75. Heyland D, Mandell LA. Gastric colonization by gram-negative bacilli and nosocomial pneumonia in the intensive care unit patient: evidence for causation. Chest 1992;101:187–193.
76. Tetteroo GW, Wagenvoort JH, Mulder PG, et al. Decreased mortality rate and length of hospital stay in surgical intensive care unit patients with successful selective decontamination of the gut. Crit Care Med 1993;21:1692–1698.
77. Hammond JM, Potgieter PD, Saunders GL, et al. Double-blind study of selective decontamination of the digestive tract in intensive care. Lancet 1992;340:5–9.
78. van Saene HK, Stoutenbeek CC, Stoller JK. Selective decontamination of the digestive tract in the intensive care unit: current status and future prospects. Crit Care Med 1992;20:691–703.
79. Becker DP, Miller JD, Ward JD, et al. The outcome from severe head injury with early diagnosis and intensive management. J Neurosurg 1977;47:491–502.
80. Stuart GG, Merry GS, Smith JA, et al. Severe head injury managed without intracranial pressure monitoring. J Neurosurg 1983;59:601–605.
81. Rosner MJ, Daughton S. Cerebral pressure management in head injury. J Trauma 1990;30:933–940.
82. Borel C, Hanley D, Diringer MN, et al. Intensive management of severe head injury. Chest 1990;98:180–189.
83. Aitkenhead AR. Analgesia and sedation in intensive care. Br J Anaesth 1989;63:196–206.
84. Pollack MH, Stern TA. Recognition and treatment of anxiety in the ICU patient. In: Rippe JM, Irwin RS, Alpert JS, et al., eds. Intensive care medicine. Boston: Little, Brown and Company, 1991;1875–1887.
85. Forzman A, Ohman R. Pharmacokinetic studies on haloperidol in man. Curr Ther Res 1976;20:319–336.
86. Christman JW, McCain RW. A sensible approach to the nutritional support of mechanically ventilated critically ill patients. Intensive Care Med 1993;19:129–136.
87. Makk LJ, McClave SA, Creech PW, et al. Clinical application of the metabolic cart to the delivery of total parenteral nutrition. Crit Care Med 1991;18:1320–1327.
88. Daly JM, Lieberman MD, Goldfine J, et al. Enteral nutrition with supplemental arginine, RNA, and

omega-3 fatty acids in patients after operation: immunologic, metabolic, and clinical outcome. Surgery 1992;112:56–67.

89. Dark DS, Pingleton SK. Nutrition and nutritional support in critically ill patients. Intensive Care Med 1993;8:16–33.

16

ALLERGIC REACTIONS

Stephen A. Vitkun

An allergic reaction may occur unpredictably after the administration of any drug. These adverse reactions to drugs are an inevitable, albeit unintended, consequence of pharmacotherapy. Untoward drug reactions are the leading cause of iatrogenic illness (1). Estimates of drug-related complications range from 6 to 15% of hospitalized patients, although allergic or immunologic reactions to drugs account for less than 25% of the total (2). Death from an allergic drug reaction is rare, with an estimated risk of one in 10,000 (1). Fortunately, most adverse reactions, although associated with some morbidity, are usually minor and transient in nature. The drug or agent responsible for eliciting an allergic reaction is termed an "allergen" or "antigen." The allergic reaction is sometimes referred to as a "hypersensitivity response" or "hypersensitivity reaction" and implies a purely quantitative response of an otherwise normal pharmacological activity (3). However, these exaggerated responses lead to destruction or injury of host tissues (1).

Some susceptible individuals, such as those with a history of atopy such as bronchial asthma, hay fever, and food allergies, are more likely to experience an allergic reaction to a drug given intravenously during the course of an anesthetic. This increased incidence is due to a genetic predisposition in these patients that causes production of increased amounts of immunoglobulin E (IgE) antibodies (4–6). Furthermore, a history of allergy and multiple exposures to the same drug or related drugs influences the incidence of developing an allergic reaction. Ideally, the same drug should not be used repeatedly for atopic patients (7). A history of an uneventful prior exposure to a drug does not eliminate the possibility of a severe allergic reaction with subsequent exposure, even in cases in which an individual has received an agent multiple times without incident. Also, a drug allergy may not be permanent. This has been demonstrated by the disappearance of penicillin sensitivity on intradermal testing (4).

Allergic reactions are more likely to occur after intravenous administration than after intramuscular administration (4). Anesthesiologists administer a many drugs that have been shown to cause allergic reactions (Table 16–1). These drugs, many of which will be discussed later in this chapter, include the intravenous induction agents, neuromuscular blocking drugs, the neuromuscular blocking antagonists, and other agents such as nitrous oxide and the potent inhalational agents. Furthermore, anesthesiologists may administer many other drugs or therapies, such as antibiotics, dextrans, or blood products, that are capable of evoking serious allergic responses. Therefore, anesthesiologists and critical care practitioners must always consider that changes in hemodynamics (3, 8, 9), electrocardiogram (10–14), or pulmonary functions (3, 9) may indicate an allergic reaction. Irrespective of the cause, an unrecognized allergic reaction may be associated with significant morbidity or mortality.

Table 16–1.　Drugs Implicated in Allergic Reactions Occurring During Anesthesia

1. Anesthetic Agents
  A. Induction Agents

Barbiturates	Benzodiazepines
Althesin	Cremophorsolubilized drugs
Etomidate	Ketamine
Propofol	

  B. Local Anesthetics

Para-aminobenzoic	Esters/Amide Type Agents (?)

  C. Narcotics

Morphine	Meperidine
Fentanyl	

  D. Muscle Relaxants

Atracurium	Doxacurium
d-Tubocurarine	Cellamine
Metocurine	Mivacurium
Pancuronium	Succinylcholine
Vecuronium	

2. Antibiotics

Aminoglycosides	Penicillin
Cephalosporins	Vancomycin
Sulfonamides	

3. Blood Products

Whole blood	Packed cells, fresh frozen
Plasma	Platelets
Cryoprecipitate	Fibrin glue
Albumin	

4. Other Agents

Atropine	Aprotinin
Antihistamines	Droperidol
Furosemide	Insulin
Bone cement (methylmethacrylate)	Chymopapain
Cyclosporine	Mannitol
Radiocontrast dyes	Dextran
Latex (natural rubber)	Vascular grafting materials
Hydroxyethyl starch	Vitamin K
Protamine	Nonsteroidal anti-inflammatory agents
Streptokinase	

Pathophysiology and Immunology of Allergic Reactions

In the early 1900s, Portier and Richet demonstrated that sublethal quantities of a sea-anemone toxin, when injected into previously sensitized animals, caused immediate convulsions and collapse. They used the term "anaphylaxis," in contrast to "prophylaxis" to describe this phenomenon. Prophylaxis indicated a benefit brought about by vaccination. Subsequently, when treating patients during a diphtheria epidemic, Pirquet and Schick discovered that a second injection of the diphtheria antitoxin could produce a delayed reaction characterized by fever and arteritis. This response is known as "serum sickness" and is now known to be mediated by circulating immune complexes (3).

THE IMMUNOGLOBULINS, MAST CELLS, AND BASOPHILS

Immunoglobulins are glycoproteins that contain less than 20% carbohydrate; the remainder is composed of polypeptides. There are two sets of polypeptide chains. One set, termed "heavy," is almost twice the size of the smaller "light" chain. There are two subgroups of light chains, called kappa and lambda, which are common to all immunoglobulin classes. Normally, one heavy chain is associated with one light chain. The immunoglobulin type is determined by the type of heavy chain. There are five major types of heavy chains called gamma, alpha, mu, delta, and epsilon, which correspond to immunoglobulin G (IgG), immunoglobulin A (IgA), immunoglobulin M (IgM), immunoglobulin D (IgD), and immunoglobulin E (IgE), respectively. Polymers of the basic monomeric antibody are made with the addition of a J chain. The J chain allows for dimers, trimers (IgA), and pentamers (IgM). There is also a "secretory component," which is associated with IgA (15, 16).

IgG makes up about 70% of the serum immunoglobulins. There are different classes of IgG molecules, depending upon differences in the gamma chain. IgD functions as a membrane receptor for lymphocytes. It has a very low concentration in the plasma. IgE is the antibody responsible for anaphylaxis and other type I reactions, which will be discussed later in this chapter. It exists in low concentrations in serum. IgE can be inactivated by heating. The constant region (Fc region) of an IgE molecule can bind to the surface of mast cells or basophils, resulting in degranulation and mediator release. IgA is the secretory antibody found in saliva and gastrointestinal and respiratory secretions. It protects against pathogenic organisms. IgA molecules resemble IgG but also contain a J chain and a secretory component. IgA constitutes about 20% of the serum immunoglobulins. IgM is the largest of the immunoglobulins. It is essentially a pentamer of IgG. IgM molecules are the first antibodies to be formed after immunization. IgM antibodies participate in ABO blood reactions because these antibodies are synthesized against blood groups not present on the

individual's own red cells (15–17). The immunoglobulins are summarized in Table 16–2.

Mast cells and basophils possess more than 100,000 membrane receptors for IgE immunoglobulins; however, they differ in their morphology, location, and biosynthetic products. Mast cells are fixed and can be found in perivascular connective tissue cells throughout the body. They also serve as sentinels on cutaneous and mucosal surfaces and around venules as they concentrate IgE on their surface, which is required for immune defense. Any given mast cell may react with a large variety of antigens. Histamine is stored in the electron-dense granules of mast cells complexed to heparin and protein enzymes. Basophils are polymorphonuclear granulocytes that make up about 1% of the circulating leukocytes. Basophils may be considered as the "circulating" mast cells. Between 5,000 and 500,000 IgE antibodies are present on a basophil. Although allergic persons have a higher average number of IgE antibodies/basophil than normal, nonallergic persons, there is a large overlap between the groups. Both cell types play a major role in immediate hypersensitivity reactions. The degranulation of mast cells may be modulated by a number of factors. Agents that decrease the level of cyclic adenosine monophosphate (c-AMP) or increase the level of guanosine monophosphate (α-adrenergic stimulation, cholinergic agents, or prostaglandin F2α) promote degranulation and release of chemical mediators. Agents that increase the level of c-AMP (epinephrine, theophylline, prostaglandins E1 and E2) inhibit mast cell degranulation. There are also a variety of nonimmunologic influences, such as cold, pressure, sunlight, heat, and exercise, that may promote mast cell degranulation (18, 19).

CHEMICAL MEDIATORS

Histamine is an imidazolylethylamine that is associated with the granules of mast cells and basophils. It affects a variety of tissue sites and is present in the parietal region of the stomach. The normal plasma concentrations

Table 16–2. A Description of the Immunoglobulins

Immunoglobulins	Components	Serum Concentration (gm/titer)	Biological Half-Life (days)	Molecular Wt	Complement Activation (Classical)	Complement Activation (Alternate)	Binding to Mast Cells	Clinical Implications and Function(s)
IgE	Epsilon heavy chain; Kappa or lambda light chains	$\geq 0.5 \times 10E\text{-}3$	2	200,000	No	Yes	Yes	Sensitize mast cells and basophils for anaphylaxis
IgM	Mu heavy chain; Kappa or lambda light chains; Possible J chain	0.5–1.5	5	900,000	Yes	No	No	Blood group antibodies; Neutralization, hemolysis, agglutination, bacteriolysis, opsonization, B-lymphocyte receptor
IgG	Gamma subtype 1–4 heavy chains; Kappa or lambda light chains	6–14	20–28	150,000	Yes	No	No	Host defenses, neutralization, opsonization, bacteriolysis, hemolysis
IgA	Alpha subtype 1 or 2 heavy chains; Kappa or lambda light chains; Possible J chain and secretory component	1–3	6	170,000 Secretory IgA (370,000)	No	Yes	No	Antibodies in saliva and secretions
IgD	Delta heavy chains; Kappa or lambda light chains	≥ 0.1	3	180,000	No	Yes	No	Membrane receptor on B-Lymphocytes

Adapted from Levy JH. Anaphylactic reactions in anesthesia and intensive care. 2nd ed. Boston: Butterworth-Heinemann, 1992; and Watkins J, Salo M. Trauma, stress and immunity in anesthesia and surgery. Boston: Butterworth Scientific, 1982.

are between 0.1 and 0.5 ng/mL. High concentrations of histamine are stored in fixed tissue mast cells of the lung, intestine, and skin. The heart also contains large amounts of histamine. The receptors in the gastrointestinal and respiratory smooth muscle cells, as well as those in the blood vessels, are termed "type H1 receptors." Stimulation of these receptors is associated with contraction of the smooth muscle and increased permeability in the blood vessels. By contrast, stimulation of H2 receptors stimulate gastric acid secretion, increase heart rate, and inhibit mediator release from basophils. Histamine is also a regulator of immune complex (type III) reactions (6, 20–23).

The eosinophil chemotactic factor of anaphylaxis (ECF-A) is present in basophils and mast cells. It is a peptide with a molecular weight of about 500 daltons. Release of this factor is associated with type I reactions and is responsible for attraction of eosinophils. Other pharmacological agents, including histamine and its metabolites, released during an immediate hypersensitivity reaction may also possess eosinophil chemotactic activity. The attraction of an eosinophil to an area of mediator release during a type I reaction may play a protective role. The eosinophil contains a number of enzymes that are capable of degrading the chemical mediators released (histamine and leukotrienes) during the immediate hypersensitivity reaction. It is not entirely clear, but the eosinophil may also function to limit the inflammatory response (6, 24, 25). During an allergic response, the neutrophil chemotactic factor of anaphylaxis (NCF-A) is also released and results in the accumulation of acute inflammatory cells, which are responsible for local edema and inflammation. The chemotactic factors are also responsible for the secondary inflammation, which occurs 3 to 6 hours after antigen challenge and produces the late-phase reactions and continued inflammation after an immediate hypersensitivity response.

The slow-reacting substance of anaphylaxis (SRS-A) and the leukotrienes (L) were initially identified in 1938 as a substance in lung perfusates that caused smooth muscle contraction. The factor was so named because it caused a gradual smooth muscle contraction of the guinea-pig ileum. After many years, it was found to be associated with the immediate hypersensitivity reaction and was subsequently called SRS-A (26, 27). In the late 1970s, while evaluating the structure of SRS-A, a new group of arachidonate-derived compounds, the leukotrienes, were identified. SRS-A was found to be composed of the leukotrienes C4, D4, and E4.

Leukotrienes were so named because they are produced by leukocytes and contain a conjugated triene molecule. Five leukotrienes identified with letters A through E and are further identified by subgroups based on the fatty acid substrate from which they were formed (6). Leukotrienes are not stored in cells. They are synthesized from arachidonic acid through the lipoxygenase pathway just before release. Prostaglandins and thromboxanes are also potent biological mediators that are derived from arachidonic acid. SRS-A is a potent bronchoconstrictor with a slower onset and longer duration of action than histamine. Studies using purified leukotrienes C4 and D4 have confirmed the prior result using SRS-A. In addition, leukotriene C4 and leukotriene D4 have been shown to be 100 to 1000 times more potent than histamine in producing bronchoconstriction in normal subjects (28–32).

Platelet-activating factor (PAF) is released from basophils and tissue mast cells. It is synthesized after IgE-dependent membrane activation of these effector cells. It promotes the release of vasoactive amines from platelets and causes platelet aggregation (6). The prostaglandins are 20-carbon unsaturated hydroxy acids. They are also synthesized from arachidonic acid through the action of the cyclooxygenase enzyme and are synthesized by virtually all tissues. Mast cells have been shown to produce prostaglandins (P) D2, E1, E2, and F2. PGE1 and PGE2 are bronchodilators, whereas PGD2 and PGF2α cause bronchoconstriction (6). Kuehl and Egan have written a detailed review of the prostaglandins (33).

Kinins are low-molecular-weight polypeptides that are cleaved from higher-molecular-weight kininogens. The larger of the two precursors exists in a complex with prekallikrein or factor XI (34). The kinins possess a variety of biological properties. They may induce contraction or relaxation of smooth muscle, increase vascular permeability, or produce pain. Bradykinin is an amino acid peptide that has been identified as a component of the anaphylactic response (35). It is responsible for vasodilation through stimulation of the endothelium-derived relaxing factor (36). The role of the kallikrein-kinin system is not well understood. Metabolism of the kinins is accomplished by a variety of enzymes, most of which are on the surface of endothelial cells in the lung (37, 38). Protamine has been shown to inhibit one of the enzymes, and this may be one possible mechanism that is responsible for protamine reactions (39). Furthermore, angiotensin-converting enzyme (ACE) inhibitors may also inhibit the breakdown of bradykinin, which may explain the severe angioedema that can occur in some patients taking ACE inhibitors (40).

Heparin is a sulfate proteoglycan that is present in the granules of mast cells found in the skin and lung. It, too, is released by immunologic activation of the mast cell. It is an anticoagulant and complement inhibitor that acts to modulate tryptase activity. Human basophils do not contain heparin but contain chondroitin 4 and 6 sulfates instead (41, 42).

Tryptase, chymase, acid hydrolases, and peroxidase are also stored in the granules of mast cells and basophils. The function of these different enzymes is uncertain. They may affect coagulation and fibrin deposition or modulate other inflammatory mediators (25, 43, 44). Tryptase is the most prominent enzyme in human lung mast cells. It is released from mast cells during IgE-mediated reactions. Tryptase levels peak at 1 to 2 hours after an antigenic reaction. This is in contrast to histamine, which peaks in minutes and can also be released by nonimmunological challenges. Because tryptase is only released from mast cells, it may provide a useful method of evaluating suspected anaphylactic reactions (25, 43–45).

IMMUNOLOGICAL HYPERSENSITIVITY REACTIONS

Normally, the immune response rapidly frees the body of invading organisms and their toxic products. This is usually brought about by phagocytosis and, in general, immunity is believed to be the ability to mount a satisfactory phagocytic attack against foreign antigens. However, it must be remembered that the initial immune response is antibody production, followed by antigen binding. This forms an immune complex that triggers an inflammatory response and complement system, which then guide the phagocytic cells to the affected area or invading organisms. Despite the lack of antibody involvement in many drug reactions, they all involve mechanisms that are conventionally associated with an expression of immunity (46).

Using the terms "anaphylactic" or "prophylactic" with a description of the rate at which the reaction occurred is not a satisfactory method of describing immunological reactions. In 1963, Gell and Coombs devised a more complete and accurate description of immunological reactions. They have provided a classification system with four types of reactions (types I through IV) depending on the antibody involved, the type of cell being modulating, the nature of the antigen, and the duration of the reaction (3).

The mechanisms responsible for allergic reactions during or after drug administration include anaphylaxis (type I hypersensitivity, immune-mediated hypersensitivity), classic pathway activation of the complement system, alternate pathway activation of the complement system, and anaphylactoid (pharmacologic, direct histamine release). Multiple mechanisms of action may be involved in an allergic reaction (4).

Type I Reactions

Type I reactions are also called "immediate hypersensitivity reactions." They are mediated by IgE antibodies, which attach to the surfaces of basophils and mast cells. When an antigenic substance binds to the IgE antibody on the surface of these cells, activation occurs, degranulation ensues, and a variety of pharmacologically active substances are released. These substance are responsible for the anaphylactic response. Not all type I reactions are anaphylactic in nature. Nonanaphylactic type I reactions may include the bee-sting reactions, extrinsic asthma, allergic rhinitis, and some penicillin allergies (17). Except for drugs given intravenously, the type I reaction is a relatively uncommon mechanism of drug hypersensitivity. However, anaphylaxis is perhaps the most common cause of death attributed to a drug allergy. Penicillin is the most common offender (1).

Clinically, type I reactions to drugs have the same clinical features as IgE-mediated reactions to other allergens. These reactions include anaphylaxis, urticaria, and/or angioedema, extrinsic asthma, rhinitis, and conjunctivitis. Immediate hypersensitivity reactions (IgE mediated) are apparent immediately after the parenteral administration of the drug or up to 6 hours after oral administration. Many drugs and other biomedical agents may produce an immediate hypersensitivity reaction. Patients who generally experience type I reactions are those who are genetically prone to produce specific types of IgE antibodies to antigens or allergens that are well tolerated by the population in general. These patients may have normally elevated concentrations of IgE in the plasma (>400 IU/mL) and are frequently termed "atopic" (7). Unfortunately, a history of allergy or atopy with or without elevated IgE levels has not proven helpful in the selection of anesthetic agents (47).

Allergic reactions to drugs are caused by interactions between the drug and the immune system. Most drugs or their metabolites, which are small organic molecules with weights of less than 1000 daltons, are haptens and are incapable of acting as a complete antigen. They may, however, react with, or bind to a carrier protein. In this way, the drug-protein complex may become a complete antigen and may stimulate the immune response. After the initial exposure, there is a latent period of 10 to 20 days during which the drug-protein complex stimulates production of a sufficient number of activated immune cells (lymphocytes) and antibodies (IgE). After this exposure or sensitization to the drug or other substance, reexposure may produce an immediate hypersensitivity reaction (2, 4).

IgE can circulate freely or bind to basophils or mast cells at specific Fc receptor sites. When cell-bound IgE combines with an antigen, characteristic type I events occur within seconds. These include release of histamine, slow-reacting substance of anaphylaxis (SRS-A), serotonin, eosinophil chemotactic factor of anaphylaxis (ECF-A), platelet activating factor (PAF), and prostaglandins from mast cells or basophils. These agents cause increased capillary permeability, vasodilation, and smooth muscle contractions. This leads to the clinical features including urticaria, angioedema, hypotension, bronchospasm, gastrointestinal spasms, and uterine contractions (15). Chemical mediators released by mast cells or basophils and their physiological effects are summarized in Table 16–3.

Type II Reactions

Type II reactions, also known as "cytotoxic" or "cytolytic" reactions, occur in response to antigens that are present on the surface of either host or foreign cells or modified host cells. The "cytotoxic antibodies" associated with this reaction are either IgG or IgM subtypes. Modification of host cells can occur as part of a viral infection. The combination of antibodies with these cellular antigens causes the demise of both cells by phagocytosis and through activation of the classical complement cascade, which leads to cell lysis. Drug-induced hemolytic anemias, ABO-in-

Table 16–3. Chemical Mediators of Allergic Reactions

Chemical Mediator	Physiological Effect(s)
Histamine	Bronchoconstriction Increased capillary permeability
Slow-reacting substance of anaphylaxis (SRS-A, leukotriene C)	Bronchoconstriction Increased capillary permeability
Eosinophil chemotactic factor of anaphylaxis (ECF-A)	Attraction of eosinophils
Neutrophil chemotactic factor of anaphylaxis (NCF-A)	Attraction of neutrophils
Leukotrienes C4, D4, E4	Smooth muscle contraction Enhanced vasopermeability
Prostaglandins PGD2, PGI2, PGE2, PGF2, thromboxanes	Variable effects on smooth muscle Contraction and vasopermeability
Heparin	Anticoagulation Inhibition of complement system activation
Platelet-activating factor (PAF)	Platelet aggregation and degranulation
Prostaglandins	Bronchoconstriction (PGD2, PGF2α) Bronchodilation (PGE1, PGE2)

compatible transfusion reactions, autoimmune hemolytic anemia, Goodpasture's syndrome, and Hashimoto's thyroiditis are examples of type II reactions (3, 7, 17). As is the case with type I reactions, the patient requires previous antigenic challenge to produce antibodies, but the antigens in this case are present on the surface of either the host or foreign cells. Type II reactions should not be confused with type IV reactions, which result in cytotoxicity by a different mechanism. Also, the distinction between type II and type III reactions should be emphasized. Although each reaction involves complement fixation, the primary reactions are different.

Type III Reactions

The Type III reaction is also called an "immune complex" reaction, "toxic-complex," reaction or "serum sickness." It is most often observed after a second injection of an antiserum, such as those used for snake bites. In this type of reaction, antibodies of IgG or IgM subtypes combine with circulating soluble antigens rather than particulate antigens. This forms an insoluble complex too small to be filtered by the liver, spleen, or macrophages of the reticuloendothelial system and results in the complexes depositing in the microcirculation. The deposition of large amounts of these complexes usually occurs in the skin, kidneys, and central nervous system. In the laboratory, the classic example of a type III reaction is the Arthus reaction. In this reaction, repeated injections of horse serum into rabbits over many days leads to a reaction at subsequent injection sites characterized by infiltration, edema, sterile abscesses, and in severe cases, gangrene. The clinical analog to the Arthus reaction is serum sickness. It was seen more commonly when heterologous serums such as equine tetanus antitoxin were used in clinical practice. The symptoms of the disease included skin lesions, fever, arthralgia, and lymphadenopathy. Similar symptoms can occur with drug allergies (15). The skin rashes and nephrotic syndromes frequently seen in systemic lupus erythematosus (SLE) and rheumatoid vasculitis originate from such complexes. A vasculitis after penicillin, drug-induced SLE, allergic granulomatous angiitis, rheumatic arteritis, periarteritis nodosa, and temporal arteritis are also examples of type III reactions. The major type of clinically severe drug reaction associated with the type III mechanism is that of a drug-induced hemolytic anemia. Many drugs can produce a type III reaction due to erythrocyte adsorption of drug-antibody complexes and include phenacetin, aspirin, sulfonamides, tetracycline, and insulin (3, 15, 17).

Type IV Reactions

Type IV reactions, also called "delayed" or "cellular" hypersensitivity reactions, are mediated by T lymphocytes and are responsible for delayed hypersensitivity, which is seen in allergic reactions to bacteria and viruses and in the rejection of transplanted tissue. Dermal sensitivity of this type is common and occurs in response to a wide range of drugs and other chemical compounds such as soaps and cosmetics. Contact dermatitis is characterized by its local nature. Erythematous lesions occur at the site of hapten fixation. The immunological reactions and their mechanisms are summarized in Table 16–4.

In classifying the hypersensitivity reactions, some believe that there are two other reactions that do not really belong in any of the four categories described. The first is called a neutralization or inactivation reaction. An example of this is a diabetic patient who develops IgG antibody reactions to the beef or pork insulin that he or she has been using. In most cases, the response is minimal and is compensated by an increase in insulin dose. It should be realized that many experts would classify this as a type II reaction. The second reaction is called a granulomatous reaction, which we have considered in our discussion as a type IV reaction. Reasons for separating granulomatous reactions from type IV reactions include morphological differences from delayed hypersensitivity reactions and differences in the kinetics of granuloma formation (15).

It is important to realize that these hypersensitivity reactions are not abnormal processes and are important in the control of various disease processes. However, it is the magnitude of the involvement in a specific reaction that gives rise to the abnormality. Furthermore, it is important to realize that it is rare for any one mechanism to be totally responsible for a hypersensitivity reaction (7).

THE COMPLEMENT SYSTEM

Only type I and type IV reactions may occur without the involvement of the complement system. The complement system is involved in type II reactions when the cell-bound antigen combines with antibody and in type III reactions after deposition of antigen-antibody complexes has taken place at the reaction site. The complement system is composed of nine major component proteins, which account for nearly 10% of the globulins present in humans. They are plasma and cell membrane proteins that lyse susceptible targets, promote phagocytosis by coating targets with complement-derived protein fragments, and generate peptides that mediate features of the inflammatory response. The system is designed to aid bodily defense processes. However, activation of the system can cause tissue damage and inflammation and often has a role in autoimmune disease processes (7, 15, 48).

Two pathways of complement activation have been defined. The first has been termed the "classical" pathway and the second is referred to as the "alternative" or "properiden" pathway. Both function through the sequential interaction of a series of complement-protein components. In most situations, the classic pathway is activated by IgG or IgM antibody-coated target particles or by IgG or IgM antigen-antibody complexes. Activation of the alternative pathway may occur in the absence of antibody if there is a suitable activating surface. Appropriate surfaces include the repeating polysaccharide chains present in many bacteria and viruses and in some parasites.

Table 16—4. Summary of Immunologic Reactions

Immunologic Reactions	Synonyms	Antibody	Mechanism(s)	Examples
Type I	Immediate Hypersensitivity, anaphylaxis	IgE	Antigen binds IgE on surface of mast cells or basophils, causing release of cell products (histamine, SRS-A, serotonin, ECF-A, PAF)	Anaphylaxis Cutaneous wheal and flair Extrinsic asthma
Type II	Cytotoxic or cytolytic	IgG or IgM	IgG, IgM binds antigen on cell membrane, complement activated, liberation of mediators, cell destruction	Transfusion reaction Hemolytic anemia Rh disease Systemic lupus erythematous Hashimoto's thyroiditis Goodpasture's syndrome
Type III	Immune complex Toxic complex Serum sickness Arthus reaction	IgG or IgM	IgG, IgM bind antigen in fluid phase, deposit in small blood vessels, complement activated, cell destruction	Serum sickness Glomerulonephritis Allergic arteritis Periarteritis nodosa Temporal arteritis
Type IV	Delayed or cellular Hypersensitivity	Not involved	Sensitized T lymphocytes bind antigen and release lymphokines	Contact dermatitis TB immunity Transplant rejection Graft-versus-host reaction

Adapted from Levy JH. Anaphylactic reactions in anesthesia and intensive care. 2nd ed. Boston: Butterworth-Heinemann, 1992; and Watkins J, Salo M. Trauma, stress and immunity in anesthesia and surgery. Boston: Butterworth Scientific, 1982.

Components of Complement Activation

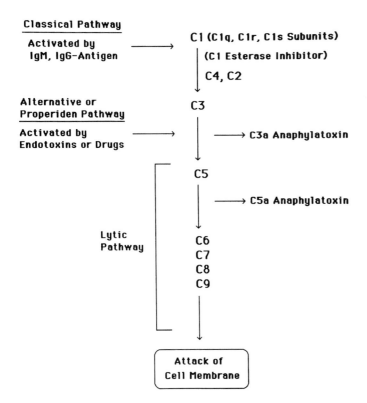

Classical Pathway

Activated by
IgM, IgG-Antigen ⟶

C1 (C1q, C1r, C1s Subunits)

(C1 Esterase Inhibitor)

C4, C2

**Alternative or
Properiden Pathway**

C3

Activated by
Endotoxins or Drugs ⟶

⟶ C3a Anaphylatoxin

C5

⟶ C5a Anaphylatoxin

**Lytic
Pathway**

C6
C7
C8
C9

Attack of
Cell Membrane

Fig. 16–1. Components of the complement activation. The diagram of activation of the complement system shows how it can be activated by immunologic as well as nonimmunologic mechanisms. Activation of the system leads to production of fragmented products that are humorally active as well as membrane attack complexes that promote cell lysis. C1 is composed of three subunits and the C1 esterase inhibitor is normally present.

In the classical pathway, the components are designated "C" followed by a number. The number sequence is not in order because the first four complements were designated before their reaction sequence was known. Also, the first complement has three subcomponents designated by the addition of letters: C1q, C1r, and C1s. IgM and IgG can bind to C1q and initiate the classical complement pathway. IgA, IgE, and IgD do not fix complement C1q. Most proteins of the alternate pathway are designated with letters (15, 48).

Both complement pathways involve sequential activation, cleavage, and assembly of protein fragments, leading to the formation of enzymes capable of cleaving protein C3, which is common to both pathways. The components and sequence of steps of complement activation are shown in Figure 16–1. The two

pathways join together at this point and then proceed through components C5, C6, C7, C8, and C9 to form a complex that is capable of acting on the membrane of the target cell to promote cell lysis (48). In contrast to type I reactions or anaphylaxis, an allergic reaction caused by classical complement system activation does not require prior sensitization and can occur on the first exposure to a drug (4).

Complement activation by either pathway produces complement proteins (C3, C4, and C5) and associated fragments. The fragments C3a, C4a, and C5a are termed "anaphylatoxins" because they stimulate the release of mediators from mast cells and basophils (49–51). Production of C5a and aggregation of neutrophils may explain the neutropenia and hypoxia, which may be associated with dialysis, and the adult respiratory distress syndrome

(ARDS) (52). It may also be responsible for the clinical manifestations of transfusion reactions (53), protamine reactions (54), and serum sickness, which may be associated with injection of streptokinase (55).

The coagulation and fibrinolytic systems have significant interaction with the classical complement system. Activation of the complement system (classical or alternative pathway) or activation of humoral amplification systems (coagulation, fibrinolysis, or kinin activation) may subsequently promote activation of surface-mediated host defense reactions (plasma contact activation) (56, 57). The Hageman factor (factor XII), factor XI, and prekallikrein may be activated by the process of contact activation (34).

NONIMMUNOLOGIC REACTIONS

There are also several nonimmunological mechanisms of allergic reactions (46). These include (a) formation of nonimmune aggregates leading to aggregate anaphylaxis, which may result from albumin or polygelatines; (b) precipitation of high concentrations of nonrelated immune complexes in patients with infection, which can occur with pentothal administration; (c) activation of the alternative complement pathway; (d) stress responses to surgery and anesthesia and psychological responses; (e) drug release of vasoactive chemicals, such as prostaglandins and kinins among others; and (f) direct activation of the coagulation and fibrinolytic systems due to collagen exposure during surgery. Although considered "nonimmune," all of these responses are associated with "immune complex" involvement. Other nonimmune responses include complement system activation. These include, specifically, C2 and C4 activation leading to enzyme defects (natural or induced), which promote vasodilation or angioedema, or excessive nonimmune alternative pathway dysfunction (C3 or C5) producing fibrinolytic enzymes leading to disseminated intravascular coagulation (DIC) or adult respiratory distress syndrome (ARDS) (46). DIC may be triggered by different mechanisms, including hypoxia, trauma, and infection. An infection and the resulting immune complexes may be potent activators of the alternative complement pathway (3). A detailed discussion of DIC and ARDS is beyond the scope of this chapter.

Nonimmunological activation of the alternative pathway occurs independent of antibodies. It may be a result of lipopolysaccharides from Gram-negative bacteria (endotoxin), teichoic acid from Gram-positive bacteria, and a variety of drugs such as althesin or radiographic contrast dye. Oxygenators used during cardiopulmonary bypass and other membranes, such as those used on dialysis equipment, are also potential nonimmunological activators of the alternative pathway (58–62).

In addition, many drugs used during anesthesia may promote histamine release from mast cells in a nonimmunologic, dose-dependent fashion. Examples of this phenomena include morphine or d-tubocurarine, which causes the release of histamine, subsequently producing vasodilation and urticaria along the vein in which the agent was administered. Intravenously administered drugs can also cause cardiovascular collapse via nonimmunologic mechanisms. These include toxicity, overdose, adverse drug interactions, and direct vasodilatory properties. These nonimmunologic reactions may seem to be an anaphylactic reaction (63–67).

Defects in the contact activation or complement system may lead to unique problems. One particular problem for the anesthesiologist or intensive care physician is hereditary angioedema. This entity is caused by an absent or defective C1 esterase inhibitor and decreased levels of C4. It manifests as intermittent attacks of deep tissue swelling. These episodes often involve the mouth, face, and larynx. Patients may have a history of attacks in response to stress. The treatment of an acute attack or prophylaxis includes fresh frozen plasma. Prophylactically, androgen derivatives such as danazol have been shown to be effective in treating hereditary angioedema because they seem to increase the hepatic synthesis of the C1 inhibitor. The dose of danazol does not correlate with body mass and must be determined empirically for each patient. Given orally, as much as 600 mg/day in three divided doses may be required. If the reaction is life threatening, tracheal intubation and other supportive measures may be necessary (57, 68).

ANAPHYLACTIC VERSUS ANAPHYLACTOID REACTIONS

Systemic anaphylaxis is the most dramatic and potentially catastrophic manifestation of immediate hypersensitivity. It has multisystem involvement and reactions range from mild pruritus and urticaria to shock and death. Anaphylactic reactions involve three factors. The first is interaction of antigen and antibody, the second is release of pharmacologically active mediators, and the last is the response of the organism. Historically, the most common antigen causing anaphylaxis in humans has been a heterologous serum such as equine tetanus antitoxin. Originally, anaphylaxis was used to describe a severe, systemic reaction to an injected substance. The term has also been used to describe the symptom complex mediated by pharmacologically active agents that occurs after the administration of an antigen to a suitably immunized subject. Anaphylactic reactions are mediated by IgE (69, 70). They require prior exposure to the inciting agent. The signs, symptoms, and differential diagnosis of anaphylaxis are summarized in Tables 16–5 and 16–6 (70, 71). Signs of anaphylaxis in an intubated (or an anesthetized patient) are presented in Table 16–7 (71). There is no definitive laboratory study to establish the presence or etiology of anaphylaxis. Hemoconcentration in a hypovolemic patient, elevated serum histamine levels, prolonged coagulation time, and reductions in complement have been observed but are not specific to a diagnosis of anaphylaxis. Anaphylaxis to intravenous agents used during anesthesia occurs every in one in 5,000 to one in 15,000 pa-

Table 16–5.   The Differential Diagnosis of Anaphylaxis

Administration of sedatives or anesthetic drugs
Asthma
Cardiogenic shock
Disconnection of overdosage of vasoactive drugs
Dysrhythmias
Pericardial tamponade
Postextubation stridor
Pulmonary edema
Pulmonary embolus
Septic shock
Tension pneumothorax
Vasovagal reactions
Venous air embolism

From Levy JH. Anaphylactic reactions in anesthesia and intensive care. 2nd ed. Boston: Butterworth-Heinemann, 1992.

tients. The reported mortality is 4 to 6%. Identification of a responsible agent is difficult because of the variety of drugs used during anesthesia. The demonstration of a specific IgE by skin testing or immunochemical analysis may provide information about the etiology of an allergen-induced reaction (72). Avoiding the use of agents to which there is a positive skin test in future anesthetics combined with a premedication regimen consisting of prednisone (50 mg orally 13 hours, 7 hours, and 1 hour before anesthesia) and diphenhydramine (50 mg orally or intramuscularly 1 hour before anesthesia) has been beneficial in treating patients who have experienced an anaphylactic reaction during induction of general anesthesia (73).

Anaphylactoid reactions are clinically indistinguishable from anaphylactic reactions. An anaphylactoid reaction involves similar chemical mediators. Anaphylactoid reactions are not mediated by IgE and do not require prior exposure to the inciting substance (69). The inciting agent may cause complement activation (classical or alternative pathway) and activation of humoral amplification systems (coagulation, fibrinolysis, or kinin activation) or may act directly on the mast cells causing mediator (histamine) release (56, 57). Activation of any of these systems may subsequently pro-

Table 16–6. Signs and Symptoms of Anaphylaxis

System	Reaction	Signs	Symptoms
Respiratory	Rhinitis	Mucosal edema	Nasal congestion and itching
	Laryngeal edema	Laryngeal stridor Vocal cord edema	Dyspnea
	Bronchospasm	Cough, wheezing, rales Respiratory distress, tachypnea	Cough, wheezing Restrosternal oppression
Cardiovascular	Hypotension	Hypotension Tachycardia	Syncope Feeling faint
	Arrhythmia	EKG changes, nonspecific ST-segment and T-wave changes, nodal rhythm, atrial fibrillation	
	Cardiac arrest	Absent pulse, EKG changes: asystole, ventricular fibrillation	
Cutaneous	Urticaria	Urticarial lesion	Pruritus, hives
	Angioedema	Edema	Nonpruritic swelling, perioral or periorbital edema
Gastrointestinal			Nausea, vomiting, abdominal pain, diarrhea
Ocular	Conjunctivitis	Conjunctival inflammation	Ocular itching/lacrimation

From Kelly JF, Patterson R. Anaphylaxis: course, mechanisms and treatment. JAMA 1974;227:1431–1436.

Table 16–7. Recognition of Anaphylaxis in Intubated Patients

System	Signs
Respiratory	Cyanosis
	Wheezing
	Increased peak airway pressure
	Acute pulmonary edema
Cardiovascular	Tachycardia
	Dysrhythmias
	Hypotension
	Pulmonary hypertension
	Decreased systemic vascular resistance
	Cardiovascular collapse
Cutaneous	Urticaria
	Flushing
	Perioral edema
	Periorbital edema

From Levy JH. Anaphylactic reactions in anesthesia and intensive care. 2nd ed. Boston: Butterworth-Heinemann, 1992.

mote activation of other systems leading to surface-mediated host defense reactions (plasma contact activation). In contrast to anaphylaxis, the anaphylactoid reaction is a nonimmunologic reaction (46), such as a rapid intravenous infusion of vancomycin causing histamine release (74–76). In European countries, anaphylactoid reactions to anesthetic agents or plasma substitutes that are either life threatening or operation disrupting have an incidence between one in 1000 and one in 10,000 (77). Overall, in many countries, the number of anaphylactoid reactions during general anesthesia has been increasing and, despite appropriate treatment, about 6% of patients who experience such a reaction die (78).

There is no way to identify an individual who has a high risk of developing an anaphylactoid response. However, for the patient who has survived an anaphylactoid reaction during anesthesia, it is essential to try to identify the drug and confirm the diagnosis to avoid a similar reaction during subsequent anesthesia (75). There are several methods of evaluating an anaphylactoid response, including measurement of plasma histamine, intradermal testing, and cellular tests and assays for specific plasma proteins (3). There are many advantages and disadvantages to each specific technique (see Table 16–8). Other specific tests to evaluate allergic reactions include complement levels, in vitro leukocyte histamine release, radioallergosorbent testing (RAST), and enzyme-linked immunoabsorbent assays (ELISA). Whereas the evaluation of complement levels can demonstrate activation of complement pathways, no information about the causative agent can be obtained (79). The in vitro leukocyte histamine release test may be used on blood from a sensitized patient. It essentially provides an in vitro method of anaphylactic challenge. It has been used to evaluate patients after reactions to pentothal, muscle relaxants, and penicillin (80–85). The leukocyte histamine release test is useful when skin testing is not possible, when confirmation of a negative or equivocal skin test is needed, and when a positive skin test does not match the case history (86). The RAST test is highly sensitive. It detects antibodies to antigen fixed to an insoluble matrix and has been shown to correlate well with skin testing and other provocation tests (87, 88). Unfortunately, the test is not widely available for drug sensitivity testing. The ELISA test is also used to detect IgE antibodies. It has been used to detect antibodies to a variety of agents, including the human immunodeficiency virus (89). Again, it is unfortunate that there are no commercially available test kits for evaluation of IgE antibodies developed in response to drugs used in anesthesia.

Skin testing is the least expensive and most widely used method of evaluating sensitivity to an allergen (75, 90). It has been used to evaluate sensitivities to barbiturates and muscle relaxants (73, 80, 91) as well as other drugs. Fisher (92) believes that intradermal testing after an anaphylactoid reaction to an anesthetic agent is the minimum investigation that should be performed. A positive intradermal test may provide useful information.

Table 16–8. Some Methods of Evaluating Allergic Responses

Technique	Advantages	Disadvantages
Plasma histamine	Direct measure of effector substance	Experimental requirements not suitable for clinical response, not useful for all reactions
Intradermal testing	Simple, only in vivo test, inexpensive	Must be carried out considerably after response, assumes immune-mediated response
Cellular tests	High sensitivity	Requires high technical skill, assumes immune-mediated response
Specific plasma protein assay	Simple, does not assume mechanism of reaction	Can only identify plasma events, poor sensitivity for marginal adverse reactions

From Watkins J, Salo M. Trauma, stress and immunity in anesthesia and surgery. Boston: Butterworth Scientific, 1982.

However, false positives may be due to local irritant effects and false negative results have also been documented (93). Therefore, a negative test does not exclude the diagnosis of an anaphylactoid reaction, even in a patient whose clinical history is doubtful. The method for skin testing has been described by Fisher (91, 92). If a patient has received several intravenous agents and has had a reaction, a positive intradermal test to one of the agents suggests that the patient should not receive that agent again (2, 75).

The Prausnitz-Küstner test is a test of passive transfer of cutaneous reactivity (anaphylaxis). It has been used to diagnose immediate-type hypersensitivity (IgE) reactions and distinguish them from IgG-initiated reactions as repeat testing with heated serum inactivates the IgE, leaving only IgG antibodies to react (79).

Laxenaire et al. (77) suggest that three tests involving both in vivo and in vitro aspects of immunity be performed 6 weeks after the anaphylactoid response, in addition to specific testing during the reaction. They include skin tests using various concentrations of the agents, the basophil degranulation test or leukocyte histamine release, and the Prausnitz-Küstner tests using both heated and untreated serum. The latter demonstrate the presence of either a specific IgE (heat labile) or IgG antibodies for specific agents.

ALLERGIC RESPONSES TO SPECIFIC AGENTS USED IN ANESTHESIA AND SURGERY

Many anesthetic agents cause hypotension and cardiovascular depression by a variety of mechanisms. Bronchospasm may occur during intubation and with lighter levels of anesthesia. Therefore, many of the clinical manifestations associated with an allergic reaction may be incorrectly attributed to adverse drug reactions. Fortunately, most allergic reactions from drugs are not serious or life threatening and are isolated cutaneous reactions or bronchospasm that respond to discontinuation of the offending agent and minimal therapeutic intervention.

Several factors may predispose a patient to experiencing an allergic reaction to an intravenously administered agent. For example, it has been shown that a history of atopy (asthma or hay fever) is present in 9 to 15% of patients who have a hypersensitivity reaction to an intravenous anesthetic. This history is even more frequent in barbiturate reactors. A history of a food or drug allergy is seen in 19% of patients who react to an intravenous anesthetic and it is suggested that this is a conservative figure (94). A history of asthma, atopy, or other food or drug allergies should alert the physician to the possibility that an unexpected reaction to an intravenous agent may represent a hypersensitivity response.

ANESTHETIC INDUCTION AGENTS

Essentially, all of the intravenous induction agents have been associated with life-threatening allergic reactions. Earlier studies indicated that allergic reactions occurred most commonly with agents that were solubilized with cremophor, such as propanidid and alphaxalone/alphadolone (Althesin), but this is mostly of historical interest because these agents are no longer widely used. Cremophor is a complex substance produced by oxyethelation of castor oil. Both unsaturated and saturated molecules are present in the preparation, which may contain as many as 60 discrete compounds. Cremophor alone, when injected into animals has a high incidence (about 75%) of pulmonary distress, hypotension, and urticaria, because it is capable of producing complement activation (3, 94). Allergic reactions after injection of alphaxalone/alphadolone or propranidid occur with a frequency of one in 1000 injections. It has been shown that cremophor enhances the immunogenicity of these drugs. There was also an increased incidence of allergic reactions to diazepam when cremophor was substituted for propylene glycol (4, 94, 95).

Sodium thiopental (pentothal) has two separate mechanisms for facilitating histamine release. There are direct effects on the mast cells to cause liberation of histamine (anaphylactoid) as well as IgE-mediated (anaphylactic) reactions. Pentothal seems to possess more than one antigenic site, and cross-reactivity with other barbiturates can occur. IgE-mediated reactions to pentothal are rare (less than one in 22,000). In skin mast cell preparations, thiopental and thiamylal caused histamine release, whereas methohexital and phenobarbi-

tal did not cause mediator release at similar concentrations. This suggests that the sulfur-containing barbiturate analogs may predispose histamine-sensitive patients (asthmatics) and "increased-histamine releasers" (atopics) to reactions and may be avoided (64). Most cases describing allergic reactions to pentothal have been in patients with a history of atopy (4). Of the reported cases of barbiturate reactions, pentothal is the agent that is implicated most commonly. The reactions are mostly cutaneous in nature, followed by cardiovascular and respiratory involvement. Although methohexital does not seem to cause direct histamine release, it has been implicated in IgE-mediated reactions (64, 94–98).

Etomidate is an imidazole derivative that is solubilized in propylene glycol. It does not cause plasma histamine release. From 1978 until 1982, there were only five cases reported of possible reactions to etomidate, and these involved cutaneous flushing or urticaria. However, the ultimate cause of these reactions was not determined. In two other cases, which involved hypotension, muscle relaxants were also given (99). In two isolated cases, etomidate was reported to have caused urticaria and severe bronchospasm leading to cardiac arrest (100) and urticaria, tachycardia, and hypotension (101). Because few reports of allergic reactions are associated with etomidate, it is considered safe for higher-risk patients such as those with a history of atopy or prior anaphylactoid reaction to an anesthetic (99).

Propofol (Diprivan) is an alkyl phenol, unrelated to other types of induction agents such as barbiturates, imidazoles, or eugenols. Initially, propofol was emulsified in a cremophor EL solution, and this solubilizing agent may have been responsible (102). Currently, it is emulsified in an aqueous solution of soybean oil, glycerol, and purified egg phosphatide, but this has not solved the problem (103). Anaphylaxis (IgE mediated) has been reported with the different propofol formulations (104, 105). In an evaluation of 14 cases of anaphylactoid reaction to propofol, Laxenaire et al. (106) reported that allergic responses occurred on the first use, especially in patients with a history of drug allergy. They also suggest that it may be prudent to avoid the use of propofol, the commercial emulsion Diprivan, in patients who experienced an anaphylactic reaction to muscle relaxants. It is believed that the IgE produced may be in response to the phenyl nucleus and the isopropyl groups that are also present in many other drugs.

Ketamine is an arylcyclohexylamine derivative of phencyclidine that can be administered intravenously or intramuscularly to produce a dissociative anesthetic state. Allergic reactions to ketamine are rare. Occasional cutaneous eruptions are related to histamine release. A 3-year-old who had previously received ketamine without incident, developed a generalized rash, without associated hypotension or wheezing. The reaction was believed to be anaphylactoid rather than anaphylactic in nature because the Prausnitz-Küstner test was negative (107, 108).

Benzodiazepines such as diazepam have been used for many years. They do not appear to cause histamine release after intravenous injection. Despite this, there have been several reports of allergic reactions other than anaphylaxis to benzodiazepines. Although hypersensitivity reactions to diazepam and other benzodiazepines are rare, they are not unreported (109). It is also possible that some of the reactions that have been reported may relate to the use of cremophor EL as the solvent. This has subsequently been changed to glycoferolalchol-benzoic acid. Benzodiazepines are generally considered safe in high-risk patients (110, 111).

NARCOTICS

Anaphylactic reactions to narcotics are extremely rare. The first reported reaction occurred in a 2½-year-old child who developed urticaria, bronchospasm, cyanosis, and hypotension within moments after the intravenous administration of meperidine. Subsequent demonstration of IgE antibodies for meperi-dine confirmed the diagnosis (112). Narcotics, most notably morphine, cause histamine release (63). This is responsible for local effects like the erythema that can occur along the vein of administration. Systemic effects such as hypotension may also occur. A correlation has been shown between the plasma histamine concentration and the reduction in systemic vascular resistance and mean arterial blood pressure after administration of intravenous morphine (113). In contrast, oxymorphone and fentanyl do not induce histamine release in human mast cell preparations. Histamine release does not seem to be related to analgesic potency, is not due to cytotoxicity, and is not related to the opioid receptors (114). In other studies, when injected intradermally in volunteers, morphine, meperidine, fentanyl, and sufentanil caused both wheal and flare responses that were significantly greater than those produced by saline. Naloxone, alfentanil, and nalbuphine did not cause wheal or flare responses (115).

Clinically, fentanyl has been associated with anaphylactic reactions during anesthesia, although these reactions are extremely rare. Bennett et al. (116) report the case of a 29-year-old patient who had an anaphylactic reaction to intravenous fentanyl that manifested as hypotension and subsequent vascular collapse without respiratory difficulty. Fentanyl was confirmed as the causative agent by intradermal skin testing 1 month later. Anaphylactic reactions to drugs administered into the epidural space are also extremely rare; however, there has also been a case report of an anaphylactic reaction to epidural fentanyl in a 35-year-old woman undergoing a repeat caesarean section. Here, too, the hypersensitivity to fentanyl was confirmed by intradermal skin testing (117). Sufentanil administered intravenously at 60 ug/minute to a dose of 15 ug/kg was not associated with histamine release in patients undergoing coronary artery bypass surgery (118). Morphine, meperidine, and codeine are the only clinically used opioids that can cause histamine release.

MUSCLE RELAXANTS

Anaphylactic and anaphylactoid reactions have been reported after administration of succinylcholine and many nondepolarizing muscle relaxants, including d-tubocurarine, gallamine, metocurine, atracurium, vecuronium, and pancuronium (4, 80, 82, 83, 119–133). Bronchospasm observed after endotracheal intubation may be related to tube placement as well as to an allergic reaction to the muscle relaxant, and distinguishing between the two diagnoses will be difficult because the events are temporally related. Intradermal skin testing has not been helpful for documentation of allergies to muscle relaxants because very low concentrations often produce a wheal-and-flare response (123). However, there are situations in which a positive intradermal test has been used as confirmatory evidence of an allergy to a muscle relaxant (4). The neuromuscular blocking agents used clinically are derived from either benzylisoquinoline (atracurium, doxacurium, d-tubocurarine, mivacurium, and metocurine), a steroid nucleus (vecuronium, pancuronium, rocuronium), or acetylcholine (succinylcholine).

Of these groups, only the benzylisoquinoline derivatives cause degranulation of cutaneous mast cells and release histamine when used clinically. The hypotension associated with administration of curare has been directly associated with increased concentrations of histamine in the plasma (65). Allergic responses to d-tubocurarine have most often been reported after a first exposure to the drug, which suggests an anaphylactoid reaction (79, 126, 127). In one report, a 3-mg dose just before intubation of the trachea resulted in generalized erythema, hypotension, and bronchospasm in a patient with no allergic history (126). In a similar fashion, decreases in blood pressure and systemic vascular resistance occur after bolus administration of 0.5 mg/kg of atracurium (132). It has been suggested that atracurium and metocurine may cause less histamine release than d-tubocurarine because of the methoxy group substitutions and, in

atracurium, carboxyl groups in the side chain. However, this may also relate to increased drug potency, allowing the administration of less drug. Most reactions to d-tubocurarine have been described after the first exposure, suggesting an anaphylactoid reaction. Papaverine is also a benzylisoquinoline analog that has a close resemblance to the side chains of atracurium. It is a potent vasodilator, and this effect may be partly due to histamine release. The benzylisoquinoline moiety may represent the specific molecular configuration responsible for the histamine release of atracurium (133).

Intradermal administration of the steroid-based muscle relaxants can also produce a wheal-and-flare response but not of the same magnitude as those produced by the benzylisoquinoline derivatives.

Anaphylactic and anaphylactoid reactions have been described in response to succinylcholine. An anaphylactic reaction has been described that is characterized by upper airway edema and generalized erythema that occurred immediately after intravenous administration of succinylcholine. The patient was allergic to penicillin. IgE levels were subsequently elevated (122). A cross-reaction between succinylcholine and penicillin is unlikely because the two drugs are not structurally related. In another report, a patient with a history of bronchial asthma developed upper airway edema, which was noted upon extubation of the trachea. This occurred without hemodynamic or pulmonary changes. It was the patient's first exposure to succinylcholine, suggesting an anaphylactoid reaction (120). Most patients who experience an allergic reaction to succinylcholine manifest bronchospasm, hypotension, and possibly generalized erythema (4). In a group of 28 patients who experienced an extreme, life-threatening sensitivity to succinylcholine reported by Youngman (134), the female/male ratio was 8/1. He observed that some patients had a reaction on the first exposure. He further noticed that most patients experienced cross-reactions to other neuromuscular blocking agents. In 50%

of these patients, circulatory collapse was the sole presenting feature.

A significant percent of patients demonstrate cross-reactivity to the muscle relaxants. In addition, 10 to 50% of patients with an allergy to a neuromuscular blocking agent exhibit cross-reactivity with other quaternary ammonium molecules with a similar structure. For example, choline functions as a hapten inhibitor and prevents the activation of IgE molecules directed against succinylcholine (82). IgE molecules directed against neuromuscular blockers can also cross-react with other agents containing a quaternary ammonium ion (133, 135), including antihistamines, neostigmine, and morphine. In addition, many foods, cosmetics, and industrial materials contain similar quaternary ammonium structures. This cross-reactivity allows sensitization to a neuromuscular blocking agent without having a previous exposure. Eighty-five percent of patients who reacted to a muscle relaxant never had a prior exposure to the drug; however, a type I hypersensitivity seems to be the most likely mechanism for life-threatening reactions to neuromuscular blocking agents (136). Muscle relaxants are often implicated in studies of anesthetic agent anaphylaxis (135).

LOCAL ANESTHETICS

Despite the extensive use of local anesthetic agents, adverse reactions are extremely rare. Most reactions are the result of accidental intravascular injection or overdose. Approximately 1% of all reactions to local anesthetic agents have an immunological cause, and these seem to be related to histamine release (137). It is important, especially with a local anesthetic reaction, to obtain a careful history about the reaction. For example, a patient who experienced urticaria and difficulty breathing probably had an allergic reaction, whereas a patient who experienced palpitations and a headache immediately after injection of the local anesthetic is probably describing an intravascular injection of an epinephrine-containing local anesthetic solution.

Ester-type local anesthetic agents are more likely than amide local anesthetics to cause an allergic reaction. This is because of their metabolism to para-aminobenzoic acid, which may cause an allergic reaction. There is one report of an allergic reaction to an amide local anesthetic in which the patient had reported an allergy to lidocaine. When skin was tested with bupivacaine, she had a systemic reaction with a decrease in the complement C4 plasma concentration, indicating that the reaction was immunologically mediated (137). The documentation of an allergic reaction to a local anesthetic usually involves intradermal testing.

Allergic reactions after the administration of a local anesthetic agent may also relate to methylparaben or similar agents used as preservatives in multidose vials (138). They are structurally similar to para-aminobenzoic acid and they may provoke an allergic reaction. Preservatives may be mixed with either ester or amide local anesthetics. Antioxidants such as bisulfite or metabisulfite also have the potential to cause allergic reactions. They are used in solutions of many different local anesthetics, which also contain vasoactive substances (139).

The toxic effects of local anesthetic agents are usually a result of an intravascular injection and include central nervous system and cardiovascular effects. Toxicity may manifest as slurred speech, euphoria, dizziness, excitement, nausea, vomiting, disorientation, or seizures. Vasovagal reactions may also occur. They present with bradycardia, sweating, and pallor. The symptoms improve significantly after the patient is placed in the supine position. Stimulation of the sympathetic nervous system may result from epinephrine in the local anesthetic solution or simply from anxiety. This may cause tremors, diaphoresis, tachycardia, and/or hypertension.

When considering a local anesthetic allergy, rather than evaluation of the allergy by intradermal skin testing, it is more practical to be sure to use a preservative-free preparation and avoid the class of local anesthetics to which the presumed reaction occurred. It is assumed that cross-reactivity between esters and amides does not occur; therefore, it is reasonable that a patient with a history of an allergy to an ester-type agent would not react adversely to an amide and vice versa (4).

ATROPINE

Atropine is used for treatment of bradycardia and drying of secretions. During the administration of anesthesia, it may also be used to prevent bradycardia during antagonism of muscle relaxants. It is an alkaloid that has been implicated rarely in allergic reactions. However, there is one case report of a 38-year-old woman who experienced anaphylactic shock that manifested as urticaria, facial edema tachycardia, and cardiovascular collapse after intravenous atropine during spinal anesthesia. Epinephrine was required to maintain the blood pressure. The patient subsequently had a positive response to intradermal testing. The Prausnitz-Küstner test was also positive, indicating the presence of specific IgE antibodies. The patient did not have a response to hyoscine (140).

ANTIBIOTICS

Anaphylactic reactions after administration of penicillin are well established. Allergic reactions to penicillin are the most common cause of anaphylaxis. In addition, penicillin allergic patients may also demonstrate a cross-reactivity to semisynthetic penicillins such as cephalosporins. Allergic reactions occur in 3 to 5% of patients treated with cephalothin (141–143). There is a 1 to 10% drug reaction rate in those without a history of penicillin allergy. In those with a prior reaction, the chance of a reaction increases from 6 to 40%. Patients with a history of a previous penicillin reaction have a fourfold to sixfold higher chance of having another reaction to penicillin than those without previous allergic history (144). Death from penicillin anaphylaxis accounts for

fatalities once in every 50,000 to 100,000 treatment cases (or approximately 400 to 800 deaths per year). Penicillin allergies may manifest as any of the four types of immunopathological reactions described earlier in this chapter. Pseudoanaphylactic reactions after inadvertent intravenous injection of procaine penicillin may occur. These are most likely related to a combination of toxic and embolic phenomena from procaine (144–146).

Penicillin itself does not cause an immune response. It must first bind to tissue macromolecules to produce hapten-protein complexes. The beta-lactam ring in penicillins opens, forming a penicilloyl group (147). It is this group that combines with proteins. This type of reaction occurs with benzylpenicillin and the semisynthetic penicillins as well. Metabolism can lead to other antigenic substances. The parenteral administration of penicillin is responsible for more allergic reactions than oral penicillin.

Cephalosporins also possess a beta-lactam ring that has some modifications from the beta-lactam ring in penicillin. Despite this, cross-reactivity between penicillin and cephalosporins has been reported (148–151). Primary cephalosporin allergies have also been observed (149). The incidence of clinically important cross-reactivity between penicillins and cephalosporins is believed to be small but the exact incidence is unknown.

Newer beta-lactam-containing antibiotics include carbapenems and monobactams, which include imipenem and aztreonam. Studies have found a high incidence of cross-reactivity between penicillin antigenic determinants and imipenem (152). However, cross-reactivity between azetreonam and other beta-lactam derivatives suggests that azetreonam may be administered safely to most patients who are allergic to penicillin (153). Allergic reactions to nonbeta-lactam antibiotics has been reviewed by Sullivan and is beyond the scope of this chapter (154).

Vancomycin, a glycopeptide antibiotic, is associated with life-threatening anaphylactoid reactions after rapid intravenous administration. When a 1-g dose is administered over 10 minutes, blood pressure has been reported to decrease 25 to 50%. The hypotension seen during rapid vancomycin administration may be accompanied by an erythematous rash (155, 156). Vancomycin also produces a dose-dependent depression of myocardial contractility (76). Hypotension was not seen when the drug was administered over 30 minutes (155). Histamine release also has been reported in some patients who experienced hypotension associated with vancomycin administration. This may be the mechanism for hypotension after the rapid administration of vancomycin (76).

APROTININ

Aprotinin is a basic polypeptide that stabilizes the platelet membrane and has been shown to decrease blood loss in patients undergoing coronary artery bypass and grafting surgery (157). It is derived from bovine lung and has the potential to cause anaphylaxis after intravenous administration. Specific IgE antibodies to aprotinin have been seen in patients who manifested hypersensitivity reactions to the drug. When used in cardiac surgery, 2 of 902 patients manifest allergic reactions with IgM or IgG antibodies (158, 159).

CONTRAST DYES

In Greenberger's study (160), the incidence of allergic reactions caused by injection of ionic contrast media is between 5 and 8%. Reactions including nausea, vomiting, flushing, or sensations of warmth range from 5 to 8%, whereas more severe reactions, including urticaria, angioedema, wheezing, dyspnea, hypotension, or death, occur in 2 to 3% of patients who receive intravenous contrast media (161). There are a variety of mechanisms, both immunologic and nonimmunologic, by which contrast dyes are believed to produce hypersensitivity reactions, but the exact mechanism is unknown. Five different types of reactions

occur: vasomotor, vasovagal, dermal, osmotic, and anaphylactoid. The most severe reactions are idiosyncratic, and history of a reaction may not predict a future response. The hyperosmolarity of the solution may have significant hemodynamic effects, or it may have direct effects on mast cells and basophils. Furthermore, other hyperosmotic agents such as mannitol may have direct effects on basophils and mast cells, causing histamine release (162). Histamine release seems to occur in some reactions, as does the activation of serum complement (160, 163). There is no evidence that IgE-mediated reactions occur in contrast dye reactions.

NONSTEROIDAL ANTI-INFLAMMATORY AGENTS

The nonsteroidal anti-inflammatory drugs (NSAIDs), including aspirin, ibuprofen, and ketorolac, among others, are inhibitors of cyclo-oxygenase. They possess analgesic and anti-inflammatory properties. These drugs are frequently reported to be the cause of adverse drug reactions. Clinical symptoms often resemble an allergy and include bronchospasm, urticaria, angioedema, and other skin manifestations. In addition, anaphylactic shock has also been observed. In asthmatic adults, NSAIDs can precipitate asthmatic attacks in approximately 8 to 20% of patients and in 60 to 85% of those who have had a prior reaction to NSAIDs. Allergic reactions to NSAIDs do not seem to be mediated by IgE antibodies. However, the mechanism of hypersensitivity is not entirely clear (164, 165). Ketorolac is the only injectable NSAID currently available in the United States. No information is available to suggest that it has any unusual characteristics that predispose hypersensitivity reactions.

FUROSEMIDE

Furosemide is a widely used intravenous diuretic. It is a sulfa compound that is related to the thiazides and sulfonamide antibiotics. An anaphylactic reaction to furosemide has been reported after administration of 20 mg intravenously. The reaction consisted of urticaria, periorbital edema, and hypotension. The allergy was confirmed by skin testing (166). Most clinical experience and widespread use indicates that furosemide is a safe drug. However, there is some evidence to suggest that there may be a group of patients who have an increased risk of allergic responses to sulfonamide-containing compounds, furosemide, and thiazides. Although the risk of a reaction seems to be low, therapy with structurally unrelated alternative drugs should be considered (166, 167).

VASCULAR GRAFTS

Vascular grafting material has been shown to cause adverse reactions manifesting as persistent decreased blood pressure and disseminated intravascular coagulation. In a report of five patients, two of three patients who had grafts replaced experienced an uneventful recovery. In the two patients in whom the grafts were not replaced, death ensued. Although the graft material Dacron is considered to be inert, the combinations of other agents used to construct the Dacron matrix are proprietary information and can vary between different companies that manufacture grafting material (168).

CHYMOPAPAIN

Chymopapain injections are used for the treatment of herniated intervertebral discs. The injection of chymopapain has been associated with allergic reactions of varying degree, including cardiovascular collapse and death. Newer preparations contain no preservatives and less extraneous protein and may pose less of a problem. Reactions seem to be more common in women and in those with multiple allergies. Previous exposure to chymopapain in meat tenderizers, cosmetics, and beer may

account for the high incidence of anaphylaxis. Chymopapain injection has significant risk because the intraoperative death rate may be 3 times higher than from general anesthesia alone. Pretreatment with antihistamines prior to injection does not inhibit or prevent anaphylaxis (169). Prevention of reactions is the best approach. However, there is no method for identifying patients at risk for the reaction. Intradermal testing is not possible as chymopapain is a proteolytic enzyme which would produce false positive results (135).

PLASMA VOLUME EXPANDERS

Anaphylactoid reactions have been reported to occur with a variety of volume expanders, including human serum albumin, dextran, and hydroxyethyl starch (170). Plasma substitutes are more likely to cause anaphylactoid rather than anaphylactic reactions or activation of the complement pathway (4). With respect to albumin, mechanisms include aggregates combining with IgG and activating complement or reaction to stabilizers. In addition, the stabilizers may alter the albumin to cause sensitization and histamine release (170, 171).

The dextrans are either low-molecular-weight or high-molecular-weight preparations. The low molecular weight is about 40,000 daltons (dextran 40) in a 10% solution and the high molecular weight is about 70,000 daltons (dextran 70) in a 6% solution. The low molecular weight preparation may be used as an intravascular volume expander and for prophylaxis against venous thrombosis. The high molecular weight solution is used only as a volume expander. Furhoff's study (172) reports 133 cases of anaphylactoid reactions to dextran occurring from 1968 until 1975. There were 113 reactions to the high-molecular-weight solution and 20 reports of reactions to the low-molecular-weight dextran 40. Reactions may be characterized by flushing or urticaria, gastrointestinal symptoms, vasodilation, hypotension, tachycardia, and cardiovascular collapse. Although relatively rare, dextran reactions are a clinical reality.

Hydroxyethyl starch is used as a plasma volume expander and in plasmapheresis. Ring and Messmer (170) reported only 14 reactions in more than 16,000 administrations. The mechanism of these anaphylactoid reactions is not entirely clear (173).

STEROIDS

As we will discuss later in this chapter, one of the many uses of corticosteroids is the treatment of anaphylactic reactions. However, anaphylactic reactions to steroids, including prednisolone and methylprednisolone sodium succinate, have been reported (174, 175). Fortunately, these reactions are rare, but the physician must always be prepared for an anaphylactic reaction to drugs used to treat anaphylactic reactions.

PROTAMINE

Protamine is a strongly basic polypeptide, derived from salmon sperm, that is primarily used to antagonize the effects of heparin anticoagulation during cardiac surgery. It may also be used to delay the absorption of some insulin preparations. A variety of adverse reactions have been reported after the administration of intravenous protamine, including urticaria, rashes, bronchospasm, hypotension, cardiovascular collapse, and death (176–180). A variety of mechanisms, both immunological and nonimmunological, have been postulated for protamine-induced reactions. Anaphylactic reactions after the first intravenous administration have been reported in diabetic patients previously treated with protamine insulin preparations. Patients receiving NPH insulin have a 50-fold increased risk (27% versus 0.5%) of developing a major protamine reaction compared to those with no history of NPH use (181). Patients with allergies to fish may also develop anaphylactic reactions after intravenous administration of protamine (182, 183).

Men who have undergone vasectomies are also at an increased risk for protamine reactions. In theory, they may develop antibodies to sperm. Normally, the testis and sperm are isolated from the immune system; however, surgical disruption of the vas deferens exposes the testis and sperm to the immune system (184–186).

The exact mechanisms by which protamine allergies occur are not fully understood. They may include complement or mast cell activation or antibody formation (135). Histamine release from mast cells does not seem to play a role, because histamine release occurs at concentrations that are much greater than those used in clinical practice (187). Protamine-heparin complexes may also activate the complement system via the classical pathway. Protamine may act in a variety of ways to cause adverse reactions. Life-threatening reactions are relatively rare and are mediated by IgG or IgE antibodies (135).

LATEX (NATURAL RUBBER)

During the past several years, there has been a dramatic increase in the awareness of anaphylaxis to latex and latex-containing products used during surgery (188). The usual immunologic response to latex is a delayed hypersensitivity or type IV reaction. Between 1988 and 1992, it is estimated that 11.8 billion examination gloves and 1.8 billion surgical latex gloves were used in the United States. During this same period, there were more than 1000 reports to the U.S. Food and Drug Administration of systemic allergic reactions to latex. These were IgE-mediated (type I) reactions (189). Prior exposure to latex and latex products may predispose an individual to an anaphylactic reaction during surgery. Patients at risk include children with spina bifida who require frequent urinary catheterization. In addition, healthcare workers and others who are exposed to latex products may also be at increased risk of developing anaphylaxis (188, 190–193). Furthermore, many people have exposure through gloves used for household cleaning, toy balloons, and latex condoms (194). However, many people seemingly develop sensitivity to latex without an apparent prior exposure. Recent reports have shown that latex dust is a component of urban air pollution and that certain food allergens may demonstrate a cross-reactivity with latex (194, 195). Natural rubber has been known to cause contact dermatitis, and rubber and plastic gloves frequently cause exacerbations of contact dermatitis. Most rubber gloves are made from latex, a milky sap derived from the rubber tree. The monomer form of natural latex is cis-1,4-polyisoprene. In addition, there are several substances added during the manufacturing process. The low-molecular-weight substances include accelerators, antioxidants, stabilizers, and vulcanizers (to improve elasticity). Some of these additives may act as haptens and cause allergic reactions (196–198). Several proteins of various sizes have been found in extracts of natural rubber latex, which seem to constitute some of the major clinically significant allergens. These include the 14-, 20- and 27-kD proteins. It is also important to realize that the amount of water-soluble proteins seems to vary from product to product and the allergenicity varies between different brands of surgical gloves. The reasons for these differences remains unclear (199).

In patients who have undergone multiple surgical procedures, the onset of an allergic reaction to latex may occur between 40 and 290 minutes after the induction of anesthesia (200). The reactions to latex may be anaphylactoid or anaphylactic in nature (196, 197, 201–203). During surgery, the lack of normal tissue barriers and the direct contact with blood, mucus membranes, and tissues can explain why the reaction may be so severe (191). Latex allergy should always be considered by the anesthesiologist when there is an allergic reaction during surgery, especially when it is without an obvious temporal relationship to administration of drugs or blood products (202). In the most difficult circumstances, allergic reactions may occur in response to more

Table 16–9. Routinely Used Medical Products That May Contain Latex

Adhesive tape	Hemodialysis equipment
Airway devices	Injection ports in i.v. tubing
Breathing bags	Penrose drains
Scented masks	Pulse oximeter sensors
Head straps	Rubber dams
Blood pressure cuffs	Rubber gloves
Breathing circuits	Rubber medication bottle
	stoppers
Condom urinary	Rubber tourniquets
collection devices	
Urinary catheters	Tooth protectors/blocks
Electrode pads	Ventilator bellows
Elastic bandages	
Elastic stockings	
Enema tubing	
Gastrointestinal tubes	

than one agent. McCormack et al. (204) reported an anaphylactic reaction to both vecuronium and latex in a 5-year-old girl with meningomyelocele.

Medical products that contain latex and are routinely used in the operating room or critical care setting are listed in Table 16–9. Patients with a history of chronic or repeated use of latex products may be at increased risk for serious allergic reactions to latex during surgery. In patients at increased risk, skin testing or other preoperative investigation may establish the diagnosis (200). Avoiding latex-containing products or using nonlatex substitutes, such as vinyl or neoprine surgical gloves, for the latex-sensitive patient is of paramount importance.

BLOOD PRODUCTS

Blood products include packed red blood cells, whole blood, fresh frozen plasma, platelets, cryoprecipitate, and fibrin glue compounds. All of these contain a variety of antigens and plasma antibodies. Several different reactions may occur after transfusion of any blood product. One of the greatest concerns associated with blood transfusions is the risk of infection. The most significant concerns are hepatitis (type B or non-A/non-B) and human immunodeficiency virus (204). In addition, several noninfectious, nonhemolytic allergic reactions can occur. Overall, about 3% of patients receiving properly cross-matched blood have an allergic reaction. This represents approximately 90% of the untoward consequences of the administration of blood products (205). Hemolytic, infectious, and transfusion reactions from ABO and Rh incompatibilities and others are beyond the scope of this chapter.

Nonhemolytic transfusion reactions include antigen-antibody reactions, which are similar to hemolytic reactions but occur between donor white cells, platelets and immunoglobulins, and the recipient's antibodies, or to problems with administration and storage of the blood product (205, 206).

Life-threatening hemolytic reactions to blood transfusion are the result of ABO incompatibility mediated by IgM antibodies. Severe and possibly life-threatening nonhemolytic allergic reactions may occur with whole blood as well as with component therapies including packed red blood cells, fresh frozen plasma, or platelets. This occurs as a result of donor antibodies against white blood cell antigens producing leukocyte agglutination (207).

Manifestations of an allergic reaction to blood products include pruritis, erythema, and urticaria, which is often accompanied by fever and eosinophilia. Laryngospasm or bronchospasm may also occur. The first manifestation may be erythema along the vein in which the blood is being administered. Mild reactions may be treated with diphenhydramine (0.5 to 1 mg/kg). If leukocyte agglutination occurs, the more serious consequences include microvascular occlusion, vascular inflammation leading to membrane damage, hypoxemia, pulmonary hypertension, and noncardiac pulmonary edema, which may manifest as adult respiratory distress syndrome. The patient will experience a high fever within 2 hours of the transfusion. It is associated with rigors, pallor, diaphoresis,

tachycardia, hypotension, and possibly cyanosis (207). More severe reactions necessitate stopping the transfusion and employing other, more aggressive therapies (4).

Immune-associated reactions involve immunoglobulins IgG, IgM, IgA, and IgE. Symptoms of these reactions include flushing, nausea, vomiting, tachycardia, and dyspnea. This results from particulate aggregates in the infusate, which causes release of histamine-like substances. IgE is the mediator of allergic symptoms. Transfusion from an allergic donor can result in transient symptoms (lasting about 30 days as the IgE is metabolized) of the same allergy in the recipient. This may account for some transient drug sensitivities such as asthma and rhinitis (205).

Platelet-associated reactions are usually febrile reactions associated with platelet transfusion. More important, however, is the development of antiplatelet antibodies in the recipient. There is no predictive test for platelet antibodies, and the best method of evaluation is reevaluation of platelet counts at 1 and 24 hours after platelet transfusion (205).

A particular group of patients with deficiency of IgA antibodies in plasma are at higher risk of transfusion reactions because they develop anti-IgA antibodies, which can provoke an anaphylactic reaction to blood products containing IgA. Washed blood products from donors with IgA deficiency may be indicated (4, 207).

CLINICAL CONSIDERATIONS AND TREATMENT OF ALLERGIC (ANAPHYLACTIC) REACTIONS

The physician is best prepared to treat an allergic reaction if prior planning has taken place. The most important aspect is obtaining a complete "allergic" history from a patient who reports a previous reaction. The history should be detailed, with a careful review of the clinical symptoms and temporal sequence of events. Old records may be very useful in this regard. If, after obtaining the history and reviewing the old records, the clinician has a high index of suspicion, the drug or class of drugs should be avoided. For example, if there is a strong suggestion of a thiobarbiturate reaction, that class of induction agents may be avoided, similarly for muscle relaxants or antibiotics. A prior reaction to aspirin or another NSAID should prompt the anesthesiologist to avoid these agents, especially if the patient has a history of nasal polyps. Also, NSAIDs should be used carefully in asthmatic patients because of the increased risk of bronchospasm. If there is a question about the causative agent, the patient may be referred for skin testing as discussed previously. If the reaction reported is severe, the patient should also be advised to wear a MedicAlert bracelet or necklace. For some drugs (such as protamine), there are no clinically available alternatives, and special considerations such as requesting an experimental agent may be necessary (208).

Many physicians use test doses to determine sensitivity to a specific agent. This practice usually is not helpful, because the test dose administered may be significant and may prompt an allergic or anaphylactic reaction. The test doses that anesthesiologists usually administer evaluate idiosyncratic effects and not allergies. For safe test dosing to assess anaphylactic reactions, very small quantities (0.05 mL) of a highly diluted drug (ug/mL or less) should be used (208).

The physician must always consider the possibility of an anaphylactic reaction. The differential diagnosis of anaphylaxis was provided in Table 16.5. The symptoms of an anaphylactic reaction are similar to those seen with many other situations that occur in the operating room or intensive care unit. The diagnosis should always be considered when hypotension with or without bronchospasm is temporally related to the parenteral administration of a drug. Although hypotension is relative to the patient's "normal" blood pressure, a good guideline is a systolic pressure less than 80 mm Hg, a mean blood pressure less than 60 mm Hg, or a decrease of at least 20% of the control (awake) value.

The pharmacology of drugs used to treat anaphylactic reactions will not be considered in this chapter. Specific agents and the rationale for their use are listed in Table 16–10. An algorithm for the management of an anaphylactic reaction is presented in Table 16–11. The initial therapy includes stopping the administration of the antigen and maintaining the airway while administering 100% oxygen. This prevents further recruitment of mast cells and basophils into the reaction process. The administration of 100% oxygen minimizes the mismatching of ventilation and perfusion that occurs from bronchospasm, pulmonary vasoconstriction, and pulmonary capillary leakage. If the trachea is not intubated, it may be necessary to do so. If there is significant laryngeal edema with distorted anatomical landmarks, a surgical airway may be necessary.

In the case of anaphylactic reactions, all anesthetic agents should be discontinued. These drugs promote hypotension. Although the inhalational anesthetics are bronchodilators, they are not the agents of choice in this situation.

Table 16–10. Drugs Used in the Treatment of Anaphylaxis

Catecholamines	Indication(s)
Epinephrine	Initial treatment
Isoproterenol	Refractory bronchospasm
Norepinephrine	Refractory hypotension
Phosphodiesterase Inhibitors	
Aminophylline	Bronchospasm
Amrinone	Pulmonary hypertension
Milrinone	Right ventricular dysfunction
Antihistamines	
Diphenhydramine	General therapy in all forms of anaphylaxis, inhibit histamine release
Cimetidine	
Ranitidine	
Corticosteroids	
Hydrocortisone	Bronchospasm
Methylprednisolone	Attenuated late-phase reactions

Table 16–11.   Treatment of Anaphylactic Reactions

Initial Therapy
1. Stop administration of suspected antigen.
2. Maintain the airway, administer 100% oxygen (consider endotracheal intubation if not already done).
3. Stop administration of anesthetics.
4. Intravascular volume expansion—consider 2 to 4 L of crystalloid/colloid (25–50 mL/kg) if hypotension exists.
5. Administer epinephrine (5–10 ug i.v. if hypotension exists, titrate to desired blood pressure); if cardiovascular collapse occurred, consider 0.5 to 1 mg i.v., repeat doses may be required.

Secondary Therapy
1. Catecholamine Infusion(s):
   Epinephrine 4–8 ug/min (0.05–0.1 ug/kg/min)
   Norepinephrine 4–8 ug/min (0.05–0.1 ug/kg/min)
   Isoproterenol 0.05–1 ug/min
   (Higher doses of epinephrine, norepinephrine, or Isoproterenol may be required)
2. Antihistamines:
   Diphenhydramine 0.5–1.0 mg/kg
3. Corticosteroids:
   Hydrocortisone 0.25–1.0 gm or methylprednisolone 25 mg/kg
4. Bicarbonate 0.5–1.0 mEq/kg
   If hypotension persists or acidosis is present
5. Reevaluate the airway before extubation

From Levy JH. Anaphylactic reactions in anesthesia and intensive care. 2nd ed. Boston: Butterworth-Heinemann, 1992.

The final initial therapies are rapid volume expansion and administration of epinephrine. The administration of volume expanders is necessary to provide replacement to the intravascular space. As much as 20 to 37% of the intravascular volume may be redistributed during anaphylactic or anaphylactoid reactions. Military antishock trousers (MAST suit) have also been helpful in treating the hypotension associated with anaphylaxis (209).

The administration of epinephrine is the mainstay of therapy. The α1-adrenergic effects make it a useful treatment for hypotension, whereas the β1 effects provide inotropic support. Furthermore, the β2 effects promote bronchodilation and inhibition of mediator release from mast cells and basophils (209).

The secondary treatment consists of anti-histamines. Although histamine is one of a number of mediators, it may account for many of the early manifestations. Diphenhydramine (1 mg/kg) is an effective H1 blocker. Norepinephrine may be used to treat persistent hypotension as adequate volume replacement is achieved. Isoproterenol, a pure β agonist, is useful in the treatment of bronchospasm and increased pulmonary vascular resistance. However, this may be at the expense of an increase in heart rate and possibly hypotension due to vasodilation. Corticosteroids are used in the treatment of severe reactions, although there is no evidence to suggest an appropriate dose or preparation. Generally, 1 gm of hydrocortisone or an equivalent is appropriate. Steroids are useful in preventing potential late-phase reactions. After the initial dose of hydrocortisone (5 to 10 mg/kg, up to 1 gm), the dose should be decreased to 2.5 mg/kg and repeated every 6 hours. Bicarbonate is used to treat acidosis if it should occur. Arterial blood gases should be followed to determine therapy (209).

ATTEMPTING TO PREVENT AN ANAPHYLACTIC OR ANAPHYLACTOID REACTION

When patients have a history that suggests that they are at a higher risk for developing an allergic reaction, it may be desirable to pretreat them in an attempt to decrease the clinical significance of a reaction if it occurs. Greenberger (160) has pretreated adult patients with a history of allergic reactions to radiographic contrast media. His protocol includes diphenhydramine 50 mg orally or intramuscularly 1 hour before the procedure and prednisone 50 mg 13 hours, 7 hours, and 1 hour before the antigen challenge. In addition, ephedrine, 25 mg orally, may be used if not contraindicated by angina, arrhythmias, or other conditions. This pretreatment regimen does not completely prevent allergic reactions. However, it seems to decrease the severity of reactions (160, 208).

SUMMARY

Allergic reactions can occur in response to any injected or intravenously administered substance, including drugs, solutions, volume expanders, and blood products. In critical care situations, the clinician must always consider an allergic reaction if hypotension, bronchospasm, or cardiovascular collapse occurs, especially if it is temporally related to the administration of any foreign substance. Anaphylactic or type I reactions, mediated by IgE, may be serious or life threatening if unrecognized or treated inappropriately. Anaphylactoid reactions, which may resemble anaphylactic reactions but are not IgE mediated, may manifest in a similar fashion and should be treated accordingly.

Patients who are young, who have a specific history of allergic reactions, asthma, or atopy, or who are pregnant may be predisposed to adverse reactions. Prevention is important and may include avoiding exposure to specific drugs or substances and making appropriate substitutions when possible. In addition, a further investigation of the allergy may be warranted. This investigation may include skin testing, leukocyte or basophil degranulation tests, or radioallergosorbent testing (RAST). In situations in which it is not possible to avoid use of a known allergen, prophylactic treatment with histamine antagonists and corticosteroids may help decrease the severity of the allergic reaction.

REFERENCES

1. DeSwarte RD. Drug allergy: an overview. Clin Rev Allergy 1986;4:143–169.
2. Patterson R, Anderson J. Allergic reactions to drugs and biologic agents. JAMA 1982;248:2637–2645.
3. Watkins J. "Hypersensitivity response" to drugs and plasma substitutes used in anaesthesia and surgery. In: Watkins J, Salo M, eds. Trauma, stress and immunology in anesthesia and surgery. London: Butterworth & Co. Ltd., 1982;254–291.
4. Stoelting RK. Allergic reactions during anesthesia. Anesth Analg 1983;62:341–356.
5. Van Arsdel PP. Diagnosing drug allergy. JAMA 1982;247:2576–2581.
6. Altman LC. Basic immune mechanisms in immediate hypersensitivity. Med Clin North Am 1981;65:941–957.
7. Watkins J. Anaphylactoid reactions to IV substances. Br J Anaesth 1979;51:51–60.
8. Hanashiro PK, Weil MH. Anaphylactic shock in man: report of two cases with detailed hemodynamic and metabolic studies. Arch Intern Med 1967;119:129–140.
9. Levy JH, Roizen MF, Morris JM. Anaphylactic and anaphylactoid reactions: a review. Spine 1986;11(3):282–291.
10. Delange C, Mullick FG, Irey NS. Myocardial lesions in anaphylaxis: a histochemical study. Arch Pathol Lab Med 1973;95:185–189.
11. Assem KSK. Anaphylactic reactions affecting the human heart. Agents Actions 1989;27:142–145.
12. Sullivan TJ. Cardiac disorders in penicillin-induced anaphylaxis. JAMA 1982;248:2161–2162.
13. Levy JH. Intravenous epinephrine therapy in anaphylaxis. JAMA 1983;249:3173.
14. Booth BH, Patterson R. Electrocardiographic changes during human anaphylaxis. JAMA 1970;211:627–631.
15. Lakin JD, Strecker RA. The immune response and classification of hypersensitivity reactions. In: Patterson R, ed. Allergic diseases: diagnosis and management. 3rd ed. Philadelphia: JB Lippincott Co., 1985;1–51.
16. Kesarwala HH, Fischer TJ. Introduction to the immune system. In: Lawlor GL, Fischer TJ, eds. Manual of allergy and immunology: diagnosis and therapy. 2nd ed. Boston: Little, Brown and Co., 1988;1–14.
17. Levy JH. Anaphylactic reactions in anesthesia and intensive care. 2nd ed. Boston: Butterworth-Heinemann, 1992;3–11.
18. Saxon A. Immediate hypersensitivity: approach to diagnosis. In: Lawlor GL, Fischer TJ, eds. Manual of allergy and immunology: diagnosis and therapy. 2nd ed. Boston: Little, Brown and Co., 1988;15–35.
19. Austen KF. Tissue mast cells in immediate hypersensitivity. Hosp Pract 1982;17:98–108.
20. Metcalfe DD. Effector cell heterogeneity in immediate hypersensitivity reactions. Clin Rev Allergy 1983;1:311–325.
21. Schleimer RP, MacGlashan DW Jr, Schulman ES, et al. Human mast cells and basophils — structure, function, pharmacology, and biochemistry. Clin Rev Allergy 1983;1:327–341.
22. Schleimer RP, MacGlashan DW Jr, Peters SP, et al. Inflammatory mediators and mechanisms of release from purified human basophils and mast cells. J Allergy Clin Immunol 1984;74:473–481.
23. Rydzynski K, Kolago B, Zaslonka J, et al. Distribution of mast cells in human heart auricles and correlation with tissue histamine. Agents Actions 1988;23:273–275.
24. Wasserman SI, Goetzl EJ, Austen KF. Preformed eosinophil chemotactic factor of anaphylaxis (ECF-A). J Immunol 1974;112:351–358.
25. Wasserman SI. Mediators of immediate hypersensitivity. J Allergy Clin Immunol 1983;72:101–115.
26. Feldberg W, Kellaway CH. Liberation of histamine and formation of lysocithin-like substances by cobra venom. J Physiol 1938;94:187–226.

27. Brocklehurst WE. The release of histamine and formation of a slow-reacting substance (SRS-A) during anaphylactic shock. J Physiol 1960;151:416–435.
28. Samuelsson B, Hammarström S, Murphy RC, et al. Leukotrienes and slow reacting substance of anaphylaxis (SRS-A). Allergy 1980;35:375–381.
29. Weiss JW, Drazen JM, Coles N, et al. Bronchoconstrictor effects of leukotriene C in humans. Science 1982;216:196–198.
30. Weiss JW, Drazen JM, McFadden ER Jr, et al. Airway constriction in normal humans produced by inhalation of leukotriene D: potency, time course, effect of aspirin therapy. JAMA 1983;249:2814–2817.
31. Drazen JM, Austen KF, Lewis RA, et al. Comparative airway and vascular activities of leukotrienes C-1 and D in vivo and in vitro. Proc Natl Acad Sci U S A 1980;77:4354–4358.
32. Smith LJ, Patterson R, Greenberger P, et al. Airway response to inhaled leukotriene D4 in man. Clin Res 1983;31:747A.
33. Kuehl FA Jr, Egan RW. Prostaglandins, arachidonic acid and inflammation. Science 1980;210:978–984.
34. Colman RW. Surface-mediated defense reactions: the plasma contact activation system. J Clin Invest 1984;73:1249–1253.
35. Eyre P, Lewis AJ. Production of kinins in bovine anaphylactic shock. Br J Pharmacol 1972;44:311–313.
36. Meier HL, Kaplan AP, Lichtenstein LM, et al. Anaphylactic release of a prekallikrein activator from human lung in vitro. J Clin Invest 1983;72:574–581.
37. Erdös EG. Kininases. In: Erdös EG, ed. Handbook of experimental pharmacology. Heidelberg: Springer-Verlag, 1979;25S:428–487.
38. Pitt BR. Metabolic functions of the lung and systemic vasoregulation. Fed Proc 1984;43:2574–2577.
39. Tan F, Jackman H, Skidgel RA, et al. Protamine inhibits plasma carboxypeptidase N, the inactivator of anaphylactoxins and kinins. Anesthesiology 1989;70:267–275.
40. Orfan N, Patterson R, Dykewicz MS. Severe angioedema related to ACE inhibitors in patients with a history of idiopathic angioedema. JAMA 1990;264:1287–1289.
41. Metcalfe DD, Lewis RA, Silbert JE, et al. Isolation and characterization of heparin from human lung. J Clin Invest 1979;64:1537–1543.
42. Metcalfe DD, Bland CE, Wasserman SI. Biochemical and functional characterization of proteoglycans isolated from basophils of patients with chronic myelogenous leukemia. J Immunol 1984;132:1943–1950.
43. Schwartz LB. Enzyme mediators of mast cells and basophils. Clin Rev Allergy 1983;1:397–416.
44. Schwartz LB. Tryptase, a mediator of human mast cells. J Allergy Clin Immunol 1990;86:594–598.
45. Schwartz LB, Yunginger JW, Miller J, et al. Time course of appearance and disappearance of human mast cell tryptase in the circulation after anaphylaxis. J Clin Invest 1989;83:1551–1555.
46. Watkins J, Thornton JA. Immunological and non-immunological mechanisms involved in adverse reactions to drugs. Klin Wochenschr 1982;60:958–964.
47. Fisher MM, Roffe DJ. Allergy, atopy and IgE: the predictive value of total IgE and allergic history in anaphylactic reactions during anaesthesia. Anaesthesia 1984;39:213–217.
48. Frank MM. Complement: a brief review. J Allergy Clin Immunol 1989;84:411–420.
49. Glovsky MM, Hugli TE, Ishizaka T, et al. Anaphylatoxin induced histamine release with human leukocytes: studies of C3a leukocyte binding and histamine release. J Clin Invest 1979;64:804–811.
50. Grant JA, Dupree E, Goldman AS, et al. Complement-mediated release of histamine from human leukocytes. J Immunol 1975;114:1101–1106.
51. Grant JA, Settle L, Whorton EB, et al. Complement-mediated release of histamine from human basophils. J Immunol 1976;117:450–456.
52. Hammerschmidt DE, Weaver LJ, Hudson LD, et al. Association of complement activation and elevated plasma C5a with adult respiratory distress syndrome. Lancet 1980;1:947–949.
53. Latson TW, Kickler TS, Baumgartner WA. Pulmonary hypertension and noncardiogenic pulmonary edema following cardiopulmonary bypass associated with an antigranulocyte antibody. Anesthesiology 1986;64:106–111.
54. Morel DR, Zapol WM, Thomas SJ, et al. C5a and thromboxane generation associated with pulmonary vaso- and bronchoconstriction during protamine reversal of heparin. Anesthesiology 1987;66:597–604.
55. Alexopoulos D, Raine AEG, Cobbe SM. Serum sickness complicating intravenous streptokinase therapy in acute myocardial infarction. Eur Heart J 1984;5:1010–1012.
56. Rosenblatt HM, Lawlor GJ. Anaphylaxis. In: Lawlor GL, Fischer TJ, eds. Manual of allergy and immunology: diagnosis and therapy. 2nd ed. Boston: Little, Brown and Co., 1988;225–232.
57. Levy JH. Anaphylactic reactions in anesthesia and intensive care. 2nd ed. Boston: Butterworth-Heinemann, 1992;51–62.
58. Fearon DT, Ruddy S, Schur PH, et al. Activation of the properdin pathway of complement in patients with gram-negative bacteremia. N Engl J Med 1975;292:937–940.
59. Lasser EC, Lang JH, Lyon SG, et al. Changes in complement and coagulation factors in a patient suffering a severe anaphylactoid reaction to injected contrast material: some considerations of pathogenesis. Invest Radiol 1980;15:S6–S12.
60. Lasser EC, Lang JH, Hamblin AE, et al. Activation systems in contrast idiosyncrasy. Invest Radiol 1980;15:S2–S5.
61. Watkins J, Clark A, Appleyard TN, et al. Immune-mediated reactions to althesin (alphaxalone). Br J Anaesth 1976;48:881–886.
62. Craddock PR, Fehr J, Brigham KL, et al. Complement and leukocyte-mediated pulmonary dysfunction in hemodialysis. N Engl J Med 1977;296:769–774.

63. Rosow CE, Moss J, Philbin DM, et al. Histamine release during morphine and fentanyl anesthesia. Anesthesiology 1982;56:93–96.

64. Hirshman CA, Edelstein RA, Ebertz JM, et al. Thiobarbiturate-induced histamine release in human skin mast cells. Anesthesiology 1985;63:353–356.

65. Moss J, Rosow CE, Savarese JJ, et al. Role of histamine in the hypotensive action of d-tubocurarine in humans. Anesthesiology 1981;55:19–25.

66. Hermens JM, Ebertz JM, Hanifin JM, et al. Comparison of histamine release in human skin mast cells induced by morphine, fentanyl, and oxymorphone. Anesthesiology 1985;62:124–129.

67. Parker CW. Drug allergy. N Engl J Med 1975;292:511–514 (Part I), 732–736 (Part II), 957–960 (Part III).

68. Poppers PJ. Anaesthetic implications of hereditary angioneurotic oedema. Can J Anaesth 1987;34:76–78.

69. Bochner BS, Lichtenstein LM. Anaphylaxis. N Engl J Med 1991;324:1785–1790.

70. Kelly JF, Patterson R. Anaphylaxis: course, mechanisms and treatment. JAMA 1974;227:1431–1436.

71. Levy JH. Anaphylactic reactions in anesthesia and intensive care. 2nd ed. Boston: Butterworth-Heinemann, 1992;135–141.

72. Sheffer AL. Continuing medical education: anaphylaxis. J Allergy Clin Immunol 1985;75:227–233.

73. Moscicki RA, Sockin SM, Corsello BF, et al. Anaphylaxis during induction of general anesthesia: subsequent evaluation and management. J Allergy Clin Immunol 1990;86:325–332.

74. Levy JH. Anaphylactic/anaphylactoid reactions during cardiac surgery. J Clin Anesth 1989;1:426–430.

75. Sage D. Intradermal drug testing following anaphylactoid reactions during anaesthesia. Anaesth Intensive Care 1981;9:381–385.

76. Levy JH, Kettlekamp N, Goertz P, et al. Histamine release by vancomycin: a mechanism for hypotension in man. Anesthesiology 1987;67:122–125.

77. Laxenaire M-C, Moneret-Vautrin DA, Watkins J. Diagnosis of the causes of anaphylactoid anaesthetic reactions. Anaesthesia 1983;38:147–148.

78. Laxenaire M-C, Moneret-Vautrin D-A, Vervloet D. The French experience of anaphylactoid reactions. Int Anesthesiol Clin 1985;23:145–160.

79. Fisher MM. Reaginic antibodies to drugs used in anesthesia. Anesthesiology 1980;52:318–320.

80. Vervloet D, Nizankowska E, Arnaud A, et al. Adverse reactions to suxamethonium and other muscle relaxants under general anesthesia. J Allergy Clin Immunol 1983;71:552–559.

81. Hirshman CA, Peters J, Cartwright-Lee I. Leukocyte histamine release to thiopental. Anesthesiology 1982;56:64–67.

82. Vervloet D, Arnaud A, Senft M, et al. Anaphylactic reactions to suxamethonium prevention of mediator release by choline. J Allergy Clin Immunol 1985;76:222–225.

83. Vervloet D, Arnaud A, Senft M, et al. Leukocyte histamine release to suxamethonium in patients with adverse reactions to muscle relaxants. J Allergy Clin Immunol 1985;75:338–342.

84. Withington DE, Leung KBP, Bromley L, et al. Basophil histamine release: a study in allergy to suxamethonium. Anaesthesia 1987;42:850–854.

85. Pienkowski MM, Kazmier WJ, Adkinson NF Jr. Basophil histamine release remains unaffected by clinical desensitization to penicillin. J Allergy Clin Immunol 1988;82:171–178.

86. Faraj BA, Gottlieb GR, Camp VM, et al. Development of a sensitive radioassay of histamine for in vitro allergy testing. J Nucl Med 1984;25:56–63.

87. Johansson SGO. In vitro diagnosis of reagin-mediated allergic diseases. Allergy 1978;33:292–298.

88. Santrach PJ, Parker JL, Jones RT, et al. Diagnostic and therapeutic applications of a modified radioallergosorbent test and comparison with the conventional radioallergosorbent test. J Allergy Clin Immunol 1981;67:97–105.

89. Roitt IM, Brostoff J, Male DK, eds. Immunology. St. Louis: CV Mosby, 1989.

90. Adkinson NF Jr. Tests for immunological drug reactions. In: Rose NR, Friedman H, Fahey JL, eds. Manual of clinical laboratory immunology. 3rd ed. Baltimore: American Society for Microbiology, 1986;692–697.

91. Fisher MM. Intradermal testing in the diagnosis of acute anaphylaxis during anesthesia — results of five years experience. Anaesth Intensive Care 1979;7:58–61.

92. Fisher M. Intradermal testing after anaphylactoid reaction to anaesthetic drugs: practical aspects of performance and interpretation. Anaesth Intensive Care 1984;12:115–120.

93. Selcow JE, Mendelson LM, Rosen JP. Anaphylactic reactions in skin test-negative patients. J Allergy Clin Immunol 1980;65:400.

94. Clarke RSJ. Adverse effects of intravenously administered drugs used in anaesthetic practice. Drugs 1981;22:26–42.

95. Beamish D, Brown DT. Adverse responses to I.V. anaesthetics. Br J Anaesth 1981;53:55–57.

96. Harle DG, Baldo BA, Smal MA, et al. Drugs as allergens: the molecular basis of IgE binding to thiopentone. Int Arch Allergy Immunol 1987;84:277–283.

97. Harle DG, Baldo BA, Smal MA, et al. Detection of thiopentone-reactive IgE antibodies following anaphylactoid reactions during anaesthesia. Clin Allergy 1986;16:493–498.

98. Etter MS, Helrich M, Mackenzie CF. Immunoglobulin E fluctuation in thiopental anaphylaxis. Anesthesiology 1980;52:181–183.

99. Watkins J. Etomidate: an "immunologically safe" anaesthetic agent. Anaesthesia 1983;38:34–38.

100. Fazackerley EJ, Martin AJ, Tolhurst-Cleaver CL, et al. Anaphylactoid reaction following the use of etomidate. Anaesthesia 1988;43:953–954.

101. Sold M, Rothhammer A. Life-threatening anaphylactoid reaction following etomidate. Anaesthetist 1985;34:208–210.

102. Briggs LP, Clarke RSJ, Watkins J. An adverse reaction to the administration of disoprofol (Diprivan). Anaesthesia 1982;37:1099–1101.

103. Laxenaire MC, Gueant JL, Bermejo E, et al.

Anaphylactic shock due to propofol. Lancet 1988;2:739–740.

104. Clarke RSJ, Dundee JW, Garrett RT, et al. Adverse reactions to intravenous anaesthetics: a survey of 100 reports. Br J Anaesth 1975;47:575–585.

105. Dye D, Watkins J. Suspected anaphylactic reaction to Cremophor EL. Br Med J 1980;280:1353.

106. Laxenaire M-C, Mata-Bermejo E, Moneret-Vautrin DA, et al. Life-threatening anaphylactoid reactions to propofol (Diprivan). Anesthesiology 1992;77:275–280.

107. Mathieu A, Goudsouzian N, Snider MT. Reaction to ketamine: anaphylactoid or anaphylactic? Br J Anaesth 1975;47:624–627.

108. Lagasse RS. Miscellaneous intravenous anesthetic agents. In: Katz RI, Vitkun SA, Eide TR, eds. Pharmacology of therapeutic agents used in anesthesia. Levittown, PA: Pharmaceutical Information Associates, Ltd., 1994;69–77.

109. Ghosh JS. Allergy to diazepam and other benzodiazepines. Br Med J 1977;1:902–903.

110. Padfield A, Watkins J. Allergy to diazepam. Br Med J 1977;1:575–576.

111. Blatchley D. Allergy to diazepam. Br Med J 1977;1:287.

112. Levy JH, Rockoff MA. Anaphylaxis to meperidine. Anesth Analg 1982;61:301–303.

113. Philbin DM, Moss J, Akins CW, et al. The use of H1 and H2 histamine antagonists with morphine anesthesia: a double-blind study. Anesthesiology 1981;55:292–296.

114. Hermens JM, Ebertz JM, Hanifin JM, et al. Comparison of histamine release in human skin mast cells induced by morphine, fentanyl, and oxymorphone. Anesthesiology 1985;62:124–129.

115. Levy JH, Brister NW, Shearin A, et al. Wheal and flare responses to opioids in humans. Anesthesiology 1989;70:756–760.

116. Bennett MJ, Anderson LK, McMillan JC, et al. Anaphylactic reaction during anaesthesia associated with positive intradermal skin test to fentanyl. Can Anaesth Soc J 1986;33:75–78.

117. Zucker-Pinchoff B, Ramanathan S. Anaphylactic reaction to epidural fentanyl. Anesthesiology 1989;71:599–601.

118. Rosow CE, Philbin DM, Keegan CR, et al. Hemodynamics and histamine release during induction with sufentanil or fentanyl. Anesthesiology 1984;60:489–491.

119. Harle DG, Baldo BA, Fisher MM. Detection of IgE antibodies to suxamethonium after anaphylactoid reactions during anaesthesia. Lancet 1984;1:930–932.

120. Cohen S, Liu KH, Marx GF. Upper airway edema — an anaphylactoid reaction to succinylcholine. Anesthesiology 1982;56:467–468.

121. Assem ESK, Ling YB. Fatal anaphylactic reaction to suxamethonium: new screening test suggests possible prevention. Anaesthesia 1988;43:958–961.

122. Ravindran RS, Klemm JE. Anaphylaxis to succinylcholine in a patient allergic to penicillin. Anesth Analg 1980;59:944–945.

123. Assem ESK, Frost PG, Levis RD. Anaphylactic-like reaction to suxamethonium. Anaesthesia 1981;36:405–410.

124. Royston D, Wilkes RG. True anaphylaxis to suxamethonium chloride. Br J Anaesth 1978;50:611–615.

125. Mandappa JM, Chandrasekhara PM, Nelvigi RG. Anaphylaxis to suxamethonium. Br J Anaesth 1975;47:523–524.

126. Cunningham Farmer B, Sivarajan M. An anaphylactoid response to a small dose of d-tubocurarine. Anesthesiology 1979;51:358–359.

127. Baldwin AC, Churcher MD. Anaphylactoid response to intravenous tubocurarine. Anaesthesia 1979;34:339–340.

128. Harle DG, Baldo BA, Fisher MM. Cross-reactivity of metocurine, atracurium, vecuronium and fazadinium with IgE antibodies from patients unexposed to these drugs but allergic to other myoneural blocking drugs. Br J Anaesth 1985;57:1073–1076.

129. Barnes PK, deRenzy-Martin N, Thomas VJE, et al. Plasma histamine levels following atracurium. Anaesthesia 1986;41:821–824.

130. Booij LHDJ, Krieg N, Crul JF. Intradermal histamine releasing effect caused by Org-NC 45: a comparison with pancuronium, metocurine and d-tubocurarine. Acta Anaesth Scand 1980;24:393–394.

131. Harle DG, Baldo BA, Fisher MM. Assays for, and cross-reactivities of, IgE antibodies to the muscle relaxants gallamine, decamethonium and succinylcholine (Suxamethonium). J Immunol Methods 1985;78:293–305.

132. Gallo JA, Cork RC, Puchi P. Comparison of effects of atracurium and vecuronium in cardiac surgical patients. Anesth Analg 1988;67:161–165.

133. Didier A, Cador D, Bongrand P, et al. Role of the quaternary ammonium ion determinants in allergy to muscle relaxants. J Allergy Clin Immunol 1987;79:578–584.

134. Youngman PR, Taylor KM, Wilson JD. Anaphylactoid reactions to neuromuscular blocking agents: a commonly undiagnosed condition? Lancet 1983;2:597–599.

135. Levy JH. Anaphylactic reactions in anesthesia and intensive care. 2nd ed. Boston: Butterworth-Heinemann, 1992;83–120.

136. Fisher MM, Munro I. Life-threatening anaphylactoid reactions to muscle relaxants. Anesth Analg 1983;62:559–564.

137. Brown DT, Beamish D, Wildsmith JAW. Allergic reaction to an amide local anaesthetic. Br J Anaesth 1981;53:435–437.

138. Aldrete JA, Johnson DA. Allergy to local anesthetics. JAMA 1969;207:356–357.

139. Simon RA. Adverse reactions to drug additives. J Allergy Clin Immunol 1984;74:623–630.

140. Aguilera L, Martinez-Bourio R, Cid C, et al. Anaphylactic reaction after atropine. Anaesthesia 1988;43:955–957.

141. Cullen DJ. Severe anaphylactic reaction to penicillin during halothane anaesthesia. Br J Anaesth 1971;43:410–412.

142. Miller R, Tausk HC. Anaphylactoid reaction to vancomycin during anesthesia: a case report. Anesth Analg 1977;56:870–872.

143. Velazquez JL, Gold MI. Anaphylactic reaction to cephalothin during anesthesia. Anesthesiology 1975;43:476–478.

144. Sogn DD. Prevention of allergic reactions to penicillin. J Allergy Clin Immunol 1986;78:1051–1052.

145. Sogn DD. Penicillin allergy. J Allergy Clin Immunol 1984;74:589–593.

146. Galpin JE, Chow AW, Yoshikawa TT, et al. "Pseudoanaphylactic" reactions from inadvertent infusion of procaine penicillin G. Ann Intern Med 1974;81:358–359.

147. Levine BB. Immunochemical mechanisms involved in penicillin hypersensitivity in experimental animals and in human beings. Fed Proc 1965;24:45–50.

148. Blanca M, Fernandez J, Miranda A, et al. Cross-reactivity between penicillins and cephalosporins: clinical and immunologic studies. J Allergy Clin Immunol 1989;83:381–385.

149. Abraham GN, Petz LD, Fudenberg HH. Cephalothin hypersensitivity associated with anti-cephalothin antibodies. Int Arch Allergy Immunol 1968;34:65–74.

150. Abraham GN, Petz LD, Fudenberg HH. Immunohaematological cross-allergenicity between penicillin and cephalothin in humans. Clin Exp Immunol 1968;3:343–357.

151. Petz LD. Immunologic cross-reactivity between penicillins and cephalosporins: a review. J Infect Dis 1978;137:S74–S79.

152. Saxon A, Beall GN, Rohr AS, et al. Immediate hypersensitivity reactions to beta-lactam antibiotics. Ann Intern Med 1987;107:204–215.

153. Adkinson NF Jr, Swabb EA, Sugerman AA. Immunology of the monobactam aztreonam. Antimicrob Agents Chemother 1984;25:93–97.

154. Sullivan TJ. Allergic reactions to antimicrobial agents: a review of reactions to drugs not in the beta lactam antibiotic class. J Allergy Clin Immunol 1984;74:594–599.

155. Newfield P, Roizen MF. Hazards of rapid administration of vancomycin. Ann Intern Med 1979;91:581.

156. Miller R, Tausk HC. Anaphylactoid reaction to vancomycin during anesthesia: a case report. Anesth Analg 1977;56:870–872.

157. Estafanous FG, Loop FD. Cardiac reoperations. In: Kaplan JA, ed. Cardiac anesthesia. 3rd ed. Philadelphia: WB Saunders Co., 1993;865–876.

158. Levy AH. Unusual reaction to Trasylol. Can Med Assoc J 1974;111:1304.

159. Dietrich W, Hahnel C, Richter JA. Routine application of high-dose aprotinin in open-heart surgery: a study on 1,784 patients. Anesthesiology 1990;73:A146.

160. Greenberger PA. Contrast media reactions. J Allergy Clin Immunol 1984;74:600–605.

161. Patterson R, DeSwarte RD, Greenberger PA, et al. Drug allergy and protocols for management of drug allergies. N Engl Reg Allergy Proc 1986;4:325–342.

162. Findlay SR, Dvorak AM, Kagey-Sobotka A, et al. Hyperosmolar triggering of histamine release from human basophils. J Clin Invest 1981;67:1604–1613.

163. Goldberg M. Systemic reactions to intravascular contrast media. Anesthesiology 1984;60:46–56.

164. Szczeklik A. Adverse reaction to aspirin and nonsteroidal anti-inflammatory drugs. Ann Allergy 1987;59:113–118.

165. Stevenson DD. Diagnosis, prevention, and treatment of adverse reactions to aspirin and nonsteroidal anti-inflammatory drugs. J Allergy Clin Immunol 1984;74:617–622.

166. Hansbrough JR, Wedner HJ, Chaplin DD. Anaphylaxis to intravenous furosemide. J Allergy Clin Immunol 1987;80:538–541.

167. Sullivan TJ. Cross-reactions among furosemide, hydrochlorothiazide, and sulfonamides. JAMA 1991;265:120–121.

168. Roizen MF, Rodgers GM, Valone FH, et al. Anaphylactoid reactions to vascular graft material presenting with vasodilation and subsequent disseminated intravascular coagulation. Anesthesiology 1989;71:331–338.

169. Bruno LA, Smith DS, Bloom MJ, et al. Sudden hypotension with a test dose of chymopapain. Anesth Analg 1984;63:533–535.

170. Ring J, Messmer K. Incidence and severity of anaphylactoid reactions to colloid volume substitutes. Lancet 1977;1:466–469.

171. Ring J, Stephan W, Brendel W. Anaphylactoid reactions to infusions of plasma protein and human serum albumin. Clin Allergy 1979;9:89–97.

172. Furhoff A-K. Anaphylactoid reaction to Dextran — a report of 133 cases. Acta Anaesth Scand 1977;21:161–167.

173. Ring J, Seifert J, Messmer K, et al. Anaphylactoid reactions due to hydroxyethyl starch infusion. Eur Surg Res 1976;8:389–399.

174. Freedman MD, Schocket AL, Chapel N, et al. Anaphylaxis after intravenous methylprednisolone administration. JAMA 1981;245:607–608.

175. Peller JS, Bardana EJ Jr. Anaphylactoid reaction to corticosteroid: case report and review of the literature. Ann Allergy 1985;54:302–305.

176. Cobb CA III, Fung DL. Shock due to protamine hypersensitivity. Surg Neurol 1982;17:245–246.

177. Vontz FK, Puestow EC, Cahill DJ. Anaphylactic shock following protamine administration. Am Surg 1982;48:549–551.

178. Chung F, Miles J. Cardiac arrest following protamine administration. Can Anaesth Soc J 1984;31:314–318.

179. Conahan TJ, Andrews RW, MacVaugh H. Cardiovascular effects of protamine sulfate in man. Anesth Analg 1981;60:33–36.

180. Horrow JC. Protamine: a review of its toxicity. Anesth Analg 1985;64:348–361.

181. Stewart WJ, McSweeney SM, Kellett MA, et al. Increased risk of severe protamine reactions in NPH insulin-dependent diabetics undergoing cardiac catheterization. Circulation 1984;70:788–792.

182. Caplan SN, Berkman EM. Protamine sulfate and fish allergy. N Engl J Med 1976;295:172.

183. Knape JTA, Schuller JL, deHaan P, et al. An ana-

phylactic reaction to protamine in a patient allergic to fish. Anesthesiology 1981;55:324–325.

184. Samuel T. Antibodies reacting with salmon and human protamines in sera from infertile men and from vasectomized men and monkeys. Clin Exp Immunol 1977;30:181–187.

185. Samuel T, Kolk AHJ, Rumke P. She immunogenicity of protamines in humans and experimental animals by means of a micro-complement fixation test. Clin Exp Immunol 1978;33:252–260.

186. Watson RA, Ansbacher R, Barry M, et al. Allergic reaction to protamine: a late complication of elective vasectomy? Urology 1983;22:493–495.

187. Sauder RA, Hirshman CA. Protamine-induced histamine release in human skin mast cells. Anesthesiology 1990;73:165–167.

188. Holzman RS. Latex allergy: an emerging operating room problem. Anesth Analg 1993;76:635–641.

189. Sussman GL, Beezhold DH. Allergy to latex rubber. Ann Intern Med 1995;122:43–46.

190. Kelly KJ, Pearson ML, Kurup VP, et al. A cluster of anaphylactic reactions in children with spina bifida during general anesthesia: epidemiologic features, risk factors, and latex hypersensitivity. J Allergy Clin Immunol 1994;94:53–61.

191. Moneret-Vautrin DA, Laxenaire MC, Bavoux F. Allergic shock to latex and ethylene oxide during surgery for spina bifida. Anesthesiology 1990;73:556–558.

192. Leynadier F, Pecquet C, Dry J. Anaphylaxis to latex during surgery. Anaesthesia 1989;44:547–550.

193. Orfan NA, Reed R, Dykewicz MS, et al. Occupational asthma in a latex doll manufacturing plant. J Allergy Clin Immunol 1994;94:826–830.

194. Raloff J. Latex allergies from right out of thin air? Science News 1995;147:244.

195. Kurup VP, Kelly T, Elms N, et al. Cross-reactivity of food allergens in latex allergy. Allergy Proc 1994;15:211–216.

196. Slater JE. Rubber anaphylaxis. N Engl J Med 1989;320:1126–1130.

197. Axelsson JGK, Johansson SGO, Wrangsjo K. IgE-mediated anaphylactoid reactions to rubber. Allergy 1987;42:46–50.

198. Spaner D, Dolovich J, Tarlo S, et al. Hypersensitivity to natural latex. J Allergy Clin Immunol 1989;83:1135–1137.

199. Alenius H, Makinen-Kiljunen S, Turjanmaa K, et al. Allergen and protein content of latex gloves. Ann Allergy 1994;73:315–320.

200. Gold M, Swartz JS, Braude BM, et al. Intraoperative anaphylaxis: an association with latex sensitivity. J Allergy Clin Immunol 1991;87:662–666.

201. Sussman GL, Tarlo S, Dolovich J. The spectrum of IgE-mediated responses to latex. JAMA 1991;265:2844–2847.

202. Gerber AC, Jorg W, Zbinden S, et al. Severe intraoperative anaphylaxis to surgical gloves: latex allergy, an unfamiliar condition. Anesthesiology 1989;71:800–802.

203. Alenius H, Turjanmaa K, Makinen-Kiljunen S, et al. IgE immune response to rubber proteins in adult patients with latex allergy. J Allergy Clin Immunol 1994;93:859–863.

204. McCormack DR, Heisser AI, Smith LJ. Intraoperative vecuronium anaphylaxis compounded by latex hypersensitivity. Ann Allergy 1994;73:405–408.

205. Gessner JS. Noninfectious complications of blood transfusions. In: Barash PG, ed. ASA refresher courses in anesthesiology. Philadelphia: JB Lippincott Co., 1993;125–133.

206. Barton JC. Nonhemolytic, noninfectious transfusion reactions. Semin Hematol 1981;18:95–121.

207. Levy JH. Allergic reactions and the intraoperative use of foreign substances. In: Barash PG, ed. ASA refresher courses in anesthesiology. Philadelphia: JB Lippincott Co., 1985;129–141.

208. Levy JH. Anaphylactic reactions in anesthesia and intensive care. 2nd ed. Boston: Butterworth-Heinemann, 1992;121–134.

209. Levy JH. Anaphylactic reactions in anesthesia and intensive care. 2nd ed. Boston: Butterworth-Heinemann, 1992;161–174.

17

METABOLIC AND ENDOCRINE DISORDERS

Stephen F. Dierdorf

Progress in cardiorespiratory monitoring and the development of new anesthetics during the past 20 years have resulted in a marked reduction in intraoperative morbidity and mortality. In fact, it is now more likely that a critical patient event will occur in the recovery room than in the operating room (1, 2). The primary reason for the shift of significant risk from the operating room to the recovery room is physiologic control. During surgery, the anesthesiologist maintains a high degree of control of the patient's cardiorespiratory systems. However, during the early postanesthesia recovery phase, patients begin to reassume control of vital organ systems. Some patients may not, for example, be able to maintain adequate ventilation and as a result develop postoperative respiratory complications. Despite the success that anesthesiologists have developed with improved intraoperative cardiorespiratory outcome, progress in the intraoperative control of metabolic disorders has been much slower (Table 17–1). Monitoring of metabolic diseases requires frequent intraoperative measurements of metabolic parameters to evaluate the effects of surgery, anesthesia, and any changes in therapy. In the past, problems caused by the time required to measure metabolic parameters prevented rapid return of results, thereby delaying intervention. Fortunately, technological improvements in laboratory equipment have provided anesthesiologists an enhanced capability for rapid measurement of metabolic parameters (Table 17–2).

Satellite laboratories in the operating room and intensive care units provide ready access to appropriate measurements. In the future, considerably more information must be acquired so efficient management of perioperative patients with metabolic disorders can be achieved. The immediate postanesthesia recovery period provides the opportunity to initiate or complete therapy for metabolic aberrations that occur in the perioperative period.

ACID-BASE DISTURBANCES

Disturbances in acid-base regulation are of considerable importance because pH changes can adversely affect a large variety of physiologic functions. The body possesses many

Table 17–1. Metabolic and Endocrine Diseases

Acid-Base Disorders:
Respiratory acidosis	Respiratory alkalosis
Metabolic acidosis	Metabolic alkalosis

Electrolyte Abnormalities:
Hypernatremia	Hyponatremia
Hyperkalemia	Hypokalemia
Hypercalcemia	Hypocalcemia
Hypermagnesemia	Hypomagnesemia

Endocrine Disorders:
Diabetes mellitus	Pheochromocytoma
Hyperthyroidism	Hypothyroidism
Hyperparathyroidism	Hypoparathyroidism
Hyperadrenocortism	Hypoadrenocorticism
Suppression of the pituitary-adrenal axis	

Table 17–2.   Normal Blood Electrolyte, Metabolic, and Endocrine Parameter Values

Normal Blood Electrolyte and Metabolic Values:

Sodium	135–145 mEq/L	135–134 mmol/L
Potassium	3.5–5.0 mEq/L	3.5–5.0 mmol/L
Chloride	98–106 mEq/L	98–106 mmol/L
Bicarbonate	18–23 mEq/L	18–23 mmol/L
Calcium (ionized)	4.0–4.6 mg/dL	1.0–1.5 mmol/L
Calcium (total)	9.0–10.5 mg/dL	2.2–2.6 mmol/L
Lactate	5–20 mg/dL	0.5–2.2 mmol/L

Normal Values of Endocrine Parameters:

Thyroid	
Thyrotropin (TSH)	0.6–4.6 uU/mL
Thyroxine (T4)	4–11 µg/dL
Triiodothyronine (T3)	75–220 ng/dL
Triiodothyronine resin uptake (RT3U)	25–35%
Parathyroid	
Parathormone	10–65 pg/mL
Calcitonin	<50 pg/mL
Adrenal	
Cortisol	
8 AM	8–24 µg/dL
4 PM	2–15 µg/dL
Corticotropin (ACTH)	20–100 pg/mL

compensatory mechanisms to maintain the pH level within a very narrow normal range. For example, hypoventilation with a significant rise in $PaCO_2$ may occur as compensation for a metabolic alkaline challenge, or profound hyperventilation can occur as compensation for an increase in metabolic acid load. In contrast, many of the physiologic effects of hypercapnia are produced by changes in pH. Carbon dioxide narcosis is produced not by the effects of an elevated carbon dioxide tension but by the acidosis and decrease in pH that is produced by hypercapnia (3).

The Henderson-Hasselbalch equation defines the basis of pH in the human (Table 17–3). The normal arterial pH is between 7.35 and 7.45, with a 20:1 ratio of the bicarbonate concentration to the carbon dioxide concentration.

Measurement of the pHa and $PaCO_2$ and plasma bicarbonate allows classification of acid-base changes as respiratory or metabolic.

Table 17–3.   Henderson-Hasselbalch Equation

$$pHa = pK + \log \frac{HCO_3}{0.03 \times PaCO_2}$$

pHa	=	negative logarithm of the arterial concentration of hydrogen ions
pH	=	6.1 at 37°C
HCO_3	=	concentration of bicarbonate, mEq · L^{-1}
$PaCO_2$	=	mm Hg

Substitution of average values for pHa (7.4) and $PaCO_2$ (40 mm Hg) results is a calculated HCO_3 concentration of 24 mEq · L^{-1}. Maintenance of a normal HCO_3 concentration relative to the concentration of carbon dioxide results in an optimal ratio of about 20:1 (24 mEq · L^{-1} divided by 1.2). This optimal ratio of 20:1 permits maintenance of a relatively normal pHa despite deviations from normal in the HCO_3 concentration.
With permission from Stoelting RK, Dierdorf SF. Anesthesia and co-existing disease. 3rd ed. New York: Churchill Livingstone, 1993.

Determination of the type of acidosis or alkalosis is extremely important because the treatments are quite different. Changes in alveolar ventilation that produce alterations in acid-base status are categorized as respiratory acidosis or alkalosis. Acid-base changes related to metabolic disturbances are described as metabolic acidosis or alkalosis. Compensatory changes to acid-base alterations are produced primarily by changes in ventilation or renal function.

Respiratory Acidosis

Alveolar hypoventilation resulting in an increase in $PaCO_2$ large enough to decrease the pHa to less than 7.35 produces respiratory acidosis. At a comparable decrease in pH, respiratory acidosis is a more potent myocardial depressant than metabolic acidosis (4). Treatment of respiratory acidosis is an increase in alveolar ventilation. Respiratory acidosis results in renal compensation within 6 to 12 hours that consists of an increase in renal secretion of hydrogen ion and an increase in plasma bicarbonate concentration. Rapid ventilatory correction of a compensated respiratory acidosis can produce metabolic alkalosis and excitation of the central nervous system (e.g., seizures). Consequently, correction of chronic respiratory acidosis (with metabolic compensation) should be performed slowly.

Respiratory Alkalosis

An increase in alveolar ventilation that decreases the $PaCO_2$ to a level resulting in a pHa greater than 7.45 is termed respiratory alkalosis. Renal compensation for respiratory alkalosis consists of decreased reabsorption of bicarbonate with a resultant loss of urinary bicarbonate and a decrease in plasma bicarbonate.

Metabolic Acidosis

The most common cause of metabolic acidosis is an accumulation of lactic acid from inadequate tissue oxygenation and anaerobic metabolism (Table 17–4). Anaerobic conditions are essential for acidosis to occur from lactate accumulation. Lactate provides an important link between aerobic and anaerobic metabolism. During aerobic conditions, increased lactate production does not produce acidosis. However, during anaerobic conditions, excess hydrogen ion cannot be reused and acidosis results (5). Lactic acidosis is defined as an arterial lactate concentration greater than 5 mmol/L and an arterial pH less than 7.25. Critically ill patients exhibiting these parameters have a high mortality rate (6). Renal failure produces metabolic acidosis by producing an accumulation of nonvolatile acids. The normal production of endogenous nonvolatile acids is 1 mEq/kg/24 hours. In the presence of renal failure, this acid load is sufficient to decrease plasma bicarbonate 1 to 2 mEq per day. Metabolic acidosis is a potent respiratory stimulant and alveolar hyperventilation is the primary means of compensation. Although the administration of sodium bicarbonate will increase pHa, the most effective treatment is correction of the underlying cause. The administration of $NaHCO_3$ for the treatment of metabolic acidosis is highly controversial. Although the administration of in-

Table 17–4. Types of Lactic Acidosis

Type A: Secondary to inadequate oxygen delivery
   1. Tissue hypoperfusion
      a. Decreased cardiac output
      b. Hypovolemia
   2. Reduced arterial oxygen content
      a. Hypoxemia
      b. Carbon monoxide poisoning
      c. Severe anemia
Type B: Not secondary to tissue hypoxia
   1. Pathologic conditions
      a. Diabetes mellitus
      b. Renal failure
      c. Hepatic failure
   2. Drug or toxin induced
      a. Biguanides (phenformin)
      b. Ethanol
      c. Methanol
      d. Ethylene glycol

travenous sodium bicarbonate increases extracellular pH, $NaHCO_3$ also increases carbon dioxide production (1 mEg/kg of intravenous bicarbonate produces 180 mL of carbon dioxide). In addition to an increase in CO_2 production, other hazards of the administration of large doses of $NaHCO_3$ include hypernatremia, increased lactate production, and exacerbation of postresuscitation or postoperative metabolic alkalosis. There is also evidence that although $NaHCO_3$ alkalinizes the plasma, it may not correct and may even exacerbate intracellular acidosis (7). Consequently, for patients with progressive metabolic acidosis when correction of the primary defect is not possible, other alkalinizing agents such as carbicarb (mixture of sodium carbonate and bicarbonate), THAM (tris hydroxymethyl amino methane, tromethamine), or dichloroacetate should be considered. Carbicarb is an equimolar solution of sodium carbonate and bicarbonate that alkalinizes blood but does not generate carbon dioxide. Animal studies of metabolic acidosis indicate that the administration of carbicarb increases arterial and intracellular pH without the potentially adverse effects produced by the administration of sodium bicarbonate (8, 9). Dichloroacetate (40 mg/kg intravenously over 60 minutes) increases pyruvate dehydrogenase activity, which accelerates the conversion of lactate to pyruvate. Dichloroacetate decreases lactate levels and increases intracellular pH. Administration of dichloroacetate has been shown to be very effective for correction of lactic acidosis occurring during liver transplantation (10). THAM (1 mg/kg) is an effective alkalinizing agent that does not contain sodium and does not generate carbon dioxide. However, THAM requires dilution in large volumes of fluid and is extremely irritating to tissues if extravasation of the solution occurs. THAM can cross the blood-brain barrier and produce cerebrospinal fluid (CSF) alkalosis, leading to apnea. Despite many years of research, THAM has not been widely recommended for routine treatment of metabolic acidosis (11, 12). Further research may establish carbicarb as a primary drug for the treatment of acidosis. Dichloroacetate and THAM may be useful for special clinical situations; however, it is unlikely that either of these drugs will be first-line drugs for the treatment of metabolic acidosis. For the present, the most effective treatment of metabolic acidosis secondary to hypoxemia or hypoperfusion is correction of the underlying cause. If urgent treatment of the acidosis is required (pH < 7.2), the judicious administration of sodium bicarbonate with frequent measurement of arterial pH is indicated until oxygenation and/or perfusion improves (13–15).

Metabolic Alkalosis

Metabolic alkalosis is caused by the loss of nonvolatile acids, most frequently by prolonged emesis or nasogastric drainage or by prolonged administration of diuretics, which leads to hypokalemia and urinary loss of hydrogen ions. The most effective treatment of metabolic alkalosis is correction of the underlying cause and the administration of potassium chloride. In rare instances, the infusion of ammonium chloride or 0.1 N hydrochloric acid is required for correction of the alkalosis. The respiratory compensation for metabolic alkalosis is alveolar hypoventilation that produces an increase in carbon dioxide tension and hydrogen ion concentration.

Acid-Base Alterations in the Recovery Room

Acid-base problems that develop intraoperatively may require ultimate correction during the immediate postoperative period. An accurate diagnosis of the precise acid-base status can be achieved by measuring pHa, $PaCO_2$, and bicarbonate concentration (Figs. 17–1, 17–2, and 17–3). The accurate diagnosis and appropriate treatment will prevent potentially dangerous interventions. For example, rapid institution of hyperventilation of a patient with hypercarbia (but a normal or compensated pH) will produce severe alkalosis. If the

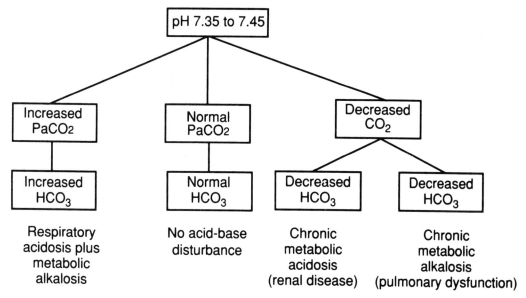

Fig. 17–1. Diagnostic approach to the interpretation of a normal arterial pH based on $PaCO_2$ and HCO_3 (bicarbonate) concentration. (With permission from Stoelting RK, Dierdorf SF. Anesthesia and co-existing disease. 3rd ed. New York: Churchill Livingstone, 1993.)

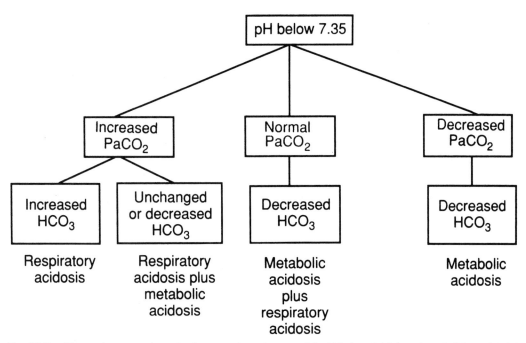

Fig. 17–2. Diagnostic approach to the interpretation of an arterial pH below 7.35 based on $PaCO_2$ and HCO_3 (bicarbonate) concentration. (With permission from Stoelting RK, Dierdorf SF. Anesthesia and co-existing disease. 3rd ed. New York: Churchill Livingstone, 1993.)

Fig. 17–3. Diagnostic approach to the interpretation of an arterial pH above 7.45 based on $PaCO_2$ and HCO_3 (bicarbonate) concentration. (With permission from Stoelting RK, Dierdorf SF. Anesthesia and co-existing disease. 3rd ed. New York: Churchill Livingstone, 1993.)

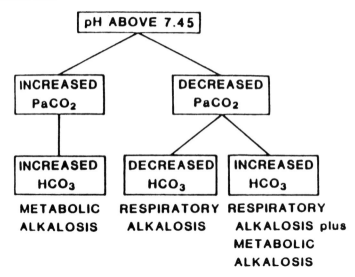

underlying cause is not readily apparent and the decrease in pH is believed to be deleterious, treatment of the alteration in acid-base status can be initiated.

The most common acid-base aberrations apparent during the immediate postoperative period are respiratory acidosis and metabolic acidosis. Acidosis interferes with a number of important physiologic functions. Acidosis depresses myocardial contractility, precipitates cardiac dysrhythmias, produces peripheral vasodilation, and decreases myocardial responses to catecholamines. Throughout the body, acidosis interferes with enzymatic functions and produces adverse effects on a number of vital organ functions. Pure respiratory acidosis (increased $PaCO_2$ and decreased pH) is caused by hypoventilation, for which there are myriad causes. Treatment of respiratory acidosis is increased alveolar ventilation, either with positive-pressure ventilation or correction of the cause (e.g., reversal of opioid-induced respiratory depression).

Metabolic acidosis in the immediate postoperative period is usually secondary to inadequate tissue perfusion. Inadequate tissue perfusion may be secondary to low cardiac output, hypovolemia, vasoconstriction, hypoxemia, or increased metabolism (e.g., malignant hyperthermia). Metabolic causes of

acidosis include renal failure, diabetic ketoacidosis, hepatic failure, cyanide toxicity, carbon monoxide poisoning, and rarely, primary lactic acidosis. Because of the severe effects of metabolic acidosis, treatment may have to be initiated before the diagnosis of the underlying cause. In some instances, the change in pH after administration of bicarbonate may be used as an indicator of the success of treatment. For example, if metabolic acidosis is a result of hypovolemia, as intravascular volume is restored, the need for exogenously administered bicarbonate diminishes. Metabolic acidosis secondary to low cardiac output and/or hypovolemia portends serious consequences in the immediate postoperative period. Aggressive therapy directed at correction of the cause and increasing cardiac output, intravascular volume, and perfusion pressure is mandated. Despite the controversy concerning the administration of $NaHCO_3$ for the treatment of metabolic acidosis, treatment of severe metabolic acidosis may be required before detection of the underlying cause and includes hyperventilation and administration of $NaHCO_3$ (16).

Less common causes of postoperative metabolic acidosis are drug related (e.g., biguanide oral hypoglycemics) or enzyme deficiencies (e.g., pyruvate dehydrogenase, pyruvate decarboxylase, lactic dehydrogenase) (17).

Respiratory alkalosis in the postanesthesia period is generally secondary to iatrogenic hyperventilation. Because most sedatives and anesthetics attenuate the ventilatory responses to hypoxemia, hypoxemia is rarely a cause of respiratory alkalosis in patients recovering from anesthesia.

Metabolic alkalosis, if it exists in the early recovery period, usually existed in the preoperative period. The most common perioperative causes of metabolic alkalosis, prolonged nasogastric suction and potassium loss secondary to diuretic therapy, rarely develop during surgery. Metabolic alkalosis, however, is relatively common in critically ill patients (18). The type of metabolic alkalosis is usually hypochloremic alkalosis. Hypochloremic alkalosis occurs when there is an imbalance in sodium and chloride ion concentrations with loss of chloride. Hypochloremic alkalosis is enhanced by loss of extracellular fluid. In the critically ill patient, chronic diuretic therapy will produce an excessive loss of chloride and contract the extracellular fluid compartment, thereby producing hypochloremic alkalosis. The presence of hypochloremic alkalosis can interfere with the process of weaning from mechanical ventilation, because the primary compensation for this type of alkalosis is hypoventilation. The primary therapy for hypochloremic alkalosis is the administration of normal saline and potassium chloride.

ELECTROLYTE ABNORMALITIES

Abnormalities in electrolyte levels are of special importance in the perioperative period because the surgical patient may have an impaired ability to regulate his or her own electrolyte intake and excretion. Perioperative changes (e.g., water absorption during transurethral resection of the prostate) may also contribute to electrolyte imbalances. Although isolated aberrations in electrolyte balance occur in the perioperative period, many patients with pathologic processes have mixed patterns of imbalance that produce multiple abnormalities.

Hyponatremia

Although hyponatremia may be secondary to a sodium deficit, hyponatremia in the surgical patient is almost always caused by an excess of free water administration and is, therefore, dilutional hyponatremia. Common causes of hyponatremia in the perioperative period include inappropriate secretion of antidiuretic hormone, intravascular absorption of large quantities of water (e.g., during TURP), and intravenous administration of solutions of free water (19). Acute reductions in the plasma sodium concentration can produce lethargy, cerebral edema, seizures, and coma.

Inappropriate secretion of antidiuretic hormone (SIADH) produces hyponatremia, an elevated urinary sodium concentration, and decreased plasma osmolarity (<280 mOsm/L). The treatment of inappropriate secretion of antidiuretic hormone (ADH) is restriction of water intake. For patients with hyponatremia secondary to inappropriate secretion of ADH, but without neurologic symptoms, fluid restriction is effective. However, if neurologic symptoms are present, the infusion of hypertonic saline (3%) is effective. However, correction of hyponatremia, especially chronic hyponatremia, should be cautious because rapid correction may result in fatal central pontine myelinolysis (20, 21). SIADH is responsible for the hyponatremia that occurs in 75% of patients with acquired immunodeficiency syndrome (AIDS) (22).

The TURP syndrome is caused by the intravascular absorption of nonelectrolyte bladder-irrigating solutions during transurethral resection of the prostate (23). The primary effects of this free water absorption are on the central nervous system and the cardiovascular system. Neurologic symptoms begin to appear when the serum sodium level decreases to 120 mEq/L; however, electroencephalogram (EEG) changes appear at higher levels of serum sodium (24). Visual disturbances that occur are most likely secondary to the absorption of glycine, which has an inhibitory effect on retinal function. Cardiovascular changes secondary to water absorption include hypervolemia, bradycardia, hypertension, angina, and congestive heart failure.

Treatment of the TURP syndrome depends on the severity of the signs and symptoms. Diuresis from the administration of furosemide (0.05 to 0.1 mg/kg) is effective for mild to moderate hyponatremia (120 to 125 mEq/L). More severe cases of hyponatremia (<120 mEq/L) may require treatment with diuretics and hypertonic saline. Recommended infusion volumes of hypertonic saline for treatment of severe hyponatremia are in the range of 100 mL of 5% saline to 200 mL of 3% saline. The goal of hypertonic saline therapy should not be complete normalization of the serum sodium level, because aggressive therapy can produce permanent neurologic sequelae. After the initial treatment with hypertonic saline, normalization of sodium levels can be achieved over 48 hours with fluid restriction. Although TURP syndrome is most commonly associated with transurethral resection of the prostate, this syndrome has also been reported after transurethral resection of bladder tumors (25).

Hypernatremia

Postoperative hypernatremia is rare and generally secondary to a body water deficit rather than a sodium excess. Causes of water deficit include diabetes insipidus or renal tubular resistance to ADH. Elderly patients may also develop dehydration because of diminished fluid intake. Laboratory abnormalities include hypernatremia, an increased blood urea nitrogen (BUN), and a urine osmolarity greater than 800 mOsm/L. Treatment is with the infusion of 5% dextrose in water. However, correction of the serum sodium level must be gradual to avoid the development of cerebral edema.

Hyperkalemia

Because most of the body's potassium is intracellular, plasma potassium levels may not be an accurate reflection of total body potassium. Consequently, hyperkalemia may be indicative of an increase in total body potassium or an alteration in the intracellular and extracellular distribution of potassium. The most common cause of an increase in total body potassium is renal failure, in which the kidneys are simply unable to excrete potassium. Hypoaldosteronism, either pathologic or drug-induced, may also produce an increase in total body potassium and hyperkalemia (26). Drugs that antagonize the effects of aldosterone, such as spironolactone and triamterene, can produce hyperkalemia. There are a considerable number of drugs and pathologic conditions that alter the distribution of potassium between the intracellullar and extracellular compartments. For example, succinylcholine can release intracellular potassium into the extracellular space and produce extreme hyperkalemia in susceptible patients. Acidosis, either respiratory or metabolic, can promote movement of potassium from the cells into the extracellular fluid space. Acute tumor lysis from chemotherapy (e.g., leukemia, lymphoma) can produce life-threatening hyperkalemia, hyperuricemia, hyperphosphatemia, and hypocalcemia (27).

Acute changes in the distribution of intracellular and extracellular potassium are more likely to cause cardiac dysrhythmias than chronic hypokalemia or chronic hyperkalemia. Electrocardiogram (ECG) changes produced by hyperkalemia include lengthening of the P-R interval, widening of the QRS complex, and peaking of the T wave (Fig. 17–4). These changes may progress to ventricular tachycardia and ventricular fibrillation.

Urgent treatment of hyperkalemia is required if there is ECG evidence of hyperkalemia or the plasma potassium concentration exceeds 6.5 mEq/L. Administration of intravenous calcium produces immediate antagonism of hyperkalemic effects on the heart and

EFFECTS OF HYPERKALEMIA

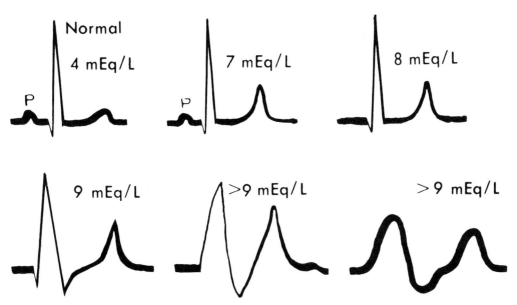

Fig. 17–4. ECG changes characteristic of progressive hyperkalemia. (With permission from Goldberger AL, Goldberger E. Clinical electrocardiography. 4th ed. St. Louis: Mosby Year Book, 1990.)

is especially effective therapy if the hyperkalemia is secondary to a transient release of intracellular potassium into the extracellular fluid compartment. It seems that calcium inhibits the effect of potassium within the myocardial cell (28). Administration of glucose and insulin promotes intracellular uptake of potassium and is effective within 15 to 30 minutes. As alkalosis shifts potassium into the cell, the administration of intravenous bicarbonate and/or hyperventilation are effective for reducing plasma potassium levels. Patients with hyperkalemia secondary to an increase in total body potassium stores usually require treatment directed at increasing potassium excretion, such as the administration of kayexelate, peritoneal dialysis, or hemodialysis.

Hypokalemia

Much like hyperkalemia, hypokalemia can be secondary to a decrease in total body potassium stores or an altered distribution of potassium between intracellular and extracellular compartments. Preoperative chronic hypokalemia is relatively common in surgical patients but rarely produces significant clinical effects in the perioperative period (29). In the perioperative period, acute hypokalemia is usually secondary to an intracellular shift of potassium. Causes of acute hypokalemia include alkalosis (respiratory or metabolic), administration of glucose and insulin, familial periodic paralysis, administration of $\beta 2$-adrenergic agonists, hypercalcemia, and hypomagnesemia. Hyperventilation during the intraoperative or immediate postoperative periods is a frequent cause of acute hypokalemia. Plasma potassium decreases 0.5 mEq/L for each 10 mm Hg reduction in $PaCO_2$. Administration of insulin to correct hyperglycemia in the perioperative period can result in hypokalemia. In fact, a decreasing plasma potassium level during insulin therapy may also reflect the onset of hypoglycemia. $\beta 2$-adrenergic agonists (epinephrine, salbutamol) are known to promote intracellular movement of potassium, which can cause hypokalemia (30). Administration of intravenous and inhaled salbutamol has been recommended for the treatment of hyperkalemia (31). Other drugs, such as theophylline, have also been reported to cause hypokalemia (32).

Depletion of total body potassium stores is generally secondary to potassium loss through the kidneys or gastrointestinal tract. Vomiting, prolonged gastric drainage, and diarrhea can result in hypokalemia. Renal potassium losses can be produced by diuretics, hyperglycemia, and increased secretion of aldosterone or cortisol. Chronic hypokalemia from administration of diuretics generally does not produce significant perioperative complications. However, patients receiving digitalis preparations who are hypokalemic may exhibit signs of increased digitalis effect if further hypokalemia develops in the perioperative period (e.g., hypokalemia secondary to respiratory alkalosis from hyperventilation).

The clinical effects of hypokalemia include skeletal muscle weakness, intestinal ileus, and cardiac conduction and contractility abnormalities. One of the earliest ECG changes that appear with hypokalemia is the appearance of a U wave. Later effects include a prolonged P-R interval, ST segment depression, and T wave inversion, ultimately leading to ventricular fibrillation (Fig. 17–5).

Treatment of hypokalemia depends on the severity of the clinical effects and the underlying cause. For example, acute hypokalemia secondary to hyperventilation can be corrected by normalizing mechanical ventilation. Because plasma potassium levels are not a good indicator of body potassium levels, correction of hypokalemia with the administration of intravenous potassium chloride may be difficult to estimate. However, small quantities of potassium may be effective for the treatment of cardiac conduction abnormalities. Administration of 0.5 to 1.0 mEq of intravenous potassium chloride every 3 to 5 minutes can be performed until the ECG normalizes. Frequent measurements of plasma potassium should be performed to avoid hyperkalemia.

Hypercalcemia

Causes of hypercalcemia include sarcoidosis, hyperparathyroidism, malignancy, vitamin D intoxication, and prolonged immobility. Malignancy produces hypercalcemia by two mechanisms: osteolysis and secretion of a parathormone-like substance by the tumor. Humorally mediated hypercalcemia is the more common mechanism of malignant hypercalcemia (33). A plasma calcium concentration greater than 5.5 mEq/L is considered abnormally high. Signs and symptoms of hypercalcemia include lethargy, vomiting, and polyuria. ECG signs of hypercalcemia include a prolonged P-R interval, widened QRS complex, and a shortened Q-T interval (Fig. 17–6). The primary treatment of hypercalcemia is hydration with normal saline and diuresis with furosemide to promote calcium excretion. Administration of plicamycin (25 ug/kg intravenously) over 4 to 6 hours will lower calcium levels within 12 hours in patients with hypercalcemia secondary to myeloproliferative disorders.

Hypocalcemia

Calcium is highly protein bound and is transported in the plasma in a protein-bound form and as an ionized fraction. The ionized fraction is physiologically active. It is relatively common that critically ill patients will have a decrease in total plasma calcium but have normal levels of ionized calcium. Normal levels of total calcium are 4.5 to 5.5 mEq/L and normal levels of ionized calcium are 1.0 to 1.25 mM/L. Causes of hypocalcemia include hypoparathyroidism, acute pancreatitis, hypomagnesemia, vitamin D deficiency, and renal failure. Signs and symptoms of hypocalcemia are generally reflected in the central nervous system, heart, and neuromuscular junction.

Acute decreases in ionized calcium levels may produce hypotension and decreased myocardial contractility. Rapid administration of whole blood or fresh frozen plasma can cause a decrease in ionized calcium secondary to

HYPOKALEMIA

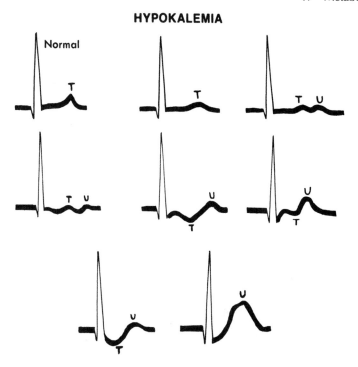

Fig. 17–5. Different ECG patterns that occur with hypokalemia. Patterns do not correlate well with specific serum potassium levels. (With permission from Goldberger AL, Goldberger E. Clinical electrocardiography. 4th ed. St. Louis: Mosby Year Book, 1990.)

complexing of calcium by citrate. The Q-T interval may be prolonged, but this is not a consistent sign of hypocalcemia (Fig. 17.6). The clinical significance of the effects of mild postoperative hypocalcemia is controversial. Mild hypocalcemia, ionized calcium 0.8 to 1.0 mM, usually does not impair cardiac function and probably does not require therapy. Severe hypocalcemia, less than 0.75 mM, is associated with depressed cardiac function and requires therapy with supplemental calcium. Treatment of hypocalcemia can be performed with 5 mL of 10% calcium chloride (1.36 mEq/mL) or 10 mL of 10% calcium gluconate (0.45 mEq/mL). After the initial administration of calcium, ionized calcium levels will increase for 1 to 2 hours. Consequently, calcium levels must be measured to ensure that calcium levels do not decrease (34).

Hypocalcemia decreases the presynaptic release of acetylcholine and can impair neuromuscular function. The effects of hypocalcemia and neuromuscular blocking drugs may be additive or synergistic and produce postoperative muscle weakness. In this clinical situation, response to peripheral nerve stimulation may be unpredictable. Ventilatory support should be provided until there is sufficient clinical evidence to indicate that spontaneous ventilation will be satisfactory.

Hypermagnesemia

Common causes of hypermagnesemia (plasma magnesium > 2.5 mEq/L) include exogenous administration of magnesium sulfate, excessive use of antacids, and chronic renal failure. Patients with a glomerular filtration rate (GFR) less than 30 mL/minute are very likely to develop hypermagnesemia when exogenous magnesium is administered. Hypermagnesemia progressing to coma reflects central nervous system depression. Cardiac depression and skeletal muscle weakness may be severe, as death from hypermagnesemia is usually caused by cardiac or respiratory arrest. Acute dysfunction produced by hypermagnesemia can be temporarily alleviated by the ad-

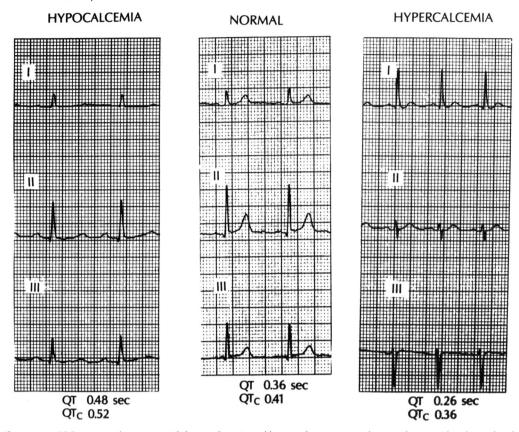

Fig. 17-6. ECG patterns that occur with hypocalcemia and hypercalcemia. Note the correlation with calcium levels and the QT interval. (With permission from Goldberger AL, Goldberger E. Clinical electrocardiography. 4th ed. St. Louis: Mosby Year Book, 1990.)

ministration of calcium. Definitive therapy for hypermagnesemia requires diuresis and, in some cases, hemodialysis. Hypermagnesemia potentiates the effects of both nondepolarizing and depolarizing muscle relaxants (35). Consequently, patients with hypermagnesemia could have persistent muscle weakness with hypoventilation during the postoperative period.

Hypomagnesemia

Only in recent years has the clinical importance of hypomagnesemia (<1.5 mEq/L) been realized. Hypomagnesemia can be secondary to renal loss, gastrointestinal loss, or endocrine disorders. A number of drugs, such as carbenicillin, gentamicin, cisplatin, cyclosporine, and loop diuretics, can produce renal loss of magnesium. Gastrointestinal (GI) abnormalities that produce malabsorption can result in hypomagnesemia. Endocrine disorders such as hyperthyroidism, hyperaldosteronism, diabetes mellitus, and diabetic ketoacidosis are associated with hypomagnesemia (36). Hypomagnesemia frequently exists with other electrolyte abnormalities, especially hypocalcemia and hypokalemia. Aggressive phosphate therapy for patients with renal failure has been reported to cause hypomagnesemia and hypocalcemia leading to vocal cord dysfunction and respiratory distress (37). Manifestations of hypomagnesemia include hyperreflexia, seizures, coma, skeletal muscle spasm, and cardiac irritability, especially digitalis-induced dysrhythmias. Dysrhythmias associated with hypomagnesemia include atrial and ventricular ectopy, ventricular tachycardia, torsade de pointes, and ventricular fibrillation. Torsade de pointes is a unique type of ventricular tachycardia that may be resistant to conventional antidysrhythmic therapy. Torsade de pointes is caused by factors that decrease the Q-T interval (hypokalemia, hypomagnesemia) and may be effectively treated with a single bolus dose of magnesium sulfate (2 grams intravenously) (38). The treatment of hypomagnesemia is with intravenous magnesium sulfate 1 gram administered over 15 minutes.

ENDOCRINE DISORDERS

The endocrine system is a closely coordinated system consisting of the hypothalamus, the pituitary gland, and target organs (e.g., thyroid gland, adrenal gland). These systems are negative feedback systems in which the increased secretion of hormones by the target organ suppresses secretion of hormones by the hypothalamus and pituitary. Hormone deficiencies may be primary (target gland failure) or secondary (lack of stimulation of the target gland). Consequently, the accurate diagnosis of endocrine gland failure must include assays of both stimulating hormones and target organ hormones (39).

The endocrine system controls many aspects of metabolism and physiology. Because the endocrine system is responsive to physiologic changes, it is logical to assume that alterations in endocrine function will occur during surgery and critical illness. There is evidence that changes in measured endocrine parameters may be very good prognosticators of outcome (40–42). Changes in thyroid and adrenal function are especially significant during critical illness. Most hospital laboratories can now measure thyroid and adrenal hormone levels in 24 to 48 hours. Measurement of such endocrine parameters will increase in the immediate future and will undoubtedly become an integral part of the evaluation of the critically ill patient during the perioperative period.

Diabetes Mellitus

There are 5.5 million patients with diabetes mellitus in the United States (2.4% of the population) and another 7 million persons with glucose intolerance. Because diabetic patients are more likely to require surgery, diabetics constitute an inordinate proportion of the total number of surgical patients. The most controversial aspect of the perioperative management of patients with diabetes mellitus is the rigidity or "tightness" of control of blood glucose levels.

ETIOLOGY AND CLASSIFICATION

Patients with diabetes mellitus can be classified into two groups: insulin-dependent diabetes mellitus (IDDM) and noninsulin-dependent diabetes mellitus (NIDDM). There is a clear genetic susceptibility to IDDM that results in an autoimmune destruction of the beta cells of the pancreas. The initial immune response may be directed against a non-β cell that is infected with a virus, which contains an amino acid sequence identical to an amino acid sequence in the β cell. Alternately, a virus may infect the β cells and expose β cells to direct attack by antiviral cytotoxic lymphocytes (43).

The etiology and pathogenesis of NIDDM is much less clear. NIDDM develops later in life (after 35 years of age) and is characterized by a gradual decline in β cell function and increased resistance of skeletal muscle and hepatic cells to the effects of insulin.

PHYSIOLOGY OF INSULIN

Humans have a continual need for energy but consume food intermittently. Consequently, in humans, an elaborate system has evolved for periodically ingesting excess amounts of calories, storing excess substrate, and breaking down these stores as energy is required. Glucose and free fatty acids are the primary circulating energy sources in humans. Glucose is stored as glycogen in skeletal muscle and the liver; free fatty acids are stored as triglycerides in adipose tissue. Small amounts of triglycerides are also stored in muscle, liver, and as circulating lipoproteins. Triglycerides are a more efficient mechanism for energy storage than glycogen. Triglycerides contain 9.5 kCal of energy per gram, whereas glycogen contains only 4 kCal per gram.

The metabolic system is extremely complex and highly regulated. The principal hormone messenger of this system is insulin. Insulin functions in concert with counterregulatory hormones such as glucagon, catecholamines, growth hormone, and glucocorticoids to maintain normoglycemia. Consequently, an insulin deficiency affects the entire nutritional and energy management system. Insulin decreases plasma glucose levels by stimulating the uptake of glucose by muscle and adipose cells and by inhibiting glycogen breakdown and gluconeogenesis. Insulin also exerts considerable influence on the regulation of protein synthesis. In diabetics with poor control (insulin deficiency), protein storage decreases and protein is degraded to release amino acids. This reduction in protein content is not uniformly distributed among different organs. For example, in patients with diabetes mellitus, the protein content of the liver increases, whereas the protein content of skeletal and cardiac muscle decreases.

TREATMENT OF DIABETES MELLITUS

Treatment of diabetes mellitus is directed at increasing the absolute levels of insulin and/or decreasing resistance to the effects of insulin. For example, weight reduction in middle-aged NIDDM patients may reduce insulin resistance and eliminate the need for exogenous insulin or oral hypoglycemic drugs. Oral hypoglycemics, such as sulfonylureas, stimulate endogenous insulin release and are effective in most patients with NIDDM. Clearly, patients with IDDM require administration of exogenous insulin.

Several insulin preparations are available. Insulin is categorized by the onset and length of action: fast acting (regular and semilente); intermediate acting (NPH and lente); long acting (PZI and ultralente). Most insulin-dependent diabetics require a combination of rapid-acting and intermediate-acting insulin preparations. Other treatment regimens, such as continuous insulin infusion pumps or pancreatic transplantations, have theoretical advantages but practical limitations have hindered widespread application.

The development of accurate and easy-to-use glucometers allow patients to monitor their own glucose levels and determine, to a large extent, how tightly their glucose levels will be regulated.

COMPLICATIONS OF DIABETES MELLITUS

Complications of long-term diabetes mellitus include accelerated atherosclerosis, ischemic heart disease, nephropathy, retinopathy, and peripheral and autonomic neuropathy. Since the initial use of insulin to treat diabetes in the 1920s, there has been a great deal of controversy concerning the relationship between "tightness" of glucose control and long-term complications. Recent evidence supports the concept that tight glucose control reduces the severity of the long-term complications of diabetes (44). However, studies comparing rigid with conventional control of glucose also report a threefold to fourfold incidence of hypoglycemia from tight control. Consequently, the short-term risks of hypoglycemia must be balanced against the long-term risks of mild to moderate hyperglycemia. Autonomic neuropathy may manifest as hypotension, tachycardia, bradycardia, and delayed gastric emptying (45–47). The cardiovascular manifestations of autonomic neuropathy are extremely varied. Increases in blood pressure during induction of anesthesia and tracheal intubation may be a manifestation of increased sensitivity to endogenously released catecholamines or decreased catecholamine clearance secondary to diminished renal function (48).

Ketoacidosis

The most serious acute complication of diabetes mellitus is diabetic ketoacidosis (DKA). There are three contributing factors producing DKA: insulin deficiency, dehydration, and increased levels of counterregulatory hormones. Insulin deficiency and an increase in catabolic hormones promote lipolysis with the increased production of free fatty acids and ketogenesis. Levels of counterregulatory hormones such as glucagon, epinephrine, and cortisol increase markedly as insulin levels decrease. Glucagon inhibits hepatic lipogenesis, which leads to a series of metabolic changes that divert fatty acids from the citric acid cycle to the formation of ketoacids (49). Clinical features of DKA include nausea, vomiting, hypovolemia, abdominal pain, and leukocytosis. Treatment of DKA includes volume replacement, administration of regular insulin (0.2 units/kg intravenously followed by 0.1 unit/kg/hour intravenously), and potassium supplementation until blood glucose levels begin to decline (Table 17–5). Bicarbonate should not be routinely administered but can be administered if the arterial pH is less than 7.2. The mortality from DKA has decreased dramatically during the past several decades.

Hyperglycemic Hyperosmolar Nonketotic State

Hyperglycemic hyperosmolar nonketotic state (HHNS) is defined by extreme hyperglycemia (>600 mg/dL), increased serum osmolarity (>330 mOsm/L), and severe dehydration without acidosis. The patient with HHNS is typically older than 55 years and, in many cases, has a precipitating factor such as vomiting, pneumonia, uremia, or a viral infection. Therapy is with insulin and rehydration.

PERIOPERATIVE MANAGEMENT OF THE DIABETIC PATIENT

The goal of metabolic management during anesthesia is to mimic normal metabolism as closely as possible while avoiding hypoglycemia, hyperglycemia, ketoacidosis, and electrolyte abnormalities. The stresses and variables encountered during surgery may make these goals difficult to achieve. The immediate postoperative period provides an opportunity to provide necessary adjustments in glucose regulation and metabolic control.

Traditionally, the perioperative management of insulin-dependent diabetics has been to initiate a glucose infusion before surgery

Table 17–5. Therapy for Diabetic Ketoacidosis (DKA)

Intravenous Fluids[a]	500–1000 mL NS per hour × 4 hr
	250–500 mL ½ NS per hour × 4 hr
	D-5% or D-10% when serum glucose <250 mg/dL
Insulin[b]	10 U regular, intravenous push
	0.1 U regular, per kg, per hour, infusion
	Double each 1–2 hr if <10% drop in glucose or no improvement in the anion gap or pH
	Reduce with glucose <250 mg/dL, if progressive improvement in anion gap and pH
Potassium[c]	40 mEq over an hour if serum K+ <3 mEq/L
	30 mEq over an hour if serum K+ <4 mEq/L
	20 mEq over an hour if serum K+ <5 mEq/L

[a] Rate of infusion may require adjustment for cardiac or renal dysfunction.
[b] The rate of insulin infusion can be doubled each 1 or 2 hours in which there is no improvement in anion gap or pH. The rate of insulin infusion can be halved when glucose levels reach 250 mg/dL and can be further reduced each 2 hours in which there is steady improvement in anion gap and pH. Infusion rates as low as 0.5 U/hr can maintain antilipolysis.
[c] In the absence of ECG changes of hyperkalemia, potassium administration is begun as soon as satisfactory urine output is documented. This replacement schedule applies to the first several hours of treatment when fluid infusion rates of 500–1000 mL/hr are needed. Smaller doses of K should be used for lower infusion rates.
NS = normal saline; D-5% = dextrose 5%; D-10% = dextrose 10%.
With permission from Fleckman AM. Diabetic ketoacidosis. Endocrinol Metab Clin North Am 1993;22:181–208.

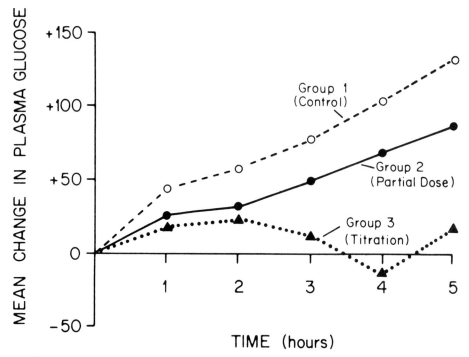

Fig. 17–7. Changes in the plasma glucose concentrations were determined during the intraoperative period in insulin-dependent adult diabetic patients. Group 1 patients received no preoperative insulin or glucose. Group 2 patients received one-fourth to one-half of their usual doses of insulin at 7:00 AM on the morning of surgery. In addition, glucose (6.25 grams/hour intravenously) was initiated at the time of insulin administration. Group 3 patients received no insulin or glucose preoperatively but were treated with regular insulin administered intravenously if the measured blood glucose concentration exceeded 200 mg/dL. (With permission from Walts LF, Miller J, Davidson MB, et al. Perioperative management of diabetes mellitus. Anesthesiology 1981;55:104–109.)

and administer subcutaneously one-half to two-thirds of the patient's morning insulin dose. The goal of this regimen was to provide insulin but avoid hypoglycemia; moderate hyperglycemia was generally acceptable. Although specific and definitive outcome studies are not available, most diabetologists agree that this approach is no longer acceptable and that tighter control of blood glucose levels is required (Fig. 17–7). The degree or "tightness" of control is, however, extremely controversial. A reasonable goal would be to maintain the glucose level between 80 and 200 mg/dL.

This approach avoids the side effects of hyperglycemia (osmotic diuresis, impaired wound healing, electrolyte disturbances) but minimizes the risk of hypoglycemia. The cornerstone to any insulin and glucose regimen, however, is the intraoperative measurement of glucose levels. Intravenous administration of insulin (intermittent or continuous infusion) can be used to maintain glucose within the desired range (50, 51) (Table 17–6).

POSTOPERATIVE MANAGEMENT

Postoperative management of the diabetic patient is an extension of intraoperative management. However, the goal of postoperative management of the patient undergoing elective surgery should be to return the patient to his or her preoperative state. Measurement of glucose levels in the recovery room can be used to manage insulin administration during the early postoperative period. The goal for

Table 17–6.   Intermittent Intravenous Insulin Injection

Intermittent Intravenous Injection During the Perioperative Period:[a]
1. Begin an infusion of glucose (5–10 g · h^{-1} i.v.) and potassium (2–4 mEq · h^{-1} i.v.) during the perioperative period.
2. Measure the blood glucose concentration every 1–2 hours during surgery and during the early postoperative period.
3. Administer regular insulin (5–10 units i.v.), if the blood glucose concentration is >250 · dL^{-1}.
4. Increase the rate of intravenous glucose infusion if the blood glucose concentration is <100 mg · dL^{-1}.

Continuous Intravenous Infusion of Regular Insulin During the Perioperative Period:[b]
1. Mix 50 units of regular insulin in 500 mL normal saline (1 unit · h^{-1} = 10 mL · h^{-1})
2. Initiate intravenous infusion at 0.5–1 unit · h^{-1}
3. Measure blood glucose concentration as necessary (usually every hour), and adjust insulin infusion rate accordingly:

<80 mg · dL^{-1}	Turn infusion off for 30 minutes
	Administer 25 mL of 50% glucose
	Remeasure blood glucose concentration
	in 30 minutes
80–120 mg · dL^{-1}	Decrease insulin infusion by 0.3
	unit · h^{-1}
120–180 mg · dL^{-1}	No change in insulin infusion rate
180–220 mg · dL^{-1}	Increase insulin infusion by 0.3 unit · h^{-1}
>220 mg · dL^{-1}	Increase insulin infusion by 0.5 unit · h^{-1}

4. Provide sufficient glucose (5–10 g · h^{-1}) and potassium (2–4 mEq · h^{-1})

[a]Data from Walts LF, Miller J, Davidson MB, et al. Perioperative management of diabetes mellitus. Anesthesiology 1981;55:104–109.
[b]Data from Hirsch IB, Magill JB, Cryer PE, et al. Perioperative management of surgical patients with diabetes mellitus. Anesthesiology 1991;74:346–359.
With permission from Stoelting RK, Dierdorf SF. Anesthesia and co-existing disease. 3rd ed. New York: Churchill Livingstone, 1993.

glucose regulation during the first 24 to 48 postoperative hours should be a return to the preoperative level of control. If the patient was poorly controlled before surgery, improved glucose regulation should be achieved over a period of several days or weeks. It is not desirable to establish rapid, tight control in patients maintained more loosely on a long-term basis.

The ability to return the patient to his or her preoperative level of control will be highly dependent on the immediate preoperative physiologic state and the extent of the surgery. The diabetic patient undergoing emergency intra-abdominal surgery may have significant preoperative aberrations in glucose regulation and a prolonged fasting period postoperatively, which will increase the difficulty of achieving metabolic homeostasis. Adjusting insulin doses based on blood glucose measurements is preferable to using urine glucose levels as a monitor for insulin administration.

Diabetic autonomic neuropathy may manifest in the immediate postoperative period as nausea and vomiting secondary to gastroparesis or as apnea as a result of abnormal ventilatory responses to hypoxia and hypercarbia (52).

Pheochromocytoma

A pheochromocytoma is a catecholamine-secreting tumor that originates most commonly in the adrenal medulla but may be found at any location along the paravertebral sympathetic chain extending from the pelvis to the skull. Only 10% of pheochromocytomas are malignant. Clinical signs and symptoms of pheochromocytoma include paroxysmal hypertension, diaphoresis, tachycardia, dysrhythmias, headache, and tremulousness. In actuality, less than 0.1% of patients with hypertension have a pheochromocytoma. However, 50% of the deaths of patients with unsuspected pheochromocytoma occur during the perioperative period or during labor and delivery (53). The diagnosis of pheochromocytoma depends on chemical confirmation of the increase in catecholamine production. Chemical confirmation can be obtained by demonstrating increased levels of catecholamines (usually norepinephrine) in the plasma or urine or as evidenced by an increase of the metabolic by-products of catecholamine degradation in the urine. A clonidine suppression test or glucogen stimulation test may be required for the diagnosis of pheochromocytoma in some patients.

Preoperative preparation of the patient with pheochromocytoma is dependent on the administration of an α-adrenergic blocker to reduce blood pressure and permit hydration. If tachycardia or cardiac dysrhythmias develop after institution of α-adrenergic blockade, β-adrenergic blockers can also be administered. Phenoxybenzamine or prazosin can be administered for α-adrenergic blockade. Intraoperative management is directed at avoiding drugs that stimulate the sympathetic nervous system. α-adrenergic blockers should be continued until the day of surgery; β-adrenergic blockers also should be continued if they were part of the preoperative regimen. Invasive monitoring consisting of an intra-arterial catheter and central venous monitoring (CVP or PA catheter) is critical for detecting hemodynamic changes that may be sudden and pronounced. Anesthesia may be induced with an intravenous agent such as thiopental, midazolam, etomidate, or propofol. After loss of consciousness, the depth of anesthesia may be increased by ventilation with a volatile anesthetic. Isoflurane, enflurane, and desflurane are suitable inhalation anesthetics. Although isoflurane and desflurane may increase the heart rate, there is usually little change in the heart rate in patients receiving opioids or adrenegic blocking agents. Halothane should be avoided because of its propensity to produce cardiac dysrhythmias when catecholamine levels are increased. Rapid acting vasodilators (e.g., nitroprusside) and β-adrenergic blockers (esmolol) should be readily available to manage any dangerous blood pressure increases that may occur during tracheal intuba-

tion or tumor manipulation. Abrupt hypotension may occur after ligation of the venous drainage of the pheochromocytoma. Hypotension may be corrected with administration of fluid or by the administration on vasoactive drugs.

POSTOPERATIVE MANAGEMENT

Invasive monitoring and careful observation of hemodynamic parameters must be continued in the postoperative period. Sudden increases and decreases in blood pressure can occur postoperatively. Approximately 50% of the patients will remain hypertensive during the postoperative period. Consequently, antihypertensive therapy may be required. The calcium channel blocker, nicardipine, administered in incremental intravenous doses of 1.25 mg may be efficacious for postoperative hypertension. Nicardipine is an effective antihypertensive agent that has no direct effect on myocardial contractility and only rarely causes hypotension.

Hypoglycemia may occur after removal of a pheochromocytoma. This is most likely secondary to the decrease in the level of circulating catecholamines. High levels of plasma catecholamines suppress insulin secretion. After excision of the pheochromocytoma, an abrupt decrease in circulating catecholamines occurs and a sudden release of insulin can produce severe protracted hypoglycemia (54, 55). Blood glucose levels should be measured frequently during the postoperative period. Delayed emergence should alert the anesthesiologist to the possibility of hypoglycemia.

Postoperative hypotension may be secondary to a number of causes. Hypovolemia must be considered as a primary cause. Consequently, invasive monitoring of cardiac filling pressures must be continued postoperatively. Appropriate administration of crystalloids, colloids, and blood can be based on hemodynamic and laboratory measurements. Some patients with pheochromocytoma develop myocarditis, possibly induced by exposure to high levels of catecholamines, and may exhibit myocardial dysfunction (56). A pulmonary artery catheter may be indicated to measure left-sided cardiac filling pressures and cardiac output. A low cardiac output with an adequate filling pressure may require the administration of inotropic agents (e.g., dobutamine, dopamine).

After excision of a pheochromocytoma, patients will require careful monitoring of hemodynamic and metabolic parameters for 48 hours after surgery.

Thyroid Disease

The effects of thyroid hormones on the metabolic activity of the body are diffuse. Thyroid hormones exert their effects on cells through the adenylate cyclase system and produce changes in biochemical reactions, energy production, and oxygen consumption. Normal daily production of thyroid hormone is 8 ug of T_3 and 90 ug of T_4. Thyroid hormone production and release are controlled by the hypothalamus and anterior pituitary glands. Thyrotropin-releasing hormone (TRH) secreted by the hypothalamus regulates thyroid-stimulating-hormone secretion from the anterior pituitary, which in turn influences thyroid hormone production and secretion by the thyroid gland.

Thyroid gland dysfunction is manifest by the overproduction or underproduction of triiodothyronine (T_3) or thyroxine (T_4). Measurements of thyroid function are directed at determining whether dysfunction is intrinsic to the thyroid gland or secondary to the dysfunction of the hypothalamic-pituitary axis (Tables 17–7 and 17–8).

Highly specific laboratory measurements of thyroid hormones and thyroid controlling hormones are available. However, the time required to analyze the samples prevents the rapid definitive diagnosis of the thyroid disorder in the immediate postoperative period. However, if the diagnosis of hyperthyroidism or hypothyroidism is suspected, blood for appropriate analysis for confirmation of the diagnosis can be obtained before initiation of therapy. This approach minimizes the possibility that therapy may interfere with diagnostic measurements.

HYPERTHYROIDISM

Increased circulating levels of T_3 or T_4 produce the signs and symptoms of hyperthyroidism, which has many causes. Hyperthyroidism may be primary when the production of excess thyroid hormone is intrinsic to the thyroid gland or may be secondary to increased stimulation from the hypothalamus or pituitary gland. The most common cause of primary hyperthyroidism is diffuse toxic goiter (Grave's disease), which is an autoimmune disease in which an IgG antibody activates thyroid-stimulating hormone (TSH) receptors on the surface of the thyroid gland (57). Other causes of primary hyperthyroidism include toxic multinodular goiter, toxic adenoma, thyroid carcinoma, and thyroiditis. Secondary causes of hyperthyroidism are much less common but can be a result of excess TSH production. All of the signs and symptoms of hyperthyroidism reflect the effect of excess amounts and T_3 and T_4 on the rate of biochemical reactions, total body oxygen consumption, and energy production. Signs and symptoms include tachycardia, anxiety, tremor, heat intolerance, fatigue, weight loss, muscle weakness, and atrial fibrillation.

Treatment of hyperthyroidism consists of antithyroid drugs, subtotal thyroidectomy, or administration of radioactive iodine. Antithyroid drugs such as propylthiouracil, carbimazole, and methimazole inhibit oxidation of inorganic iodine and produce euthyroidism in most patients in 1 to 6 months. Side effects of antithyroid drugs include agranulocytosis, hepatitis, and a lupus-like syndrome.

THYROID STORM

Thyroid storm is a sudden episode of hyperthyroidism that produces hypermetabolism and exaggerated cardiovascular activity. In fact, thyroid storm occurring in the perioperative period can mimic malignant hyperthermia (58). The initial treatment of thyroid

Table 17–7.   Tests of Thyroid Gland Function

Test	Purpose
Total plasma thyroxine (T$_4$) level	Detects >90% of hyperthyroid patients; influenced by level of T$_4$-binding globulin
Resin triiodothyronine uptake (RT$_3$U)	Clarifies whether changes in T$_4$ level are due to thyroid gland dysfunction or alterations in T$_4$-binding globulin
Total plasma triiodothyronine (T$_3$) level	Confirm diagnosis of hyperthyroidism; may be low in absence of hypothyroidism in patients who are cirrhotic, uremic, or malnourished
Thyroid-stimulating hormone (TSH) level	Confirms diagnosis of primary hypothyroidism; may be increased before T$_4$ level is decreased
Thyroid scan	Demonstrates iodide-concentrating capacity of thyroid gland; functioning thyroid gland tissue is rarely malignant
Ultrasonography	Discriminates between cystic (rarely malignant) and solid (may be malignant) nodules
Antibodies to thyroid gland components	Distinguishes Hashimoto's thyroiditis from cancer

With permission from Stoelting RK, Dierdorf SF. Anesthesia and co-existing disease. New York: Churchill Livingstone, 1993.

storm is a rapid-acting β-adrenergic blocker such as esmolol to maintain an acceptable heart rate. Supportive therapy includes administration of cooled intravenous solutions and corticosteroids. Administration of antithyroid medications should be initiated; however, the effects will not be immediate (Table 17–9).

INTRAOPERATIVE MANAGEMENT

The development of specific tests of thyroid activity has significantly improved the diagnostic specificity of hyperthyroidism. Consequently, it is not very likely that patients with poorly controlled hyperthyroidism will present for elective surgery. Patients with hyperthyroidism should not undergo elective surgery until they are euthyroid and have their hyperdynamic cardiovascular system con-

trolled with β-adrenergic antagonists. The preoperative treatment of hyperthyroid patients with methimazole and potassium iodide, or propranolol alone or in combination with potassium iodide, virtually eliminates the likelihood of postoperative thyroid storm. Inorganic iodine (Lugol's solution or potassium iodide) inhibits the release of thyroid hormone for several days and may be useful for the preoperative preparation of the hyperthyroid patient or as treatment for thyroid storm (59). If emergent surgery is required before control of hyperthyroidism, a continuous infusion of esmolol (100 to 300 μg/kg/minute) can be used to establish cardiovascular control (60). Although thiopental may have antithyroid activity because of its chemical structure, it is unlikely that this antithyroid activity is of clinical significance. Other induction agents such

Table 17–8.   Differential Diagnosis of Thyroid Gland Dysfunction

Condition	T$_4$	RT$_3$U	T$_3$	TSH
Hyperthyroidism	Increased	Increased	Increased	Normal
Primary hypothroidism	Decreased	Decreased	Decreased	Increased
Secondary hypothroidism	Decreased	Decreased	Decreased	Decreased
Pregnancy	Increased	Decreased	Normal	Normal

See Table 7–7 for definitions.
With permission from Stoelting RK, Dierdorf SF. Anesthesia and co-existing disease. 3rd ed. New York: Churchill Livingstone, 1993.

Table 17–9. Treatment of Thyroid Storm

Treatment of cardiovascular effects of thyroid hormone
  β-adrenergic blockade
    Propranolol: 2–5 mg i.v. q 4 hours
    Esmolol: loading dose of 250–500 μg/kg i.v. followed by continuous i.v. infusion at 50–100 μg/kg/min
  Corticosteroids: 300 mg hydrocortisone i.v.
  Treatment of atrial dysrhythmias
  Vasoactive drugs for congestive heart failure
Anti-thyroid gland treatment
  Inhibition of thyroid hormone synthesis
    Propylthiouracil
      Loading dose: 600–1000 mg
      Maintenance dose: 200–250 mg q 4 hours
    Methimazole
      20 mg q 4 hours
  Inhibition of thyroid hormone release
    Inorganic iodine (oral administration)
      Lugol's solution: 8 drops every 6 hours
      Potassium iodide: 5 drops every 6 hours
Treatment of systemic effects
  Active cooling if hyperthermic
  Hydration

as propofol and midazolam are suitable for patients with thyroid dysfunction. Ketamine, however, may produce excessive tachycardia and hypertension (61). The use of volatile, halogenated anesthetics for hyperthyroid patients is controversial. There is animal evidence and some anecdotal human evidence suggesting that there is an increased likelihood of hepatic damage in hyperthyroid subjects after exposure to halogenated agents, especially halothane (62, 63). However, there is little evidence that exposure to such agents is dangerous for patients rendered euthyroid before surgery (64). Monitoring during the perioperative period is directed at early recognition of increased thyroid activity.

POSTOPERATIVE MANAGEMENT

Monitoring for evidence of increased thyroid activity must be continued into the immediate postoperative period. If evidence of hyperthyroidism develops, cardiovascular dysfunction should initially be controlled with esmolol until therapy with longer-acting β-adrenergic blockers, as well as antithyroid therapy, can be instituted.

Patients undergoing subtotal thyroidectomy for hyperthyroidism have experienced complications such as incomplete control of hyperthyroidism, recurrent laryngeal nerve damage, and tracheal compression. Unilateral recurrent laryngeal nerve damage is characterized by hoarseness with a paralyzed vocal cord. Bilateral recurrent laryngeal nerve damage produces bilateral vocal cord paralysis with airway obstruction. Laryngeal edema may mimic recurrent laryngeal nerve injury. Consequently, it may be advisable to evaluate vocal cord function at the conclusion of surgery. Chronic pressure of an enlarged thyroid against the tracheal wall can produce tracheomalacia, which is manifest as airway obstruction after tracheal extubation. An anterior cervical hematoma can also produce tracheal compression and airway obstruction postoperatively. Although hypoparathyroidism after subtotal thyroidectomy due to accidental parathyroidectomy is extremely rare, hypocalcemia can be manifest as laryngeal stridor 24 to 72 hours after surgery but may occur as early as 1 to 3 hours postoperatively. Treatment consists of the administration of calcium chloride or calcium gluconate.

HYPOTHYROIDISM

Decreased circulating levels of T_3 and T_4 produce hypothyroidism. Primary hypothyroidism may be caused by chronic thyroiditis (Hashimoto's disease), thyroidectomy, irradiation of the neck, excessive antithyroid drugs, or dietary iodine deficiency. Hashimoto's thyroiditis is an autoimmune disease in which antibodies are formed against thyroid peroxidase. This type of thyroiditis is the most common cause of primary hypothyroidism in the United States (65). Secondary hypothyroidism is caused by hypothalamic or anterior pituitary dysfunction.

Many of the signs and symptoms of hypothyroidism are very gradual in onset and can be difficult to recognize. The signs and symptoms are a reflection of a generalized decrease in metabolic activity. Cardiac output is decreased secondary to bradycardia and decreased stroke volume. The decreased cardiac output in conjunction with increased systemic vascular resistance produces a long circulation time and a decreased pulse pressure. Manifestations of hypothyroidism that mimic congestive heart failure include cardiomegaly, pericardial effusion, pleural effusion, ascites, and peripheral edema. Adrenal cortical atrophy with decreased cortisol production is also associated with hypothyroidism and may contribute to the clinical manifestations of hypothyroidism.

Myxedema coma is a rare manifestation of hypothyroidism that presents with profound lethargy or coma, hypothermia (<35°C), hypoventilation, and congestive heart failure. Treatment is with intravenous T_3 and cortisol. Treatment with thyroid hormone must be initiated cautiously, because too aggressive therapy may increase metabolism and oxygen demand too rapidly and unmask ischemic heart disease.

Treatment of hypothyroidism is the oral administration of thyroid hormone (T_4) until the signs and symptoms of hypothyroidism are alleviated and plasma levels of TSH have normalized.

INTRAOPERATIVE MANAGEMENT

Although elective surgery should be postponed in patients with symptomatic hypothyroidism until they have been rendered euthyroid, most patients with mild to moderate hypothyroidism are not at increased risk for major perioperative complications (66). Minor postoperative complications that may occur in hypothyroid patients include gastrointestinal side effects and a decreased ability to develop a fever secondary to postoperative infection (67). Clinical experience indicates that hypothyroid patients are sensitive to inhaled anesthetic drugs and opioids, have a prolonged recovery period, and have a higher incidence of perioperative cardiac complications. There are no specifically contraindicated anesthetic drugs. Adequate monitoring can guide the administration of anesthetics and neuromuscular blocking drugs to reduce the likelihood of adverse cardiovascular effects or prolonged neuromuscular blockade. Hypothyroid patients undergoing cardiac surgery may be at increased risk for manifestations of hypothyroidism and may require levothyroxine intraoperatively. Non-β-adrenergic vasopressors such as amrinone may be indicated for the treatment of decreased cardiac output secondary to hypothyroidism (68).

POSTOPERATIVE MANAGEMENT

Potential postoperative complications in the patient with hypothyroidism are secondary to impaired physiologic responses and delayed drug metabolism. The severity of the hypothyroidism will determine the rapidity for treatment. Myxedema coma, although very rare, is a medical emergency with 50% mortality and has been reported in the postoperative period (69). If myxedema is suspected, blood samples for T_3, T_4, and thyrotropin levels should be obtained. Treatment, however, must be initiated before a definitive diagnosis is made. Treatment can be initiated with intravenous l-thyroxine (T_4), 300 to 500 μg. Hemodynamic parameters must be carefully monitored as thyroid replacement may in-

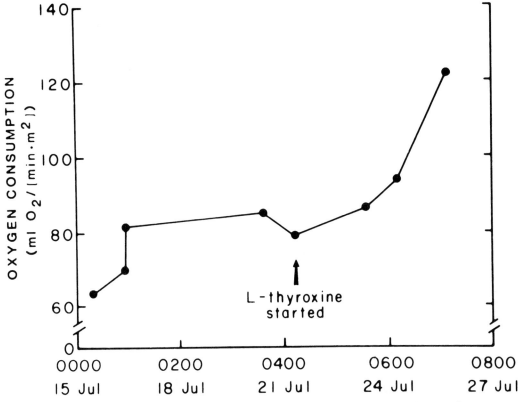

Fig. 17–8. Oxygen consumption in a patient with unsuspected hypothyroidism who underwent elective surgery complicated by hypotension and the need for postoperative mechanical ventilation. Administration of thyroxine restored vital signs, ventilation, and oxygen consumption to normal. (With permission from Levelle JP, Jopling MW, Sklar GS. Perioperative hypothyroidism: an unusual postanesthetic diagnosis. Anesthesiology 1985;63:195–197.)

crease oxygen consumption and cardiac demand with resultant myocardial ischemia. Hydrocortisone (100 mg intravenously) may also be administered, although adrenal insufficiency associated with severe hypothyroidism is rare. Postoperative ventilatory support is of critical importance as hypoventilation is a consistent feature of severe hypothyroidism. Hypoventilation may be aggravated by residual effects of anesthetics and neuromuscular blockers (70). Hypothermia is also a very common manifestation of myxedema, but rewarming should be performed very gradually to avoid hypotension from vasodilation.

More typically, postoperative manifestations of hypothyroidism may be very subtle and include mild hypotension, hypothermia, and hypoventilation (71) (Fig. 17–8). A high index of suspicion for hypothyroidism must be maintained when a postsurgical patient has this type of clinical complex.

Parathyroid Disorders

The parathyroid glands secrete parathormone, which maintains a normal blood calcium level (4.5 to 5.5 mEq/L). Parathormone secretion is stimulated by hypocalcemia and suppressed by hypercalcemia. Parathormone modulates calcium levels by its actions on the gastrointestinal tract, the renal tubules, and bone.

HYPERPARATHYROIDISM

Hyperparathyroidism is caused by a functioning benign adenoma in 90% of the patients but may also be caused by parathyroid hyperplasia or cancer. Secondary hyperparathyroidism is a compensatory response of the parathyroid glands to a hypocalcemia. For example, chronic renal disease produces hypocalcemia and secondary parathyroid hyperplasia. Decreased renal degradation of parathormone from renal failure also results in increased parathormone levels in uremic patients. Increased parathormone levels inhibit erythropoiesis and contributes to the anemia of renal failure (72). Ectopic hyperparathyroidism is caused by the secretion of a parathormone-like substance by a variety of malignant tumors (lung, breast, pancreas, kidney).

The hallmark of hyperparathyroidism is hypercalcemia (>5.5 mEq/L), which produces skeletal muscle weakness, renal stones, anemia, and ECG changes (prolonged P-R interval, shortened Q-T interval). Symptomatic hypercalcemia is treated with diuresis with furosemide and administration of normal saline. Calcitonin produces a prompt reduction in plasma calcium concentrations, but its effects are transient. Plicamycin (25 ug/kg/day) produces a sustained decrease in calcium levels by inhibiting the osteoclastic activity of parathormone. Preoperatively calcium levels should be reduced before elective surgery. Goals for intraoperative management include adequate hydration and diuresis. The response to neuromuscular blocking drugs is unpredictable. There are reports of sensitivity to succinylcholine and resistance to atracurium (73).

Postoperative Management

Postoperative abnormalities are secondary to hypercalcemia and include muscle weakness, somnolence, hypertension, and ECG changes. Postoperative muscle weakness from hypercalcemia may be aggravated by the residual effects of neuromuscular blocking drugs.

If symptomatic weakness is present, providing mechanical ventilation until calcium levels are reduced and neuromuscular blockers have been excreted may be the safest course of action.

HYPOPARATHYROIDISM

Parathormone deficiency is most commonly secondary to inadvertent parathyroidectomy as may occur during thyroidectomy. A plasma calcium concentration less than 4.5 mEq/L is the usual sign of hypoparathyroidism. Clinical signs and symptoms of hypocalcemia depend, to a great extent, on the rapidity with which hypocalcemia develops. Acute hypocalcemia that may occur after surgical parathyroidectomy is manifest by restlessness and neuromuscular irritability (positive Chvostek or Trousseau signs). A positive Chvostek sign is present when facial muscle twitching occurs after manual tapping of the tissue over the facial nerve. A positive Trousseau sign occurs when carpal spasm occurs after 3 minutes of arm ischemia as produced by a tourniquet. Inspiratory stridor with airway obstruction secondary to irritability of the laryngeal muscles may occur soon after parathyroidectomy or as late as 72 hours after parathyroidectomy.

Disorders of the Adrenal Cortex

The adrenal cortex produces three groups of hormones: glucocorticoids, mineralocorticoids, and androgens. Cortisol is the principal glucocorticoid produced by the adrenal cortex; normal daily endogenous cortisol production is 20 to 30 mg. The physiologic effects of cortisol are diverse and essential to life. Cortisol regulates epinephrine production in the adrenal medulla and thereby contributes to the maintenance of cardiovascular stability. Metabolic effects of cortisol include gluconeogenesis and inhibition of the peripheral uptake of glucose.

HYPERADRENOCORTICISM

Excess production of cortisol can be caused by increased secretion of adrenocorticotropic hormone (ACTH) by the pituitary, overproduction of cortisol by an adrenal tumor, ectopic production of ACTH by a malignant tumor (lung, kidney, pancreas), or exogenous administration of cortisol. Typical signs and symptoms of hyperadrenocorticism include hypertension, hyperglycemia, obesity, moon facies, osteoporosis, poor wound healing, and increased susceptibility to infection. Anesthetic management for the patient with increased cortisol production is directed primarily at the complications of increased cortisol activity such as hypertension and hyperglycemia. If the surgical procedure is to remove the source of increased cortisol secretion, postoperative management will be concerned with the likelihood of the patient developing acute cortisol deficiency.

Postoperative Management

If the side effects of excess cortisol production are well controlled preoperatively, it is unlikely that significant postoperative complications will develop. If the source of the excess cortisol production has been surgically removed, the patient may require postoperative administration of corticosteroids (hydrocortisone, 100 mg/day). If a pituitary tumor is removed, there is the possibility of postoperative diabetes insipidus.

HYPOADRENOCORTICISM

Causes of hypoadrenocorticism include destruction of the adrenal cortex by hemorrhage, malignancy, or granulomatous disease, suppression of the pituitary-adrenal axis (exogenous administration of corticosteroids), ACTH deficiency. Signs and symptoms of adrenal insufficiency include nausea and vomiting, weight loss, skeletal muscle weakness, hypotension, and increased skin pigmentation. Adrenal insufficiency may be life threat-ening and should be treated with hydrocortisone 100 mg intravenously.

Postoperative Management

Adrenal insufficiency may be difficult to diagnose intraoperatively. The usual intraoperative manifestation is hypotension that is resistant to usual therapy (e.g., fluid administration, administration of vasopressors, decreasing depth of anesthesia). If the diagnosis of adrenal insufficiency is suspected, the intravenous administration of hydrocortisone will produce a dramatic effect on the blood pressure. In addition to hypotension, hyponatremia, hyperkalemia, and hypoglycemia may also be present. Measurement of cortisol and ACTH levels will help confirm the diagnosis and suggest whether the adrenal insufficiency is primary or secondary.

SUPPRESSION OF THE PITUITARY ADRENAL AXIS

The patient that has been receiving corticosteroid supplementation may have suppression of the pituitary adrenal axis to the extent that they cannot produce cortisol in response to stress (e.g., surgery). The duration of this suppression is controversial but may be as long as 12 months after steroid therapy (74). Consequently, these patients may require exogenous corticosteroids during the postoperative period. The amount of steroid required is, however, quite controversial. Because corticosteroids have significant side effects, such as retardation of healing, susceptibility to infection, and gastrointestinal hemorrhage, the minimally effective dose of steroid is desired. It has been estimated that the maximal cortisol requirement after major surgery is 75 to 150 mg/day (Fig. 17–9). Consequently, a reasonable dose would be 25 mg of hydrocortisone with induction of anesthesia followed by the intravenous administration of 100 mg of hydrocortisone every 12 to 24 hours (75). This regimen would ensure adequate cortisol for the most physiologically stressful surgical procedures.

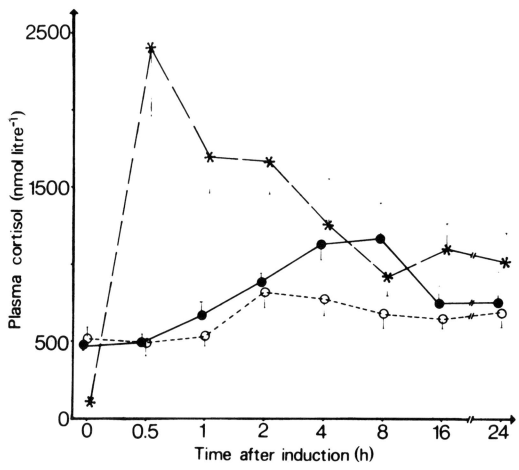

Fig. 17–9. Plasma cortisol levels were measured before and after induction of anesthesia for elective surgery in three groups of patients. Control patients (group I: solid circles) had never been treated with corticosteroids. Group II (open circles) consisted of patients receiving long-term corticosteroid treatment in whom normal increases in plasma concentrations of cortisol were manifest in response to preoperative administration of adrenocorticotrophic hormone. These patients, as well as the control patients, did not receive exogenous corticosteroids during the perioperative period. Group III (asterisks) consisted of patients receiving long-term corticosteroid treatment in whom subnormal changes in plasma concentrations of cortisol were manifest in response to preoperative administration of adrenocorticotrophic hormone. These patients received low-dose cortisol substitution during the perioperative period, consisting of intravenous cortisol (25 mg) after induction of anesthesia, plus continuous intravenous infusions of cortisol (100 mg) during the next 24 hours. Time courses for changes in the plasma concentrations of cortisol were similar in groups I and II, except at 4 hours and 8 hours after induction of anesthesia, when plasma concentrations were greater in group I patients ($P < .05$). Control plasma concentrations of cortisol were significantly lower in group III, compared with the other two groups ($P < .001$). After intravenous administration of cortisol, plasma concentrations increased markedly and significantly above the values present in groups I and II for the next 2 hours ($P < .01$). Thereafter, mean values for the plasma concentrations were similar to those present in the other two groups. (With permission from Symreng T, Karlberg BE, Kagedal B, et al. Physiological cortisol substitution of long-term steroid treated patients undergoing major surgery. Br J Anaesth 1981;53:949–953.)

REFERENCES

1. Tiret L, Desmonts JM, Hatton F, et al. Complications associated with anaesthesia — a prospective survey in France. Can Anaesth Soc J 1986;33:336–344.
2. Orkin FK. Practice standards: the Midas touch or the emperor's new clothes? Anesthesiology 1989;70:567–571.
3. Nunn JF. Applied respiratory physiology. 4th ed. Oxford: Butterworth, 1993;518–528.
4. Steenbergen C, Deleeuw G, Rich T, et al. Effects of acidosis and ischemia on contractility and intracellular pH of rat heart. Circ Res 1977;41:849–858.
5. Mizock BA. Controversies in lactic acidosis. JAMA 1987;258:497–501.
6. Hindman BJ. Sodium bicarbonate in the treatment of subtypes of acute lactic acidosis: physiologic considerations. Anesthesiology 1990;72:1064–1076.
7. Ritter JM, Doktor HS, Benjamin N. Paradoxical effects of bicarbonate on cytoplasmic pH. Lancet 1990;335:1243–1246.
8. Bersin RM, Arieff AI. Improved hemodynamic function during hypoxia with carbicarb, a new agent for the management of acidosis. Circulation 1988;77:227–233.
9. Blecic S, DeBacker D, Deleuze M, et al. Correction of metabolic acidosis in experimental CPR: a comparative study of sodium bicarbonate, carbicarb, and dextrose. Ann Emerg Med 1991;20:235–238.
10. Shangraw RE, Winter R, Hromco J, et al. Amelioration of lactic acidosis with dichloroacetate during liver transplantation in humans. Anesthesiology 1994;81:1127–1138.
11. Minuck M, Sharma GP. Comparison of THAM and sodium bicarbonate in resuscitation of the heart after ventricular fibrillation in dogs. Anesth Analg 1977;56:38–45.
12. Yoshida K, Marmarou A. Effects of tromethamine and hyperventilation on brain injury in the cat. J Neurosurg 1991;74:87–96.
13. Wetterberg T, Sjoberg T, Steen S. Effects of buffering in hypercapnia and hypercapneic hypoxemia. Acta Anesthesiol Scand 1993;37:343–349.
14. Von Planta M, Bar-Joseph G, Wiklund L, et al. Pathophysiologic and therapeutic implications of acid-base changes during CPR. Ann Emerg Med 1993;22(2):404–410.
15. Arieff AI. Indications for use of bicarbonate in patients with metabolic acidosis. Br J Anaesth 1991;67:165–177.
16. Domino KB, Hlastala MP. Hyperventilation in the treatment of metabolic acidosis does not adversely affect pulmonary function. Anesthesiology 1994;81:1445–1453.
17. Dierdorf SF, McNiece WL. Anaesthesia and pyruvate dehydrogenase deficiency. Can Anaesth Soc J 1983;30:413–416.
18. Fencl V, Rossing TH. Acid-base disorders in critical care medicine. Annu Rev Med 1989;40:17–29.
19. Arieff AI. Hyponatremia, convulsions, respiratory arrest, and permanent brain damage after elective surgery in healthy women. N Engl J Med 1986;314:1529–1535.
20. Sterns RH, Thomas DJ, Herndon RM. Brain dehydration and neurologic deterioration after correction of hyponatremia. Kidney Int 1989;35:69–75.
21. Ayus JC, Krothapalli RK, Arieff AI. Treatment of symptomatic hyponatremia and its relation to brain damage: a prospective study. N Engl J Med 1987;317:1190–1197.
22. Perazella MA, Brown E. Electrolyte and acid-base disorders associated with AIDS. J Gen Intern Med 1994;9:232–236.
23. Jensen V. The TURP syndrome. Can J Anaesth 1991;38:90–97.
24. Reddy RV, Moorthy SS, Dierdorf SF. Electroencephalographic changes from hyponatremia during transurethral resection of the prostate. J Urol 1993;149:1144–1145.
25. Hahn RG. Transurethral resection syndrome after transurethral resection of bladder tumours. Can J Anaesth 1995;42:69–72.
26. Doman K, Perlmutter JA, Muhammedi M, et al. Life-threatening hyperkalemia associated with captopril administration. South Med J 1993;86:1269–1272.
27. Malik IA, Abubakar S, Alam F, et al. Dexamethasone-induced tumor lysis syndrome in high-grade non-Hodgkin's lymphoma. South Med J 1994;87:409–411.
28. Bisogno JL, Langley A, Von Dreele MM. Effect of calcium to reverse the electrocardiographic effects of hyperkalemia in the isolated rat heart: a prospective, dose-response study. Crit Care Med 1994;22:697–704.
29. Hahn RG, Lofgren A, Nordin AM. Health status and the preoperative change in serum potassium concentration. Acta Anesthesiol Scand 1993;37:329–333.
30. DuPlooy WJ, Hay L, Kahler CP, et al. The dose related hyper- and hypokalemic effects of salbutamol and its arrhythmogenic potential. Br J Pharmacol 1994;111:73–76.
31. McClure RJ, Prasad VK, Brocklebank JT. Treatment of hyperkalemia using intravenous and nebulized salbutamol. Arch Dis Child 1994;70:126–128.
32. Flack JM, Ryder KW, Strickland D, et al. Metabolic correlates of theophylline therapy: a concentration-related phenomenon. Ann Pharmacother 1994;28:175–179.
33. Wysolmerski JJ, Broadus AE. Hypercalcemia of malignancy: the central role of parathyroid hormone related protein. Annu Rev Med 1994;45:189–200.
34. Prielipp R, Zaloga GP. Calcium action and general anesthesia. Adv Anesth 1991;8:241–278.
35. Ghoneim MM, Long JP. The interaction between magnesium and other neuromuscular blocking agents. Anesthesiology 1970;32:23–27.
36. Whang R, Hampton EM, Whang DD. Magnesium homeostasis and clinical disorders of magnesium deficiency. Ann Pharmacother 1994;28:220–226.
37. Lye WC, Leong SO. Bilateral vocal cord paralysis secondary to treatment of severe hypophosphatemia in a continuous ambulatory peritoneal dialysis patient. Am J Kidney Dis 1994;23:127–129.
38. Banai S, Tzivoni D. Drug therapy for torsade de pointes. J Cardiovasc Electrophysiol 1993;4:206–210.

39. Vance ML. Hypopituitarism. N Engl J Med 1994;330:1651–1662.

40. Rothwell PM, Lawler PG. Prediction of outcome in intensive care patients using endocrine parameters. Crit Care Med 1995;23:78–83.

41. Rothwell PM, Udwadia ZF, Lawler PG. Thyrotropin concentration predicts outcome in critical illness. Anaesthesia 1993;48:373–376.

42. Schein RMH, Sprung CL, Marcial E, et al. Plasma cortisol levels in patients with septic shock. Crit Care Med 1990;18:259–263.

43. Atkinson MA, Maclaren NK. The pathogenesis of insulin-dependent diabetes mellitus. N Engl J Med 1994;331:1428–1436.

44. The Diabetes Control and Complications Trial Research Group. The effect of intensive treatment of diabetes on the development and progression of long-term complications in insulin-dependent diabetes mellitus. N Engl J Med 1993;329:977–986.

45. Burgos LG, Ebert TJ, Asiddao C, et al. Increased intraoperative cardiovascular morbidity in diabetics with autonomic neuropathy. Anesthesiology 1989;70:591–597.

46. Vohra A, Kumar S, Charlton AJ, et al. Effect of diabetes mellitus on the cardiovascular responses to induction of anaesthesia and tracheal intubation. Br J Anaesth 1993;71:258–261.

47. Ishihara H, Singh H, Giesecke AH. Relationship between diabetic autonomic neuropathy and gastric contents. Anesth Analg 1994;78:943–947.

48. Kirvela M, Scheinin M, Lindgren L. Haemodynamic and catecholamine responses to induction of anaesthesia and tracheal intubation in diabetic and non-diabetic uraemic patients. Br J Anaesth 1995;74:60–65.

49. Fleckman AM. Diabetic ketoacidosis. Endocrinol Metab Clin North Am 1993;22:181–207.

50. Hirsch IB, Magill JB, Cryer PE, et al. Perioperative management of patients with diabetes mellitus. Anesthesiology 1991;74:346–359.

51. Walts LF, Miller J, Davidson MB, et al. Perioperative management of diabetes mellitus. Anesthesiology 1981;55:104–109.

52. Tasch MD. Endocrine disease and implications for management of anesthesia. Adv Anesth 1985;2:103–166.

53. Kirkendall WM, Leighty RD, Culp DA. Diagnosis and treatment of patients with pheochromocytoma. Arch Intern Med 1965;115:529–536.

54. Costello GT, Moorthy SS, Vane DW, et al. Hypoglycemia following bilateral adrenalectomy for pheochromocytoma. Crit Care Med 1988;16:562–563.

55. Levin H, Heifetz M. Phaeochromocytoma and severe protracted postoperative hypoglycemia. Can J Anaesth 1990;37:477–478.

56. Bravo EL, Gifford RW. Pheochromocytoma. Endocrinol Metab Clin North Am 1993;22:329–341.

57. Klein I, Becker DV, Levey GS. Treatment of hyper-

thyroid disease. Ann Intern Med 1994;121:281–288.

58. Peters KR, Nance P, Wingard DW. Malignant hyperthyroidism or malignant hyperthermia? Anesth Analg 1981;60:613–615.

59. Franklyn JA. The management of hyperthyroidism. N Engl J Med 1994;330:1731–1738.

60. Thorne AC, Bedford RF. Esmolol for perioperative management of thyrotoxic goiter. Anesthesiology 1989;71:291–294.

61. Kaplan JA, Cooperman LH. Alarming reactions to ketamine in patients taking thyroid medication: treatment with propranolol. Anesthesiology 1971;35:229–230.

62. Berman ML, Kuhnert L, Phythyon JM, et al. Isoflurane and enflurane induced hepatic necrosis in triiodothyronine pretreated rats. Anesthesiology 1983;58:1–5.

63. Hubbard AK, Roth TP, Gandolfi AJ, et al. Halothane hepatitis patients generate an antibody response toward a covalently bound metabolite of halothane. Anesthesiology 1988;68:791–796.

64. Seino H, Dohi S, Aiyoshi Y, et al. Postoperative hepatic dysfunction after halothane or enflurane anesthesia in patients with hyperthyroidism. Anesthesiology 1986;64:122–125.

65. Rapoport B. Pathophysiology of Hashimoto's thyroiditis and hypothyroidism. Annu Rev Med 1991;42:91–96.

66. Weinberg AD, Brennan MD, Gorman CA, et al. Outcome of anesthesia and surgery in hypothyroid patients. Arch Intern Med 1983;143:893–897.

67. Ladenson PW, Levin AA, Ridgway EC, et al. Complications of surgery in hypothyroid patients. Am J Med 1984;77:261–267.

68. Whitten CW, Latson TW, Klein KW, et al. Anesthetic management of a hypothyroid cardiac surgical patient. J Cardiothorac Vasc Anesth 1991;5:156–159.

69. Ragallen M, Quintel M, Bender HJ, et al. Myxedema coma: a rare postoperative complication. Anaesthetist 1993;42:179–183.

70. Miller LR, Benumof JL, Alexander L, et al. Completely absent response to peripheral nerve stimulation in an acutely hypothyroid patient. Anesthesiology 1989;71:779–781.

71. Levelle JP, Jopling MW, Sklar GS. Perioperative hypothyroidism: an unusual postanesthetic diagnosis. Anesthesiology 1985;63:195–197.

72. Klahr S, Slatopolsky E. Toxicity of parathyroid hormone in uremia. Annu Rev Med 1986;37:71–78.

73. Al-Hohaya S, Naguib M, Abdelatif M, et al. Abnormal responses to muscle relaxants in a patient with primary hyperparathyroidism. Anesthesiology 1986;65:554–556.

74. Libertino JA. Surgery of adrenal disorders. Surg Clin North Am 1988;68:1027–1033.

75. Symreng T, Karlberg BE, Kagedal B, et al. Physiological cortisol substitution of long term steroid treated patients undergoing major surgery. Br J Anaesth 1981;53:949–953.

18

SPECIAL CONSIDERATIONS IN THE GERIATRIC POPULATION

Susan W. Krechel

Previous chapters have addressed many of the common postanesthesia care unit (PACU) problems in detail, from the perspective of surgical populations as a whole. In this chapter, I will look once again at many of these common problems and discuss how and why the geriatric patient may need special consideration, because the elderly have a higher mortality rate than younger patients undergoing the same procedure. Table 18–1 delineates the common postanesthesia care unit (PACU) problems that will be discussed in this chapter.

HYPERTENSION/HYPOTENSION

Hypertension

In reviewing 443 patients admitted to their PACU, Zelcer and Wells (1) noted a 10% incidence of vascular instability (hypertension/hypotension). Although patients of all ages were included in this study, all cases of hypertension occurred in patients older than 60 years of age. These findings suggest that hypertension in the PACU is more likely to occur in the elderly patient. Specific physiologic and pharmacologic changes occurring during the aging process make the occurrence of hypertension (which, for the purposes of this discussion, is defined as systolic blood pressure greater than 160 to 170 mm Hg) more common in the elderly.

There are two distinct populations of elderly patients: the healthy elderly person who

has taken especially good care of his or her body by paying special attention to optimum nutrition and exercise; and the more commonly encountered elderly patient, who has cardiovascular disease, who is often malnourished (either emaciated or obese) and is frequently relatively sedentary. Early investigators chose to study elderly patients without consideration for the presence or absence of diseases not necessarily related to the aging process itself. Consequently, when looking at data pertaining to the elderly, it is important to determine from which subgroup of elderly patients the data are derived.

Table 18–2 delineates the physiologic changes associated with aging that might be expected to increase the prevalence of postoperative hypertension in elderly patients.

Table 18–1. Common Recovery Room Problems

Problem	Occurrence Rate (%)
Hypotension/hypertension	10
Delayed arousal	9
Pain	9
Ischemia/dysrhythmias	8
Nausea/vomiting	5
Agitation/dysphoria	3
Oliguria	1
Hypoxemia	1
Hypercarbia	1
Laryngeal spasm	0.7
Hypothermia	0.5

Data from Zelcer J, Wells DG. Anesthetic related recovery room complications. Anaesth Intensive Care 1987; 15:168–174.

Table 18–2. Physiologic Changes of Aging Associated with the Prevalence of Postoperative Hypertension in Elderly Patients

Preexisting hypertension[a] (secondary to):
   Arterial stiffening and increased pulse wave
      velocity[b] (5)
   Increased Norepinephrine levels[a] (6)
      (not cause effect) (5)
Reduced baroreflex sensitivity[a,b] (7,8)

[a] All elderly
[b] Healthy elderly

Hypertension occurs commonly in elderly individuals. Stephen found that 46.6% of 1000 elderly patients evaluated preoperatively had preexisting hypertension (2). Physicians have long recognized diastolic hypertension as a cause of cardiovascular mortality. It is, however, only recently that we have come to realize that isolated systolic hypertension, which is so prevalent in the elderly, is actually a very potent contributor to cardiovascular mortality and morbidity (3, 4). The cause of systolic hypertension in the elderly, according to Lakatta, is arterial stiffening and the associated increase in pulse wave velocity (5). Although an association between increases in norepinephrine levels in the elderly and increased blood pressure has been noted (6), this is believed to be a casual relationship rather than one of cause and effect (5). The normal aging process is associated with a decreased sensitivity of the baroreflex, which may result in labile blood pressure (7, 8).

The causes of postoperative hypertension are listed in Table 18–3. Many of these conditions are found more commonly in elderly individuals. Data from both Prys-Roberts (9) and Goldman and Caldera (10) suggest that postoperative hypertension is more common in patients with a history of preoperative hypertension, regardless of whether hypertension is brought under control by medications preoperatively. Several commonly performed surgical procedures are associated with postoperative hypertension. These procedures include both neck dissection (11) and carotid

endarterectomy, presumably because of carotid sinus denervation associated with the surgical procedure (12). It has further been noted that hypertension secondary to carotid sinus denervation occurs immediately after surgery; the average onset time is 1.4 hours and the average duration is 5 to 6 hours (11, 13). Fluid overload certainly can be a cause of postoperative hypertension as is seen after transurethral resection of the prostate, in which large volumes of irrigant fluid are absorbed through open venous sinuses in the bladder. A full bladder alone may cause postoperative hypertension (15). Hypothermia may cause hypertension by virtue of an increase in systemic vascular resistance or by causing shivering with its concomitant increase in sympathetic nervous system activity and circulating norepinephrine levels (16). Sympathetic overactivity with resultant hypertension and tachycardia is seen in 40% of patients sustaining an acute anterior myocardial infarction (17). The acute withdrawal of antihypertensive medications preoperatively is associated with rebound hypertension (18). This is especially true after withdrawal of cloni-

Table 18–3. Causes of Postoperative Hypertension

Preexisting hypertension[a]
   (treated or untreated) (9,10)
Related to surgical procedure
   Neck dissection (carotid sinus denervation)[a] (11)
   Carotid endarterectomy (carotid sinus denervation)[a]
      (12)
   Vascular surgery[a] (14)
   TURP—volume overload[a]
Pain
Hypercarbia
Volume overload
Full bladder (15)
Hypothermia[a] (16)
Hypoxia[a]
Wrong cuff size or transducer height
Myocardial infarction[a] (17)
Acute withdrawal of antihypertensive agents[a] (18)
   (e.g., clonidine or β blockers) (19,20)
ICP—(Cushing reflex)

[a] Conditions found more commonly in elderly than in younger patients.

dine (19) or β blockers (20). Although the causes of postoperative hypertension listed in Table 18–3 are listed in order of the most common to the least common according to the authors' experience, it must be emphasized that both hypoxia and hypercarbia must be ruled out before other possible causes are entertained.

TREATMENT

After the cause of postoperative hypertension is identified, a plan of treatment should be considered. If the cause is hypoxia or hypercarbia, the treatment may be as simple as the administration of oxygen and ventilation. If the cause of hypertension is a full bladder, it can be easily and efficiently relieved by the insertion of a urinary bladder catheter. The administration of analgesics to alleviate pain is effective in controlling hypertension caused by pain. It is important to correctly identify the cause of the hypertension before initiating treatment. For example, the treatment of hypertension caused by a full bladder with an antihypertensive drug is an invitation for disaster. If an antihypertensive drug is administered and the bladder is then relieved, severe hypotension may occur.

To Treat or Not to Treat

Allowing hypertension to persist even though it is expected to be short lived (for example, hypertension secondary to carotid sinus denervation) may be hazardous. The bleeding and hematoma formation that may result are especially hazardous when they occur in the neck. In addition, there is always the fear of subendocardial ischemia related to increased myocardial work and pulmonary edema caused by acute left ventricular failure or cerebral vascular accidents. Conversely, there is evidence that the treatment of hypertension may also be deleterious. Perhaps the first indication that the treatment of postoperative hypertension could be detrimental came from the work of Fremes (14). In studying

hypertension after aortocoronary bypass operations and its treatment with sodium nitroprusside, the authors noted that the treatment of patients to a mean arterial blood pressure of 92 to 120 mm Hg was beneficial in terms of myocardial performance and compliance; however, the further lowering of mean arterial pressure to 80 mm Hg was associated with increased lactate production and decreased compliance. These investigators were, in essence, describing the J-curve phenomenon as it was dubbed by later investigators. Using meta analysis, Farnett determined that lowering diastolic blood pressure levels below 85 mm Hg was associated with an increased risk of cardiac morbidity (21). In a prospective study of hypertensive males with a history of ischemia or hypertrophy, Lindblad et al. noted that the lowering of diastolic blood pressure below 95 mm Hg was associated with an increased risk of acute myocardial infarction (22). In a large study of 2287 patients, Madhavan et al. (23) noted that patients with isolated systolic hypertension, i.e., a wide pretreatment pulse pressure, were at the greatest risk of myocardial infarction from either too large or too small a fall in diastolic pressure, i.e., a curvilinear or J-curve phenomenon. The exact mechanism by which the lowering of diastolic blood pressure below critical levels causes an increase in myocardial complications, especially myocardial infarction, is unknown. A decreased coronary flow secondary to lowered diastolic blood pressure may cause ischemia in a hypertrophied ventricle with its increased myocardial demand. Alternatively, the excessive lowering of diastolic blood pressure leads to low coronary flow, increased blood viscosity, and platelet adhesiveness potentiating thrombosis, ischemia, infarction, and/or dysrhythmias (21). Unfortunately, we do not know the critical level of diastolic pressure required for any given patient.

Which Drugs

After it has been decided to treat postoperative hypertension that is not due to an easily treatable cause such as a full bladder or pain, we must decide which drugs to use. Theoretically, β blockers should be relatively ineffective for elderly patients because of a decreased β receptor responsiveness (5) and a low renin state (24). Nevertheless, β blockers have been shown to be effective for elderly patients (25). Although labetalol is a combined α and β blocker shown to be effective for elderly patients (26), it must be kept in mind that labetalol is mainly a β-blocking drug. Le Bret et al. have shown, using transesophageal echocardiography, that the principal effect of labetalol is negative inotropism (27).

The author has found the use of sublingually administered nifedipine to be extremely useful for the reduction of blood pressure in elderly patients in the postanesthesia recovery area. A gel capsule can be pierced and the fluid can be applied under the tongue. Nifedipine is mainly a vasodilator and has little myocardial depressant and atrioventricular nodal activity (28). Drugs with α-blocking side effects such as droperidol or thorazine may also be used. For short duration only, either nitroglycerin or nitroprusside may be used. Nitroglycerin, which is primarily a venous dilator, is sometimes associated with a less than desired fall in blood pressure in younger patients. In contrast, conscious elderly patients have an exaggerated hypotensive response to nitroglycerin (29). This finding is not surprising in view of the fact that elderly patients are far more dependent than younger patients on preload, especially during exercise (5). Likewise, in a recent study, Wood (30) suggested that a lower dose of nitroprusside should be used in elderly patients to achieve the same effect. Sodium nitroprusside, in contrast, works primarily on the resistance side of the vascular tree. Although the reason for the increased sensitivity to the drug in elderly patients is unknown, it may be secondary to diminished baroreflex activity, resistance of cardiac adrenergic receptors to catecholamine stimulation, or to other as yet unexplained mechanisms (30).

Hypotension

At the other extreme of the vascular pendulum is hypotension. Physiologic changes associated with aging may also put the elderly patient at greater risk for hypotension in the postoperative period. Table 18–4 delineates the physiologic changes of aging associated with postoperative hypotension. The baroreflex is particularly important in maintaining cardiovascular homeostasis, especially when the system is stressed, as in hemorrhage or sudden postural changes, both of which are likely in the postoperative period. In most cases, the elderly patient arriving in the recovery room has hemorrhaged to some extent in the operating room and then has been moved briskly to a different bed and to the PACU. In addition, the elderly patient has an altered ability to regulate extracellular fluid volume, secondary to a 30 to 50% reduction in basal and stimulated levels of renin and aldosterone. Increased levels of atrial natriuretic peptide also have been measured in healthy elderly individuals, promoting salt wasting and additional difficulty in maintaining extra cellular volume (31).

Elderly individuals are more dependent on preload than their younger counterparts. Also, physical changes in the myocardium cause a

Table 18–4. Physiologic Changes of Aging Associated with the Prevalence of Postoperative Hypotension in Elderly Patients

Reduced baroreflex activity[a,b] (7,8)
Altered ability to regulate extracellular volume[b] (24)
   30–50% reductions in basal and stimulated levels of renin and aldosterone[b]
   Increased levels of atrial naturetic peptide[b] (31)
Greater dependence on preload[b] (5)
   Highly dependent on atrial kick[b] (32)
Reduced β-receptor affinity for agonists[b] (35)
   Decreased response to β-adrenergic stimulation[b] (34)
Decreased intrinsic heart rate[b] (36)
Decreased resting heart rate[b] (37)
Decreased heart rate response to exercise[b] (37)
Increased myocardial relaxation time[a,b] (42)

[a]All elderly
[b]Healthy elderly

prolongation of the isovolumetric relaxation period and early left ventricular diastolic filling is impaired. Despite this, diastolic volume and cardiac output are well preserved in the healthy elderly through enhanced atrial contraction during late diastole. Elderly individuals are highly dependent on the "atrial kick" (32). Consequently, anything that reduces venous return is apt to result in hypotension in elderly patients, and dysrhythmias such as atrial fibrillation can be devastating.

An additional reason for enhanced susceptibility to hypotension in elderly individuals is decreased responsiveness to β-adrenergic stimulation, presumably due to a reduced β-receptor affinity for agonists (33, 34). The changes in adrenergic responsiveness may be compounded in postsurgical patients, as suggested by Marty et al., who found that β-adrenergic receptor function was acutely altered in surgical patients (35).

Healthy elderly individuals display a decreased intrinsic heart rate, which was clearly demonstrated by Jose (36). After administration of propranolol and atropine to block both the sympathetic and the parasympathetic systems, intrinsic heart rates were determined in patients of various ages. Between 15 and 70 years of age, a linear regression equation was defined in which intrinsic heart rate equaled $117.2 - (0.53 \times age)$ (36). In another study, Rodeheffer et al. noted a decrease in resting heart rate with age and an age-related decrease in heart rate response to exercise (37). The protocol was controlled rigorously to include only patients who showed no cardiac abnormalities, i.e., (a) no clinical evidence of cardiac disease, (b) a normal resting electrocardiogram, (c) a normal exercise treadmill test conducted according to a rigorous protocol in which the subject was required to reach 90% of the predicted mean age-specific heart rate with no evidence of ischemia, (d) a normal maximum exercise thallium test, (e) an ejection fraction of greater than 0.5 at rest, and (f) no abnormal wall motion during exercise on a gated blood pool scan (Fig. 18–1).

In addition to the normal physiologic changes associated with aging, there are pathophysiologic changes associated with aging that also contribute to the likelihood of hypotension in the recovery room. The aging myocardium requires an increased length of time to achieve full relaxation (42). Evidence derived from animal data suggests that this slower relaxation might be related to the rate at which calcium is accumulated (43). More oxygen and energy are required for relaxation than for contraction. Consequently, this is the vulnerable period for hypoxia and ischemia. The stage is set for diastolic dysfunction that may result in heart failure. Beginning in the fifth decade of life, the incidence of congestive heart failure doubles among men every 10 years and every 7 years among women. Seventy five percent of these cases are secondary to hypertension or coronary artery disease (39).

Also related to the prevalence of coronary artery disease is the increased risk of myocardial infarction in the perioperative period. It is important to keep in mind that parasympathetic overactivity and hypotension occur in 65% of patients suffering an acute myocardial infarction (17).

In addition, Coriat et al. have shown that elderly patients with known coronary artery disease who have open cholecystectomies suffer significant declines in left ventricular ejection fraction in the immediate postoperative period (40). This finding may be due to the increased cardiac work associated with the early recovery period.

DIFFERENTIAL DIAGNOSIS

The important causes of postoperative hypotension that must be considered before deciding how best to treat an individual episode are listed in Table 18–5.

The causes can be divided easily into problems of preload, afterload, and intrinsic cardiac dysfunction. The most frequently seen preload problem is hypovolemia. Severe acidosis, leading to decreased afterload, may manifest as hypotension in the PACU. Acidosis, how-

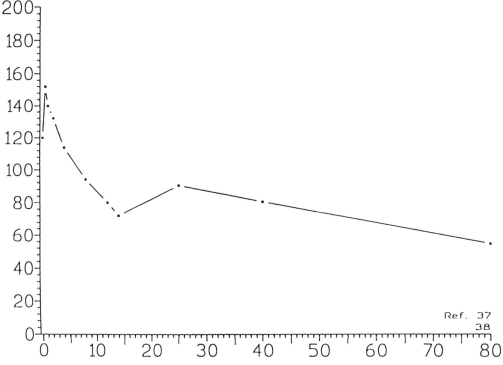

Fig. 18–1.   Effect of age on resting pulse rate. (Data from Rodeheffer RJ, Gerstenblith G, Becker LC, et al. Exercise cardiac output is maintained with advancing age in healthy human subjects: cardiac dilatation and increased stroke volume compensate for a diminished heart rate. Circulation 1984;69:203–213; and Shinbourne EA. Growth and development of the cardiovascular system: functional development. In: Davis JA, Dobbing J, eds. Scientific Foundations of Pediatrics. London: Heinemann, 1982;198–213.)

ever, is more often a result of a more serious problem, such as hypovolemia or ischemia.

Hypotension in the elderly patient is most often secondary to intrinsic myocardial dysfunction. The immediate postoperative period is associated with numerous factors likely to either increase myocardial oxygen demand or decrease oxygen supply. For example, oxygen demand may be increased by tachycardia and hypertension associated with pain and/or anxiety. Shivering increases oxygen demand fivefold. Oxygen supply may be decreased by hypoxemia and anemia, both common in the early postoperative period. In addition, tachycardia not only causes increased demand but may also decrease supply by virtue of decreasing coronary perfusion time. The elderly patient with coronary artery disease is especially vulnerable.

TREATMENT

It is important to treat hypotension rapidly in the elderly patient if one is to avoid such devastating complications as myocardial infarction, stroke, and renal failure. Even the healthy elderly patient is also at risk, albeit slightly less, if hypotension is left untreated.

The treatment obviously depends on the etiology of the hypotension. Most treatments are not specific to elderly patients and are discussed elsewhere.

Congestive heart failure, which is so common in the elderly, is often treated inappropriately. Force of contraction (systolic function) remains perfectly normal in most older patients. Even in patients older than 80 years of age with diagnosed heart failure, systolic function is normal in more than 50% of cases

Table 18–5.   Causes of Postoperative Hypotension

Preload Problems
Hypovolemia
  1. Blood loss
    a. Recorded
    b. Occult
  2. Inadequate fluid replacement
  3. Diuresis
  4. Bowel prep—unreplaced losses
Pharmacologic Sympathectomy
  1. regional anesthesia
  2. nitroglycerin, etc.
Histamine Release
  1. Drugs, e.g., morphine
  2. Blood products
Anaphylaxis
Sepsis
Tension pneumothorax or excessive airway pressures
Abdominal mass or tense ascites
Pulmonary embolus

Afterload Problems
Pharmacologic sympathectomy
  1. Regional anesthesia
  2. Nitroprusside, etc.
Severe acidosis
Anaphylaxis
Sepsis
Corticosteroid insufficiency

Intrinsic Cardiac Problems
Dysrhythmias[a]
Ischemia[a]
  —with left ventricular dysfunction
Decreased myocardial contractility[a]
  1. Intrinsic age, associated[a]
  2. Acute myocardial infarction[a]
  3. Residual drug effect[a]
    a. inhalation agents
    b. propofol
    c. β blockers
Cardiac Tamponade
Valvular Heart Disease
  e.g., acute regurgitation
    (possibly ischemic related)[a]
    (or myocardial infarction related)[a]

[a] Conditions found more commonly in the elderly.

(41). Instead, diastolic dysfunction is the primary cause of heart failure in the elderly (42). The treatment of diastolic dysfunction should be aimed at improving ventricular filling and relaxation rather than decreasing preload and flogging the heart with inotropes (the appropriate treatment for systolic dysfunction). Calcium channel blockers, β blockers, and angiotensin-converting enzyme inhibitors all have been useful for patients who have isolated diastolic dysfunction.

DELAYED AROUSAL

Delayed arousal is the second most common recovery room problem noted by Zelcer and Wells (1) (Table 18–1).

Although there is no specific evidence that delayed arousal is more common in elderly individuals, many of the physiologic changes in the central nervous system that occur with aging seem to support this concept (Table 18–6). Despite the substantial loss of neurons, synapses, and neurotransmitters and the increased destruction of neurotransmitters, the elderly individual functions quite well in an unstressed state. The central nervous system, like other organ systems, lacks *reserve capacity*. Because anesthesia and surgery are major causes of stress, one should anticipate that elderly patients may display central nervous system dysfunction. This dysfunction may be manifest by delayed arousal or confusional states (discussed later in this chapter). It is, however, imperative that the clinician also consider other causes of delayed arousal when faced with an elderly patient in the PACU who is unresponsive.

Table 18–6.   Physiologic Changes[a] in the Central Nervous System Associated with Aging

Decreased cerebral blood flow
Slowing of electroencephalographic alpha frequency
25–50% loss of neurons
Significant synapse loss
Decreased dopamine levels
  (as well as decreased precursors tyrosine hydroxylase and dopa decarboxylase)
Decreased choline acetytransferase
  (synthesizing enzyme of acetylcholine)
Increased activity of catabolic enzymes, monoamine oxidase, and catechol-o-methyl transferase

[a] All data from healthy elderly patients.

Differential Diagnosis

The differential diagnosis of delayed arousal is listed in Table 18–7. The most common cause of delayed arousal in the PACU is prolonged action of anesthetic drugs. Prolonged action of all drugs is common in elderly patients. Minimal alveolar concentration (MAC) for inhalation agents is decreased in

Table 18–7.   The Differential Diagnosis of Delayed Arousal

Prolonged action of anesthetic drugs
  Inhalation agents[a]
  Intravenous agents[a]
  Muscle relaxants[a]
Metabolic encephalopathy
  Hypoglycemia[a]
  Hyperglycemia[a] (68)
  Hypothyroidism[a] (67)
  Hyponatremia[a]
  Hypernatremia[a]
    (secondary to dehydration)
  Hypocalcemia
  Hypercalcemia
  Hypoxemia
  Hypercarbia
  Adrenal insufficiency
  Hypothermia[a]
  Acidosis
  Hypophosphatemia
  Hypermagnesemia
  Hypomagnesemia
  Nutritional deficiencies (cofactors)[a]
    B_{12}
    Niacin
    Folate
    Thiamine
    B_{16}
  Hepatic failure (ammonia)
  Renal failure (uremia)
Neurologic injury
  Cerebral ischemia[a]
    Hypotension
    Obstruction to flow
    (head position)
    Hemorrhage
      hypertension[a]
      anticoagulation[a]
  Cerebral embolism
  Seizures and postictal state
Delirium

[a] Conditions found more commonly in elderly patients.

Table 18.8   The Physiologic and Pharmacokinetic Changes of Normal Aging Effecting Intravenous Drug Distribution and Elimination

Distribution
  Decreased initial volume of distribution[a] (50–52)
  Increased free drug levels
  Decreased albumin[a,b] (53,54)
  Increased free drug levels
  Increased α-1, acid glycoprotein[a] (53)
  (No change in healthy elderly) (54)
  Decreased lean body mass[a] (49)
  Increased body fat[a] (49)

Elimination
  Decreased hepatic mass[b] (57)
  Decreased hepatic blood flow[a] (57)
  Decreased renal blood flow[a] (58)
  Decreased glomerular filtration[a] (58)

[a] All elderly
[b] Healthy elderly

an almost linear fashion from youth to senescence (45, 46). Electroencephalographic evidence suggests that there is, at least in the case of isoflurane, an increased cortical sensitivity to inhalation agents in elderly patients (47). Inadvertent overdose is a real possibility. In addition, age alters the pharmacokinetics of inhaled anesthetics (48). Recovery from inhaled agents proceeds more slowly in the elderly than in younger subjects. The changes observed are compatible with decreased tissue perfusion and the increase in fat/lean body mass known to occur as a function of the normal aging process (49).

The pharmacokinetic profile of intravenously administered drugs is also altered significantly. A decrease in the dose required and an increase in the duration of action is common in elderly patients. The normal age-related physiologic and pharmacokinetic changes that alter intravenous drug distribution and elimination are delineated in Table 18–8. Smaller initial volumes of distribution (50–52) lead to higher levels of free drug in the plasma. This is especially important with the centrally acting drugs. In addition, because many drugs are protein-bound, alterations in protein binding affect the pharmacokinetics and pharmacodynamics of many commonly used drugs. Drugs bound to proteins are not free to act at specific receptor sites. Mainly acidic drugs are bound to serum albumin. Among the most important of these, from the standpoint of delayed arousal in the PACU, are the benzodiazepines. Midazolam has been shown to be 94% protein bound (55). In this instance, if there is a 20% reduction in albumin, the amount of drug free in the plasma is increased fourfold. A dose that is perfectly acceptable in a young person may represent a fourfold overdose in an elderly individual. Basic drugs are bound to α-1 acid glycoprotein. Local anesthetics and narcotics are important members of this group. α-1-glycoprotein levels are unchanged in healthy elderly patients (54) but tend to increase in patients with diseases such as malignancy, rheumatoid arthritis, and myocardial infarction (56). Intravenous drug clearance decreases in elderly patients as a result of diminished functioning of the two most important organs responsible for elimination, the liver (57) and the kidney (58).

The action of muscle relaxants also may be prolonged in aged patients. Residual muscle paralysis may be mistaken for delayed arousal. The following muscle relaxants have been shown to exhibit a prolonged effect in elderly patients as compared to younger patients: pancuronium (59), vecuronium (60), d-tubocurare and metacurine (61), rocuronium (62), doxacurium (63), and mivacurium (64). This effect is not seen with atracurium. Although atracurium clearance via the liver and kidney is decreased in elderly patients, clearance via Hoffman elimination and ester hydrolysis is increased (65). Consequently, no net change in the duration of action of atracurium between old and young patients is noted. Likewise, the duration of action of pipercuronium does not seem to be altered by age (66).

A less common cause of delayed arousal in elderly patients is some form of metabolic encephalopathy. Hypothyroidism (67) and hyperglycemia (68) are two of the more common potential causes of delayed arousal that

often go undiagnosed until some precipitating event, such as anesthesia and surgery, bring these conditions to light.

Although a high percentage of elderly patients presenting for surgery have cerebrovascular disease (2), fewer than 1% suffer postoperative cerebrovascular accidents (2, 69). Nonetheless, this and other types of neurologic injury must be ruled out when an elderly patient fails to arouse from general anesthesia.

Delirium may also present as a reduced level of consciousness and psychomotor activity. This subject is discussed in detail later in this chapter.

Diagnosis and Treatment

Finding the true cause of delayed arousal among the many causes set forth in Table 18–7 requires a complete neurologic examination, evaluation of the neuromuscular junction, arterial blood gases, electrolytes, and a full metabolic assessment. It is prudent and certainly more economical to consider reversal of the possible effects of anesthetic agents before doing a battery of laboratory tests.

Naloxone, a specific narcotic antagonist, may be useful to reverse not only the general somnolence associated with narcosis but also any concomitant hypercarbia and hypoxemia that may be associated. Naloxone also has been noted to reverse new postoperative hemiplegia (70). It must be noted, however, that naloxone is associated with adverse effects that are potentially very harmful to an elderly patient. These detrimental effects include severe hypertension (71), rupture of a cerebral aneurysm (72), pulmonary edema (73–75), and sudden death (76).

Flumazenil is a specific benzodiazepine antagonist that is apparently safe and effective for reversing excessive somnolence secondary to benzodiazepines (77). The duration of action of flumazenil, however, is short enough (0.7 to 1.8 hours) that resedation may occur (78).

If anticholinergic effects of a centrally active drug such as scopolamine or atropine is suspected, physostigmine is a useful antagonist (79, 80). It must be noted that elderly patients are particularly prone to this anticholinergic syndrome (81).

PAIN

Postoperative pain occurred in 9% of recovery room patients studied by Zelcer and Wells (1) (Table 18–1).

Despite the fact that postoperative pain has been associated with an increased incidence of nausea and/or vomiting (82), acute confusional states (83), and postoperative complications such as atelectasis (84) in elderly patients, pain remains largely undertreated (85).

Acute pain assessment and treatment of elderly patients received little attention in the literature before the 1990s. In 1992, the United States government focused attention on acute pain management. The U.S. Department of Health and Human services, in conjunction with the Public Health Service and Agency for Health Care Policy and Research, published a clinical practice guideline (86) with the proclaimed goals of (*a*) reducing the incidence and minimizing the severity of postoperative and posttraumatic pain; (*b*) educating patients about the importance of communicating unrelieved pain to facilitate prompt evaluation and treatment; (*c*) promoting patient comfort and satisfaction; (*d*) reducing the frequency of potential postoperative complications and possibly decreasing the length of hospital stay after surgical procedures.

Evidence suggests that although elderly patients report more pain relief after analgesic administration (87, 88), they actually perceive pain initially to the same degree as their younger counterparts (89). The important pharmacokinetic differences between old and young patients with respect to commonly used analgesic drugs are shown in Table 18–9. The volume of distribution is consistently lower in elderly patients than in the younger ones, which means that more drug is available to cross the blood-brain barrier and exert its effect on the brain. Consequently, brain recep-

Table 18–9. Analgesic Pharmacokinetics: Young versus Old

	YOUNG	OLD
MORPHINE		
Volume of distribution (L/kg)	2.12 (90)	1.16 (90)
Elimination half-time (minutes)	104 (91)	270 (92)
Clearance (mL/min/kg)	23 (91)	12 (92)
FENTANYL (93)		
Volume of distribution (L/kg)	2.27	1.36
Elimination half-time (minutes)	133	103
Clearance (mL/min/kg)	13.9	13.1
SUFENTANIL (52)		
Volume of distribution (L/kg)	4.1	2.5
Elimination half-time (minutes)	141	156
Clearance (mL/min/kg)	21	12.7
BUPIVACAINE (epidural) (94)		
Elimination half-time (minutes)	457	585
Clearance (mL/min)	514	332

tor saturation may be greater in elderly patients, accounting for the observed need for a lower dose of analgesic (95). Longer elimination half-times and slower clearances account for the fact that elderly patients remain pain free for longer periods of time after analgesic administration (96).

Veering et al. have shown that epidural doses of bupivacaine achieve a higher level and faster onset in elderly patients as opposed to younger patients. The physiologic changes associated with aging may help explain this phenomenon. Sclerotic intervertebral foramina may limit the lateral escape of anesthetic solution. In addition, like the brain, the spinal cord loses neurons steadily with advancing age, resulting in faster saturation of the neuronal population in elderly patients. If lateral escape of anesthetic solution is limited, duration also would be expected to increase with age. It is surprising that this study did not demonstrate an increased duration of action of epidural anesthesia in elderly patients, because the investigators demonstrated delayed plasma clearance of bupivacaine (94).

Older patients do get consistently better pain relief of longer duration at the same dose (70 µg/kg) of epidural morphine appropriate for younger patients (89). Smaller doses (2 mg) administered to older patients have been found to be as effective as larger doses (5 mg) administered epidurally to younger patients (97). The physiologic factors noted above may explain this phenomenon.

PACU management of pain begins with a full assessment. It is important that the patient participate in the initial and subsequent assessments because nurse and patient assessments differ significantly, with the nurse consistently reporting lower scores (98). Although the simple act of asking the patient if he or she has pain is helpful, it is also important to quantify the amount of pain perceived by the patient. Several instruments have been described for use with elderly patients (99). These include the visual analog scale (ranging from no pain to worst pain), a numerical rating scale (least, 0; worst, 10), a numerical descriptor scale (0, no pain; 1, mild pain; 2, distressing pain; 3, severe pain; 4, horrible pain; 5, excruciating pain), and an observational behavioral faces scale. Of these scales, only the latter is appropriate for use with the patient who is unable to communicate or cooperate in the assessment procedure.

Although physicians may order sufficient doses of pain medication, nurses consistently give less than half of the amount ordered. A recent survey of intensive care units revealed that patients continued to be in pain despite the administration of pain treatment (30 to 36% of the ordered amount) (100). This underscores the fact that pain must be reassessed after the therapeutic intervention to ensure adequate control.

When narcotics are administered in the recovery room, either by intravenous bolus, by patient-controlled analgesia devices, or intramuscularly, respiratory depression can and does occur (101). Additional side effects of opioids include central nervous system effects (sedation, confusion, hallucinations, etc.) and gastrointestinal effects (nausea, vomiting, constipation). Nonsteroidal anti-inflammatory drugs (NSAIDs) are frequently used in the elderly postoperative patient for their narcotic sparing effect (102). The elderly patient, however, may be more susceptible to adverse side effects of NSAIDs, renal impairment, bleeding problems, and hepatotoxicity. Studies to confirm or deny this supposition in healthy elderly patients have yet to be reported.

ISCHEMIA/DYSRHYTHMIAS

Zelcher and Wells (1) note electrocardiographic evidence of ischemia or dysrhythmias in 8% of patients during their recovery room stay (Table 18–1).

Ischemia

Coronary artery disease is frequent in elderly patients (103). In men, the incidence increases in a linear fashion from 50 to 80 years of age and then levels off (104). This phenomena is delayed in women until after the menopause.

Hollenberg et al. (The Study of Perioperative Ischemia Research Group) have noted coronary artery disease to be one of the factors predictive of postoperative myocardial ischemia in patients undergoing noncardiac surgery (105). Additional factors identified include left ventricular hypertrophy, hypertension, diabetes mellitus, and digoxin use. These investigators noted the incidence of postoperative myocardial ischemia to vary between 22% for patients with none of the five predictors and 97% for patients with four of the five predictors.

Most ischemia episodes among elderly patients in the postoperative period are silent, that is, not associated with perceived pain (106). The reason for this seems to be twofold: first, silent ischemia is more common in elderly patients (107); secondly, the pain may not be perceived because narcotics given for postsurgical pain may mask its presence or the intensity of the postsurgical pain may overshadow the pain associated with myocardial ischemia. Evidence suggests that postoperative ischemia is associated with adverse cardiac outcome, including myocardial infarction and death (106). Of additional interest is the fact that, of those who survive a myocardial infarction, 63% will suffer another ischemic episode in the months after surgery (108, 109).

Given this information, it seems perfectly obvious that such ischemic events should be avoided or promptly treated. Mangano et al. (The Study of Perioperative Ischemia Research Group) (106) have noted that silent postoperative ischemia is related to chronically elevated heart rate. Presumably, tachycardia increases myocardial oxygen demand, thereby disrupting the delicate balance between myocardial oxygen supply and demand. Simple postoperative maneuvers such as prompt pain control, prevention of hypoxia, hypercarbia, and hypothermia, as well as close attention to fluid balance, may decrease the incidence of tachycardia and thereby the incidence of postoperative myocardial ischemia.

TREATMENT

Nitroglycerin is the most commonly used drug for the treatment of myocardial ischemia; however, the conscious elderly patient may have an exaggerated hypotensive response to nitroglycerin (29). Specific features of additional therapeutic agents such as β blockers and calcium channel blockers have been discussed previously in this chapter.

Table 18–10. Anatomic Changes[a] in the Hearts of Healthy Elderly Subjects

Decreased muscle in the sinoatrial node (113)
  (half that of younger subjects)
Increased fibrosis in internodal tracts (113)
  (twice that of younger subjects)
Increased interstitial fibrosis (114)
Amyloidosis (114)
  Pancardic   (23% of specimens)
  Atrial only   (43% of specimens)

[a] Changes believed to be responsible for the observed increase in all dysrhythmias.

Dysrhythmias

Even when patients are carefully screened to exclude coronary artery disease, the incidence of all dysrhythmias increases in frequency with advancing age (110). Of the tachydysrhythmias, only atrial fibrillation seems to have any effect on mortality in patients free of coronary or valvular heart disease. In the case of atrial fibrillation, embolic phenomena seem to be the cause of this increased mortality. Premature ventricular contractions occur in 70 to 80% of otherwise healthy elderly patients (111, 112). Asymptomatic ventricular tachycardia occurs in 4% of these patients. None of the bradydysrhythmias have a known independent effect on mortality (110).

Postmortem studies have defined specific anatomic changes associated with the normal aging process (113, 114) (Table 18–10). These changes are believed to be responsible for the observed increase in all dysrhythmias in healthy elderly individuals.

Not all dysrhythmias observed in elderly patients in the postoperative period are the result of the normal aging process. The common pathologic, potentially treatable causes of dysrhythmias are listed in Table 18–11.

TREATMENT

Causes listed in Table 18–11 are, in most cases, best treated directly rather than by suppression of the secondary dysrhythmia.

Table 18–11.   Pathologic Causes of Dysrhythmias Seen in Elderly Recovery Room Patients

Coronary artery disease
  Ischemia
  Infarction
Electrolyte abnormalities
  Hypokalemia
  Hypomagnesemia
Hypoxia
Hypercarbia
Drugs
  (e.g., digitalis, cholinesterase inhibitors, local anesthetics, β blockers, methylxanthines, etc.)
Intracardiac catheters
Severe poorly compensated pulmonary disease
  (multifocal atrial tachycardia)
Pulmonary embolus
  (atrial fibrillation)

The Study of Perioperative Ischemia Research Group suggests that ventricular dysrhythmias occurring postoperatively, in patients at high risk for ischemia (those with known coronary artery disease or at high risk for coronary artery disease), need not be aggressively monitored or treated unless other symptoms suggestive of myocardial infarction are present (116).

In instances in which drug therapy is chosen for dysrhythmia suppression, specific attention must be paid to the age-related changes in the pharmacology of the various antiarrhythmic drugs (Table 18–12).

NAUSEA AND VOMITING

Data from Zelcer and Wells (1) (Table 18–1) indicate that the incidence of nausea and vomiting in PACU patients is 5%. More recent data collected from a larger group of patients suggest that this incidence is higher, 9.8% (120).

Several studies suggest that the incidence of nausea and vomiting is actually less in elderly patients than in younger patients (83, 121, 122). The reason for this is unknown.

On the other hand, the most worrisome sequela of early postoperative nausea and vomiting, i.e., aspiration, may be more of a risk in elderly patients. Protective airway reflexes, evaluated by ammonia inhalation, are blunted with increasing age (123). Also, gastric pH increases with increasing age (124) (Fig. 18–2). These findings suggest that although aspiration is more common in elderly patients, it is potentially less serious.

AGITATION/DYSPHORIA

Zelcer and Wells (1) (Table 18–1) found a 3% incidence of agitation/dysphoria in the 443 PACU patients they studied. With respect to the elderly, the more common terms for this condition are "delirium" or "acute confusional state."

Delirium or acute confusional states are global disorders of cognition and attention that are characterized by an acute reduction in the level of consciousness, attention, perception, thinking, and memory; an abnormally increased or decreased level of psychomotor activity; and disturbed sleep-wake cycles. This is one of the most common forms of psychopathology in the elderly (125), occurring in 2.2 to 41% of patients undergoing

Table 18–12.   Age-Related Changes in the Pharmacology of Various Antiarrhythmic Drugs

DRUG	AGE-RELATED PHARMACOKINETIC CHANGES	RECOMMENDED THERAPEUTIC ALTERATIONS
Digoxin	Increased elimination half-life	Reduce maintenance dose; monitor serum levels
Quinidine	Increased elimination half-life Decreased clearance	Reduce maintenance dose
Lidocaine	Increased elimination half-time Decreased clearance	Reduce maintenance dose
Propranolol	Decreased clearance	Reduce maintenance dose

Fasting Gastric pH and Protective Airway Reflexes

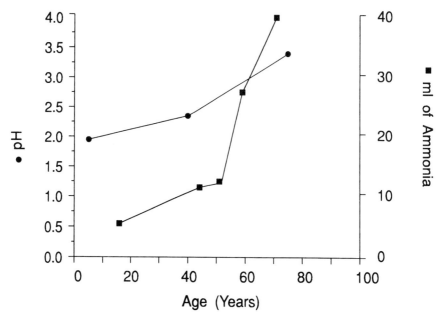

Fig. 18–2. Combined plots of protective laryngeal reflexes versus age. (Data from Pontoppidan H, Beecher HK. Progressive loss of protective reflexes in the airway with the advance of age. JAMA 1960;174:2209–2213; and Manchikanti L, Colliver JA, Marrero T, et al. Assessment of age-related acid aspiration risk factors in pediatric, adult, and geriatric patients. Anesth Analg 1985;64:11–17.)

anesthesia and surgery (2, 126–128). The presence of delirium is associated with significant morbidity and mortality. For example, delirious patients spend twice as many days in the hospital as nondelirious patients (129, 130, 134). Patients who are delirious upon admission to the hospital have been noted to have a 25% mortality rate (131). This high mortality may be secondary to the fact that delirium is often the presenting symptom of some life-threatening systemic disorder, such as bowel perforation, malignancy, heart failure, or uremia.

Some aspects of cognitive function decline with normal aging. For example, short-term memory, immediate memory, and divided and sustained attention all decline with advancing age, as does speed of central processing. This leads to difficulty in comprehension of complex material and problem solving (44, 132,

133). Again, this reduced reserve capacity may make the elderly patient more prone to cognitive dysfunction in the postoperative period.

Differential Diagnosis

Table 18–13 depicts the potentially reversible causes of delirium. Depression is an important risk factor for the development of postoperative delirium (134, 135). Tryptophan is a precursor of serotonin, the neurotransmitter involved in such functions as aggressive, impulsive behavior, mood, motor activity, and sleep. Tryptophan levels have been noted to be decreased in some situations in which postoperative delirium is common, such as after cardiac procedures (136). Almost any systemic illness may be associated with delirium, especially in elderly patients, but that of the endocrinopathies is potentially revers-

Table 18–13. Potentially Reversible Causes of Delirium

D	E	L	I	R	I	U	M
Depression (134,135)	Endocrinopathies Hypothyroidism Hyperthyroidism Hypercalcemia Hypoglycemia Hyperglycemia (130)	Lack of *nutrition*,[a] (137) especially subclinical *deficiency*[a] (138)	Infirmities *Hearing loss*[a] *Visual impairment*[a]	*Rx*: Scopolamine Narcotics (144) Benzodiazepines (142) Anticholinergics (134,138,141,142)	*Ischemia* (137,143,145) Cerebral: *TIAs*[a,b] *Strokes*[a] Cardiovascular: *MI*[a] *Dysrythmias*[a] *CHF*[a] Hypotension Hyperventilation Hypoxia (145,148)	Unrelenting pain (83) associated with trauma, surgical or environmental	Metabolic (130,137) *Hyponatremia*[a] *Hypernatremia*[a] *Azotemia*[a] *Acid-base imbalance*[a]
Decreased trace elements (Tryptophan) (136)	Environmental change (137,138) (*hospitalization*)[a]		*Impaction (fecal)*[a]	Digitalis (142) Anesthetics (140) Ketamine Barbiturates (142) Antihistamines (137)	*Infection*[a] Sepsis	*Urinary retention*[a]	Hepatic failure

[a] Commonly occurring in elderly patients.
[b] TIA, transient ischemic attack; MI, myocardial infarction; CHF, congestive heart failure.

423

ible. Environmental change (e.g., hospitalization) is a frequent cause of delirium in aged patients (137, 138). Goodwin et al. (139) have found a link between malnutrition and cognitive dysfunction. Infirmities of aging, hearing loss, and visual impairment may add to the effects of environmental change, especially when corrective lens and hearing aids are taken from the patient preoperatively. Fecal impaction and urinary retention, which are common in the elderly, are associated with delirium. Drugs are perhaps the most common causes of postoperative delirium. Anticholinergics such as scopolamine and atropine are well-known causes of delirium in elderly patients (134, 140–142). It is important to realize that anticholinergic activity is also possessed by other drugs commonly used in the perioperative period, for example, promethazine, diphenhydramine, chlorpromazine, meperidine, thiopental, and flurazepam (137, 142, 144). Cerebral ischemia is an important cause of delirium in the postoperative period. This ischemia may be of primary vascular origin as in transient ischemic attacks (TIAs) and strokes or may be secondary to hypotension, hyperventilation, or hypoxia (137, 143, 145, 147). Infection (sepsis) is another systemic illness commonly associated with delirium. Although narcotics, especially meperidine, can be associated with cognitive dysfunction in the elderly postoperative patient, Duggleby and Lander (83) found that pain rather than the administration of analgesics was more predictive of mental status decline. Finally, common metabolic abnormalities are also associated with delirium (130, 137).

Prevention

A study by Gustafson et al. (147) suggests that acute confusional states of elderly individuals, such as delirium, can be prevented. Anesthesiologists were successful in preventing a significant number of such events by careful preoperative and postoperative assessments, oxygen therapy, early scheduling of surgery, prevention and treatment of perioperative blood pressure declines, and prompt treatment of other postoperative complications. Total hospital stays in the intervention group were also shorter than in the nonintervention group.

Treatment

If a specific cause is identified, specific treatment of that cause is warranted, i.e., oxygen administration for hypoxemia or correction of metabolic abnormalities. When environmental factors are believed to be the cause, effective treatment may be as simple as returning a hearing aid or eye glasses or bringing familiar objects or family members into the environment.

Delirium caused by anticholinergic drugs or those with anticholinergic properties can be reversed by physostigmine. Patients may also be treated symptomatically with haloperidol. Although haloperidol is the least sedating and exhibits the least anticholinergic properties among neuroleptic drugs, it is associated with extrapyramidal side effects.

OLIGURIA

Oliguria is a clinically significant problem in 1% of recovery room patients (1) (Table 18–1).

Oliguria (urine output of less than 400 mL/day or an output of less than 0.5 mL/kg/hour) and acute renal failure (ARF) are more common in elderly patients (148, 149). The important age-related changes that affect renal function are listed in Table 18–14.

The 28% loss in renal mass seen in healthy elderly patients is primarily cortical. Medullary mass is spared. The 50% decrease in renal blood flow seen by 80 years of age is not simply proportional to the decrease in renal mass, because flow per gram of tissue falls progressively after the fourth decade. Although glomerular filtration rate (GFR) declines in two-thirds of the elderly population (149), serum creatinine may remain normal in elderly individuals until significant renal

Table 18–14.   Effect of Aging on the Renal System

Decreased renal mass (28% loss by eighth decade[b]
Diverticulae formation in distal nephron[b]
Sclerotic changes in walls of large renal vessels, arteriolar
   sparing[b]
Decreased renal blood flow (50% loss by 80 years of age[b]
   Medullary blood flow well preserved
   Decreased flow is largely cortical
   Decreased glomerular filtration rate (GFR)[a] (150,151)
   Decreased creatinine clearance[a] ($\downarrow$ of 8 ml/min/1.74
      m2/decade after the 4th decade (149)
   Decreased (30–50%) basal renin levels[a] (149)
      as a result
   Decreased (30–50%) plasma aldosterone concentra-
      tions (149)

[a] All elderly
[b] Healthy elderly

function is lost, because the muscle mass from which creatinine is derived declines to approximately the same degree as GFR. A simple formula that allows for the computation of creatinine clearance from creatinine values is

$$\text{Creatinine clearance} \atop \text{(mL/min)} = \frac{140 - \text{age (yr) (body weight) kg}}{72 \text{ (serum creatinine) mg/dL}}$$

For women multiply by 0.85

Creatinine clearance typically declines in a linear fashion beyond the fourth decade of life (149).

Although oliguria is not a completely reliable sign of impending ARF (152), it is the most serious ramification. Age is an independent risk factor for the development of ARF (153). Other predictive factors include preoperatively elevated serum creatinine or blood urea nitrogen, preoperative renal dysfunction, and left ventricular dysfunction (153). Aortic reconstructive surgery is also associated with a decline in renal function (154), which could progress to ARF, depending on the patient's preoperative renal function status. Renal hypoperfusion secondary to hypovolemia is a well known precipitant of ARF in elderly patients (155). Elderly patients frequently enter the hospital in a dehydrated state as a result of a disease process and associated symptoms

such as vomiting or diarrhea, poor fluid intake, or impaired renal ability to concentrate urine and conserve sodium (Table 18–14). Intragenically induced hypovolemia is another critical factor. Patients are sometimes kept NPO for a series of tests and then subjected to enemas as part of preoperative preparation. Unless careful attention is paid to fluid balance, ARF may result. In addition, the elderly patient encounters a number of nephrotoxic agents during any routine hospital stay. Hyperosmolar contrast material used for radiology studies may be especially damaging to the kidneys of elderly patients (155). Antibiotics of nearly every type have been implicated in ARF (155). Of more recent concern is the widespread use of parenteral nonsteroidal acute inflammatory drugs such as ketorolac. Renal dysfunction associated with these drugs is more common in elderly patients (156).

Differential Diagnosis and Treatment

When oliguria presents, a specific cause must be identified before appropriate treatment can be initiated. Postrenal causes should be ruled out first. Catheter obstruction caused by kinks or sludge should be sought. Irrigation is often sufficient to solve this problem. In the absence of a urinary bladder catheter, the elderly are especially prone to obstructive causes of oliguria. Elderly men are subject to bladder outlet obstruction secondary to enlarged prostate glands. Fecal impaction may cause outlet obstruction in patients of either sex. Additional causes of outlet obstruction include anticholinergic drugs and neuraxial narcotic administration (157). The latter two causes are treated easily by the insertion of a urinary bladder catheter. The former two outlet obstruction causes are also curable by the insertion of a catheter; however, insertion may be difficult and a suprapubic catheter may be necessary.

After catheter obstruction and bladder neck obstruction have been ruled out, the next most common cause of oliguria in elderly patients is hypovolemia. Tests of urine osmolality, urea nitrogen, and sodium may be of some diagnostic help; prerenal causes of oliguria are associated with high osmolality (>500 mOsmol/kg) and low sodium (<20 mOsmol/L). If the oliguria is secondary to renal causes (i.e., ARF), osmolality is not so high <350 mOsmol/kg) and urine sodium is high (>40 mmol/L).

After oliguria secondary to hypovolemia is diagnosed or suspected, consideration should be given to the insertion of a central venous pressure (CVP) or pulmonary artery catheter for the measurement of central pressures. This will help establish the diagnosis and guide therapy to improve the volume status without risking fluid overload, another potentially serious complication in the aged patient.

A fluid challenge of 200 to 500 mL should cause filling pressures to rise 2 to 3 mm Hg. If this rise is sustained, normovolemia is implied; if it falls to baseline in a space of a few minutes, hypovolemia is implied. A large (>3 mm Hg) sustained rise in central pressures with such therapy implies hypervolemia (155).

Some authors suggest a small test dose (0.1 mg/kg) of furosemide to help differentiate ARF from prerenal oliguria. This practice should be discouraged, however (155), because not only is there no evidence that it is beneficial, but further hypovolemia may ensue, increasing the risk that ARF will develop.

After prerenal and postrenal causes have been ruled out, we are left with the diagnosis of ARF. Here, large doses (1 to 2 mg/kg) of furosemide may be beneficial (159, 160). It must be remembered, however, that in high doses, furosemide itself may be nephrotoxic as well as ototoxic (155). Mannitol may be a better choice to establish a diuresis in an attempt to convert oliguric renal failure into nonoliguric renal failure. This may be especially important for elderly patients because fluid balance is much easier to maintain and mortality rates are lower in nonoliguric renal failure (161). Additional therapy with renal dose dopamine and vasodilators is also recommended (158).

Aggressive therapy of ARF may be associated with both pulmonary and cardiovascular complications. Pulmonary edema is a risk of excessive volume loading, whereas myocardial ischemia may result if left ventricular end-diastolic pressure is maintained too high. Elderly patients have an increased risk of both of these complications as a result of their reduced reserve capacity (see *Cardiovascular and Respiratory* section).

HYPOXEMIA/HYPERCARBIA

Hypoxemia and hypercarbia each occur in 1% of PACU patients according to the data of Zelcer and Wells (1) (Table 18–1).

Although hypoxemia and hypercarbia may occur separately, they often occur together. The ensuing discussion largely considers these two entities together.

Age-Associated Changes in Respiratory System Function

Table 18–15 lists age-associated changes in respiratory system function. Here, perhaps more than in any other area of study, little is known about functional changes resulting from age alone. The ubiquitous presence of cigarette smoking and environmental pollutants makes the identification of large groups of older unexposed individuals difficult.

When corrected for height, which tends to decrease in elderly individuals because of collapse of intervertebral spaces, total lung capacity (TLC) remains largely unchanged with increasing age (162). As the chest wall becomes stiffer and the lung parenchyma become less able to recoil because of changes in elastic fibers within the airway, residual volume (RV) increases. Functional residual capacity (FRC) also tends to increase, depending on the balance between these two opposing factors (163). Airflow rates are decreased in the elderly compared to younger patients (163). Consequently, they may have a limited ability to cough and clear secretions, leaving

Table 18–15. Age-Associated Changes[a] in Respiratory System Function

Volumes and capacities		
Total lung capacity	No change	(when corrected for height)
Residual volume	↑	(10–20 mL/yr beyond 20 years of age) (160)
Vital capacity	↓	(20–30 mL/yr beyond 20 years of age (162)
Functional residual capacity (FRC)	No change to ↑	(depending on compliance factors)
Compliance (163)		
Chest wall compliance	↓	(stiffening and calcification of costal cartilage)
Static lung compliance	↑	(decreased elastic recoil)
Airflow		
Forced expiratory volume (1 sec)	↓	($4\frac{1}{2}$ L/sec at 20 years of age ($2\frac{1}{2}$ L/sec at 80 years of age)
Maximum midexpiratory flow rate	↓	
Airway closure		
Closing capacity (CC)	↑	(CC exceeds supine FRC by 44 years of age and sitting FRC by 65 years of age (164) (leads to maldistribution of ventilation relative to perfusion)
Arterial oxygen tension (165,166)	↓	(see Fig. 18.3) (decreases 4 mm Hg per decade beyond 20 years of age 20) (165)
Control of breathing		
Ventilatory response to hypoxemia and hypercapnia	↓	(25% and 40%, respectively)
Sleep apnea (171) (central and obstructive)	↑	
Reserve capacity (162)		
Maximal voluntary ventilation	↓	(declines from 12× basal at 20 years of age to 7× basal by 90 years of age)

[a] All data from elderly patients.

them vulnerable to hypoxemia and hypercarbia in the postoperative period. Among the most common causes of hypoxemia in the postoperative period is maldistribution of ventilation relative to perfusion. In elderly individuals, compared to young individuals, this maldistribution begins secondary to the increase in closing capacity, which is a direct result of decreased elastic recoil of alveoli (164). The progressive decline in arterial oxygen tension with increasing age is illustrated in Figure 18–3 (165, 166). Typical ventilatory responses to hypoxemia in different age groups are depicted in Figure 18–4 (167, 169, 170). In response to hypoxia, the elderly adult increases ventilation only 25% of that of the middle-aged adult. Likewise, elderly individuals show a significantly reduced ventilatory response to hypercapnia (168). This altered response may explain the high incidence of both central and obstructive apneas noted in elderly individuals (171). Ventilatory reserve declines significantly with age. Maximum voluntary ventilation declines to 7× basal at 90 years age

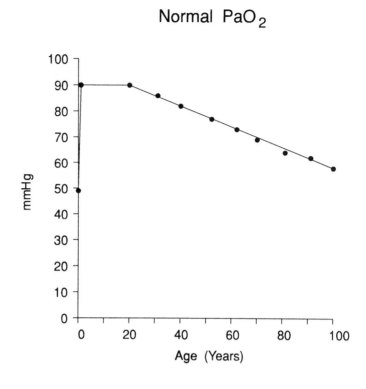

Fig. 18–3. Change in arterial oxygen tension versus age. (Data from Sorbini CA, Grassi V, Solina E, et al. Arterial oxygen tension in relation to age in healthy subjects. Respiration 1968;25:3–13; and Klaus M. Respiratory function and pulmonary disease in the newborn. In: Klaus M. Pediatrics. 15th ed. New York: Appleton Century Crofts, 1972;1255–1273.)

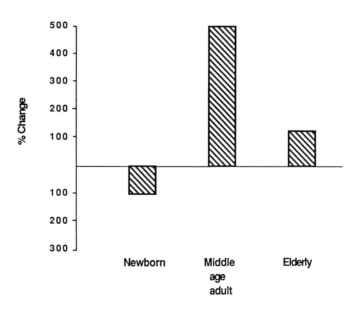

Fig. 18–4. Ventilatory response to hypoxemia in various age groups. Data from Kronenberg RS, Drage CW. Attenuation of the ventilatory and heart rate responses to hypoxia and hypercapnia with aging in normal men. Clin Invest 1973;52:1812–1819; Bryan AC, Bryan MH. Control of respiration in the newborn. In: Thibeault PW, Gregory GA, eds. Neonatal pulmonary care. 2nd ed. Norwalk, CT: Appleton Century Crofts, 1986;33–48; and Campbell EJ, Lefrak SS. Physiologic process of aging in the respiratory system. In: Krechel SW, ed. Anesthesia and the geriatric patient. Orlando, FL: Grune & Stratton Inc., 1984;23–43.)

from 12× basal at 20 years of age (162). It is important to remember that under conditions of upper abdominal or thoracic surgical stress, infection (sepsis) or other causes of hypermetabolism (e.g., prolonged high glucose loads during hyperalimentation), this reserve may be insufficient.

Respiratory System Functional Changes Associated with Anesthesia Surgery

Changes in pulmonary function occur with anesthesia and surgery (163, 172). These changes are more common in elderly individuals (171). Vital capacity, FRC, arterial oxygen tension, and compliance all decrease in the immediate postoperative period (172). These changes accentuate those that are associated with age (Table 18–15). In addition, residual anesthesia (0.05 to 0.1 MAC) levels of inhalation agents depress both hypoxic and hypercapnic ventilatory drive (175–178). Consequently, elderly patients, more so than their younger counterparts, are likely to suffer hypoxemia and/or hypercarbia during the immediate PACU stay and are less able to compensate for these adverse events.

DIFFERENTIAL DIAGNOSIS AND TREATMENT

Steps taken to diagnose and treat hypoxemia and/or hypercarbia in elderly patients are not different from those taken in younger patients and are discussed elsewhere in this text.

Laryngeal Spasm

Laryngeal spasm was noted to occur in 0.7% of PACU patients in the Zelcer and Wells study (1) (Table 18–1). Although specific data pertaining to the incidence of laryngospasm in elderly individuals are unavailable, clinical experience suggests that it is a rare occurrence. Figure 18–2 illustrates the fact that protective airway reflexes evaluated by ammonia inhala-

tion and most often manifest by laryngeal spasm are blunted with increasing age (124).

Hypothermia

Hypothermia, defined as core body temperature <36°C, is the final common PACU complication to be discussed. Zelcer and Wells (1) observed a 0.5% incidence in their study population (Table 18–1).

It has been observed that elderly patients arrive in postanesthesia recovery areas with lower body temperature than younger patients (179–181). Also, elderly patients remain hypothermic nearly twice as long as young patients (180, 181).

The age-related physiologic changes predisposing elderly patients to postoperative hypothermia are listed in Table 18–16. Basal metabolic rate decreases with age (182); consequently, elderly patients are not able to generate heat at the same rate as the young. Collins et al. (183) have demonstrated an impaired sensory perception of cold in individuals free of disease. Possibly the most relevant factor is the impaired thermoregulatory vasoconstriction capacity observed in the aged (185). Sessler et al. have determined that thermoregulatory vasoconstriction decreases cutaneous metabolic heat loss by 25% (188). Several investigators have demonstrated that during anesthesia, elderly patients are less able than young patients to respond with this protective thermoregulatory mechanism (186, 187).

Hypothermia may be especially hazardous for elderly individuals. The harmful effects of hypothermia that are most detrimental to el-

Table 18–16. Age-Related Physiologic Changes Predisposing Postoperative Hypothermia

Decreased basal metabolic rate[a] (181)
Impaired sensory perception of cold[b] (183)
Impaired thermoregulatory vasoconstriction capacity[a] (184,186,187,189)

[a]All elderly
[b]Healthy elderly

Table 18–17.   Negative Effects of Hypothermia: Special Relevance to Elderly Patients

Negative Effect	Relevance to Elderly
Shivering (O$_2$ consumption 5× basal) (189)	Reduced reserve capacity of respiratory and cardiovascular systems demand greater than supply (tissue hypoxemia).
Myocardial ischemia (190) (not related to shivering)	Elderly more prone to various degrees of coronary artery occlusion.
Increased muscle protein breakdown (191)	Increased postoperative catabolism leading to even longer recovery time.
Delayed awakening (192)	Arousal often slow in elderly patients without added effects of hypothermia.
Increased mortality (193)	Mortality rates high in elderly patients without adding additional risks.

derly patient are listed in Table 18–17. Shivering, which occurs postoperatively as the body attempts to rewarm itself, carries a very high metabolic cost. Oxygen consumption is increased fivefold (189). As previously noted in this chapter, the reduced reserve capacity of both the cardiovascular and respiratory systems may not be able to meet this excessive demand, and tissue hypoxemia may result.

Unrelated to shivering is the increased incidence of myocardial ischemia noted in patients whose core temperatures were allowed to fall below 35°C (190). Because aging is associated with varying degrees of coronary occlusion, such episodes of hypothermia-induced ischemia can be expected to be even more prevalent and perhaps more serious for elderly patients. Catabolism, as measured by muscle protein breakdown, is enhanced by perioperative hypothermia (191). The greater the degree of catabolism, the longer the recovery time. Finally, mortality is increased in patients admitted to the intensive care unit in a hypothermic state (193). Even in the absence of this added stress, elderly patients suffer a higher mortality rate than younger patients (194).

TREATMENT

The specific treatment of perioperative hypothermia is not different for elderly patients and is discussed elsewhere in this text.

CONCLUSION

E.A. Rovenstein, one of the pioneers of our specialty, stated that (195): "Anesthesia for those in the extremes of life was developed and improved for pediatric surgery earlier than for geriatric surgery. In pediatric surgery it was soon learned that from the anesthetist's point of view the infant was not a small adult. More recently there is the realization that, similarly, the aged are not to be considered merely as individuals of prolonged maturity" (195). Although these words were first published nearly 40 years ago, we are still discovering how true they are.

REFERENCES

1. Zelcer J, Wells DG. Anaesthetic-related recovery room complications. Anaesth Intensive Care 1987;15:168–174.
2. Stephen CR. The risk of anesthesia and surgery in the geriatric patient. In: Krechel SW, ed. Anesthesia and the geriatric patient. New York: Grune and Stratton, 1984;231–246.
3. Kannel WB, Dawber TR, McGee DL. Perspectives on systolic hypertension. The Framingham Study. Circulation 1980;61:1179–1182.
4. Psaty BM, Furberg CD, Kuller LH, et al. Isolated systolic hypertension and subclinical cardiovascular disease in the elderly. JAMA 1992;268:1287–1291.
5. Lakatta E. Normal changes of aging. In: The Merck manual of geriatrics. Newark, NJ: Merck and Company Inc., 1990;310–325.
6. Palmer GJ, Ziegler MG, Lake CR. Response of norepinephrine and blood pressure to stress increases with age. J Gerontol 1978;33:482–487.
7. Gribbin B, Pickering TG, Sleight P, et al. Effect of age and high blood pressure on baroreflex sensitivity in man. Circ Res 1971;29:424–431.

8. Duke PC, Wade JG, Hickey RF, et al. The effects of age on baroreceptor reflex function in man. Can Anaesth Soc J 1976;23:111–124.

9. Prys-Roberts C. Hypertension and anesthesia—fifty years on. Anesthesiology 1979;50:281–284.

10. Goldman L, Caldera DL. Risks of general anesthesia and elective operation in the hypertensive patient. Anesthesiology 1979;50:285–292.

11. McGuirt WF, May JS. Postoperative hypertension associated with radical neck dissection. Arch Otolaryngol Head Neck Surg 1987;113:1098–1100.

12. Wade JG, Larson CP Jr, Hickey RF, et al. Effect of carotid endarterectomy on carotid chemoreceptor and baroreceptor function in man. N Engl J Med 1970;282:823–829.

13. Bove EL, Fry WJ, Gross WS, et al. Hypotension and hypertension as consequences of baroreceptor dysfunction following carotid endarterectomy. Surgery 1979;85:633–637.

14. Fremes SE, Weisel RD, Baird RJ, et al. Effects of postoperative hypertension and its treatment. J Thorac Cardiovasc Surg 1983;86:47–56.

15. Gal TJ, Cooperman LH. Hypertension in the immediate postoperative period. Br J Anaesth 1975;47:70–74.

16. Morrison RC. Hypothermia in the elderly. Int Anesthesiol Clin 1988;26:124–133.

17. Pantridge JF, Adgey AAJ, Geddes JS, et al. In: The acute coronary attack. New York: Grune Stratton, Inc., 1975.

18. Parker M, Atkinson J. Withdrawal syndromes following cessation of treatment with antihypertensive drugs. Gen Pharmacol 1982;13:79–85.

19. Geyskes GG, Boer P, Dorhout Mees EJ. Clonidine withdrawal. Mechanism and frequency of rebound hypertension. Br J Clin Pharmacol 1979;7:55–62.

20. Hannson L. Clinical aspects of blood pressure crisis due to withdrawal of centrally acting antihypertensive drugs. Br J Clin Pharmacol 1983;15:485S–489S.

21. Farnett L, Mulrow CD, Linn WD, et al. The J-curve phenomenon and the treatment of hypertension. Is there a point beyond which pressure reduction is dangerous? JAMA 1991;265:489–495.

22. Lindblad U, Rastam L, Ryden L, et al. Control of blood pressure and risk of first acute myocardial infarction: Skaraborg hypertension project. Br Med J 1994;308:681–686.

23. Madhavan S, Ooi WL, Cohen H, et al. Relation of pulse pressure and blood pressure reduction to the incidence of myocardial infarction. Hypertension 1994;23:395–401.

24. Crane MG, Harris JJ. Effects of aging on renin activity and aldosterone excretion. J Lab Clin Med 1976;87:947–959.

25. Wikstrand J, Westergren G, Berglund G, et al. Antihypertensive treatment with metoprolol or hydrochlorothiazide in patients aged 60-75 years. JAMA 1986;255:1304–1310.

26. Abernathy DR, Schwartz JB, Plachetka JR, et al. Comparison in young and elderly patients of pharmacodynamics and disposition of labetalol in systemic hypertension. Am J Cardiol 1987;60:697–702.

27. Le Bret F, Gosgnach M, Baron JF, et al. Transesophageal echocardiographic assessment of left ventricular function in response to labetalol for control of postoperative hypertension. J Cardiothorac Vasc Anesth 1992;6:433–437.

28. Tjoa HI, Kaplan NM. Treatment of hypertension in the elderly. JAMA 1990;264:1015–1018.

29. Cahalan MK, Hashimoto Y, Aizawa K, et al. Elderly, conscious patients have an accentuated hypotensive response to nitroglycerin. Anesthesiology 1992;77:646–655.

30. Wood M, Hyman S, Wood AJJ. A clinical study of sensitivity to sodium nitroprusside during controlled hypotensive anesthesia in young and elderly patients. Anesth Analg 1987;66:132–136.

31. Haller BGD, Zust H, Shaw S, et al. Effects of posture and ageing on circulating atrial natriuretic peptide levels in man. J Hypertens 1987;5:551–556.

32. Bryg RJ, Williams GA, Labovitz AJ. Effects of aging in left ventricular diastolic filling in normal subjects. Am J Cardiol 1987;59:971–974.

33. Feldman RD, Limbird LE, Nadeau J, et al. Alterations in leukocyte β-receptor affinity with aging. A potential explanation for altered β-adrenergic sensitivity in the elderly. N Engl J Med 1984;310:815–819.

34. Kuramoto K, Matsushita S, Kuwajima I, et al. Comparison of hemodynamic effects of exercise and isoproterenol infusion in normal young and old men. Jpn Circ J 1979;43:71–76.

35. Marty J, Nimier M, Rocchiccioli C, et al. β-adrenergic receptor function is acutely altered in surgical patients. Anesth Analg 1990;71:1–8.

36. Jose AD. Effect of combined sympathetic and parasympathetic blockade on heart rate and cardiac function in man. Am J Cardiol 1966;18:476–478.

37. Rodeheffer RJ, Gerstenblith G, Becker LC, et al. Exercise cardiac output is maintained with advancing age in healthy human subjects: cardiac dilatation and increased stroke volume compensate for a diminished heart rate. Circulation 1984;69:203–213.

38. Shinbourne EA. Growth and development of the cardiovascular system: functional development. In: Davis JA, Dobbing J, ed. Scientific foundations of pediatrics. London: Heinemann, 1982;198–213.

39. McKee PA, Castelli WP, McNamara PM, et al. The natural history of congestive heart failure: the Framingham study. N Engl J Med 1971;285:1441–1446.

40. Coriat P, Mundler O, Bousseau D, et al. Response of left ventricular ejection fraction to recovery from general anesthesia. Anesth Analg 1986;65:593–600.

41. Luchi RJ, Snow E, Luchi JM, et al. Left ventricular function in hospitalized geriatric patients. J Am Geriatr Soc 1982;30:700–705.

42. Wei JY. Age and the cardiovascular system. New Engl J Med 1992;327:1735–1739.

43. Lakatta EG. Alterations in the cardiovascular system that occur in advanced age. Fed Proc 1979;38:163–167.

44. Katzman R, Terry R. Normal aging of the nervous system. In: Katzman R, Terry R, eds. The neurology of aging. Philadelphia: FA Davis, 1983;15–50.

45. Gregory GA, Eger EI, Munson ES. The relationship between age and halothane requirement in man. Anesthesiology 1969;30:488–491.
46. Stevens WC, Dolan WM, Gibbons RT, et al. Minimum alveolar concentrations (MAC) of isoflurane with and without nitrous oxide in patients of various age. Anesthesiology 1975;42:197–200.
47. Schwartz AE, Tuttle RH, Poppers PJ. Electroencephalographic burst suppression in elderly and young patients anesthetized with isoflurane. Anesth Analg 1989;68:9–12.
48. Strum DP, Eger EI II, Unadkat JD, et al. Age affects the pharmacokinetics of inhaled anesthetics in humans. Anesth Analg 1991;73:310–318.
49. Novak LP. Aging. Total body potassium, fat free mass and cell mass in males and females between ages 18-85 years. J Gerontol 1972;27:438–443.
50. Homer TD, Stanski DR. Effect of increasing age on thiopental disposition and anesthetic requirement. Anesthesiology 1985;62:714–724.
51. Berkowitz BA, Ngai SH, Yang J, et al. Disposition of morphine in surgical patients. Clin Pharmacol Ther 1975;17:629–635.
52. Matteo RS, Ornstein E, Young WL, et al. Pharmacokinetics of sufentanil in the elderly. Anesth Analg 1986;65:S94.
53. Verbeeck RK, Cardinal J-A, Wallace SM. Effects of age and sex on the plasma binding of acidic and basic drugs. Eur J Clin Pharmacol 1984;27:91–97.
54. Veering BT, Burm GL, Souverijn HM, et al. The effect of age on serum concentrations of albumin and α_1-acid glycoprotein. Br J Clin Pharmacol 1990;29:201–206.
55. Allonen H, Zeigler G, Klotz U. Midazolam kinetics. Clin Pharmacol Ther 1981;30:653–661.
56. Wood M. Plasma drug binding: implications for anesthesiologists. Anesth Analg 1986;65:786–804.
57. Wynne HA, Cope LH, Mutch E, et al. The effect of age upon liver volume and apparent liver blood flow in healthy man. Hepatology 1989;9:297–301.
58. Davies DF, Shock NW. Age changes in glomerular filtration rate, effective renal plasma flow and tubular excretory capacity in adult males. J Clin Invest 1950;29:496–507.
59. Duvaldestin P, Saada J, Berger JL, et al. Pharmacokinetics, pharmacodynamics and dose-response relationships of pancuronium in control and elderly subjects. Anesthesiology 1982;56:36–40.
60. Lien CA, Matteo RS, Ornstein E, et al. Distribution elimination and action of vecuronium in the elderly. Anesth Analg 1991;73:39–42.
61. Matteo RS, Backus WW, McDaniel DD, et al. Pharmacokinetics and pharmacodynamics of d-tubocurarine and metocurine in the elderly. Anesth Analg 1985;64:23–39.
62. Matteo RS, Orstein E, Schwartz AE, et al. Pharmacokinetics and pharmacodynamics of rocuronium (Org 9426) in elderly surgical patients. Anesth Analg 1993;77:1193–1197.
63. Koscielniak-Nielsen ZJ, Law-Min JC, Donati F, et al. Dose-response relations of doxacurium and its reversal with neostigmine in young adults and healthy elderly patients. Anesth Analg 1992;74:845–850.
64. Maddineni VR, McCoy EP, Mirakhur RK, et al. Mivacurium in the elderly: comparison of neuromuscular and hemodynamic effects with adults. Anesthiology 1993;79:A964.
65. Kitts JB, Fisher DM, Canfell C, et al. Pharmacokinetics and pharmacodynamics of atracurium in the elderly. Anesthesiology 1990;72:272–275.
66. Ornstein E, Matteo RS, Schwartz AE, et al. Pharmacokinetics and pharmacodynamics of pipecuronium bromide (Arduan) in elderly surgical patients. Anesth Analg 1992;74:841–844.
67. Sawin CT, Castelli WP, Hershman JM, et al. The aging thyroid. Thyroid deficiency in the Framingham Study. Arch Intern Med 1985;45:1386–1388.
68. Davidson MB. The effect of aging on carbohydrate metabolism: a review of the english literature and a practical approach to the diagnosis of diabetes mellitus in the elderly. Metabolism 1979;28:688–705.
69. Djokovic JL, Hedley-Whyte J. Prediction of outcome of surgery and anesthesia in patients over 80. JAMA 1979;242:2301–2306.
70. Krechel SW, Orr RM, Couper NB, et al. Naloxone: report of a beneficial side effect. J Neurosurg Anesthesiol 1989;1:346–351.
71. Azar I, Turndorf H. Severe hypertension and multiple atrial premature contractions following naloxone administration. Anesth Analg 1978;58:524–525.
72. Estilo AE, Cothrell JE. Naloxone, hypertension and ruptured cerebral aneurysm. Anesthesiology 1981;54:352.
73. Flacke JW, Flacke WE, Williams GD. Acute pulmonary edema following naloxone reversal of high dose morphine anesthesia. Anesthesiology 1977;47:376–378.
74. Partridge BL, Ward CF. Pulmonary edema following low dose naloxone administration. Anesthesiology 1986;65:709–710.
75. Prough DS, Raymond R, Bumgarner J, et al. Acute pulmonary edema in healthy teenagers following conservative doses of intravenous naloxone. Anesthesiology 1984;60:485–486.
76. Andree RA. Sudden death following naloxone administration. Anesth Analg 1980;59:782–784.
77. Geller E, Halpern P, Chernilas J, et al. Cardiorespiratory effects of antagonism of diazepam sedation with flumazenil in patients with cardiac disease. Anesth Analg 1991;72:207–211.
78. Klotz U, Zeigler G, Ludwig L, et al. Pharmacodynamic interaction between midazolam and a specific benzodiazepine antagonist in humans. J Clin Pharmacol 1985;25:400–406.
79. Duvoisin RC, Katz R. Reversal of central anticholinergic syndrome in man by physostigmine. JAMA 1968;206:1963–1965.
80. Holzgrafe RE, Vondrell JJ, Mintz SM. Reversal of postoperative reactions to scopolamine with physostigmine. Anesth Analg 1973;52:921–925.
81. Smith DS, Orkin FK, Gardner SM, et al. Prolonged sedation in the elderly after intraoperative atropine administration. Anesthesiology 1979;41:348–349.
82. Quinn AC, Brown JH, Wallace PG, et al. Studies

in postoperative sequelae. Nausea and vomiting-still a problem. Anaesthesia 1994;49:62–65.

83. Duggleby W, Lander J. Cognitive status and post-operative pain: older adults. J Pain Symptom Manage 1994;9:19–27.

84. Puntillo K, Weiss SJ. Pain: its mediators and associated morbidity in critically ill cardiovascular surgical patients. Nurs Res 1994;43:31–36.

85. Brockopp G, Warden S, Colclough G, et al. Nursing knowledge: acute postoperative pain management in the elderly. J Gerontol Nurs 1993;19:31–37.

86. Acute Pain Management Guideline Panel. Acute pain management: operative or medical procedures and trauma. Clinical Practice Guideline AHCPR Pub. No. 92-0032. Rockville, MD: Agency for Health Care Policy and Research Public Health Service, U.S. Department of Health and Human Services, 1992.

87. Bellville JW, Forrest WH Jr, Miller E, et al. Influence of age on pain relief from analgesics. JAMA 1971;217:1835–1841.

88. Moore AK, Vilderman S, Lubenskyi W, et al. Differences in epidural morphine requirements between elderly and young patients after abdominal surgery. Anesth Analg 1990;70(3):316–320.

89. Harkins SW, Price DD, Martelli M. Effects of age on pain perception: thermonociception. J Gerontol 1986;41:58–63.

90. Owen JA, Sitar DS, Berger L. Age-related morphine kinetics. Clin Pharmacol Ther 1983;34:364–368.

91. Murphy MR, Hug CC Jr. Pharmacokinetics of intravenous morphine in patients anesthetized with enflurane-nitrous oxide. Anesthesiology 1981;54:187–192.

92. Stanski DR, Greenblatt DJ, Lowenstein E. Kinetics of intravenous and intramuscular morphine. Clin Pharmacol Ther 1978;24:52–59.

93. Singleton MA, Rosen JI, Fisher DM. Pharmacokinetics of fentanyl in the elderly. Br J Anaesth 1988;60:619–622.

94. Veering BT, Burm AGL, van Kleef JW, et al. Epidural anesthesia with bupivacaine: effects of age on neural blockade and pharmacokinetics. Anesth Analg 1987;66:589–593.

95. Scott JC, Stanski DR. Decreased fentanyl and alfentanil dose requirements with age. A simultaneous pharmacokinetic and pharmacodynamic evaluation. J Pharmacol Exp Ther 1987;240:159–166.

96. Burns JW, Hodsman TTC, McLintock GW, et al. The influence of patient characteristics on requirements for postoperative analgesia. Anaesthesia 1989;44:2–6.

97. Ready LB, Chadwick HS, Ross B. Age predicts effective epidural morphine dose after abdominal hysterectomy. Anesth Analg 1987;66:1215–1218.

98. Bowman JM. Perception of surgical pain by nurses and patients. Clin Nurs Res 1994;3:69–76.

99. Ferrell BA. Pain management in elderly people. J Am Geriatr Soc 1991;39:64–73.

100. Tittle M, McMillan SC. Pain and pain-related side effects in an ICU and on a surgical unit: nurses' management. Am J Crit Care 1994;3(1):25–30.

101. Etches RC. Respiratory depression associated with patient-controlled analgesia: a review of eight cases. Can J Anaesth 1994;41:87–90.

102. Smallman JMB, Powell H, Wart MC, et al. Ketorolac for postoperative analgesia in elderly patients. Anaesthesia 1992;47:149–152.

103. Tejada C, Strong JP, Montenegro MR, et al. Distribution of coronary and aortic atherosclerosis by geographic location, race, and sex. Lab Invest 1968;18:49–66.

104. Lakatta EG, Fleg JL. Aging of the adult cardiovascular system. In: Stephen CR, Assaf RAE, eds. Geriatric anesthesia. Boston: Butterworth, 1985;1–26.

105. Hollenberg M, Mangano DT, Browner WS, et al. Predictors of postoperative myocardial ischemia in patients undergoing noncardiac surgery. JAMA 1992;268:205–209.

106. Mangano DT, Hollenberg M, Fegert G, et al. Perioperative myocardial ischemia in patients undergoing noncardiac surgery. I: incidence and severity during the 4 day perioperative period. J Am Coll Cardiol 1991;17:843–850.

107. Miller PF, Sheps DS, Bragdon EE, et al. Aging and pain perception in ischemic heart disease. Am Heart J 1990;120:22–30.

108. Mangano DT, Browner WS, Hollenberg M, et al. Association of perioperative myocardial ischemia with cardiac morbidity and mortality in men undergoing noncardiac surgery. N Engl J Med 1990;323:1781–1788.

109. Mangano DT, Browner WS, Hollenberg M, et al. Long-term cardiac prognosis following noncardiac surgery. JAMA 1992;268:233–239.

110. Fleg JL. Arrhythmias and conduction disorders. In: Abrams WB, Berkow R, Fletcher AJ, eds. The Merck manual of geriatrics. Newark, NJ: Merck & Co., 1990;370–379.

111. Camm AJ, Evans KE, Ward DE, et al. The rhythm of the heart in active elderly subjects. Am Heart J 1980;99:598–603.

112. Fleg JL, Kennedy HL. Cardiac arrhythmias in a healthy elderly population. Detection by 24-hour ambulatory electrocardiography. Chest 1982;81:302–307.

113. Davies MJ, Pomerance A. Quantitative study of ageing changes in the human sinoatrial node and internodal tracts. Br Heart J 1972;34:150–152.

114. Klima M, Burns TR, Chopra A. Myocardial fibrosis in the elderly. Arch Pathol Lab Med 1990;114:938–942.

115. Owens WD, Waldbaum LS, Stephen CR. Cardiac dysrhythmia following reversal of neuromuscular blocking agents in geriatric patients. Anesth Analg 1978;57:186–190.

116. O'Kelly B, Browner WS, Massie B, et al. Ventricular arrhythmias in patients undergoing noncardiac surgery. JAMA 1992;268:217–221.

117. Drayer DE, Lorenzo B, Werns S, et al. Plasma levels, protein binding, and elimination data of lidocaine and active metabolites in cardiac patients of various ages. Clin Pharmacol Ther 1983;34:14–22.

118. Abernathy DR, Greenblatt DJ. Impairment of lidocaine clearance in elderly male subjects. J Cardiovasc Pharmacol 1983;5:1093–1096.

119. Cusson J, Nattel S, Matthews C, et al. Age-dependent lidocaine disposition in patients with acute myocardial infarction. Clin Pharmacol Ther 1985;37:381–386.

120. Hines R, Barash PG, Watrous G, et al. Complications occurring in the postanesthesia care unit: a survey. Anesth Analg 1992;74:503–509.

121. Bellville JW. Postanesthetic nausea and vomiting. Anesthesiology 1961;22:773–780.

122. Cohen MM, Duncan PG, DeBoer DP, et al. The postoperative interview: assessing risk factors for nausea and vomiting. Anesth Analg 1994;78:7–16.

123. Pontoppidan H, Beecher HK. Progressive loss of protective reflexes in the airway with the advance of age. JAMA 1960;174:2209–2213.

124. Manchikanti L, Colliver JA, Marrero T, et al. Assessment of age-related acid aspiration risk factors in pediatric, adult, and geriatric patients. Anesth Analg 1985;64:11–17.

125. Lipowski ZJ. Delirium in the elderly patient. N Engl J Med 1989;320:578–582.

126. Millar HR. Psychiatric morbidity in elderly surgical patients. Br J Psychiatry 1981;138:17–20.

127. Cryns AG, Gorey KM, Goldstein MA. Effects of surgery on the mental status of older persons. A meta-analytic review. J Geriatr Psychiatry Neurol 1990;3:184–191.

128. Williams-Russo P, Urquhart BL, Sharrock NE, et al. Post-operative delirium: predictors and prognosis in elderly orthopedic patients. J Am Geriatr Soc 1992;40:759–767.

129. Thomas RI, Cameron DJ, Fahs MC. A prospective study of delirium and prolonged hospital stay. Arch Gen Psychiatry 1988;45:937–1040.

130. Marcantonio ER, Goldman L, Mangione CM, et al. A clinical prediction rule for delirium after elective noncardiac surgery. JAMA 1994;271:134–139.

131. Berggren D, Gustafson Y, Eriksson B, et al. Postoperative confusion after anesthesia in elderly patients with femoral neck fractures. Anesth Analg 1987;66:497–504.

132. Rabins PV, Folstein MF. Delirium and dementia: diagnostic criteria and fatality rates. Br J Psychiatry 1982;140:149–153.

133. Knoefel JE, Albert ML. Neurologic changes in the elderly. In: Kathic MR, ed. Geriatric surgery comprehensive care of the elderly patient. Munich: Urban & Schwarzenberg, 1990;153–164.

134. Goodnick P, Gershon S. Chemotherapy of cognitive disorders in geriatric subjects. J Clin Psychiatry 1984;45:196–209.

135. Folks DG, Freeman AM III, Sokol RS, et al. Cognitive dysfunction after coronary artery bypass surgery. South Med J 1988;81:202–206.

136. van der Mast RC, Fekkes D, Moleman P, et al. Is postoperative delirium related to reduced plasma tryptophan? Lancet 1991;338:851–852.

137. Jones MJT. The influence of anesthetic methods on mental function. Acta Chir Scand Suppl 1989;550:169–176.

138. Kuroda S, Ishizu H, Ujike H, et al. Senile delirium with special reference to situational factors and recurrent delirium. Acta Med Okayama 1990;44:267–272.

139. Goodwin JS, Goodwin JM, Garry PJ. Association between nutritional status and cognitive functioning in a healthy elderly population. JAMA 1983;249:2917–2921.

140. Smith RJ, Roberts NM, Rodgers RJ, et al. Adverse cognitive effects of general anaesthesia in young and elderly patients. Int Clin Psychopharmacol 1986;1:253–259.

141. Simpson KH, Smith RJ, Davies LF. Comparison of the effects of atropine and glycopyrrolate on cognitive function following general anaesthesia. Br J Anaesth 1987;59:966–969.

142. Tune LE, Bylsma FW. Benzodiazepine-induced and anticholinergic-induced delirium in the elderly. Int Psychogeriatr 1991;3:397–408.

143. Tune LE, Holland A, Folstein MF, et al. Association of postoperative delirium with raised serum levels of anticholinergic drugs. Lancet 1981;11:650–653.

144. Tune LE. Postoperative delirium. Int Psychogeriatr 1991;3:325–332.

145. Aakerlund LP, Rosenberg J. Postoperative delirium: treatment with supplementary oxygen. Br J Anaesth 1994;72:286–290.

146. Rosenberg J, Kehlet H. Postoperative mental confusion-association with postoperative hypoxemia. Surgery 1993;114:76–81.

147. Gustafson Y, Brannstrom B, Berggren D, et al. A geriatric-anesthesiologic program to reduce acute confusional states in elderly patients treated for femoral neck fractures. J Am Geriatr Soc 1991;39:655–662.

148. Abreo K, Moorthy V, Osborne M. Changing patterns and outcome of acute renal failure requiring hemodialysis. Arch Intern Med 1986;146:1338–1341.

149. Rowe JW. Renal systems. In: Abrams WB, Barkow R, Fletcher AJ. The Merck manual of geriatrics. Newark, NJ: Merck & Co., 1990;598–607.

150. Jose PA, Stewart CL, Rina LU, et al. Renal Disease. In: Avery GB, ed. Neonatology. 3rd ed. Philadelphia: JB Lippincott Co., 1987;795–849.

151. Rowe JW, Andres R, Tobin JD, et al. Age-adjusted standards for creatinine clearance. Ann Intern Med 1976;84:567–569.

152. Kellen M, Aronson S, Roizen MF, et al. Predictive and diagnostic tests of renal failure: a review. Anesth Analg 1994;78:134–142.

153. Novis BK, Roizen MF, Aronson S, et al. Association of preoperative risk factors with postoperative acute renal failure. Anesth Analg 1994;78:143–149.

154. Awad RW, Barham WJ, Taylor DN, et al. The effect of infrarenal aortic reconstruction on glomerular filtration rate and effective renal plasma flow. Eur J Vasc Surg 1992;6:362–367.

155. Seymor G. Kidney function and fluid balance in the elderly surgical patient. In: Medical assessment of the elderly surgical patient. Rockville, MD: Aspen Publications, 1986;189–223.

156. Mather LE. Do the pharmacodynamics of the non-steroidal anti-inflammatory drugs suggest a role in the management of postoperative pain? Drugs 1992;44:(Suppl 5):1–12.

157. Jacobson L, Chabal C, Brody MC. A dose-response study of intrathecal morphine: efficacy, duration, optimal dose and side effects. Anesth Analg 1988;67:1082–1088.
158. Prough DS, Zaloga GP. management of acute oliguria in the elderly patient. Int Anesthesiol Clin 1988;26:112–118.
159. Cantarovich F, Galli C, Benedetti L, et al. High dose furosemide in established acute renal failure. Br Med J 1973;4:449–450.
160. Mimuth AN, Terrell JB, Suki WN. Acute renal failure: a study of the course and prognosis of 104 patients and the role of furosemide. Am J Med Sci 1976;271:317–324.
161. Anderson RJ, Tinas SL, Berns AS, et al. Non oliguric acute renal failure. N Engl J Med 1977;296:1134–1138.
162. Smith TC. Respiratory effects of aging. Semin Anesthesia 1986;5:14–22.
163. Wahba WM. Influence of aging on lung function-clinical significance of changes from age twenty. Anesth Analg 1983;62:764–776.
164. Tockman MS. The effects of age on the lung. In: Abrams WB, Berkow R, Fletcher AJ, eds. The Merck manual of geriatrics. Newark, NJ: Merck & Co., 1990;423–432.
165. Sorbini CA, Grassi V, Solina E, et al. Arterial oxygen tension in relation to age in healthy subjects. Respiration 1968;25:3–13.
166. Klaus M. Respiratory function and pulmonary disease in the newborn. In: Pediatrics. 15th ed. New York: Appleton Century Crofts, 1972;1255–1273.
167. Kronenberg RS, Drage CW. Attenuation of the ventilatory and heart rate responses to hypoxia and hypercapnia with aging in normal men. J Clin Invest 1973;52:1812–1819.
168. Brischetto MJ, Millman RP, Peterson DD, et al. Effect of aging on ventilatory response to exercise and CO_2. J Appl Physiol 1984;56:1143–1150.
169. Bryan AC, Bryan MH. Control of respiration in the newborn. In: Thibeault PW, Gregory GA, eds. Neonatal pulmonary care. 2nd ed. Norwalk, CT: Appleton Century Crofts, 1986;33–48.
170. Campbell EJ, Lefrak SS. Physiologic process of aging in the respiratory system. In: Krechel SW, ed. Anesthesia and the geriatric patient. Orlando, FL: Grune Stratton, Inc., 1984;23–43.
171. Pack AI, Millman RP. Changes in control of ventilation, awake and asleep, in the elderly. J Am Geriatr Soc 1986;34:533–544.
172. Seymor G. The respiratory system in the elderly surgical patient. In: Medical assessment of the elderly surgical patient. Rockville, MD: Aspen Publications, 1986;24–77.
173. Nunn JF. Anesthesia and the lung. Anesthesiology 1980;52:107–108.
174. Knill RL, Gelb AW. Ventilatory responses to hypoxia and hypercapnia during halothane sedation and anesthesia in man. Anesthesiology 1978;49:244–251.
175. Knill RL, Manninen PH, Clement JL. Ventilation and chemoreflexes during enflurane sedation and anaesthesia in man. Can Anaesth Soc J 1979;26:353–360.
176. Knill RL, Clement JL. Variable effects of anaesthetics on the ventilatory response to hypoxemia in man. Can Anaesth Soc J 1982;29:93–99.
177. Knill RL, Kieraszewicz HT, Dodgson BG. Chemical regulation of ventilation during isoflurane sedation and anaesthesia in humans. Can Anaesth Soc J 1983;30:607–614.
178. Dahan A, Berkenbosch A, DeGoede J, et al. Effects of subanesthetic halothane on the ventilatory responses to hypercapnia and acute hypoxia in healthy volunteers. Anesthesiology 1994;80:727–738.
179. Goldberg MJ, Roe CF. Temperature changes during anesthesia and operations. Arch Surg 1966;93:365–369.
180. Vaughan MS, Vaughan RW, Cork RC. Postoperative hypothermia in adults: relationship of age, anesthesia, and shivering to rewarming. Anesth Analg 1981;60:746–751.
181. Frank SM, Beattie C, Christopherson R, et al. Epidural versus general anesthesia, ambient operating room temperature, and patient age as predictors of inadvertent hypothermia. Anesthesiology 1977;77:252–257.
182. Guyton AC. Body temperature, temperature regulation and fever. In: Textbook of medical physiology. 7th ed. Philadelphia: WB Saunders, 1986;849.
183. Collins KJ, Exton-Smith AN, Dore C. Urban hypothermia: preferred temperatures and thermal perception in old age. Br Med J 1981;282:175–177.
184. Collins KJ, Dore C, Exton-Smith AN, et al. Accidental hypothermia and impaired temperature homeostasis in the elderly. Br Med J 1977;1:353–356.
185. Richardson D, Tyra J, McCray A. Attenuation of the cutaneous vasoconstrictor response to cold in elderly men. J Gerontol 1992;47:211–214.
186. Kurz A, Plattner O, Sessler DI, et al. The threshold for thermoregulatory vasoconstriction during nitrous oxide/isoflurane anesthesia is lower in elderly than in young patients. Anesthesiology 1993;79:465–469.
187. Frank SM, Shir Y, Raja SN, et al. Core hypothermia and skin-surface temperature gradients. Anesthesiology 1994;80:502–508.
188. Sessler DI, Moayeri A, Stoen R, et al. Thermoregulatory vasoconstriction decreases cutaneous heat loss. Anesthesiology 1990;73:656–660.
189. Horvath SM, Spurr GB, Hutt BK, et al. Metabolic cost of shivering. J Appl Physiol 1956;8:595–602.
190. Frank SM, Beattie C, Christopherson R, et al. Unintentional hypothermia is associated with postoperative myocardial ischemia. Anesthesiology 1993;78:468–476.
191. Cali F, Itiaba K. Effect of heat conservation during and after major abdominal surgery on muscle protein breakdown in elderly patients. Br J Anaesth 1986;58:502–507.
192. Flacke JW, Flacke WC. Impaired thermoregulation and perioperative hypothermia in the elderly. Clin Anesthesiol 1986;4:859–880.
193. Slotman GJ, Jed EH, Burchard KW. Adverse effects of hypothermia in postoperative patients. Am J Surg 1985;149:495–501.
194. Tompkins RG, Welch CE. Surgery: preoperative evaluation and intraoperative and postoperative

cure. In: Abrams WB, Berkow R, Fletcher AJ, eds. The Merck manual of geriatrics. Newark, NJ: Merck & Co., 1990;225–229.

195. Rovenstine EA. Geriatric anesthesia. Geriatrics 1956;1:46–53.

19

SPECIAL CONSIDERATIONS FOR THE PEDIATRIC PATIENT

Steven C. Hall

Most children receive surgical, anesthetic, and nursing care in institutions that care for both children and adults. Only a minority of children receive surgical care in specialized children's hospitals. For this reason, the provision of postanesthesia care units (PACUs) that are capable of caring for pediatric surgical patients is an important part of improving pediatric care in general. This involves facility and staff preparation, education, and ongoing reeducation.

One of the most common mottoes of pediatric healthcare professionals is "children are *not* small adults!" Several studies (1–5) have shown that the pattern of complications in the PACU is different for pediatric patients than for adult patients. These studies have also shown significant differences between children of different ages. For an institution's PACU to be able to care for children of all ages, the facility and its staff must understand the unique challenges and requirements of pediatric patients.

SETUP OF THE PEDIATRIC PACU UNIT

A PACU that is properly arranged, equipped, and staffed for pediatric patients can be an invaluable resource for the institution (6). The postanesthetic period is a crucial time for surgical patients; without the facilities and staff to monitor and treat pediatric patients, the total health care delivered to those

children is in jeopardy. A well-run PACU not only ensures a high level of care for these diverse patients but is also a positive public relations tool for pleasing families and attracting additional business to the institution. The PACU that is prepared to care for children can also serve as a backup to the pediatric intensive care unit (ICU), as well as a triage area for pediatric trauma, an overflow area for pediatric patients who need overnight admission, a procedure area for functions such as cardioversion, and diagnostic or therapeutic pain management procedures.

The PACU should be physically near the operating room suites to minimize the time required for transport of children. There is the possibility for airway obstruction, vomiting, loss of body heat, and other complications during the transport period (7). By ensuring that transport time is short, it is possible to minimize the chance that a significant complication will occur in a setting in which the anesthesiologist is not equipped to provide proper care. One aspect of the transport to the PACU that was often overlooked in older facilities was the space requirement of corridors and doorways on the trip from the operating suite to the PACU. Although a crib or bed will usually fit through the corridor with ease, it may be necessary to use additional equipment, such as a freestanding cart with monitors and gases, to assist with the transport. The equipment, along with the accompanying personnel, must have adequate room to maneuver and have ready access to the patient throughout the move. If the corridor, elevator, or doorway is crowded, this represents a potential hazard to patient care.

A second concern about the distance from the PACU to the operating suites is the availability of emergency personnel. If physicians and/or additional nurses are needed for an emergency in the PACU, proximity of the PACU allows rapid response from operating room personnel. The PACU must have a means of rapid communication with operating room personnel to allow summoning of additional help. An intercom or audible paging system should be designed to guarantee that the needed personnel will clearly hear the call for help. Although telephone and paging systems can be used, they often are not as fast as an audible intercom system in alerting multiple personnel.

The physical space in the PACU should be arranged to allow easy access to each patient without interrupting care to other patients. Not only should there be adequate space between patients, but there should also be a means of providing privacy for each patient. Although individual recovery rooms or cubicles provide the maximum of privacy and noise reduction, they reduce access to the individual patient, as well as flexibility in the use of the PACU space. For these reasons, most PACUs have an open architecture with curtains or partitions between bed spaces. This is especially useful if a critically ill child requires an increased amount of equipment (ventilator, electroencephalogram monitor, multiple intravenous pumps, etc.) and personnel at the bedside. If parents are allowed into the PACU, there must be provision for the parents to stand or, preferably, sit while the bedside nurse has unimpeded access to the child.

The number of bed spaces in the PACU is determined by a several factors. Numbers as high as two or three bed spaces per operating suite have been suggested (8). A state regulatory requirement usually exists for the minimum number of acceptable bed spaces per operating suite. In the state of Illinois, the requirement is that there be one bed space per operating room. If the surgery schedule is composed of large numbers of short cases, such as ear tube surgeries and herniorrhaphies, the PACU may quickly fill with patients who stay in the unit longer than the time it takes for the next patient to have their surgery and be transported to the PACU for recovery. This "bunching" of patients can put a temporary, but significant, strain on the bed space availability. It is a common problem with pediatric patients because of the short nature of many pediatric procedures. Although the most common response to this is to build additional spaces, there are other alternatives. One effective alternative is creative scheduling of the operating room; there is agreement among surgeons, anesthesiologists, and operating room nurses that short cases will be interspersed with longer cases to allow the short cases to be recovered and discharged. Another alternative is to speed discharge of healthy patients to other, intermediate areas, such as the area from which the patient was admitted. This strategy works only if there are adequately trained staff and facilities in those areas. A third alternative is to cluster children who have awakened but are not yet ready for discharge in one section of the PACU with less space and nursing coverage than in the area where patients are initially admitted.

Each bed space should be designed to provide adequate monitoring of the patient, as well as therapeutic intervention (6). Every site should have equipment and monitors that are suitable for the age and size of the full range of patients that may be recovered. There must be a reliable source of oxygen at each bedside; this is usually piped-in oxygen from a central source in most institutions. PACU personnel must be instructed in the location and use of the emergency shut-off valve in case of fire. There should also be backup source of oxygen that is at least the equivalent of an "E" cylinder. If preterm (<37 weeks gestation) and expreterm infants will be recovered in the unit, there may be a need to administer enriched oxygen at levels less than 100% to minimize the risk of retinopathy of prematurity. For these sites, there should be an additional source of air or nitrogen that mixes with oxygen in a blender and is then measured by an oxygen analyzer before going through a flowmeter to the administering device.

The oxygen source will usually be attached to an appropriately sized mask or nasal prongs. However, there must be readily available self-inflating resuscitation bags of appropriate size that are capable of delivering >90% oxygen when attached to the oxygen source. Because of the range of sizes of pediatric patients, at least two different sizes of bag are needed; this usually consists of a neonatal/infant bag and a child/adolescent bag. It may be desirable to have other, additional means of delivering oxygen and positive airway pressure if the staff prefers using them. A Jackson-Rees, Bain, or other similar circuit may be selected because of staff familiarity with these circuits. Each bedside must be equipped with an array of ventilating mask and oral and nasal airways that are appropriate for each age of child that will be cared for at the site. Lastly, a ventilator should be readily available in case a child needs prolonged mechanical ventilation. The operation of the ventilator should be familiar to the staff.

Other equipment that should be available at the bedside includes suction and various sizes of suction catheters. Because of the significant incidence of vomiting in patients and the consequent risk of aspiration, it is useful to keep the suction active during the working day, with a tonsil or other rigid suction tube attached. Other considerations include adequate lighting and electrical outlets. A minimum of the lighting and outlets must be attached to dedicated emergency power circuits to allow evaluation and treatment of the patient in the event of an institution-wide power failure. Each PACU should have adequate numbers of heating lights, heating blankets, and fluid warmers (9, 10), as well as intravenous fluid pumps, pediatric intravenous fluid administration sets, and protective bed pads (for combative patients).

Each bedside should be equipped with monitors and probes or electrodes that are age appropriate (Table 19–1). A pediatric variety of blood pressures cuffs, pulse oximeter probes, temperature probes, and capnograph leads should be available and the staff should be familiar with their use. Standard monitoring of the PACU patient should include con-

Table 19–1. Equipment for Pediatric PACU

Monitors
 Pulse oximeter with pediatric/neonatal probes
 Blood pressure cuffs—neonatal through adult cuffs
 Doppler probe/monitor (for blood pressure measurement)
 Electrocardiogram
 Thermometer
 Capnograph or chemical CO_2 detector
Airway equipment
 Clear ventilation masks, neonatal to adult size
 Full range of oral and nasal airways
 Self-inflating resuscitation bag capable of administering >90% oxygen
 Two laryngoscope handles with variety of pediatric blades (minimum of Miller nos. 0 and 1, Macintosh nos. 2 and 3)
 Oxyscope blades (optional) for delivering O_2 during laryngoscopy
 Uncuffed endotracheal tubes (2.5 to 6.5 mm i.d.)
 Cuffed endotracheal tubes (5.5 to 8.0 mm i.d.)
 Stylets for all sizes of endotracheal tubes
 Cricothyrotomy set
 Suction catheters of all sizes
 Oxygen/air blender with appropriately sizes masks
 Ultrasonic mist generator
Cardiac equipment
 Pediatric fluid administration sets
 Pediatric intravenous catheters (20, 22, 24 gauges)
 Pediatric defibrillation paddles
 Bone marrow needles
 Cutdown tray
Other equipment
 Blood warmer
 Heating lights
 Cellophane film or other protective covering
 Warm blankets
Medications
 Standard resuscitation drug set
 Racemic epinephrine
 Dexamethasone
 Albuterol inhaler
Written list of drug doses for pediatric patients

tinuous pulse oximetry. Pulse oximetry has been shown to be accurate for all ages of children, including newborns (11–13). It has also been shown to be of great benefit in detecting hypoxemia in children (14, 15). Intermittent blood pressure can be accomplished by using a standard cuff or automated devices (16, 17). Temperature is often initially measured using an axillary temperature. However, core measurements should be used if there is any chance that the patient may be hypothermic (18, 19). Electrocardiogram (ECG) monitoring is used commonly for pediatric patients and should be readily available (20). However, it may not be as useful for the pediatric patient as for the adult patient. Myocardial ischemia and subsequent ECG changes are rare in children; although dysrhythmias can occur in children, the abnormal rate or rhythm can usually be initially detected by attention to the pulse oximeter. The ECG monitor is particularly useful when the patient is critically ill or at risk for dysrhythmias. It is also useful to measure and display waveform data if the child has intra-arterial, central venous, or intracranial catheters in place.

The nursing staff must be familiar not only with the use of monitors in children of different ages and sizes but also must understand the ranges of values expected at different ages (21–23).

Lastly, a resuscitation cart should be available. In addition to the normal equipment found in standard resuscitation carts, special attention should be paid to pediatric-specific equipment. There should be a variety of uncuffed and cuffed endotracheal tubes, stylets that will fit the different sizes of tubes, laryngoscope blades, masks, and oral and nasal airways (Table 19–2). There should also be pediatric fluid administration sets, 22- and 24-gauge intravenous catheters, a bone marrow needle, and pediatric paddles for the defibrillator. It should be noted that adult electrode paddles are more effective than pediatric paddles when the child weighs more than 10 kg (24). There should also be a device that is capable of detecting exhaled carbon dioxide,

Table 19–2. Recommended Endotracheal Tube Sizes

Patient Age	Internal Diameter (mm)	Type of Tube
Premature newborn	2.5–3.0	Uncuffed
Full-term newborn	3.0–3.5	Uncuffed
3 months	3.5	Uncuffed
1 year	4.0	Uncuffed
2 years	4.5	Uncuffed
4 years	5.0	Uncuffed
6 years	5.5	Uncuffed
8 years	6.0	Cuffed or uncuffed
10 years	6.5	Cuffed
12 years	7.0	Cuffed

such as a capnograph or chemical carbon dioxide detector (25, 26). There should be a protocol on the resuscitation cart that lists appropriate pediatric drug dosages and endotracheal tube sizes. Although barrier precautions should be used for all patients (27, 28), special consideration should be given to the potential for latex allergy in certain pediatric patients (29, 30). For this reason, consideration should be given to having only latex-free gloves, tourniquets, and fluid administration sets on all resuscitation carts. Unfortunately, latex is indigenous in the medical environment; multidose vials, dressings, and even flexible pulse oximeter leads can contain latex. Although it is a considerable challenge to eliminate latex-containing equipment from the environment, efforts should be directed to reducing the amount of exposure.

There is another part of the resuscitation cart that should be part of every pediatric critical care setting — a bone marrow or intraosseous needle. Intraosseous administration of fluid and drugs can be lifesaving when adequate vascular access is difficult (31–33). The most accessible site in children usually is the flat surface of the anterior (medial) tibia about an inch inferior to the epiphyseal plate. After insertion into the marrow, fluid administration is started. Care is taken to observe the leg to ensure that there is not extravasation. Through this access, it is possible to give all drugs used in resuscitation or general anesthesia, as well as crystalloid and colloid. This method of administration can be established quickly and allow emergency treatment of the patient until other vascular access is obtained.

Lastly, a chart that lists the doses needed for resuscitative drugs by weight should be included on the resuscitation cart. Because pediatric patients can be as small as less than a kilogram to adult size, drug doses must be tailored to the individual patient (34).

Staffing of the PACU in which children are recovered is crucial. Children come to the PACU with a wide variety of potential problems. Nursing staff must be familiar with the unique problems of pediatric patients if they are to effectively monitor and manage them. Children should have one-on-one coverage during their initial recovery phase so that the nurse can place close attention to the airway, respiratory, and cardiac status of the patient. As the patient regains consciousness, reflexes, and ability to maintain the airway, the need for close observation decreases. In the last phases of recovery, it may be possible for a single nurse to effectively observe more than a single patient. This must be performed only if the nursing staff is convinced that the children involved will not need closer observation.

What nurses should be assigned to pediatric patients? There are a couple of alternatives for institutions that admit both adult and pediatric patients to ensure that the nursing staff is adequately trained. The first alternative is to have an ongoing program of training and education for all PACU staff about the principles of safe pediatric care. This should be the joint responsibility of the nursing and anesthesia staffs and include materials that convey not only general pediatric medicine principles but also the proper role and responsibilities of nursing staff in the care of children. A second alternative is to hire personnel with specific pediatric training and assign them to these patients exclusively. In a busy unit, this may be a reasonable choice. However, most units will not be busy enough or have a consistent enough flow of pediatric patients throughout

the day to ensure that only the trained pediatric nurses care for all pediatric patients. On the other hand, these specially trained nurses can serve as a valuable resource and source of education and consultation for the unit. A third alternative is to cross-train nursing personnel in pediatric care and use them in the PACU when needed. The two likely other areas that use pediatric nurses are the outpatient admission area for the operating rooms and the pediatric intensive care unit. If outpatient nurses are used, a system can be employed in which the admitting nurse follows the child throughout the admission and recovery processes. From a nursing standpoint, this continuity of care is considered desirable. However, it does provide some logistic problems, the greatest of which is the inability of the nurse to consistently care for more than one child at a time because of the need to move with the assigned child from one unit to another as the child progresses through the system. If ICU nurses are used, they bring a great deal of capability and experience of caring for the sickest of patients. Because routine procedures are performed on most pediatric surgical patients, these patients need nursing care that recognizes their unique requirements, but they do not require the equivalent of intensive care nursing. However, in an institution in which few children are treated, the extra safety of trained intensive care nurses may be beneficial.

Parental Presence

Parental presence in the PACU is a controversial area. The needs and desires of the nursing and medical staff may be at odds with those of the parents and child. Many nursing and medical staff members believe that close observation of the child, the ability to deal with complications and emergencies, access to the patient, and traffic control in the PACU are best accomplished without the presence of parents. On the other hand, some nursing and medical staff believe that parental participation in the recovery process can calm the child, reduce the anxiety of the parents, and help reduce the workload of nursing staff. There are little data other than personal experience to provide guidance in this area. However, several trends seem to be growing.

The traditional prohibitions against parental presence seem to be relaxing. Increasingly, parents are allowed to at least visit their child in the PACU after the child has regained consciousness. This is permitted only after the nursing staff is assured that therapeutic interventions such as support of a marginal airway are not likely. Because parents often desire to see their child as soon as they know that the surgery is completed, it is useful to explain to parents before the surgery starts that they will be able to visit after an initial period of stabilization, not immediately after arrival in the PACU. It is also useful to have established and clearly explained rules and protocols about parents' presence in the PACU (Table 19–3).

Table 19–3.   Parental Presence in the PACU — Special Considerations

Physical Preparation
    Enough space at each bed space for parent
    Side rails on each bed/crib
    Chair for parent
    Curtain or other barrier to provide privacy

Policy Decisions
    Who screens parent for suitability for visit?
    Can parent visit any child in PACU?
    Can more than one parent visit at a time?
    Can parent stay until patient is discharged from PACU?
    Can parent hold/feed awake child?

    Limitations if PACU busy
    Limitations if extra nursing staff are not available
    Limitations if critically ill patient in PACU
    Limitations if procedure or resuscitation in process
    Who removes parent if parent is uncooperative/disruptive?

Parental Instructions
    Parents must agree to comply with all nursing requests, including a request to leave
    Parents must sit if holding/feeding child
    Parents must be instructed not to:
        Talk with other parents or nurses
        Leave bed space area
        Visit other bed spaces
        Inquire about other patients or parents

In many units, policies have changed to allow parents to visit and then stay with the child until the child is discharged from the PACU. This is more problematic; it increases congestion in the PACU and limits healthcare staff access to the patient. If parents stay, they will be more observant not only of their own child's care but also of the care of other children. The noise level in the PACU, the presence of other sick children, and space constraints may be distressing to the parents. It is the responsibility of the nursing staff to be observant of this and explain the situation to the parents. If an emergency arises in the PACU or if the parents are becoming increasingly distressed, the nursing staff should calmly, but firmly, request that the parents return to the waiting area.

It is commonly recognized that there is a subset of patients that definitely benefit from parental presence. Patients with handicaps, such as blindness, deafness, or mental retardation, often have difficulty communicating with nursing staff effectively. Because the lack of communication can lead to combative and disruptive behaviors, parents can be especially useful in communicating with these patients after the patient has reached a level of consciousness that allows communication. These parents are helpful not only in calming their child but also in initiating the taking of oral fluids, assessing the need for pain medication, and determining the preexisting functional level of the patient.

ROUTINE RECOVERY OF CHILDREN

The routine emergence and recovery of a pediatric patient is a dynamic process that is affected not only by the age of the child but also by the procedure performed, underlying medical conditions, and perioperative complications. In general, initial return of reflexes, ventilation, and airway patency occurs in the operating room before transfer to the PACU. It is the responsibility of the anesthesiologist to ensure that the patient is stable and able to maintain ventilation, oxygenation, and cardiovascular hemodynamics before leaving the operating suite.

Most children will have an independently maintained airway for transport from the operating suite to the PACU. After extubation, the airway should be checked and any secretions or blood should be removed. It is common for infants and small children to demonstrate a small amount of intermittent soft tissue obstruction of the upper airway during the early phase of recovery due to blunting of tone of the glossopharyngeal muscle by anesthetic agents. This is more common in pediatric patients (35). Although this soft tissue obstruction is often treated in adults by performing a chin lift, applying pressure under the tip of the mandible, this can actually increase soft tissue obstruction of the pediatric airway because of the relatively large tongue (36). A more useful maneuver is to perform a jaw thrust, advancing the soft tissue of the upper airway forward, opening the posterior pharynx. If this maneuver is not adequate, consideration should be given to turning the patient on their side. The airway often is not only less obstructed in this position, but secretions or blood in the pharynx are less likely to obstruct the airway.

If neither of these maneuvers are successful in maintaining a patent airway, the anesthesiologist should consider the use of an oral or nasal airway. However, there is a significant danger of laryngospasm if the airway is stimulated by an artificial airway in a child who is partially anesthetized. The clinician must closely balance the need for artificial airway support and the potential for airway irritation.

Before discontinuing operating room monitoring, the anesthesiologist should assess ventilation and oxygenation of the child. Specifically, the pulse oximetry determinations of oxygen saturation on room air are determined. If the patient is not able to maintain adequate oxygenation on room air, the reason for this should be investigated. Children have a greater tendency toward desaturation with airway obstruction or hypoventilation than

adults because, although their functional residual capacity (FRC) is the same as adults on a volume/body weight basis, their ratio of FRC to oxygen consumption is much less because of the child's higher metabolic rate. If the anesthesiologist determines that the child needs supplemental oxygen, this should be provided during transport. In this situation, oxygen usually can be provided by a portable oxygen tank connected via flowmeter to a simple mask. However, if there is concern about the potential for hypoventilation, a self-inflating resuscitation bag should be used for administration.

Most children recover reflexes quickly in the operating suite and do not require either oxygen support or special monitoring for transport to the PACU. It is a common and wise practice to keep a precordial stethoscope on the patient and to use this for the short trip to the PACU. The precordial stethoscope is particularly useful because it not only monitors effectiveness of airway and ventilation (adequate breath sounds) but also heart rate, rhythm, and strength of tones. The anesthesiologist experienced with this monitor can gather a great deal of continuous information from its use. However, if the patient is unstable, other monitoring may be needed for the transport to the PACU. Portable monitors are available that fit easily on the bed, such as the battery-powered Propaq monitor (Protocol Systems, Beaverton, OR), and provide electrocardiography, pulse oximetry, and invasive pressure monitoring capability with both numeric and waveform readouts. Alternatively, a portable cart can be built that houses not only a portable monitor but also air and oxygen tanks connected through a blender to a flowmeter and storage space for airway equipment and drugs.

Children should be transported in a cart that has side rails and can be tilted, if needed. The anesthesiologist in charge of the transport should be at the head of the patient, while another member of the operating room team, such as a member of the surgical team, provides the steering and pulling of the cart. If an emergency occurs, this person can provide needed assistance. If the patient is critically ill, a third person may be needed during the transport to either help with patient care or to obtain needed supplies or equipment.

Rarely, the patient must be transported for long distances to reach the PACU. This is becoming more common as anesthesiologists are asked more often to provide services outside the traditional operating room environment (37). This is particularly true for pediatric patients; anesthesia services are often asked to help with sedation or anesthesia for children in the magnetic resonance scanner, the angiography suite, and the cardiac catheterization laboratory. The anesthesia service must decide whether it is best to provide recovery services in the traditional PACU or at the site where the anesthetic is provided. If the child is to be transported back to the PACU, it is prudent to provide monitoring and emergency equipment similar to what would be used if the patient is critically ill (see above). The longer time needed for these transports increases the potential for unexpected complications. Also, there are physical hazards associated with long transports; some of these include sloping floors, crowded corridors, raised floor expansion joints ("speed bumps"), slow elevators, and interactions with other personnel and visitors to the institution. The anesthesiologist must not only prepare for these transports but also ensure that personnel assisting with the transport is qualified to help care for the patient in these unusual settings.

Admission to the PACU

When the child is brought to the PACU by the anesthesiologist, the patient is immediately evaluated by both the anesthesiologist and the assigned nurse. This starts with inspection of the patient, with special attention to level of consciousness, patency of the airway, depth and rate of ventilation, and color. Initial vital signs include heart rate, blood pressure, respiratory rate, temperature, and oxygen saturation. Breath signs are auscultated, and a

peripheral pulse is palpated. If the patient has an intra-arterial or central venous line left in place, the anesthesiologist must determine whether they should be connected to a monitor for continuous observation. After initial evaluation of the patient, vital signs are checked a minimum of every 5 minutes until the patient is ready for discharge. Vital signs should be recorded on a sheet that is a part of the permanent record. The nursing staff should also record level of consciousness, medications, fluids, and any other pertinent data on this sheet.

It is useful for the vital signs and patient status to be part of a systematic approach to patient evaluation. There are several recovery scoring systems in use, although most are based on the work of Aldrete. His original score was based on the evaluation of the five functions of activity, respiration, circulation, consciousness, and color (38). Steward developed a similar score that was designed specifically for children (39). In our institution, a preprinted form is used that not only has a recovery score based on consciousness, ventilation, and movement but also has specific spaces for listing vital signs in a graphic, time-based manner; intake and output, with running totals; presence of drains, invasive monitors, and other equipment; x-rays and other tests; medications; and a comments section. By using a record that encourages the recording of information in a uniform manner, it is easier to consistently find information on an individual patient.

The anesthesiologist must give a report to the assigned nurse as soon as possible. The report should start with the patient's age and a short description of any pertinent medical history. This can be especially important for patients with diabetes, heart disease, seizures, mental retardation, allergies, etc. The surgical procedure and, if appropriate, the reason for the surgery are reported. Any significant surgical or anesthetic complications should be mentioned, as well as any potential postoperative complications or concerns. The anesthesiologist should mention what has been given to the patient to minimize postoperative pain and what plans have been made, if any, for further pain management. The anesthesiologist is responsible for the care of their patient throughout the recovery period. The patient is left in the care of the nursing staff only after ensuring that the patient is stable and unlikely to experience complications. The nursing staff must know how to contact the anesthesiologist quickly if there are questions about the patient's status or plans for further management. It is also the responsibility of the anesthesiologist to ensure that assistance can be provided in the PACU if an emergency arises.

It is common to administer supplemental oxygen by mask or nasal prongs to all children admitted to the PACU. The reason for this has been the finding that a drop in oxygen saturation is common in the first minutes after leaving the operating suite and that desaturation is usually not easily detected by visual inspection (40). Several studies have demonstrated that children arriving in the recovery room have oxygen saturation values lower than preoperative values (41–48). In most studies, the lower saturations are found in children who continue to sleep in the PACU. However, it has been shown that the oxygen saturation values do not correlate with a standardized recovery room score, indicating that level of awareness and movement is not necessarily predictive of ability to maintain adequate oxygenation (40). It is important to remember that clinical examination is not an effective method of determining hypoxemia and that pulse oximetry of other monitoring is needed to accurately determine oxygenation (14, 49).

Children who are recovering from a general anesthetic do not respond to hypoxemia in the same fashion as an adult. Motoyama and Glazener (43) demonstrated that children do not increase ventilation to an appropriate degree, possibly because of depression of chemoreceptors by the anesthetic. Other factors in infants include a relatively compliant chest wall, small alveolar bed, and a decreased functional residual capacity/metabolic rate ratio. Children suffering or recovering from an up-

per respiratory tract infection also demonstrate relative hypoxemia in the PACU because of lower respiratory tract swelling and secretions (42).

The routine use of oxygen should be an institutional decision so that the initial administration or monitoring is consistently practiced. It is our practice to routinely administer oxygen to all patients on admission to the PACU and, as the patient awakens, to monitor the child without oxygen for periods of time, using the pulse oximeter as a guide. If the child is able to maintain oxygen saturations above 95% without supplemental oxygen, the oxygen is discontinued. However, all patients are continuously monitored with pulse oximetry until discharge. A child who is not able to maintain an oxygen saturation at or above 95% on room air, but is otherwise suitable for discharge, is sent to the floor with oxygen therapy. Oxygen saturations are then continuously monitored until the child is able to maintain adequate saturations without supplemental oxygen.

The only patients who do not routinely receive mask oxygen on admission at our institution are those who are wide awake and apparently ready for discharge on admission to the PACU. This is frequently the case in infants and small children who have undergone short procedures such as ear tubes or suture removals. Other patients who do not receive supplemental oxygen routinely are preterm infants under 48 weeks of gestation. There is question about whether they may be at some risk for retinopathy of prematurity after prolonged supplemental oxygen administration (50–52). The time course needed for this to be a factor is unclear. Our routine is to first check room air saturations on the infant and then use supplemental oxygen if the saturations are below 93 to 94%. The reason this level was chosen is that it approximates the normal range for otherwise healthy sleeping preterm infants (53).

It should be mentioned that the need for oxygen beyond the recovery room recently has been called into question (54). Tyler et al. recently studied otherwise healthy children who received postoperative analgesia with intravenous, intramuscular, or epidural narcotics (55). Using the percent of time when the child had oxygen saturations under 95 and 90% as a measure, they compared these values to matched pairs preoperatively. They found no difference in the patterns between preoperative and postoperative overnight recordings. There was no difference in either the frequency or severity of episodes of desaturation between the preoperative and postoperative studies. These data were used to conclude that children undergoing opioid therapy, in a variety of modalities, are not at risk for greater periods of desaturation than preoperatively.

The emergence of children from anesthesia in the PACU may include a period of agitation or restlessness. This is a normal part of recovery, although it may be worse in children with pain, hypoxemia, a distended bladder, or hypoglycemia. The nursing staff must first ensure that there is no evidence of clinical deterioration of the patient; the staff must then make a judgment regarding whether therapy such as additional pain medication is needed or if this is a normal part of emergence that will respond to comforting of the patient. Parental presence is often instrumental in soothing a frightened child.

Emergence and New Anesthetic Agents

In recent years, we have seen the introduction of many new anesthetic agents. Several of the intravenous and volatile agents have been promoted as ideal drugs for the pediatric population. Because most pediatric surgeries can be performed on a same-day-surgery basis, anesthetic techniques that promote rapid emergence and discharge from the institution are an advantage.

Propofol has been studied extensively because of its characteristics of rapid emergence and potential antiemetic activity (56–58). It has found to be useful not only in the operating suite but also in settings such as the cardiac catheterization laboratory (59) and the magnetic resonance imaging suite (60–61). Although most studies have shown that propofol is associated with rapid emergence characteristics, it has not been proven universally to be superior to other anesthetic techniques, such as isoflurane anesthesia (62–63). Despite its favorable profile, some practitioners have found that its use is limited by the need to establish intravenous access before induction. Modalities such as EMLA cream can help remove some of the difficulty with this task (64, 65).

The new volatile inhalation agents desflurane (66, 67) and sevoflurane (68–70) have also been promoted as desirable for pediatric anesthesia. They are associated with rapid emergence. Although this may mean that the child is awake faster than with halothane or isoflurane anesthesia, the difference in time to initial awakening is often small; time to discharge from the PACU and, if an outpatient, from the institution may not be significant.

There is little evidence that the new agents are associated with a significant benefit in terms of the quality of emergence. In some cases, the rapid awakening may be associated with agitation (see *The Child with Emergence Delirium* section). There is also little evidence that the new agents are associated with a marked shortening of the total recovery period. More prospective studies must be performed to establish whether there is any significant difference between agents and emergence and discharge characteristics.

Discharge from the PACU

Some institutions have instituted policies about minimum length of stay for pediatric patients. If the PACU nurses are not very familiar with the care of children, the establishment of minimum times of recovery can be a guide. Purely on the basis of physiology and pharmacology, there should not be a minimum time required for recovery. Most children undergoing short procedures recover quickly and commonly are ready for discharge in 15 minutes or less. However, there are many reasons that emergence from anesthesia may be delayed, such as length of surgery, underlying medical conditions, preoperative sleep deprivation, and the use of long-acting anesthetic medications.

As with all patients potentially experiencing delayed awakening, a determination of the cause must be made (Table 19–4). This examination is age-dependent, because the recovery characteristics vary by age. The newborn patient is least like an adult in terms of evaluation. Newborns spend most of their day sleeping, so natural, arousable sleeping is normal at this age. On the other hand, a limp or poorly responsive newborn should be assessed quickly for adequacy of airway, breathing, and cardiac function. After this initial assessment, sources of delayed awakening such as hypothermia, hypoglycemia, and low cardiac output are investigated. The newborn is especially susceptible to swings in blood sugar related to fluid management and surgical stress (71). A bedside check of the glucose level will quickly establish the likelihood of this being a concern. Intravascular status is evaluated not only by vital signs but also by mucosal and skin turgor, capillary refill, and fullness of the fontanel (6). If there is concern about the intravascular status, prompt treatment is important to restore core circulation. It is reasonable, in this situation, to administer an initial bolus of 10 mL/kg of balanced salt solution, followed by crystalloid or colloid infusions if indicated by the clinical situation. Lastly, surgical and anesthetic-related causes of delayed awakening are considered. Continued fluid or blood loss, pneumothorax, or prolonged drug effect can decrease cardiac output and contribute to delayed emergence.

Because of the variations in recovery time based on both the type of surgery and interventions in the PACU, some institutions have developed "rules of thumb" based on their clinical experiences. It is not unusual to keep patients who have undergone either long surgical procedures or those associated with a higher risk of airway (laser excision of laryngeal papilloma) or pulmonary (scoliosis surgery) complications for at least 1 hour in the PACU. Likewise, patients who have undergone a craniotomy, thoracotomy, or an extensive intra-abdominal procedure are often arbitrarily kept at least 1 to 2 hours. Children who have received parenteral narcotics are often observed for at least 30 minutes before discharge to ensure that the pain is effectively treated and that the combination of the narcotic's direct effect and the relief of pain has not resulted in hypoventilation.

The criteria for discharge from the PACU is dependent on where the child will go after being discharged. Most children will go to either a short-stay unit or a floor bed, although some institutions will discharge patients home directly from the PACU. It is assumed that a patient transferred out of the PACU will be able to maintain an adequate airway, is ventilating and oxygenating well, is hemodynamically stable, has normal protective reflexes, and is easily arousable. The standardized recovery score is a tool to ensure that there is consistent evaluation of the important components of patient evaluation. Other tools, such as motion-detecting platforms to detect stability (72, 73), have been used, as has the ability of ambulatory patients to ambulate easily. If

Table 19–4. Delayed Awakening in the Pediatric Patient

Hypoxemia
Hypercarbia
Hypovolemia
Acidosis
Hypothermia
Residual anesthetic agent
Residual narcotic
Residual muscle relaxant
Hypoglycemia
Hyperglycemia
Postictal
Increased intracranial pressure
Neonate, especially preterm (normally sleeps 90% of day)
Sleep deprivation

there is question about the patient's status, the patient should be kept in the PACU until the status improves or arrangements have been made to care for the child in an ICU or special unit capable of monitoring and treating an unstable patient.

If the child is to be discharged home, more stringent criteria are used. The patient should be able to maintain normal cardiopulmonary function and should have returned to their preanesthetic level of consciousness. It is common for children to nap during the recovery phase, but they should be awake and alert at the time of discharge from the institution. If they have received a regional anesthetic, they should have normal motor and sensory function (with the exception of pain) before discharge. Although it may be common to require adults to void before discharge from the institution, this is not common with children (74). There has been a reevaluation of the need for the child to drink fluids before discharge. Although it was previously common to require drinking before discharge (75), recent work (76, 77) has demonstrated that there is no difference in outcome if children drink or do not drink before discharge. It is assumed, however, that patients have received enough intravenous fluids during the procedure and recovery period to replace fasting losses and any losses from the procedure. Pediatric practitioners have found that if fluids are "pushed" on a child who is not thirsty or desirous of fluids, the common response is vomiting.

Rarely, a patient scheduled for discharge from the institution will have complications that require reevaluation for potential admission to the hospital. If the child has persistent vomiting, bleeding, agitation, or postintubation stridor, the anesthesia and surgical services should examine the child and decide together what course is appropriate. If there is question about either the patient's status or the ability of the parents to deal with the child and potential complications, discharge from the institution should be delayed. Although infrequent, it is expected that a same-day surgery patient will occasionally require admission to the institution.

A routine part of the discharge process is ensuring that the parents are prepared for undertaking the care of the child at home. Infants and small children should be transported home only through the use of a car seat. The parents should clearly understand what to expect in terms of patient behavior, pain management, and potential complications. We explain to the parents that the child will often be sleepy or nap more than usual for the next 12 hours. Parents are instructed about slowly advancing feedings, examining wound dressings, assessing the need for additional pain medication, and advancing the activity of the child only when the child demonstrates a return of normal coordination. Parents must be given a phone number to call any time during the next day if they have questions about the patient's status or what should be done about complications such as fever, vomiting, or bleeding. A follow-up phone call should be made the next day to not only ensure that the child and parents are doing well, but also to answer questions and record data that become part of the quality assurance activity of the institution.

Recovery Outside the PACU

If general anesthesia or deep sedation has been provided in a setting outside the operating suite, the patient will need postanesthesia recovery. If the decision is made for the child to recover in the area where the anesthetic was given, the same level of care should be provided as in the PACU. Nursing staff should be of the same caliber and training as found in the PACU, and similar protocols and approaches should be used (78). The site should have the same equipment and monitors as the PACU. Recently, the American Society of Anesthesiologists published guidelines for provision of anesthetic care outside the operating room environment (79). These guidelines are useful to review as part of the site evaluation that must be performed before agreeing to provide service outside the traditional setting and ensuring that there are adequate facilities for recovery. These matters should be investigated and the site should be prepared before the first anesthetic is given.

Special attention should be given to the presence of an appropriate resuscitation cart, adequate space for patient access during the recovery phase, a means of rapid two-way communication, and protocols for recovery parameters, physician involvement in care, and discharge criteria (37). It is useful to have nursing personnel spend time in the PACU not only as initial training but as a periodic retraining in current care patterns. If recovery services are provided outside the traditional PACU, care in these areas should be subject to the same quality assurance monitoring as the PACU.

COMPLICATIONS

The PACU staff is responsible not only for monitoring the normal recovery of patients but also for recognizing and initially treating complications in these patients. For this reason, it is imperative that the anesthesiologist inform the nursing staff about the underlying medical status of the patient, as well as any anticipated complications related to the surgery or anesthesia. This will prepare the nursing staff to identify and treat potential problems as quickly as possible.

THE CHILD WITH EMERGENCE DELIRIUM

It is common for infants and small children to intermittently waken and then nap during the initial recovery period (80), with the periods of wakefulness increasing during the recovery process. Most children show some degree of crying, uncoordinated movement, and thrashing during the early stages of emergence from anesthesia. This is usually of short duration, and children respond to reassurance. Care is taken to ensure that the child does not

injure himself; the use of pads along the length of the bed rail can be helpful in preventing injury. It is also important, especially in younger children, to securely tape intravenous catheters in place with, if possible, the use of a padded arm or foot board, to prevent accidental dislodgement of the catheter during emergence. A reassuring voice and cuddling or other physical reassurance is normally enough to calm most children.

However, a child will occasionally demonstrate unusual agitation or delirium upon emergence from anesthesia. In this situation, it is the responsibility of the anesthesia and nursing staff to examine the patient and determine whether there is a treatable cause of the agitation. Unexpected combative behavior can be due to potentially hazardous conditions, such as hypoxemia, hypotension, hypoventilation, acidosis, or increased intracranial pressure. The potential for these conditions causing the agitation are ruled out first. After the patient's safety has been ensured, other causes of agitation should be investigated. Pain is a common cause of agitation and should be treated as aggressively as for adult patients. If the staff members do not feel that the child is experiencing significant pain, unusual agitation can be related to the anesthetic agents themselves. It is believed, for instance, that there is a higher incidence of postanesthetic excitement with anticholinergic medication, especially scopolamine (81). Although treatment of patients with physostigmine (0.02 to 0.05 mg/kg) has been suggested as a specific antidote for scopolamine-induced delirium, most children pass through emergence quickly without the need for therapeutic intervention. Ketamine also has been suggested as a cause of postanesthetic agitation in adults (82), but agitation is less common in children and usually responds to recovery in a quiet, dimly lit environment.

Lastly, awakening in a new environment can be sufficient cause to induce agitation, especially in small children or patients with mental retardation. An alternative at this point is to expedite parental presence. Parental presence is most helpful in calming the child when recovery has progressed to the point that the child recognizes the voice of the parent. It is occasionally necessary to encourage and remind parents to be soothing and comforting in manner, minimizing their own anxiety in the presence of the child.

Extreme agitation in the PACU can be disturbing to the nursing staff, other patients, and parents. It is the responsibility of the recovery staff to evaluate the patient and rule out both potentially hazardous conditions and the need for pain medication, as well as to protect and restrain the child as needed. Most agitation will pass quickly, especially when treated with reassurance and comforting of the child. If the agitation persists, the staff must reconsider the potential for physiologic disturbances such as hypoxemia, increased intracranial pressure, or underappreciated pain.

Short-acting anesthetics have become extremely popular in current pediatric practice. As discussed earlier, most of the newest agents have a pharmacodynamic profile that provides quick awakening at the end of the procedure. However, the anesthesiologist must remember that a potential disadvantage of rapid elimination of anesthetic drug is removal of analgesia and sleepiness that can help provide a slow transition to awareness. The young child may suddenly find themselves in pain, awake, and in a strange surroundings. This can promote agitation and combative behaviors. Excitatory movements have been described in children during recovery from propofol anesthesia, for instance (83, 84). As we increasingly use these short-acting agents to promote rapid emergence and discharge, it is incumbent on the anesthesiologist to provide adequate pain relief for the immediate postanesthetic period and to understand that the analgesic and sedative effects of longer-acting drugs may help some patients awaken in a more peaceful and less disruptive manner.

PAIN MANAGEMENT

Pain in children is one of the most overlooked areas in modern anesthesia. For years,

practitioners have undertreated painful conditions in children. It was not unusual for no pain medication to be given after painful surgical procedures, with the exception of the occasional acetaminophen suppository. Many myths and misunderstandings have contributed to this unfortunate state. For instance, it has been written that children do not feel, remember, or respond to pain in the same degree as adults (85, 86). Because of these attitudes, practitioners often have not treated pain as aggressively as they would for adult patients. Good evidence now exists that this truly is not the case. Children, including preterm newborns, have intact and functional pain pathways and do feel pain (87–90). Pediatric patients of all ages also have significant stress responses to pain. These stress responses include not only increased heart rate, blood pressure, and respiratory rates but also significant stress hormone release (90–100). Newborns, for instance, may also respond to pain by breath-holding, apnea, and hypoxemia (101). There has even been the suggestion that, in the neonatal cardiac population, outcome as measured by survival can be increased by more aggressive management aimed at blunting pain and stress responses (102).

There are also myths about treating pain in children with techniques that either have limited effectiveness or present significant risk of complications. There has been great reluctance to give narcotics to children, especially young children and infants. It has been feared that children of all ages are "sensitive" to narcotics and would be at great risk for hypoventilation and hypotension. There are animal data that young rats (in the first days of life) are particularly sensitive to the respiratory depressant effects of narcotics (103). This has been used as justification that narcotics are more dangerous for younger children. Older data from humans confirmed an increased risk for ventilatory depression, as measured by depression of carbon dioxide response curves, after morphine or meperidine in infants (104). However, more recent human data have changed our understanding of narcotics in children.

It has been demonstrated that infants, especially younger than 10 weeks of age, have a lower clearance and longer elimination half-life of morphine, compared with adults (105–108). However, infants develop kinetics comparable to adults by 5 to 6 months of age (109–111). In an important recent clinical study, Lynn et al. examined the clinical implications of this difference (112). They found that in children between 2 days and 570 days of age, there was no difference in the ventilatory depression when the administration of infusions of morphine was altered to produce the same blood level of drug. When the blood level reached 20 ng/mL, significant respiratory depression was seen. The importance of this article is that it demonstrates that if the pharmacokinetics are understood and accounted for in dosing, it is possible to safely administer potential analgesics to children of all ages.

Lastly, practitioners have not been particularly skilled at evaluating the signs and symptoms of pain in children. The type of surgery is sometimes the only factor considered in estimating the degree of pain likely to be experienced. There are several other potential causes of pain; significant irritation can be produced by a tight cast or bandage, intravascular lines, bladder catheter, gastrostomy or nasogastric tube, chest tube, and surgical drains under tension, etc. Staff must not only estimate the potential for pain but also observe the child for evidence of distress. Grimacing, splinting, crying, restlessness, and refusal to interact with nurses or parents are among the signs that can be used to detect distress. Vital signs such as unexpected tachycardia, tachypnea, and hypertension may also be indicative. Older children may verbalize their discomfort, especially if specifically asked. Lastly, there are visual analog scales that have been used to estimate changing levels of pain in children (113, 114). These have been developed to account for age and language problems associated with children. They range from a series of smiling/ frowning/crying cartoon faces to a series of actual pictures of children in various degrees of pain and comfort. Analog scales are used more commonly after the initial recovery period but can be used if the staff is familiar with their use and interpretation.

The first step in providing effective pain relief for children in the PACU begins in the operating room. Postoperative pain relief should be an integral part of the planning of each anesthetic. Intraoperative medications can include intravenous narcotics or nonsteroidal analgesics, as well as rectal medications, especially acetaminophen. By administering these medications during the anesthetic, it is possible to have adequate blood levels during the recovery period as well as to titrate incremental doses to effect. This has the advantages of ensuring adequate analgesia but also fostering a more calm and less traumatic awakening. This must be balanced against the potential for delaying emergence and recovery. Although there has been concern that providing pain relief with potent agents such as narcotics would delay discharge from the PACU and the institution, clinical experience has demonstrated that effective use of potent agents not only produces a less stressful recovery but also does not delay discharge.

Regional anesthesia has been increasing in popularity for pediatric anesthesia. As practitioners become more familiar and comfortable with these techniques, they are used to provide both intraoperative and postoperative benefit. Regional blocks have been used as both the sole anesthetic for a variety of procedures, and as an adjunct for both intraoperative and postoperative pain relief (115–119). The clear advantage of regional anesthesia for pain relief is the provision of analgesia without attendant sedation, nausea, or respiratory depression. This can be especially useful for neonates and infants if there is concern about the depressant actions of parenteral agents. On the other hand, the lack of sedation may not be desirable in some patients. Appropriate techniques include epidural, caudal, and other regional blocks, such as brachial plexus blocks.

Interestingly, it has also been demonstrated that either wound infiltration (120) or simple instillation of local anesthetic into the wound (and allowed to sit for a few minutes) can produce analgesia during the PACU period that is almost the equivalent of a regional block (121).

One block that has become increasingly popular is the caudal block (122–126). This block is particularly easy to perform in children because of the easy-to-palpate landmarks. The caudal block can provide significant pain relief for most operations below the diaphragm and is most often used as an adjunct for lower limb, inguinal, bladder, and umbilical procedures. In our institution, it is common to administer either 0.25 or 0.125% bupivacaine with 1/200,000 epinephrine at 0.75 to 1 mL/kg (20 mL maximum). For longer procedures, a continuous caudal or epidural technique is applicable, although it is possible to use a single-shot technique at the beginning of the procedure and then again at the end. Continuous techniques or those that use narcotics in addition to local anesthetics are usually reserved for patients who will stay at the institution at least overnight, such as those having a pectus repair, bowel anastomosis, or exstrophy repair (127–131). If the block is given at the end of the procedure to provide postoperative pain relief, 0.125% bupivacaine is administered to minimize the risk of sensory or motor block. Although the pharmacokinetics of local anesthetics would suggest that these blocks should last for only a few hours, it is not unusual for children to experience several hours of effective analgesia after caudal administration.

If the patient arrives in pain or develops pain in the PACU, early intervention is not only humane but is also more likely to be effective than waiting until the pain gets worse. Acetaminophen is commonly used in oral or, more commonly, rectal suppository form in the PACU (132). The advantage of acetaminophen is its lack of side effects; its primary disadvantages are slow onset and limited effectiveness against moderate or severe pain. The normal dose of 10 to 15 mg/kg is currently undergoing reevaluation because of concern that the blood levels achieved with this dose are below the therapeutic range (133). Rectal ibuprofen in a dose of 10 mg/kg also has been used successfully (134). There has been some interest in injectable nonsteroidal agents, specifically ketorolac, in pediatric patients (135). This has the advantage of pain relief without sedation or nausea. However, because of the concern about its antiplatelet activity and the potential for promoting bleeding (133), ketorolac has not found wide acceptance in many centers. This may change as our experience with the agent increases.

Narcotics are the most commonly used agents for significant pain in the PACU, producing effective analgesia in a short period of time (136–141). Morphine and fentanyl tend to be the agents of choice, although codeine and meperidine are also advocated. Whenever narcotics are administered, the patient should be closely observed for signs of excess sedation or hypoventilation. Narcotics can not only produce dose-dependent hypoventilation but also dilate the capacitance vessels of the vascular system. Although narcotic administration is usually associated with limited cardiovascular change, dilation can lead to hypotension in patients who are hypovolemic or who have rapid positional changes. Small doses of intravenous drug are usually titrated instead of using a single, larger dose or intramuscular injection, with doses repeated at 10- to 15-minute intervals. Although intramuscular injection may provide a longer period of analgesia with less of a peak effect, it is difficult to titrate the dose to effect in the individual patient. Morphine is often given in boluses of 0.05 to 0.1 mg/kg, whereas fentanyl is often given in doses of 0.5 to 1 μg/kg. Although it is possible to use narcotics in patients younger than 1 month of age, special attention is directed to titrating in smaller doses than normal and observing the patient's response, keeping in mind the longer action of drug in these newborn patients.

Continuous infusions of narcotics have been used in the postoperative period (142–145) but are not commonly used in the PACU unless it is part of patient-controlled analgesia (PCA). PCA has become popular in pediatric patients, providing analgesia under the control of the patient (85, 146–150). Although there has been hesitancy to use PCA for younger patients, there has been a trend to use this modality for patients as young as 3 years of age and for patients who demonstrate the ability to understand the concept of PCA. There is controversy about the advantage of a continuous background infusion of narcotic with the demand function (151, 152). Although some authors have demonstrated better pain relief with both a demand and continuous function, others have found more nausea, sedation, and episodes of hypoxemia. In our institution, we have found that PCA is most effectively used if the concept is explained and demonstrated to both the patient and parent before the surgical procedure. This facilitates the starting of the PCA in the PACU, establishing the parameters of its use and the comfort of both the child and parents with the modality. Initial analgesia is usually established with bolus narcotics, but use of PCA is encouraged toward the end of the patient's stay in the PACU so that the patient can see how the machine works and the expected effect under nursing supervision.

NAUSEA AND VOMITING

Although it is common to discuss nausea and vomiting as a single entity, children rarely complain of nausea during the early phases of recovery. As a child becomes more awake, they may or may not notice a feeling of nausea associated with vomiting. Vomiting is the most common postoperative event in children during the first 3 days (153). Although some of this vomiting occurs in the PACU, it has been demonstrated that most vomiting actually occurs after discharge from the PACU (76). The overall incidence of vomiting varies tremendously between studies, ranging from 9 to 80% of patients (153–155). In general, the incidence of vomiting seems to be about double that seen in adults for equivalent surgeries (156). Several factors are recognized as being associated with a higher incidence of vomiting. There is a higher rate with children older than 4 years of age (especially adolescents) and those who undergo longer surgeries, strabismus surgery, intra-abdominal surgery, tonsil or adenoid surgery, narcotic use, mask ventilation, a history of motion sickness, and early administration of fluids.

Vomiting is rarely a cause of significant fluid loss. However, it is distressing to the child, as well as the parents and nursing staff. There is the potential for aspiration of gastric contents and pneumonitis, although this has not been a commonly recognized problem in the PACU. Aspiration is, however, a significant concern if the there is recurrent vomiting or if the child has poor protective reflexes secondary to an underlying medical or surgical condition or related to depth of residual sedation or anesthesia. The retching associated with active vomiting may also put undue pressure on suture lines, as well as increase intraocular and intracranial pressures.

The best treatment of nausea and vomiting is prevention. The preanesthetic history is an opportunity to identify patients with a past history of vomiting or reflux, as well as a history of motion sickness. These patients, and those undergoing procedures associated with a high incidence of postoperative vomiting, may benefit from planning and prospective attention to the possibility of vomiting. Although it is not usually possible to change the intended surgical procedure, there are measures that can be taken by the anesthesiologist to minimize the risk of vomiting.

Mask ventilation has been shown to result in an association with an increased risk of vomiting (155). Although narcotics are also a risk factor, this must be balanced against the known tendency of pain to increase the incidence of vomiting (157). There is increasing evidence that the anesthetic agent regimen used also has an effect on the incidence of vomiting. In particular, propofol seems to be associated with a lower incidence of postoperative vomiting in children, given either alone or in combination with other anesthetic agents (158–163). This includes one study in which there was a lower incidence of vomiting with propofol and a narcotic (possibly increasing the chances of vomiting) than with thiopental and halothane (164). Of all available anesthetic agents, propofol clearly offers some advantage if the object is to decrease (but not eliminate) the incidence of vomiting. Although there has been some concern about the ability of nitrous oxide to increase vomiting, recent work indicates that this is not the case (165). Lastly, providing adequate intravenous hydration during the case and delaying oral fluids can be an effective strategy to minimize vomiting (76).

A wide variety of antiemetics are available that have been shown to be effective for children. Belladonna drugs, specifically scopolamine (166), and the phenothiazine derivatives, such as promethazine and prochlorperazine, have commonly been used, especially by pediatricians (167). They have the advantage of being well known and inexpensive, but they are associated with a significant incidence of sedation and other side effects, as well as not being the most efficacious agents available. Droperidol has a long history of use for both prophylactic and therapeutic administration. The recommended doses have varied widely, from 5 to 100 μg/kg (168–170). Droperidol has the disadvantages of prolonged sedation and, occasionally, extrapyramidal side effects (171). Metoclopramide has found some usefulness as an antiemetic, particularly in a dose of 0.25 mg/kg (172–174). Most recently, ondansetron has become extremely popular as an antiemetic (175–177). An intravenous dose of 50 μg/kg is an effective dose for minimizing the incidence and frequency of vomiting in children (178).

With all antiemetics, the question has been raised whether it is prudent and cost effective to give antiemetics prophylactically. Several issues are raised with this question. Antiemet-ics decrease but do not eliminate the incidence of vomiting; they also have side effects of their own, such as sedation. These risks, as well as the cost of the agents, must be balanced against the desired effect of decreased vomiting and decreased chance of patient hospital admission, as well as patient and parent dissatisfaction. In formulating a strategy for antiemetic use, it is reasonable to balance these concerns with the knowledge that there are patients who are at higher risk for vomiting who may benefit from prophylaxis (179).

If a patient is vomiting, should there be a delay in discharging the patient from the PACU and the institution (if an outpatient)? Clinical experience has shown that patients who vomit tend to fall into one of two groups. The large group will vomit once or twice in the PACU. If these patients are allowed to rest quietly and receive intravenous but not oral fluids, they usually stop vomiting and can be discharged. There is a much smaller group that will have recurrent vomiting despite these measures. These patients benefit from continued intravenous fluids, antiemetic medication, and if needed, overnight observation and therapy. As anesthesiologists and nurses have become less aggressive about pushing oral fluids, the incidence of admission for overnight hydration has become very small.

RESPIRATORY COMPLICATIONS

Respiratory complications are the most common serious complications in the immediate postoperative period in children (5). Cohen et al. found that after vomiting, the most common PACU complications were airway obstruction, including laryngospasm, and other respiratory problems. The incidence of respiratory problems in the Winnipeg study was higher than all other problems (excepting vomiting) combined (1). Morray et al. also found that respiratory events were prominent in the closed-claim evaluation of malpractice claims for pediatric cases in the United States (2). These studies emphasize the nature and severity of airway and ventilatory problems in pediatric patients. Respiratory problems can be divided into upper airway obstruction, lower airway obstruction, and hypoventilation.

Upper Airway Obstruction

The most common cause of difficulty is upper airway obstruction. Soft-tissue obstruction is common in the recently anesthetized child for several reasons. Children, especially those under 8 years of age, have qualitative differences in their upper airway (36, 180). They have a relatively large tongue, a long and floppy epiglottis, abundant and loose soft tissue, and hypertrophied lymphoid tissue. There is some evidence that control of the tongue is lost at lower levels of anesthesia than in adults (35), making upper airway obstruction more common in infants and small children emerging from anesthesia. When children develop soft-tissue obstruction, they characteristically demonstrate inspiratory stridor, intercostal and suprasternal retractions, paradoxical ("rocking boat") chest movements, and with time, desaturation. This obstruction usually responds to a jaw thrust or positioning the child in the lateral or prone position (181).

If the patient is still partially anesthetized, they may require more aggressive treatment if the tongue and soft tissue continue to obstruct the airway. An oral airway can be of use in this situation by displacing the tongue forward and opening any seal that may have developed between the tongue and soft palate. The appropriately sized oral airway is one in which the tip ends just before the angle of the mandible; one smaller than this will not effectively hold the soft tissue forward, whereas a larger one can obstruct the airway and induce laryngospasm. The proper size can be determined by placing the airway next to the child's face to check landmarks before insertion. Most children will not tolerate an oral airway after waking up enough to develop pharyngeal reflexes. The airway must be removed at this point to prevent induction of laryngospasm.

Although nasal airways are occasionally helpful, they must be used with caution because of potential bleeding from friable nasal mucosa or hypertrophied adenoid tissue.

Laryngospasm may develop if pain is induced in a partially anesthetized patient (182–185). This should not happen in the PACU if the patient was properly awakened and extubated in the operating suite. However, it does occur rarely in the PACU. Laryngospasm is diagnosed by its characteristic high-pitched whistling sound, along with other signs of airway obstruction. Treatment must start immediately with positive airway pressure with 100% oxygen. This will relieve the obstruction in most cases. All PACU staff must not only be able to diagnose laryngospasm and soft-tissue airway obstruction but also should know the proper use of a self-inflating bag and mask to apply airway pressure and restore a clear airway. If positive pressure by mask does not rapidly relieve the obstruction, intravenous succinylcholine is given. Neither a full intubating dose of succinylcholine (25% or 50% of the intubating dose) nor intubation is usually needed to clear the airway. Controlled mask ventilation is used as long as partial paralysis is present. If laryngospasm recurs after the succinylcholine wears off, the oral pharynx should be suctioned of any blood, secretions, or foreign material that may be irritating the vocal cords.

Rarely, patients may display recurrent upper airway obstruction, even after awakening. This is most commonly seen in infants with congenital micrognathia, such as Pierre Robin or Treacher Collins syndrome. These infants have incomplete muscular control of the tongue until about 3 months of age, leading to airway obstruction even when awake. Maneuvers such as nursing in the prone position are occasionally effective, but more aggressive measures such as a nasopharyngeal airway may be needed. If patients have undergone intraoral procedures such as glossectomy or extensive cleft palate repairs, the surgeon may leave a silk suture through the tongue to facilitate pulling the tongue forward and clearing the airway. Rarely, tongue or palate swelling can be so severe that an endotracheal tube or tracheostomy is needed (186). These patients should be recovered and observed in an intensive care setting.

Postintubation croup is a more common presenting sign in children than in adults; the incidence is between 1 and 6% of pediatric cases. In the preadolescent child, the narrowest area of the airway is at the level of the cricoid, the first complete ring. Pressure from an endotracheal tube on the mucosa at this level can cause significant swelling and obstruction of air flow. In an infant's airway, 1 mm of edema at this level can reduce airflow in the newborn by as much as 75% (187). Edema becomes progressively less significant in older children, explaining why postintubation croup is uncommon after 4 years of age. Croup is more likely after traumatic or repeated intubations, coughing or "bucking" on the tube, intubation for more than 1 hour, surgery in a position that requires movement, and an endotracheal tube fit that prevents an air leak until pressures above 25 cm H_2O are used (188). Young children with congenital narrowing of the larynx, such as those with Down's syndrome or congenital subglottic stenosis, are at special risk.

Postintubation croup usually becomes symptomatic within the first hour after extubation but may develop later. The maximal edema usually occurs at 4 hours after extubation and resolves by 24 hours (189). Croup characteristically presents with a "barky" cough, intercostal retractions, and tachypnea; cyanosis, a muffled voice, and patient anxiety are signs of significant compromise. Although postintubation croup usually resolves without significant impairment of the airway, the obstruction can worsen. Therapy usually starts with humidified oxygen by face mask to sooth the airway. Nebulized racemic epinephrine (0.5 mL of 2.25% epinephrine in 2.5 mL saline) can be given by face mask to vasoconstrict the laryngeal mucosa. After racemic epinephrine administration, improvement in the stridor is usually noticed immediately (189). Be-

cause of the limited length of action of the vasoconstriction, the patient must be reexamined after 1 hour to determine whether there has been a continuation of the subglottic edema and obstruction. Although a single racemic treatment is usually adequate, it can be repeated at hourly intervals, rarely limited by the development of tachycardia. In cases of extreme obstruction, helium/oxygen mixtures have been used to decrease airway resistance and increase flow (190). The efficacy of steroids is controversial because the bulk of research has been on viral laryngotracheobronchitis, not postintubation croup (191, 192). Most recent studies have indicated that dexamethasone does decrease signs in viral croup but must be given in large doses and takes 4 to 6 hours for maximum effect (Table 19–5).

Rarely, the obstruction is severe enough to justify prolonged observation in the PACU or ICU by personnel equipped to provide immediate airway support. Patients that continue to have a barky cough but do not have other signs of respiratory distress may be difficult to assess. Discharge to home can be reasonable if both the physicians and parents are in agreement that the croup is very mild and does not represent a threat to the child. The parents are instructed to observe the child frequently through the night and to bring the child back to the institution immediately if there are any signs of respiratory distress. If there is any doubt by either the medical staff or parents about the advisability of discharge, the child should be admitted for observation overnight.

Lower Airway Obstruction

Lower airway obstruction can be due to a variety of causes. These causes may be directly related to the surgical procedure, such as a hemothorax or pneumothorax, an underlying medical condition, such as asthma, or complications during the case, such as aspiration pneumonitis. Initial evaluation should assess the adequacy of the airway, ventilation, and

Table 19–5.   Therapy for Postintubation Croup

Initial evaluation
   Adequacy of airway—need for urgent intubation?
Monitoring
   Pulse oximetry
   Arterial blood gas—if unsure of status
Humidified oxygen
   Ultrasonic mist may soothe inflamed tissue
Racemic epinephrine
   0.25 to 0.5 mL of 2.25% racemic epinephrine in 2-mL saline given by nebulization
   May substitute with *half* the amount of epinephrine
   Obstruction may be worse (because of underlying process) when racemic wears off after an hour. Must be reex-
      amined an hour after administration.
   May be repeated; watch for tachypnea/dysrhythmias
Parenteral steroids
   Controversial
   Dexamethasone, 0.5 to 1 mg/kg i.v.
   Effect seen over 1 to 4 hours
Airway intervention
   Intubation if significant obstruction persists
   Strongly consider direct laryngoscopy/bronchoscopy to evaluate degree/source of obstruction
Continued observation
   If symptomatic, consultation with otolaryngologist to consider need for admission for observation/further therapy

oxygenation. If the child does not need immediate airway or ventilatory intervention, further diagnostic work can be performed to de-
lineate the problem.

Many of the causes of lower airway obstruction are similar to those seen in the adult.
Aspiration pneumonitis, atelectasis, lung contusion, hemothorax, and pneumothorax are
diagnosed and treated the same as in adults.
However, two conditions are more common
in pediatric patients that deserve mention:
asthma and postobstructive pulmonary
edema.

Approximately 10% of all children are diagnosed as being asthmatic at some time in their
pediatric life. Some children will have a history
that is minimal, with a single episode of
wheezing during a pneumonia many years
ago. Other children will have a more extensive
and recent history of bronchospasm. Of those
patients with known reactive airway disease,
most will be stable on bronchodilator medication, although some patients are either in poor
control at the time of surgery or develop an
exacerbation after the stress of the procedure
(193).

If the patient is symptomatic in the PACU,
therapy depends on the degree of wheezing
and functional impairment. In the recent past,
standard treatment for asthma was based on
oral aminophylline and intravenous theophylline. However, these drugs had significant toxicity that ranged from irritability, tachycardia,
and vomiting to cardiac dysrhythmias, hypokalemia from diuresis, and seizures. The
proper dose was difficult to maintain because
the metabolism differs not only with the age
of the child but also because of other medications or accompanying medical conditions.
Measuring theophylline levels could guide
therapy but was not practical in the acute setting of bronchospasm in the PACU.

Current bronchodilator therapy is based on
the $\beta 2$ agonists, such as albuterol and meta-
proterenol (193, 194). They can be given by
oral, subcutaneous, intravenous (salbutamol),
and inhalation methods, as well as by metered-
dose inhaler for the conscious, cooperative pa-

tient. These drugs have a large safety margin. Albuterol is our current drug of choice in the PACU, with a dose of 0.25 mL given in 2.5 mL of saline by nebulization over approximately 15 minutes. Children with severe wheezing may benefit from the addition of steroids intravenously. (In our institution, the allergists currently provide known moderate or severe asthmatics with 3 days of oral prednisone before elective surgery to prevent any potential adrenal insufficiency and to enhance the action of other bronchodilators at the time of surgery.)

If the bronchospasm does not respond to nebulized albuterol, consideration is given to adding a theophylline infusion. However, if the bronchospasm is severe enough to cause significant, life-threatening hypoxemia, terbutaline (5 to 10 μg/kg subcutaneously) or epinephrine (5 to 10 μg/kg subcutaneously or intravenously) is given to immediately improve gas exchange. If the bronchospasm continues, consideration is given to endotracheal intubation and ventilation, accompanied by continuous nebulized albuterol until the bronchospasm improves.

The other cause of lower airway obstruction more commonly seen in children than adults is postobstructive pulmonary edema. Acute pulmonary edema can appear after an episode of acute upper airway obstruction. This can be induced by laryngospasm, obstruction of an endotracheal tube, or soft tissue obstruction of the airway (195, 196). The time between the acute obstruction and appearance of the pulmonary edema may be very short or delayed, with no known relationship between the degree of obstruction and the time course (197). However, the edema usually appears within a few minutes of relief of the obstruction. This edema usually is seen in patients who are attempting to breathe against a closed or obstructed airway; the assumption is that there is a massive increase in transpleural pressure and subsequent alveolar membrane disruption (198).

The treatment of postobstructive pulmonary edema is reintubation of the airway and positive end-expiratory pressure with an enriched oxygen supply. This is usually adequate to relieve the edema, although positive-pressure ventilation and diuresis occasionally are added. The edema resolves quickly, and although it may be possible to extubate the child in a short period of time, positive pressure is often continued in an intensive care setting for several hours. No sequelae are expected from this self-limited event as long as it is recognized and treated promptly.

Hypoventilation

Hypoventilation in the absence of airway obstruction can be secondary to a variety of reasons in children. Residual anesthetic, residual muscle relaxant, splinting, and hypothermia are common causes. The evaluation and treatment of these conditions are essentially the same as for adults, with a few caveats.

The evaluation of muscle relaxant reversal is more difficult for newborns and infants than for older children or adults. For small infants, it may not be possible to adequately see a reliable twitch with a standard blockade monitor (199). In this situation, the anesthesiologist must depend on physical examination to make a determination about adequacy of reversal of relaxants. Newborns are diaphragmatic breathers with poor intercostal muscle development, so that the pattern of chest expansion is not helpful. On the other hand, anything that impedes diaphragmatic function, such as gastric distension, can significantly hinder ventilation. Although the clinical sign of a head lift for 5 seconds is easy to elicit in adults, a newborn patient may not cooperate. Another sign that is commonly seen in newborns and correlates with adequate reversal is the ability to lift the hips off the table. It is useful to note that preterm newborns have a trait normally not seen in full-term newborns or infants; when stressed, the preterm newborn may develop fatigue of the diaphragm and consequent hypoventilation. This is not a trait usually seen in full-term newborns.

Hypothermia is a frequently missed source of hypoventilation or delayed emergence. Newborns and infants are especially susceptible to hypothermia because of their lack of shivering and vasoconstrictive capability (200–203). The hypothermic infant will not only hypoventilate but also will not respond, as older children, to hypoxemia with tachypnea (204). The combination of hypothermia and hypoxemia or respiratory acidosis may actually decrease the central respiratory drive in newborns. Consequently, it is important that newborns and infants be monitored frequently for core temperature. Every effort should be made to minimize heat loss in the PACU, including the use of protective coverings like cellophane film, heating lights and blankets, warm room temperature, and nursing in an incubator or radiant warmer-equipped bed. Because rewarming a hypothermic infant will take substantial time, intubation and ventilatory support should be provided until the infant is rewarmed if there is significant hypoventilation secondary to hypothermia.

Although the workup of hypoventilation is similar to that seen in adults, there is one recognizable source of apnea that is unique to infancy. The "apnea of prematurity" has been defined as apneic spells in preterm infants that either last longer than 15 or 20 seconds or are accompanied by bradycardia (205). The etiology of these spells seems to be primarily central (approximately 70%) but with some incidence of obstructive or mixed origins in others (206, 207). It is assumed that these spells are potentially life threatening, but there are no outcome data related to surgery that provides definitive support for the magnitude of the problem. Although apneic spells rarely have been reported in full-term infants (208–210), this seems to primarily be a problem with infants who were preterm at birth.

Steward first described the finding that preterm infants had an extraordinary incidence of respiratory complications, especially apnea, after herniorrhaphies (211). This procedure is probably the most common surgical procedure routinely performed on preterm infants in the first months of life. Since that report, many papers have described experiences with preterm infants (205, 212–218). Multiple authors have tried not only to describe their experiences but also to offer advice about what patients are at risk and how that risk could be minimized.

There is some general agreement among most authors on some issues. It is usually agreed that the incidence decreases with advancing gestational and postconceptual ages. It is generally agreed that apneic spells usually appear during the first 12 hours after surgery and that patients should be observed and monitored in-house for at least 12 hours after surgery or after their last spell, whichever is later. Because patients undergoing hernia repairs often are outpatients, this requires a change in institutional policy. Beyond this, there have been several areas of disagreement between authors.

There has not been general agreement about which patients are at risk. Authors have noticed different apnea rates in the PACU and hospitalization, ranging from 5 to 49% (207). Authors have disagreed about which patients should be monitored in-house; recommendations range from 46 to 60 weeks postconceptual age (205, 219). There is disagreement about whether there is any correlation with previous medical history or apneic spells (205, 207, 219, 220). Lastly, Welborn et al. have suggested that administration of 10 mg/kg of caffeine intravenously decreases the incidence of apneic spells in susceptible patients (221).

Caffeine and theophylline have been used by neonatologists for years to increase ventilatory drive in newborns (222). By increasing the central respiratory drive, the incidence of apnea and hypoventilation is decreased. Caffeine, in the dose used, does not cause noticeable cardiovascular changes and lasts many hours. One practical note about the use of caffeine is that if it is to be used for preterm infants, it must be specially prepared because commercially prepared caffeine comes with concentrations of sodium benzoate that are too high to be given to preterm infants.

Cote et al. recently published an analysis of the current work on the apnea of prematurity after herniorrhaphy (207). In addition to noting the substantial differences between methodologies of the different studies and the small number of total patients studied, they statistically evaluated the studies and made several conclusions. It was confirmed that anemia, in itself, is a separate risk factor for apnea (223). The rest of the data were then presented in a form not commonly seen in the anesthesia literature. Instead of giving an absolute cutoff for admission of the preterm for overnight observation, they presented probabilities of apnea occurring. They stated that in nonanemic infants free of PACU apneic spells, the probability of apnea is not less than 5% (with 95% statistical confidence) until the postconceptual age was 48 weeks (gestational age, 35 weeks) or 50 weeks (gestational age, 32 weeks.) Similar data were given for a 1% probability of apnea. This method of analyzing and presenting data changes the way a problem is addressed by allowing the practitioner to choose what risk they are willing to take for a rare event to occur.

The overall incidence and distribution of the apnea of prematurity is still uncertain. Therapeutic modalities such as caffeine or the use of regional anesthesia (220, 224, 225) have been proposed, but there is much that has still not been proven. Lastly, the significance of apneic spells, with or without bradycardia, has not been delineated clearly. This unique problem will benefit from further investigation.

CARDIOVASCULAR COMPLICATIONS

Cohen et al. found that cardiovascular complications were much less common than respiratory complications, were usually seen under a year of age, and primarily manifested as hypotension (1). Hypotension is relatively rare in the PACU in children. When it does

occur, the causes are usually related to blood or fluid loss (203, 226), although hypotension can be caused by hypothermia, tension pneumothorax, air embolism, and other similar etiologies. Initial evaluation is similar to that followed for adults, as is treatment. One difference between infants and older children or adults is the infant's dependence on heart rate for adequate cardiac output. The ventricles of the neonatal heart (227) are relatively stiff and do not increase stroke volume when there is a decrease in heart rate. Bradycardia is associated, then, with a proportionate decrease in cardiac output in these patients. Although the use of atropine or epinephrine may speed the heart rate, the anesthesiologist should determine the cause of the bradycardia and correct it as soon as possible instead of just driving the heart rate up. Before pulse oximetry was commonly used, it was a maxim in pediatric anesthesia that "bradycardia means hypoxemia (until proven otherwise)." After hypoxemia is ruled out, potential abnormalities causing the bradycardia, such as hypothermia, hypovolemia, respiratory or metabolic acidosis, or electrolyte abnormalities, should be investigated and corrected.

Low cardiac output can be associated with specific problems related to congenital heart disease, including poor myocardial contractility, sudden increases in pulmonary hypertension, dysrhythmias, valvular obstruction, septal obstruction (IHSS), intracardiac shunting, and congestive heart failure (227–230). However, these causes are rare and beyond the scope of this chapter.

SUMMARY

Although many of the concerns, practices, and protocols used for recovering children from anesthesia are similar to those used for adult patients, there are many unique differences. Emergence from anesthesia is a particularly dangerous time in the life of any child. Children are dependent on adults to provide the vigilance and care needed to ensure that they pass through this period without harm.

A properly designed and operated PACU not only is prepared for routine care and emergencies but has policies and procedures in place to minimize pain and psychological upset of the child and restore the child to the parents' care as soon as possible. This requires an understanding of the unique anatomic, physiologic, pharmacologic, and psychologic differences between children of different ages, with special attention to newborns and infants. Close communication and cooperation between nursing and physician staff members are essential for this partnership to provide the best in pediatric care.

REFERENCES

1. Cohen MM, Cameron CB, Duncan PG. Pediatric anesthesia morbidity and mortality in the perioperative period. Anesth Analg 1900;70:160–167.
2. Morray JP, Geiduschek JM, Caplan RA, et al. A comparison of pediatric and adult anesthesia closed claim malpractice claims. Anesthesiology 1993;78:461–467.
3. McConachie IW, Day A, Morris P. Recovery from anaesthesia in children. Anaesthesia 1989;44:986–990.
4. Tiret L, Nivoche Y, Hatton F, et al. Complications related to anaesthesia in infants and children. A prospective survey of 240 anaesthetics. Br J Anaesth 1988;61:263–269.
5. Van Der Walt JH, Sweeney DB, Runciman WB, et al. Paediatric incidents in anaesthesia: an analysis of 2000 incident reports. Anaesth Intensive Care 1993;21:655–658.
6. Hall SC. Perioperative pediatric care. In Vender JS, Spiess BD, eds. Acute postoperative care. Philadelphia: WB Saunders, 1992;256–267.
7. Besag FMC, Singh MP, Whitelaw AGL. Surgery of the ill, extremely low birthweight infant: should transfer to the operating theatre be avoided? Acta Paediatr Scand 1984;73:594–595.
8. Cauldwell CB. Induction, maintenance, and emergence. In: Gregory GA, ed. Pediatric anesthesia. 3rd ed. New York: Churchill Livingstone, 1994;227–259.
9. Goudsouzian NG, Morris RH, Ryan JF. The effects of a warming blanket on the maintenance of body temperatures in anesthetized infants and children. Anesthesiology 1973;39:351–353.
10. Stothers JK. Head insulation and heat loss in the newborn. Arch Dis Child 1981;56:530–534.
11. Hay WW, Brockway JM, Eyzaguirre M. Neonatal pulse oximetry: accuracy and reliability. Pediatrics 1989;83:717–722.
12. Smith DC, Canning JJ, Crul JF. Pulse oximetry in the recovery room. Anaesthesia 1989;44:354–358.
13. Brooks TD, Gravenstein N. Pulse oximetry for early detection of hypoxemia in anesthetized infants. J Clin Monit 1985;1:135.
14. Cote CJ, Goldstein EA, Cote MA, et al. A single-blind study of pulse oximetry in children. Anesthesiology 1988;68:184–188.
15. Cote CJ, Rolf N, Liu LMP, et al. A single-blind study of combined pulse oximetry and capnography in children. Anesthesiology 1991;74:980–987.
16. Mather CMP. Paediatric blood pressure and anaesthesia. Anaesthesia 1991;46:381–382.
17. Friesen RH, Lichtor JL. Indirect measurement of blood pressure in neonates and infants utilizing an automatic noninvasive oscillometric monitor. Anesth Analg 1981;60:742–745.
18. Nilsson K. Maintenance and monitoring of body temperature in infants and children. Paediatr Anaesth 1991;1:13–20.
19. Gauntlett I, Barnes J, Brown TCK, et al. Temperature maintenance in infants undergoing anaesthesia and surgery. Anaesth Intensive Care 1985;13:300–304.
20. Ehrenwerth J, Eisenkraft JB. Anesthesia equipment; principles and applications. St. Louis: CV Mosby, 1993;537–564.
21. Nielsen PE, Clausen LR, Olsen CA, et al. Blood pressure measurement in childhood and adolescence: international recommendations and normal limits of blood pressure. Scand J Clin Lab Invest Suppl 1989;192:7–12.
22. Hegyi T, Carbone MT, Anwar M, et al. Blood pressure ranges in premature infants. I. The first hours of life. J Pediatr 1994;124:627–633.
23. Park MK, Lee D, Johnson GA. Oscillometric blood pressures in the arm, thigh, and calf in healthy children and those with aortic coarctation. Pediatrics 1993;91:761–765.
24. Atkins DL, Kerber RE. Pediatric defibrillation: current flow is improved by using "adult" electrode paddles. Pediatrics 1994;94:90–93.
25. Bhende MS, Thompson AE. Evaluation of an end-tidal CO_2 detector during pediatric cardiopulmonary resuscitation. Pediatrics 1995;95:395–399.
26. Ping STS, Mehta MP, Symreng T. Accuracy of the FEF CO_2 detector in the assessment of endotracheal tube placement. Anesth Analg 1992;74:415–419.
27. Gerberding JL. Management of occupational exposures to blood-borne viruses. N Engl J Med 1995;332:444–451.
28. Tobin MJ, Stevenson GW, Hall SC. A simple, cost-effective method of preventing laryngoscope handle contamination. Anesthesiology 1995;82:790.
29. Holzman RS. Latex allergy: an emerging operating room problem. Anesth Analg 1993;76:635–641.
30. Gerber AC, Jorg W, Zbinden S, et al. Severe intraoperative anaphylaxis to surgical gloves: latex allergy, an unfamiliar condition. Anesthesiology 1989;71:800–802.
31. Spivey WH. Intraosseous infusions. J Pediatr 1987;111:639–643.
32. Stewart FC, Kain ZN. Intraosseous infusion: elective use in pediatric anesthesia. Anesth Analg 1992;75:626–629.
33. Vidal R, Kissoon N, Gayle M. Compartment syndrome following intraosseous infusion. Pediatrics 1993;91:1201–1202.
34. Tendler C, Grossman S, Tenenbaum J. Medication

dosages during pediatric emergencies: a simple and comprehensive guide. Pediatrics 1989;84:731–735.

35. Ochiai R, Guthrie RD, Motoyama EK. Differential sensitivity to halothane anesthesia of the genioglossus, intercostals, and diaphragm in kittens. Anesth Analg 1992;74:338–344.

36. Borland LM. The pediatric airway. Int Anesthesiol Clin 1988;26:1–88.

37. Hall SC. Anesthesia outside the operating room. In: Gregory GA, ed. Pediatric anesthesia. 3rd ed. New York: Churchill Livingstone, 1994;813–835.

38. Aldrete JA, Kroulik D. A postanesthetic recovery score. Anesth Analg 1970;49:924–934.

39. Steward DJ. A simplified scoring system for the post operative recovery room. Can Anaesth Soc J 1975;22:111–113.

40. Soliman IE, Patel RI, Ehrenpreis MB, et al. Recovery scores do not correlate with postoperative hypoxemia in children. Anesth Analg 1988;67:53–56.

41. Kataria BK, Harnik EV, Mitchard R, et al. Postoperative arterial oxygen saturation in the pediatric population during transportation. Anesth Analg 1988;67:280–282.

42. DeSoto H, Patel RI, Soliman IE, et al. Changes in oxygen saturation following general anesthesia in children with upper respiratory infection signs and symptoms undergoing otolaryngological procedures. Anesthesiology 1988;68:276–279.

43. Motoyama EK, Glazener CM. Hypoxemia after general anesthesia in children. Anesth Analg 1986;65:267–272.

44. Pullerits J, Burrows FA, Roy WL. Arterial desaturation in healthy children during transfer to the recovery room. Can J Anaesth 1987;34:470–473.

45. Patel R, Norden J, Hannallah RS. Oxygen administration prevents hypoxemia during postanesthetic transport in children. Anesthesiology 1988;69:616–618.

46. Lanigan CJ. Oxygen desaturation after dental anaesthesia. Br J Anaesth 1992;68:142–145.

47. Vijayakumar HR, Matriyakool K, Jewell MR. Effects of 100% oxygen and a mixture of oxygen and air on oxygen saturation in the immediate postoperative period in children. Anesth Analg 1987;66:181–184.

48. Laycock GJA, McNicol LR. Hypoxaemia during recovery from anaesthesia — an audit of children after general anaesthesia for routine elective surgery. Anaesthesia 1988;43:984–987.

49. Margolis PA, Ferkol TW, Marsocci S, et al. Accuracy of the clinical examination in detecting hypoxemia in infants with respiratory illness. J Pediatr 1994;124:552–560.

50. Lucey JF, Dangman B. A reexamination of the role of oxygen in retrolental fibroplasia. Pediatrics 1984;73:82–96.

51. Gibson DL, Sheps SB, Uh SH, et al. Retinopathy of prematurity-induced blindness: birth weight-specific survival and the new epidemic. Pediatrics 1990;86:405–412.

52. Merritt JC, Sprague DH, Merritt WE, et al. Retrolental fibroplasia: a multifactorial disease. Anesth Analg 1981;60:109–111.

53. Richard D, Poets CF, Neale S, et al. Arterial oxygen saturation in preterm neonates without respiratory failure. J Pediatr 1993;123:963–968.

54. Kurth CD. Postoperative arterial oxygen saturation: what to expect (editorial). Anesth Analg 1995;80:1–3.

55. Tyler DC, Woodham M, Stocks J, et al. Oxygen saturation in children in the postoperative period. Anesth Analg 1995;80:14–19.

56. Paut O, Suidon-Attali C, Viviand X, et al. Pharmacodynamic properties of propofol during recovery from anaesthesia. Acta Anaesthesiol Scand 1992;36:62–66.

57. Hannallah RS, Britton JT, Schafer PG, et al. Propofol anaesthesia in paediatric ambulatory patients: a comparison with thiopentone and halothane. Can J Anaesth 1994;41:12–18.

58. Sharples A, Shaw EA, Meakin G. Recovery times following induction of anaesthesia with propofol, methohexitone, enflurane or thiopentone in children. Paediatr Anaesth 1994;4:101–104.

59. Lebovic S, Reich DL, Steinberg LG, et al. Comparison of propofol versus ketamine for anesthesia in pediatric patients undergoing cardiac catheterization. Anesth Analg 1992;74:490–494.

60. Martin LD, Pasternak LR, Pudimat MA. Total intravenous anesthesia with propofol in pediatric patients outside the operating room. Anesth Analg 1992;74:609–612.

61. Frankville DD, Spear RM, Dyck JB. The dose of propofol required to prevent children from moving during magnetic resonance imaging. Anesthesiology 1993;79:953–958.

62. Larsen LE, Gupta A, Ledin T, et al. Psychomotor recovery following propofol or isoflurane anaesthesia for day-care surgery. Acta Anaesthesiol Scand 1992;36:276–282.

63. White PF, Stanley TH, Apfelbaum JL, et al. Effects on recovery when isoflurane is used to supplement propofol-nitrous oxide anesthesia. Anesth Analg 1993;77:S15–S20.

64. Robieux I, Kumar R, Radhakrishnan S, et al. Assessing pain and analgesia with a lidocaine-prilocaine emulsion in infants and toddlers during venipuncture. J Pediatr 1991;118:971–973.

65. Chang PC, Goresky GV, O'Connor G, et al. A multicentre randomized study of single-unit dose package of EMLA patch vs EMLA 5% cream for venepuncture in children. Can J Anaesth 1994;41:59–63.

66. Davis PJ, Cohen IT, McGowan FX, et al. Recovery characteristics of desflurane versus halothane for maintenance of anesthesia in pediatric ambulatory patients. Anesthesiology 1994;80:298–302.

67. Taylor RH, Lerman J. Induction, maintenance and recovery characteristics of desflurane in infants and children. Can J Anaesth 1992;39:6–13.

68. Sarner JB, Levine M, Davis PJ, et al. Clinical characteristics of sevoflurane in children. Anesthesiology 1995;82:38–46.

69. Piat V, Dubois M, Johanet S, et al. Induction and recovery characteristics and hemodynamic responses to sevoflurane and halothane in children. Anesth Analg 1994;79:840–841.

70. Naito Y, Tamai S, Shingu K, et al. Comparison between sevoflurane and halothane for paediatric ambulatory anaesthesia. Br J Anaesth 1991;67:387–389.
71. Larsson LE, Nilsson K, Niklasson A, et al. Influence of fluid regimens on perioperative blood-glucose concentrations in neonates. Br J Anaesth 1990;64:419–424.
72. Hiller A, Pyykko I, Saarnivaara L. Evaluation of postural stability by computerised posturography following outpatient paediatric anaesthesia. Comparison of propofol/alfentanil/N₂O anaesthesia with thiopentone/halothane/N₂O anaesthesia. Acta Anaesthesiol Scand 1993;37:556–561.
73. Steward DJ, Volgyesi G. Stabilometry: a new tool for the measurement of recovery following general anaesthesia for outpatients. Can Anaesth Soc J 1978;25:4–6.
74. Fisher QA, McComiskey CM, Hill JL, et al. Postoperative voiding interval and duration of analgesia following peripheral or caudal nerve blocks in children. Anesth Analg 1993;76:173–177.
75. Steward DJ. Anesthesia for pediatric outpatients. In: White PF, ed. Outpatient anesthesia. New York: Churchill Livingstone, 1990;173.
76. Woods AM, Berry FA, Carter BJ. Strabismus surgery and post-operative vomiting: clinical observations and review of the current literature; a medical opinion. Paediatr Anaesth 1992;2:223–229.
77. Schreiner MS, Nicolson SC, Martin T, et al. Should children drink before discharge from day surgery? Anesthesiology 1992;76:528–533.
78. Committee on Drugs, American Academy of Pediatrics. Guidelines for monitoring and management of pediatric patients during and after sedation for diagnostic and therapeutic procedures. Pediatrics 1992;89:1110–1115.
79. American Society of Anesthesiologists. Guidelines for nonoperating room anesthetizing locations. Park Ridge, IL: American Society of Anesthesiologists, 1994.
80. Chinyanga HM, Vandenberghe H, MacLeod S, et al. Assessment of immediate post-anaesthetic recovery in young children following intravenous morphine infusions, halothane and isoflurane. Can Anaesth Soc J 1984;31:28–35.
81. Greene LT. Physostigmine therapy of anticholinergic-drug depression in postoperative patients. Anesth Analg 1971;50:222–226.
82. Friesen RH, Morrison JE. The role of ketamine in the current practice of paediatric anaesthesia. Paediatr Anaesth 1994;4:79–82.
83. Borgeat A, Wilder-Smith OHG, Despland PA, et al. Spontaneous excitatory movements during recovery from propofol anaesthesia in an infant: EEG evaluation. Br J Anaesth 1993;70:459–461.
84. Reynolds LM, Koh JL. Prolonged spontaneous movement following emergence from propofol/nitrous oxide anesthesia. Anesth Analg 1993;76:192–193.
85. Yaster M, Deshpande JK. Management of pediatric pain with opioid analgesics. J Pediatr 1988;113:421–429.
86. Yaster M, Tobin JR, Fisher QA, et al. Local anesthetics in the management of acute pain in children. J Pediatr 1994;124:165–176.
87. Moss R, Conner H, Yee WPH, et al. Human beta-endorphin-like immunoreactivity in the perinatal/neonatal period. J Pediatr 1982;101:443–446.
88. Pasternak GW, Zhang AZ, Tecott L. Developmental differences between high and low affinity opiate binding sites: their relationship to analgesia and respiratory depression. Life Sci 1980;27:1185–1190.
89. Tobin AJ, Khrestchatisky M, MacLennan AJ, et al. Structural, developmental and functional heterogeneity of rat GABAA receptors. Adv Exp Med Biol 1991;287:365–374.
90. Kinney HC, White WF. Opioid receptors localize to the external granular cell layer of the developing human cerebellum. Neuroscience 1991;45:13–21.
91. Anand KJS, Hickey PR. Pain and its effects in the human neonate and fetus. N Engl J Med 1987;317:1321–1329.
92. Anand KJS, Ward-Platt MP. Neonatal and pediatric stress responses to anesthesia and operation. Int Anesthesiol Clin 1988;26:218–225.
93. Anand KJS, Brown MJ, Bloom SR, et al. Studies on the hormonal regulation of fuel metabolism in the human newborn infant undergoing anesthesia and surgery. Horm Res 1985;22:115–128.
94. Anand KJS, Brown MJ, Causon RC, et al. Can the human neonate mount an endocrine and metabolic response to surgery? J Pediatr Surg 1985;20:41–48.
95. Schmeling DJ, Coran AG. The hormonal and metabolic response to stress in the neonate. Pediatr Surg Int 1990;5:307–321.
96. Yaster M. Analgesia and anesthesia in neonates. J Pediatr 1987;111:394–396.
97. Anand KJS, Sippell WG, Aynsley-Green A. Randomized trial of fentanyl anaesthesia in preterm babies undergoing surgery: effects on the stress response. Lancet 1987;1:243–248.
98. Quinn MW, Wild J, Dean HG, et al. Randomized double-blind controlled trial of effect of morphine on catecholamine concentrations in ventilated preterm babies. Lancet 1993;342:324–327.
99. Anand KJS, Sippell WG, Schofield NM, et al. Does halothane anaesthesia decrease the stress response of newborn infants undergoing operation? Br Med J 1988;296:668–672.
100. Emhardt JD, Vasko MR. Do neonates need anesthesia? Adv Anesth 1990;7:45–81.
101. Pokela M. Pain relief can reduce hypoxemia in distressed neonates during routine treatment procedures. Pediatrics 1994;93:379–383.
102. Anand KJS, Hickey PR. Halothane-morphine compared with high-dose sufentanil for anesthesia and postoperative analgesia in neonatal cardiac surgery. N Engl J Med 1992;326:1–9.
103. Zhang AZ, Pasternak GW. Ontogeny of opioid pharmacology and receptors: high and low affinity site difference. Eur J Pharmacol 1981;73:29–40.
104. Way WL, Costley EC, Way EI. Respiratory sensitivity of the newborn infant to meperidine and morphine. Clin Pharmacol Ther 1965;6:454–461.
105. Bhat R, Chari G, Gulati A, et al. Pharmacokinetics of a single dose of morphine in preterm infants

during the first week of life. J Pediatr 1990;117:477–481.

106. Lynn AM, Slattery JT. Morphine pharmacokinetics in early infancy. Anesthesiology 1987;66:136–139.

107. Koren G, Butt W, Chinyanga H, et al. Postoperative morphine infusion in newborn infants: assessment of disposition characteristics and safety. J Pediatr 1985;107:963–965.

108. Hartley R, Green M, Quinn M, et al. Pharmacokinetics of morphine infusion in premature neonates. Arch Dis Child 1993;69:55–58.

109. Choonara A, McKay P, Hain R, et al. Morphine metabolism in children. Br J Clin Pharmacol 1989;28:599–604.

110. Olkkola KT, Maunuksela EL, Korpela R, et al. Kinetics and dynamics of postoperative intravenous morphine in children. Clin Pharmacol Ther 1988;44:128–136.

111. Dahlstrom B, Bolme P, Feychting H, et al. Morphine kinetics in children. Clin Pharmacol Ther 1979;26:354–365.

112. Lynn AM, Nespeca MK, Opheim KE, et al. Respiratory effects of intravenous morphine infusions in neonates, infants, and children after cardiac surgery. Anesth Analg 1993;77:695–701.

113. Schecter NL, Berde CB, Yaster M. Pain in infants, children, and adolescents. Baltimore: Williams & Wilkins, 1993;145–171.

114. Maunuksela E, Olkkola KT, Korpela R. Measurement of pain in children with self-reporting and behavioral assessment. Clin Pharmacol Ther 1987;42:137–141.

115. Lee JJ, Rubin AP. Comparison of a bupivacaine-clonidine mixture with plain bupivacaine for caudal analgesia in children. Br J Anaesth 1994;72:258–262.

116. Holthusen H, Eichwede F, Stevens M, et al. Preemptive analgesia: comparison of preoperative with postoperative caudal block on postoperative pain in children. Br J Anaesth 1994;73:440–442.

117. Lloyd-Thomas AR. Pain management in paediatric patients. Br J Anaesth 1990;64:85–104.

118. Swinhoe CF, Pereira NH. Intrapleural analgesia in a child with a mediastinal tumour. Can J Anaesth 1994;41:427–430.

119. Chambers FA, Lee J, Smith J, et al. Post-circumcision analgesia: comparison of topical analgesia with dorsal nerve block using the midline and lateral approaches. Br J Anaesth 1994;73:437–439.

120. Schindler M, Swann M, Crawford M. A comparison of postoperative analgesia provided by wound infiltration or caudal analgesia. Anaesth Intensive Care 1991;19:46–49.

121. Casey WF, Rice LJ, Hannallah RS, et al. A comparison between bupivacaine instillation versus ilioinguinal/iliohypogastric nerve block for postoperative analgesia following inguinal herniorrhaphy in children. Anesthesiology 1990;72:637–639.

122. Rice LJ, Pudimat MA, Hannallah RS. Timing of caudal block placement in relation to surgery does not affect duration of postoperative analgesia in paediatric ambulatory patients. Can J Anaesth 1990;37:429–431.

123. Dalens B. Regional anesthesia in children. Anesth Analg 1989;68:654–672.

124. Spear RM. Dose-response in infants receiving caudal anaesthesia with bupivacaine. Paediatr Anaesth 1991;1:47–52.

125. Wolf AR, Valley RD, Fear DW, et al. Bupivacaine for caudal analgesia in infants and children: the optimal effective concentration. Anesthesiology 1988;69:102–106.

126. Yaster M, Maxwell LG. Pediatric regional anesthesia. Anesthesiology 1989;70:324–338.

127. Wolf AR, Hughes D, Hobbs AJ, et al. Combined morphine-bupivacaine caudals for reconstructive penile surgery in children: systemic absorption of morphine and postoperative analgesia. Anaesth Intensive Care 1991;19:17–21.

128. Maunuksela LB, Loper KA, Nessly M, et al. Postoperative epidural morphine is safe on surgical wards. Anesthesiology 1991;75:452–456.

129. Rosen KR, Rosen DA. Caudal epidural morphine for control of pain following open heart surgery in children. Anesthesiology 1989;70:418–421.

130. Valley RD, Bailey AG. Caudal morphine for postoperative analgesia in infants and children: a report of 138 cases. Anesth Analg 1991;72:120–124.

131. Wolf AR, Hughes D, Wade A, et al. Postoperative analgesia after paediatric orchidopexy: evaluation of a bupivacaine-morphine mixture. Br J Anaesth 1990;64:430–435.

132. Howard CR, Howard FM, Weitzman ML. Acetaminophen analgesia in neonatal circumcision: the effect on pain. Pediatrics 1994;93:641–646.

133. Rusy LM, Houck CS, Sullivan LJ, et al. A double-blind evaluation of ketorolac tromethamine versus acetaminophen in pediatric tonsillectomy: analgesia and bleeding. Anesth Analg 1995;80:226–229.

134. Maunuksela E, Ryhanen P, Janhunen L. Efficacy of rectal ibuprofen in controlling postoperative pain in children. Can J Anaesth 1992;39:226–230.

135. Munro HM, Riegger LQ, Reynolds PI, et al. Comparison of the analgesic and emetic properties of ketorolac and morphine for paediatric outpatient strabismus surgery. Br J Anaesth 1994;72:624–628.

136. Hendrickson M, Myre L, Johnson DG, et al. Postoperative analgesia in children: a prospective study of intermittent intramuscular injection versus continuous intravenous infusion of morphine. J Pediatr Surg 1990;25:185–191.

137. Sfez M, Mapihan YL, Gaillard JL, et al. Analgesia for appendectomy: comparison of fentanyl and alfentanil in children. Acta Anaesthesiol Scand 1990;34:30–34.

138. Doyle E, Mottart KJ, Marshall C, et al. Comparison of different bolus doses of morphine for patient-controlled analgesia in children. Br J Anaesth 1994;72:160–163.

139. Berde CB, Beyer JE, Bournaki M, et al. Comparison of morphine and methadone for prevention of postoperative pain in 3- to 7-year-old children. J Pediatr 1991;119:136–141. 140. Knight JC. Post-operative pain in children after day case surgery. Paediatr Anaesth 1994;4:45–51.

141. Campbell WI. Analgesic side effects and minor sur-

gery: which analgesic for minor and day-case surgery? Br J Anaesth 1990;64:617–620.

142. McNichol R. Postoperative analgesia in children using continuous s.c. morphine. Br J Anaesth 1993;71:752–756.

143. Hendrickson M, Myre L, Johnson DG, et al. Postoperative analgesia in children: a prospective study of intermittent intramuscular injection versus continuous intravenous infusion of morphine. J Pediatr Surg 1990;25:185–191.

144. Farrington EA, McGuinness GA, Johnson GF, et al. Continuous intravenous morphine infusion in postoperative newborn infants. Am J Perinatol 1993;10:84–87.

145. Lynn AM, Opheim KE, Tyler DC. Morphine infusion after pediatric cardiac surgery. Crit Care Med 1984;12:863–866.

146. Berde CB, Lehn BM, Yee JD, et al. Patient-controlled analgesia in children and adolescents: a randomized, prospective comparison with intramuscular administration of morphine for postoperative analgesia. J Pediatr 1991;118:460–466.

147. Gaukroger PB, Chapman MJ, Davey RB. Pain control in paediatric burns — the use of patient-controlled analgesia. Burns 1991;17:396–399.

148. Irwin M, Gillespie JA, Morton NS. Evaluation of a disposable patient-controlled analgesia device in children. Br J Anaesth 1992;68:411–413.

149. Mackie AM, Coda BC, Hill HF. Adolescents use patient-controlled analgesia effectively for relief from prolonged oropharyngeal mucositis pain. Pain 1991;46:265–269.

150. Rodgers BM, Webb CJ, Stergios D, et al. Patient-controlled analgesia in pediatric surgery. J Pediatr Surg 1988;23:259–262.

151. Doyle E, Robinson D, Morton NS. Comparison of patient-controlled analgesia with and without a background infusion after lower abdominal surgery in children. Br J Anaesth 1993;71:670–673.

152. Doyle E, Harper I, Morton NS. Patient-controlled analgesia with low dose background infusions after lower abdominal surgery in children. Br J Anaesth 1993;71:818–822.

153. Kermode J, Walker S, Webb I. Postoperative vomiting in children. Anaesth Intensive Care 1993;23:196–199.

154. Patel RI, Hannallah RS. Anesthetic complications following pediatric ambulatory surgery: a 3-year study. Anesthesiology 1988;69:1009–1012.

155. Lerman J. Surgical and patient factors involved in postoperative nausea and vomiting. Br J Anaesth 1992;69:24S–32S.

156. Vance JP, Neill RS, Norris W. The incidence and aetiology of post-operative vomiting in a plastic surgical unit. Br J Plast Surg 1973;26:336–339.

157. Anderson R, Krohg K. Pain as a major cause of postoperative nausea. Can Anaesth Soc J 1976;23:366–369.

158. Watcha M, Simeon RM, White PF, et al. Effect of propofol on the incidence of postoperative vomiting after strabismus surgery in pediatric outpatients. Anesthesiology 1991;75:204–209.

159. Snellen FT, Vanacker B, Van Aken H. Propofol-nitrous oxide versus thiopental sodium-isoflurane-nitrous oxide for strabismus surgery in children. J Clin Anesth 1993;5:37–41.

160. Smith I, White PF, Nathanson M, et al. Propofol. An update on its clinical use. Anesthesiology 1994;81:1005–1043.

161. Martin TM, Nicolson SC, Bargas MS. Propofol anesthesia reduces emesis and airway obstruction in pediatric outpatients. Anesth Analg 1993;76:144–148.

162. Weir PM, Munro HM, Reynolds PI, et al. Propofol infusion and the incidence of emesis in pediatric outpatient strabismus surgery. Anesth Analg 1993;76:760–764.

163. Runcie CJ, MacKenzie SJ, Arthur DS, et al. Comparison of recovery from anaesthesia induced in children with either propofol or thiopentone. Br J Anaesth 1993;70:192–195.

164. Larsson S, Asgeirsson B, Magnusson J. Propofol-fentanyl anesthesia compared to thiopental-halothane with special reference to recovery and vomiting after pediatric strabismus surgery. Acta Anaesthesiol Scand 1992;36:182–186.

165. Splinter WM, Roberts DJ, Rhine EH, et al. Nitrous oxide does not increase vomiting in children after myringotomy. Can J Anaesth 1995;42:274–276.

166. Horimoto Y, Tomie H, Hanzawa K, et al. Scopolamine patch reduces postoperative emesis in paediatric patients following strabismus surgery. Can J Anaesth 1991;38:441–444.

167. Hannallah RS, Patel RI. Pediatric considerations. In: Twersky RS, ed. The ambulatory anesthesia handbook. St. Louis: CV Mosby, 1995;160–161.

168. Grunwald Z, Schreiner MS, Parness J, et al. Droperidol decreases the incidence and the severity of vomiting after tonsillectomy and adenoidectomy in children. Paediatr Anaesth 1994;4:163–167.

169. Christensen S, Farrow-Gillespie A, Lerman J. Incidence of emesis and postanesthetic recovery after strabismus surgery in children: a comparison of droperidol and lidocaine. Anesthesiology 1989;70:251–254.

170. Abramowitz MD, Oh TH, Epstein BS, et al. The antiemetic effect of droperidol following outpatient strabismus surgery in children. Anesthesiology 1983;59:579–583.

171. Nicolson SC, Kaya KM, Betts EK. The effect of preoperative oral droperidol on the incidence of postoperative emesis after paediatric strabismus surgery. Can J Anaesth 1988;35:364–367.

172. Lin DM, Furst SR, Rodarte A. A double-blinded comparison of metoclopramide and droperidol for prevention of emesis following strabismus surgery. Anesthesiology 1992;76:357–361.

173. Broadman LM, Ceruzzi W, Patane PS, et al. Metoclopramide reduces the incidence of vomiting following strabismus in children. Anesthesiology 1990;72:245–248.

174. Ferrari LR, Donlon JV. Metoclopramide reduces the incidence of vomiting after tonsillectomy in children. Anesth Analg 1992;75:351–354.

175. Splinter WM, Baxter MRN, Gould HM, et al. Oral ondansetron decreases vomiting after tonsillectomy in children. Can J Anaesth 1995;42:277–280.

176. Ummenhofer W, Frei FJ, Urwyler A, et al. Effects of ondansetron in the prevention of postoperative nausea and vomiting in children. Anesthesiology 1994;81:804–810.

177. Furst SR, Rodarte A. Prophylactic antiemetic treatment with ondansetron in children undergoing tonsillectomy. Anesthesiology 1994;81:799–803.

178. Watcha MF, Bras PJ, Cieslak GD, et al. The dose-response relationship of ondansetron in preventing postoperative emesis in pediatric patients undergoing ambulatory surgery. Anesthesiology 1995;82:47–52.

179. Lerman J. Are antiemetics cost-effective for children? (editorial). Can J Anaesth 1995;42:263–266.

180. Westhorpe RN. The position of the larynx in children and its relationship to the ease of intubation. Anaesth Intensive Care 1987;15:384–388.

181. Lioy J, Manginello FP. A comparison of prone and supine positioning in the immediate postextubation period of neonates. J Pediatr 1988;112:982–984.

182. Laffon M, Plaud B, Dubousset AM, et al. Removal of laryngeal mask airway: airway complications in children, anaesthetized versus awake. Paediatr Anaesth 1994;4:35–37.

183. Olsson GL. Laryngospasm during anaesthesia. A computer incidence study of 136,929 patients. Acta Anaesthesiol Scand 1984;28:567–575.

184. Roy WL, Lerman J. Laryngospasm in paediatric anaesthesia. Can Anaesth Soc J 1988;35:93–98.

185. Pounder DR, Blackstock D, Steward DJ. Tracheal extubation in children: halothane versus isoflurane versus awake. Anesthesiology 1991;74:653–655.

186. Patane PS, White SE. Macroglossia causing airway obstruction following cleft palate repair. Anesthesiology 1989;71:995–996.

187. Koka BV, Jeon ISA, Andre JM, et al. Postintubation croup in children. Anesth Analg 1977;56:501–505.

188. Kemper KJ, Benson MS, Bishop MJ. Predictors of postextubation stridor in pediatric trauma patients. Crit Care Med 1991;19:352–355.

189. Maze A, Bloch E. Stridor in pediatric patients. Anesthesiology 1979;50:132–145.

190. Kemper KJ, Ritz RH, Benson MS, et al. Helium-oxygen mixture in the treatment of postextubation stridor in pediatric trauma patients. Crit Care Med 1991;19:356–359.

191. Kairys SW, Olmstead EM, O'Connor GT. Steroid treatment of laryngotracheitis: a meta-analysis of the evidence from randomized trials. Pediatrics 1989;83:683–693.

192. Super DM, Cartelli NA, Brooks LJ, et al. A prospective randomized double-blind study to evaluate the effect of dexamethasone in acute laryngotracheitis. J Pediatr 1989;115:323–329.

193. Spear RM, Deshpande JK, Davis PJ. Systemic disorders in pediatric anesthesia. In: Motoyama EK, Davis PJ, ed. Smith's anesthesia for infants and children. St. Louis: CV Mosby, 1990;781–785.

194. Schuh S, Parkin P, Rajan A, et al. High- versus low-dose, frequently administered, nebulized albuterol in children with severe, acute asthma. Pediatrics 1989;83:513–518.

195. Warner LO, Martino JD, Davidson PJ, et al. Negative pressure pulmonary oedema: a potential hazard of muscle relaxants in awake infants. Can J Anaesth 1990;37:580–583.

196. Wilder RT, Belani KG. Fiberoptic intubation complicated by pulmonary edema in a 12-year-old child with Hurler syndrome. Anesthesiology 1990;72:205–207.

197. Lynch M, Underwood S. Pulmonary oedema following relief of upper airway obstruction in the Pierre-Robin syndrome: a consequence of early palatal repair? Br J Anaesth 1991;66:391–393.

198. Oswalt CE, Gates GE, Holmstrom FM. Pulmonary edema as a complication of acute airway obstruction. Rev Surg 1977;34:346–347.

199. Gwinnutt CL, Meakin G. Use of the post-tetanic count to monitor recovery from intense neuromuscular blockade in children. Br J Anaesth 1988;61:547–550.

200. Bach V, Bouferrache B, Kremp O, et al. Regulation of sleep and body temperature in response to exposure to cool and warm environments in neonates. Pediatrics 1994;93:789–796.

201. Antonen H, Puhakka K, Niskanen J, et al. Cutaneous heat loss in children during anaesthesia. Br J Anaesth 1995;74:30–310.

202. Bissonnette B, Sessler DI. Mild hypothermia does not impair postanesthetic recovery in infants and children. Anesth Analg 1993;76:168–172.

203. Hall SC. Neonatal surgical emergencies. Adv in Anesthesia 1992;9:27–64.

204. Stebbens VA, Poets CF, Alexander JR, et al. Oxygen saturation and breathing patterns in infancy. I. Full term infants in the second month of life. 2. Preterm infants at discharge from special care. Arch Dis Child 1991;66:569–578.

205. Liu LMP, Cote CJ, Goudsouzian NG, et al. Life-threatening apnea in infants recovering from anesthesia. Anesthesiology 1983;59:506–510.

206. Barrington KJ, Finer NN. Periodic breathing and apnea in preterm infants. Pediatr Res 1990;27:118–121.

207. Cote CJ, Zaslavsky A, Downes DJ, et al. Postoperative apnea in former preterm infants after inguinal herniorrhaphy. Anesthesiology 1995;82:809–822.

208. Andropoulos DB, Heard MB, Johnson KL, et al. Postanesthetic apnea in full-term infants after pyloromyotomy. Anesthesiology 1994;80:216–219.

209. Karayan J, LaCoste L, Fusciardi J. Postoperative apnea in a full-term infant (letter). Anesthesiology 1991;75:375.

210. Cote CJ, Kelly DH. Postoperative apnea in a full-term infant with a demonstrable respiratory pattern abnormality. Anesthesiology 1990;72:559–561.

211. Steward DJ. Preterm infants are more prone to complications following minor surgery than are term infants. Anesthesiology 1982;56:304–306.

212. Sims C, Johnson CM. Postoperative apnea in infants. Anaesth Intensive Care 1994;22:40–45.

213. Cox RG, Goresky GV. Life-threatening apnea following spinal anesthesia in former premature infants. Anesthesiology 1990;73:345–348.

214. Watcha MF, Thach BT, Gunter JB. Postoperative apnea after caudal anesthesia in an ex-premature infant. Anesthesiology 1989;71:613–615.

215. Kurth CD, LeBard SE. Association of postoperative

apnea, airway obstruction, and hypoxemia in former premature infants. Anesthesiology 1991;75:22–26.

216. Malviya S, Swartz J, Lerman J. Are all preterm infants younger than 60 weeks postconceptual age at risk for postanesthetic apnea? Anesthesiology 1993;78:1076–1081.

217. Melone JH, Schwartz MZ, Tyson KRT, et al. Outpatient inguinal herniorrhaphy in premature infants: is it safe? J Pediatr Surg 1992;27:203–208.

218. Poets CF, Samuels MP, Noyes JP, et al. Home event recordings of oxygenation, breathing movements, and heart rate and rhythm in infants with recurrent life-threatening events. J Pediatr 1993;123:693–701.

219. Kurth CD, Spitzer AR, Broennle AM, et al. Postoperative apnea in preterm infants. Anesthesiology 1987;66:483–488.

220. Welborn LG, Rice LJ, Hannallah RS, et al. Postoperative apnea in former preterm infants: prospective comparison of spinal and general anesthesia. Anesthesiology 1990;72:838–842.

221. Welborn LG, Hannallah RS, Fink R, et al. High-dose caffeine suppresses postoperative apnea in former preterm infants. Anesthesiology 1989;71:347–349.

222. Aranda JV, Gorman W, Bergsteinsson H, et al. Efficacy of caffeine in the treatment of apnea in low-birth-weight infant. J Pediatr 1977;90:467–472.

223. Welborn LG, Hannallah RS, Luban NLC, et al. Anemia and postoperative apnea in former preterm infants. Anesthesiology 1991;74:1003–1006.

224. Krane EJ, Haberkern CM, Jacobson LE. Postoperative apnea, bradycardia, and oxygen desaturation in formerly premature infants: prospective comparison of spinal and general anesthesia. Anesth Analg 1995;80:7–13.

225. Cox RG, Goresky GV. Life-threatening apnea following spinal anesthesia in former premature infants. Anesthesiology 1990;73:345–348.

226. Coran AG, Drongowski RA. Body fluid compartment changes following neonatal surgery. J Pediatr Surg 1989;24:829–832.

227. Salem RM, Hall SC, Motoyama EK. Anesthesia for thoracic and cardiovascular surgery. In: Motoyama EK, Davis PJ, eds. Smith's anesthesia for infants and children. St. Louis: CV Mosby, 1990;463–544.

228. Burrows FA, Klinck JR, Rabinovitch M, et al. Pulmonary hypertension in children: perioperative management. Can Anaesth Soc J 1986;33:606–628.

229. Moorthy SS, Dierdorf SF, Krishna G, et al. Transient hypoxemia from a transient right-to-left shunt in a child during emergence from anesthesia. Anesthesiology 1987;66:234–235.

230. Hall SC. Children with congenital heart disease undergoing noncardiac surgery. Semin Anesth 1993;12:8–17.

20

SPECIAL CONSIDERATIONS FOR AMBULATORY SURGICAL PATIENTS

Charles B. Hickok, Herbert D. Weintraub

Ambulatory surgery has undergone tremendous growth during the past decade and it will continue to grow well into the 21st century. Dr. J. Nicoll, of the Glasgow Royal Hospital for Sick Children (1), and Dr. R. Waters, of the Down-Town Anesthesia Clinic in Sioux City, Iowa (2), were among the pioneers in the field of ambulatory surgery and anesthesia at the beginning of the 20th century. The field grew slowly during the mid-1900s until the establishment of the first hospital-based ambulatory surgical unit at the University of California at Los Angeles in 1962 (3). This was followed by the opening of a discrete hospital-based unit at George Washington University, Washington, DC in 1966 (4). The Phoenix Surgicenter in Phoenix, Arizona (5) opened in 1970 and was the first successful freestanding ambulatory surgical facility. It is from units such as these that much of our information on the recovery of the ambulatory surgical patient has been derived.

Today's ambulatory postanesthesia care unit (PACU) is vitally important in the success of an ambulatory surgical facility. The ability of the staff to facilitate recovery and discharge patients to home in a caring and timely manner is an important aspect of ambulatory perioperative care. Issues that are currently handled in the ambulatory PACU include recovery from various anesthetic agents and techniques, appropriate pain management, treatment of postoperative nausea and vomiting, and discharging the patient in the company of a responsible person as early as feasible without placing the patient at any increased risk. Additionally, complications of various types do occur in the ambulatory PACU as they do with inpatients. All of these issues will be discussed in the following text.

PHYSICAL PLANT

Postanesthesia care of the ambulatory patient differs from that provided to the inpatient, and the organization and layout of the ambulatory PACU should reflect this difference. Most centers now divide the recovery of the ambulatory patient into phase I and phase II. Phase I represents the initial recovery immediately after the operating room. All of the equipment and personnel required to respond to an emergency should be readily available. Phase I may be part of the main recovery room used for inpatients, although it is desirable to separate outpatients from inpatients. This is because the outpatients tend to be more alert and aware of their surroundings and may be disturbed by inpatients who have undergone more extensive surgical procedures. Nursing care and philosophy also differs for these two groups of patients, and again, their separation promotes increased nursing efficiency.

Phase II typically includes a reclining lounge chair for the patient to continue recovery until the time of discharge. Many institutions require the patient to ambulate from phase I to phase II recovery areas. Having already demonstrated hemodynamic stability and continuing recovery, this ambulation serves as another milestone in the recovery process. The reclining chair provides a comfortable position, but it also provides the capability to be placed nearly flat if the patient experiences hypotension. A beverage and crackers may be offered in phase II, which is yet another step toward discharge from the unit. Voiding and the lack of significant nausea will serve as additional steps toward discharge. Some institutions encourage family members to stay with the patient in phase II. The presence of family members can encourage recovery and enhance postoperative teaching while possibly lightening some of the nursing duties. This is especially true with the pediatric population. Discharge instructions are usually given to the patient and the responsible adult who takes the patient home in phase II, just before departure.

The location of the phase I and II recovery areas ideally should be near the operating room. This not only provides a short transit for the patient to the PACU but also provides ready access by members of the anesthesia and surgical staff in the event of an emergency or simply for the convenience of dealing with routine postoperative issues. Patient lockers, changing areas, restrooms, and family waiting areas should also be located nearby to facilitate patient flow and communication with family members. Consideration also must be given to the location of support services such as laboratory, laundry, etc.

Finally, consideration must be given to the decor of the unit. Ambulatory patients are more alert and aware of their surroundings than their inpatients. Therefore, the environment should project a pleasant, friendly feeling and not the typical emotionless hospital gray or beige walls. As the marketplace becomes more competitive, it is important not only to provide a quality service but to make the experience as pleasant as possible to our increasingly consumer-oriented society.

SPECIAL NEEDS OF THE OUTPATIENT IN THE PACU

As the goals of the inpatient PACU are different from the goals of the ambulatory PACU, so are the needs of these two patient groups. Patients who are scheduled for admission postoperatively can usually be discharged to a hospital room once they have demonstrated a stable cardiopulmonary status, have relatively good pain control and have recovered sufficiently from anesthesia. These inpatients may be discharged from the PACU with significant levels of sedation and requirements for ongoing pain control as well as an inability to ambulate. This is not the case for the ambulatory patient. The ambulatory patient must exceed the requirements established for the inpatient.

"Home readiness" is the term commonly used to refer to the ambulatory patient who can to be safely discharged. The patient who is home ready should be stable and have near preoperative levels from a cardiopulmonary standpoint. This patient also should have little psychomotor impairment, be able to think relatively clearly, and be able to ambulate in an unassisted fashion (unless interdicted by the type of surgery). There should be good pain control that can be maintained at home. The absence of marked nausea or vomiting is currently used as a discharge requirement at most institutions, as is the ability to micturate before discharge (except for rectal surgery patients who may not be able to micturate) and to tolerate oral fluids. The latter two requirements are somewhat controversial and will be discussed later in this chapter.

Two major anesthetic reasons for an unanticipated hospital admission are persistent nausea and vomiting and pain that cannot be controlled adequately on an outpatient basis. The overall incidence of unanticipated admissions ranges from 0.68 to 4.1%. There is a lower incidence at freestanding ambulatory centers, whereas hospital-affiliated and university-based ambulatory units tend to have higher rates of unanticipated admission (6).

Although the problems of nausea and pain can be addressed specifically in the PACU, the impact of the anesthetic technique on recovery and discharge should be examined as well.

Intraoperative Management and PACU Care

The appropriate, rational choice of an anesthetic for a particular case may have a far greater impact on the recovery and timely discharge of that patient than any plan that can be implemented in the PACU after the fact.

For example, a spinal or epidural may eliminate or decrease the need for parenteral sedatives or narcotics, which can contribute to psychomotor impairment and result in a delayed discharge. Additionally, this regional technique will provide excellent initial pain relief, but analgesia should be maintained as the block resolves. However, if a spinal or an epidural is chosen for a very short case, the above advantages may be offset by the disadvantage of a delayed discharge while waiting for resolution of the block to the point at which the patient is ambulatory. Additionally, urinary retention can complicate the recovery after a spinal or epidural. Upper extremity blocks, on the other hand, can provide good operative anesthesia as well as good postoperative analgesia while usually causing no delay in discharge of the ambulatory patient, as long as there is no contraindication to discharging the patient with a residual upper extremity block. A simple alternative may be an intravenous regional technique (Bier block), because it can provide good intraoperative anesthesia but is associated with rapid return of motor and sensory function. The commonly used regional techniques are associated with a decreased incidence of nausea and vomiting when not augmented with narcotics. Occasionally, however, nausea and vomiting may occur as a result of hypotension related to the sympathectomy associated with spinal or epidural anesthesia.

Conscious sedation is associated with a low complication rate in the ambulatory setting and a reduced PACU. Therefore, this technique can minimize PACU problems such as nausea and vomiting and may allow for a quicker recovery of psychomotor function leading to a timely discharge from the ambulatory unit.

General anesthesia, although associated with a higher incidence of nausea and vomiting than regional and conscious sedation techniques, may be the anesthetic of choice in many cases. The issue of nausea and vomiting can be addressed by identifying patients "at risk" for postoperative nausea and vomiting and taking appropriate precautions to decrease the likelihood of its occurrence. Although the initial psychomotor impairment may be greater than that associated with neuroaxial blockade, the ability to meet discharge criteria after short general cases may be faster than that associated with a spinal or epidural if the patient is expected to ambulate without assistance postoperatively.

The pharmaceutical methodology of the anesthesiologist is ever increasing and provides the practitioner with a wide variety of choices. Many of the recently developed drugs have improved pharmacodynamics and pharmacokinetic profiles, providing highly titratable agents with rapid onset and offset and minimal side effects. These characteristics are especially desirable for ambulatory surgical patients. The wide selection of agents can improve the quality of the recovery.

Propofol, approved for use in the United States in 1989, is one such agent that is highly desirable in the ambulatory population, because it provides rapid intravenous induction and smooth maintenance and is associated with a rapid, clearheaded emergence and recovery when used as part of a general anesthetic (7). Along with the rapid return of psychomotor function, propofol has a low incidence of nausea and vomiting associated with its use (8).

Desflurane is one of the newer volatile agents with a low blood gas partition coefficient that allows for rapid uptake and rapid emergence, thus also possibly providing more rapid recovery of preoperative function and perhaps earlier discharge from the ambulatory unit.

NAUSEA AND VOMITING

Postoperative nausea and vomiting (PONV) can be a major problem for ambulatory surgical patients. PONV is the primary anesthetic reason for unplanned hospital admission in the ambulatory patient population. Currently, most discharge criteria call for a patient to be free of nausea and vomiting before discharge.

The act of vomiting is coordinated by the emetic center, which is believed to be located in the lateral reticular formation close to the tractus solitarius in the brainstem (9,10). The chemoreceptor trigger zone (CTZ) located in the area postrema is activated by multiple chemical stimuli carried via the blood or cerebrospinal fluid. Many endogenously occurring substances (serotonin, histamine, dopamine, and muscarinic and cholinergic agents) are capable of stimulating the CTZ. Opioids and other analgesic agents seem to be capable of stimulating the CTZ. Afferent input from the visual and vestibular centers, pharynx, gastrointestinal tract, and the mediastinum may directly stimulate the emetic center. Therefore, the cause of PONV is multifactorial in nature and as such there is, as yet, no single solution to this problem.

There are a number of patient factors that may place a patient at increased risk for PONV. Identifying these factors preoperatively and modifying the anesthetic plan accordingly may reduce the incidence of PONV. Age less than 14 years, female gender, obesity, stage of menstrual cycle, anxiety, gastroparesis, and a history of PONV or motion sickness have been implicated as patient risk factors (11).

The surgical site also plays a role in determining the incidence of PONV. Laparoscopic ovum retrieval procedures and laparoscopies in females are associated with a 54% and 35% incidence of postoperative emesis,

respectively. These procedures account for the highest incidence of PONV in the adult population (12). In the pediatric population, strabismus surgery, orchiopexy, and ear, nose, and throat surgery are procedures that are likely to be associated with PONV. These procedures are usually performed on an ambulatory basis.

The choice of the anesthetic technique and/or agents may influence the incidence of PONV after outpatient anesthesia. This section will briefly explore several agents that are used commonly for general anesthesia and their potential impact on PONV. Propofol is the least likely of the induction agents to be associated with PONV. Conversely, etomidate has a high incidence of postoperative emesis associated with its use as an induction agent while methohexital and thiopental are intermediate between these two. Narcotics are associated with PONV, especially the longer-acting narcotics such as morphine and meperidine. There are conflicting reports regarding the incidence of emesis after the use of the various semisynthetic opioids (fentanyl, sufentanil, alfentanil) (13–19). However, it has been demonstrated that the use of a nitrous oxide opioid-relaxant technique has a higher incidence of postoperative emesis than an inhalational technique (20–24). This evidence would seem to incriminate narcotics. Controversy exists regarding the role of nitrous oxide in contributing to PONV. Early studies found a correlation between the use of nitrous oxide (plus a volatile anesthetic) and the incidence of PONV. More recently, studies have questioned any correlation between nitrous oxide and PONV (25–28).

Consideration should also be given to the role of neuromuscular blocker reversal agents. The increased muscarinic effects created by the use of an anticholinesterase may increase gastrointestinal motility, which may lead to increased PONV. White demonstrated a decreased incidence of PONV in ambulatory patients receiving general anesthesia for laparoscopic tubal ligation when mivacurium was used without reversal agents versus mivacurium with antagonism using neostigmine and glycopyrrolate (29).

Apart from the consideration of antiemetic prophylaxis in selected "at risk" patients, any patient could benefit from a wise choice of anesthetic technique. PONV is generally less common with regional techniques than with general anesthesia, but this difference may not be obvious if large doses of intravenous agents are given for sedation and/or amnesia. Because of the sympathectomy and potential for hypotension, central neuroaxial blockade is more likely to be associated with nausea and vomiting than peripheral nerve block.

Prevention and Treatment

Considering the saying, "an ounce of prevention is worth a pound of cure," one naturally wonders about the role of routine prophylactic antiemetic administration in the ambulatory patient. Fewer than 30% of all postoperative patients will experience PONV, and of that 30%, most will be of limited duration and severity not requiring treatment. Considering the fact that the commonly used antiemetics can be associated with side effects such as sedation, extrapyramidal symptoms and dysphoria, and increased expense, the routine administration of prophylactic antiemetics to all ambulatory patients is not warranted. However, prophylaxis may be appropriate for patients who are at greater risk for PONV. Those at increased risk include patients with a history of PONV and/or motion sickness, females undergoing gynecological procedures, and pediatric patients undergoing emetogenic procedures such as strabismus surgery, otoplasty, tonsilloadenoidectomy, and orchiopexy (11, 30, 31).

Postoperative pain has been reported to be a cause of PONV. Anderson and Krohg demonstrated that it was unusual to have complete relief of pain without simultaneous relief of nausea when the two occurred concomitantly (32). In this study, only 10% of the patients complained about nausea without having accompanying pain. Therefore, effective postop-

erative analgesia may contribute to a decreased incidence of emesis. Small doses of intravenous narcotic (fentanyl, 25 μg) or regional techniques may help provide this analgesia in the ambulatory PACU.

Sudden movements or position changes have been implicated as contributing to the problem. The literature suggests that opioids sensitize the vestibular system to motion-induced nausea and vomiting (33, 34).

Anesthetic maneuvers such as avoiding excessive positive pressure during mask ventilation will help prevent insufflation of the stomach, which may contribute to PONV. The lower esophageal sphincter will be forced open by pressure greater than 20 cm of water pressure. Decompression of the stomach with a gastric tube after intubation and before extubation may also help decrease the incidence of PONV.

Antiemetic Agents

Pharmacologic antiemetic agents can be divided into five categories: antihistamines (hydroxyzine), phenothiazine (prochlorperazine), anticholinergics (scopolamine), butyrophenones (droperidol), and dopamine antagonists (metoclopramide). An additional group recently added is the serotonin antagonist group (ondansetron). It is speculated that the serotonin antagonist agents will have fewer sedative, cardiovascular, or extrapyramidal side effects that can be associated with many of the classical antiemetics.

Anticholingeric agents are most efficacious in the treatment of motion sickness. In the perioperative setting, scopolamine has been delivered primarily with the transdermal patches (TDS). The efficacy of TDS in preventing PONV has been evaluated in several studies. TDS was found to be ineffective in treating PONV. In addition, scopolamine can have a high incidence of anticholinergic side effects.

Droperidol, 75 μg/kg, is very effective prophylaxis for pediatric patients undergoing strabismus repair. However, recovery time is excessively long because of marked sedation, which prevents these children from meeting home discharge criteria (35). Droperidol, in doses of 7 to 14 μg/kg, is probably the most commonly used antiemetic in the adult surgical population. Studies generally support its effectiveness when compared to placebo. Higher adult doses are likely to be associated with excessive sedation, possibly leading to delayed discharge from the ambulatory unit. Postoperative dysphoria or restlessness for up to 24 hours has also been reported for outpatients given even small doses of droperidol in the perioperative setting (36).

Metoclopramide is another commonly used antiemetic. It is generally believed to be less sedating than droperidol but may be associated with extrapyramidal symptoms if given in higher doses. The commonly used dose of 10 mg intravenously for a 70-kg adult is usually well tolerated, although dystonic reactions are possible (37, 38). There are varying results on the efficacy of metoclopramide. Cohen compared low-dose droperidol to metoclopramide in ambulatory patients and noted a lack of antiemetic effect of the metoclopramide-treated group in ambulatory patients. However, this group was able to sit, walk, and be discharged sooner than either the control or droperidol-treated groups (39). Doze et al. demonstrated the effectiveness of the combination of metoclopramide (10 to 20 mg intravenously 20 minutes before induction) and droperidol (0.5 to 1.0 mg intravenously 6 minutes before induction) to be more effective than droperidol alone and resulted in shorter PACU times (40).

Ondansetron, the first serotonin antagonist introduced, originally was found to be effective as an antiemetic agent during cancer chemotherapy treatments. Studies in the perioperative setting showed ondansetron to be more effective than placebo (and metoclopramide, droperidol) in preventing or treating nausea and vomiting after the administration of a balanced general anesthetic (41, 42). Equally significant is ondansetron's lack of side effects.

The use of intramuscular ephedrine 25 to 50 mg or 5 to 10 mg intravenously in the adult have been used as a treatment for PONV with some success (43).

Therefore, a logical approach to the issue of PONV in the ambulatory patient population would be one of risk stratification. Prophylaxis is not appropriate for all patients, but it should be considered for certain high-risk patients. These at-risk patients should be given an anesthetic with a low potential of contributing to PONV as well as receiving some form of prophylaxis. Finally, any patient with significant PONV should be treated promptly.

POSTOPERATIVE PAIN MANAGEMENT FOR THE AMBULATORY PATIENT

Postoperative pain is second only to postoperative nausea and vomiting as a reason for prolonged discharge times and unanticipated hospital admission from an ambulatory facility. This is more of an issue currently than in the past for three reasons. First, new anesthetic agents allow patients to come to the PACU more awake, clearheaded, and aware of their environment and, consequently, their pain. Second, more extensive surgical procedures are being performed on an ambulatory basis than in the past, leading to increased requirements for analgesia and the use of more potent analgesic agents both intraoperatively and postoperatively. Lastly, as acute pain management has emerged as a major issue in medicine, patients have greater expectations for good analgesia during the postoperative period, particularly in the ambulatory care setting.

As the mechanism of pain has become better understood recently, our ability to effectively treat and/or prevent pain has improved. It is now clear that the prevention or very early treatment of pain is desirable. Prevention or early treatment results not only in a more satisfied patient, but less total analgesic agent will be required. Therefore, the sedative and respiratory depressant effects are likely to be less,

Table 20–1. Opioids

Opioid	Comments
Morphine	Slow onset
Meperidine	Difficult to titrate
Alfentanil	Too short duration of action
Fentanyl	Easily titrated
Sufentanil	Too potent
NSAIDs	Effective for mild to moderate postoperative pain
Local anesthetics	Used for specific nerve block, wound infiltration or wound splash

thereby possibly preventing prolonged recovery stays. The subject of preemptive analgesia is receiving increasing attention and may have potential implications for the ambulatory population as this area of study unfolds.

The major form of treatment of acute pain in the ambulatory PACU is pharmacologic and consists of opioids, nonsteroidal anti-inflammatory drugs, and local anesthetics (see Table 20–1).

Opioids

A variety of opioids and routes of administration have been investigated for use in the outpatient surgical setting.

The ideal opioid for this purpose would provide rapid, reliable, and complete pain relief while being devoid of side effects such as sedation, respiratory depression, and nausea. Small (25 μg) incremental doses of intravenous fentanyl would be the best choice as an opioid analgesic in the ambulatory PACU. It should be administered early when pain is first noted or perhaps as pain is anticipated.

Morphine and meperidine should not be used in the ambulatory PACU as they have a slow onset and are difficult to titrate to relief of acute pain. Alfentanil, on the other hand, has a very rapid onset (2 to 3 minutes), but its duration of action is so short that it cannot provide lasting analgesia. Additionally, alfentanil may contribute to nausea and vomiting. Sufentanil, presumably because of its potency,

has not received much investigation in the ambulatory PACU setting.

Opioid agonist-antagonists have been evaluated for their ability to produce analgesia while having fewer μ-receptor-related side effects. The theoretically attractive features of the opioid agonist-antagonists are that they are less likely to produce significant respiratory depression as modulated by μ-2 receptors. These agents are said to have a "ceiling effect," such that increasing the dose beyond a certain point will not increase the effect. These drugs display a ceiling for respiratory depression, but they often have a low ceiling effect for analgesia, which may limit their ability to prevent and/or relieve postoperative pain. Nalbuphine (0.25 mg/kg), which is an agonist-antagonist equal in potency to morphine as an analgesic agent, produced better postoperative analgesia than fentanyl (1.5 μg/kg) when given immediately before termination of pregnancy; however, it was associated with prolonged psychomotor impairment and significant nausea and vomiting (44). Butorphanol, another agonist-antagonist (20 μg/kg intravenously), immediately before induction for inpatients undergoing general anesthesia for laparoscopic tubal ligation, proved no better than fentanyl (2 μg/kg) intravenously before induction in relieving pain postoperatively (45).

Another form of intravenous opioid administration that is in its early stages of development for outpatients is patient-controlled analgesia (PCA) in the ambulatory PACU. Zelcer et al. reported good pain scores for patients undergoing oocyte retrievals with conscious sedation using intravenous PCA with alfentanil (46). The pain and comfort scores of these patients were comparable to the control group in which the anesthesiologist administered alfentanil boluses of 5 mcg/kg. There is a possible role for intravenous PCA in the ambulatory PACU and perhaps beyond.

Other Systemic Opioid Routes

Whereas the use of early, small doses of intravenous fentanyl would seem to be the most appropriate treatment of acute pain in the PACU, other routes of administration do exist and may have advantages in selected settings. The intramuscular route, although not novel, is mentioned here only to discourage its use in this patient population as the absorption is unreliable and the onset is slow.

Transdermal therapeutic system (TTS) of fentanyl has undergone evaluation in the surgical population. This system employs a patch applied to the skin that is able to continuously deliver fentanyl at rates of 25 to 100 µg/hour (depending on the surface area of the patch) for up to 72 hours. Several problems exist with this system. Although blood levels are measurable after the first 2 hours of administration, 8 to 16 hours may be required until full clinical effect is noted. This presents some logistical problems for the ambulatory surgical patient as far as when and how to obtain the patch and when to start its use. Because of fentanyl deposition in the skin, plasma levels will decline only by 50% in 16 hours after patch removal, which may be an unacceptably long duration of offset. The need for additional opioid in patients using the fentanyl TTS, as judged by intravenous PCA requirements, is variable. Sevarino et al. demonstrated no opioid sparing effect of the TTS for fentanyl in female inpatients after abdominal gynecologic surgery (47). Caplan et al., however, reported significant opioid sparing effects in a similar patient population (48). The most significant drawback to the fentanyl TTS is the incidence of nausea and vomiting as high as 70%, which makes its use in the ambulatory surgical population less feasible as demonstrated in the studies by Sevarino and Caplan.

One of the more novel ways of opioid administration is via the internasal route using fentanyl and meperidine. Inpatient studies have demonstrated pain relief as effective as that obtained with intravenous fentanyl (49). The future application of this in the ambulatory patient requires further investigation. Also requiring further evaluation is the use of the fentanyl lollipop or the oral transmucosal fentanyl lozenge, which provides rapid and effective analgesia (50). The future of these products still must be defined, especially because they may have significant abuse potential.

The literature abounds with reports of intrathecal and epidural administration of opioids in inpatients with generally good postoperative analgesia for a variety of surgical procedures (51). Concerns about respiratory depression have limited the use of intrathecal or epidural opioids in ambulatory patients and to date there are no published data on this subject.

In contrast, however, there is an increasing use of intra-articular morphine in patients undergoing outpatient arthroscopic knee surgery. This seems to provide a good quality of postoperative analgesia, especially when combined with dilute local anesthetic (52).

Nonsteroidal Anti-Inflammatory Drugs

Nonsteroidal anti-inflammatory drugs (NSAIDs) have the ability to block the enzyme cyclooxygenase, thereby preventing the conversion of arachidonic acid to prostaglandin E_2, which is a mediator of pain. These agents have been studied most extensively in patients undergoing gynecologic or orthopedic procedures and seem to decrease narcotic requirements. Narcotics can have side effects such as sedation, respiratory depression, nausea, vomiting, and urinary retention. Because NSAIDs are devoid of these side effects, it is desirable, in certain cases, to substitute NSAIDs for narcotics or supplement narcotics with NSAIDs.

Ibuprofen, 800 mg orally 1 hour before induction of anesthesia, has been reported to be more effective than fentanyl with regard to postoperative analgesia in patients undergoing laparoscopic surgery. A low incidence of nausea and vomiting was also reported (53). Ketorolac, a parenteral NSAID, has been reported to be equipotent to 12 mg of morphine for postoperative analgesia (54). Ketorolac and indomethacin were found to be equally efficacious and better than placebo for the relief of minor postoperative pain in women undergoing gynecological or breast surgery on an ambulatory basis (55). Conversely, Higgins et al. reported no difference in pain scores or opioid requirements in patients undergoing laparoscopic Yoon ring tubal ligation who received either placebo, intramuscular ketorolac, or oral ibuprofen preoperatively (56). In evaluating ketorolac for intraoperative analgesia as opposed to postoperative analgesia, White found ketorolac alone to be less effective than fentanyl 50 to 100 μg alone or the combination of fentanyl 50 to 100 μg plus ketorolac 30 to 60 mg intravenously (57). NSAIDs may be contraindicated for patients with significant renal disease, because of the drugs' ability to reversibly alter renal blood flow, as well as for patients who are at increased risk for either gastrointestinal or surgical bleeding.

Local Anesthetics and Intra-Articular Narcotics

Local anesthetics can play an important role in reducing postoperative analgesic requirements in the ambulatory patient. Extremity nerve blocks, such as interscalene, axillary, and ankle or popliteal blocks, can provide both intraoperative anesthesia as well as postoperative analgesia. Such blocks may be used alone or in conjunction with general anesthesia or conscious sedation. In most cases, patients can be discharged from the unit with residual block still present, as long as the patient is aware of the need to protect the extremity.

The use of local anesthetic infiltrated or even "splashed" into a wound before closure of the skin can reduce postoperative pain (58). Infiltration of the mesosalpinx during laparoscopic tubal ligation can be performed to improve the quality of analgesia in the PACU and at home (59, 60).

Finally, intra-articular injection of local anesthetics with or without morphine has been shown to reduce supplementary analgesia requirements while demonstrating improved visual analog scores for pain when compared to placebo in patients undergoing knee arthroscopy.

In conclusion, the management of postoperative analgesia is best addressed preoperatively with an evaluation of the proposed surgical procedure and its associated postoperative pain. Then, an anesthetic plan can be decided upon to maximize analgesia as the patient is admitted to the PACU. This may take the form of a particular general anesthetic or regional technique or a combination of the two techniques. The intraoperative participation of the surgeon should always be considered in relation to the administration of local anesthetics and/or opiates directly to the operative site. After the patient is in recovery, fentanyl (in 25-μg increments) may be titrated carefully to provide analgesia while avoiding excessive sedation. The early and prompt treatment of postoperative pain may decrease the total dose of narcotic needed overall and thereby minimize side effects. Oral medication such as oxycodone and acetaminophen (Percocet) or acetaminophen with codeine can be used for pain not requiring parenteral narcotics. The early use of such oral analgesic agents will help overcome the slower onset associated with orally administered medications, as well as allowing one to evaluate the efficacy of pain control of the chosen oral agent. Likewise, these oral agents can be used in conjunction with fentanyl to provide a longer duration of analgesia. NSAID agents such as ketorolac can be administered in the PACU although they are probably more effective if given intraoperatively or even preoperatively.

ADDITIONAL ISSUES IN THE AMBULATORY PACU

Other problems can arise that can delay or prevent discharge from the unit. More extensive surgery than anticipated may dictate the need for hospitalization either because of the extent of the surgery or the need for analgesia that cannot be met at home. This is less of a logistical problem at a hospital-based facility than it is at a freestanding facility.

Social reasons, such as failure of a responsible adult to escort the patient home, will occasionally delay or prevent a discharge. This source of delayed discharge is best avoided by thorough preoperative instructions and by ensuring that the patient has made appropriate arrangements for discharge at the time of admission to the facility.

One issue that has yet to be addressed by the medical community is the adequacy of home care that the patient will receive. As more extensive procedures are performed on an ambulatory basis and as a larger percentage of the population are defined as elderly, the ability of a patient to receive adequate home care will become more of an issue.

Unanticipated bleeding is a reason for unplanned admission. Under such a circumstance, it would be unwise to discharge such a patient to home, especially if he/she lives some distance from the facility.

Ambulatory patients are not immune to complications that may befall any other surgical patients. Complications, such as laryngospasm, bronchospasm, suspected aspiration, hypoxemia, hypotension, etc., should all be treated as they normally would in any postoperative patient. Only after the problem has been thoroughly evaluated and corrected should discharge be considered.

MORBIDITY AND MORTALITY AFTER DISCHARGE

Major morbidity and mortality within 1 month of ambulatory surgery and anesthesia was studied by Warner et al. In a follow-up of 38,598 patients aged 18 years or older undergoing 45,090 ambulatory procedures and anesthetics, this group found that the overall morbidity and mortality rate was very low. Thirty-three patients either experienced major morbidity or died. Of the four patients who died, two died of myocardial infarctions and two died of automobile accidents. Approximately two-thirds of all major morbidities oc-

curred within 48 hours of surgery. The remaining one-third occurred during the following 28 days (61).

DISCHARGE CRITERIA

The appropriate and timely discharge of ambulatory patients is essential to the efficiency of the PACU and the ambulatory surgical unit. Patients who are inappropriately discharged prematurely are more likely to have postoperative complications or to suffer injuries due to psychomotor impairment. Discharging patients after an inappropriately long stay will begin to create a backlog of patients, which eventually will affect the operating suites because there no recovery beds are available. Therefore, an effective system of judging recovery is required.

The recovery period can be divided into several stages. Early recovery is synonymous with emergence and the ability to protect and maintain one's airway. Intermediate recovery deals with the achievement of certain milestones in the PACU, culminating in discharge from the surgical facility. It is at this intermediate recovery stage that the anesthesiologist and PACU personnel play the most important role to ensure a safe and timely passage through the facility. Full recovery refers to the patient's resumption of normal daily activities, which may require days to weeks.

Several tests are available to evaluate a patient's psychomotor recovery after anesthesia. These tests, however, are used mostly for research purposes and do not lend themselves to practical clinical use as standard determinants of discharge readiness. As these tests are used to determine effects of various anesthetic agents on the intermediate recovery phase, they will be discussed briefly. Perceptual speed tests require the patients to recognize a specific letter or number in a long line of letters or numbers and circle or cross out that specific number or letter wherever it appears during a 2- or 3-minute period. The digit symbol substitution test (DSST) requires the patient to replace random digits (0 through 9) with

Table 20–2.   Guidelines for Safe Discharge after Ambulatory Surgery

Patient's vital signs must have been stable for at least 1 hour.

Patient must have no evidence of respiratory depression.

Patient must be:

   oriented to person, place, and time.

   able to maintain orally administered fluids.[a]

   able to void.[a]

   able to dress himself or herself.

   able to walk without assistance.

Patient must not have:

   more than minimal nausea or vomiting.

   excessive pain.

   bleeding.

Patients must be discharged by a member of the postanesthesia care team and the person who performed surgery or by their designees. Written instructions for the postoperative period at home, including a contact place and person, must be reinforced.

Patients must have a responsible "vested" adult escort them home and stay with them at home.

[a] The role of these variables as criteria for discharge remains to be established.

Modified from Korttila K. Recovery period and discharge. In: White P, ed. Outpatient anesthesia. New York: Churchill Livingstone, 1990; 369–395.

a symbol that is given in a key. The DSST is one of the most sensitive writing tests for the detection of residual anesthetic effects. The Maddox wing test detects imbalance of extraocular muscles but is not a good measure of cognitive or psychomotor recovery. A force platform can be used to measure body sway as a measure of psychomotor recovery, which correlates with a patient's ability to ambulate safely.

Safe discharge from the ambulatory facility requires not only the return of vital signs to near a baseline level but also requires the patient to be free of significant cognitive or psychomotor impairment. Other desirable discharge criteria are presented in Table 20–2 (62). To help judge recovery and movement toward meeting discharge criteria, some scoring systems have been proposed. The Aldrete scoring system, which is one of the earliest, mimics the Apgar scoring system and is useful for evaluating recovery of patients who are to

be discharged to the hospital ward (63). The Aldrete system is not appropriate for the ambulatory patient because it does not address the level of hydration, the ability to tolerate oral fluids (controversial), or the ability to ambulate.

Dr. F. Chung has developed the Postanesthesia Discharge Scoring system (PADS) to specifically address the intermediate recovery phase of the ambulatory patient. This system more accurately assesses the areas of importance in the ambulatory patient: (a) vital signs, (b) activity and mental status, (c) pain, nausea, vomiting, (d) surgical bleeding, and (e) intake and output (see Table 20–3) (64). PADS allows patients to be discharged significantly earlier than those of clinical criteria alone. Such a numeric scoring system not only provides a rapid and accurate means of assessing a patient's recovery progress but also provides medicolegal documentation. Therefore, the appropriate application of a scoring system designed for the ambulatory patient should efficiently and safely move patients through the

Table 20–3.   Postanesthesia Discharge Scoring System (PADSS)

Vital signs

   2 = within 20% of preoperative value

   1 = 20% to 40% of preoperative value

   0 = 40% of preoperative value

Ambulation and mental status

   2 = oriented × 3 and has a steady gait

   1 = oriented × 3 or has a steady gait

   0 = neither

Pain or nausea and vomiting

   2 = minimal

   1 = moderate

   0 = severe

Surgical bleeding

   2 = minimal

   1 = moderate

   0 = severe

Intake and output

   2 = has had oral fluids and has voided

   1 = has had oral fluids or has voided

   0 = neither

Note: Maximum total score is 10; patients scoring 9 or 10 are considered fit for discharge home. "× 3" means that the patient is oriented sufficiently to know his name, his location, and the time.

PACU. The ability to tolerate oral fluid and to micturate are controversial and not universally accepted as guidelines for discharge. Research has suggested that requiring a patient to take fluids before that patient feels ready may increase the incidence of PONV and thereby prolong the PACU stay. The emerging opinion is that if a patient has received adequate intravenous hydration and has no or minimal nausea, then he may be discharged without taking fluids before discharge. The inability to void after surgery is multifactorial in nature. It is a common problem in surgery involving the rectum, genitalia, and inguinal area. Reflex urethral spasm and detrusor muscle dysfunction are some of the causes. These can be precipitated by rectal pain and/or distention, altered autonomic input to the bladder after major conduction anesthesia, or systemically administered drugs and/or a bladder, which has become overdistended intraoperatively.

Realizing that the ability to tolerate fluids and void are not universally accepted as guidelines, Dr. Chung developed a modified PADS that deleted these two requirements. The modified PADS also separated the mental status and activity section, which were combined in the original PADS (see Table 20–4) (64). The deletion of these requirements for fluids and voiding allowed a shorter time to discharge in the patient group evaluated with the modified PADS system. There was no increase in the readmission or complication rate when using the modified PADS system.

Therefore, it may be reasonable to relax some of the discharge requirements that had been set forth originally. The original guidelines were developed largely on an empiric basis. The application of a modified PADS system could allow better use of PACU space and staffing especially in an era of increasing medical-economic restraints as long as there continues to be no adverse effect on patient outcome.

UNANTICIPATED HOSPITAL ADMISSION

The reasons for unanticipated hospital admission from an ambulatory unit may be surgi-

Table 20–4. Modified Postanesthesia Discharge Scoring System (Modified PADSS)

Vital signs
  2 = within 20% of preoperative value
  1 = 20% to 40% of preoperative value
  0 = 40% of preoperative value
Ambulation
  2 = steady gait/no dizziness
  1 = with assistance
  0 = non ambulatory or dizziness
Nausea and vomiting
  2 = minimal
  1 = moderate
  0 = severe
Pain
  2 = minimal
  1 = moderate
  0 = severe
Surgical bleeding
  2 = minimal
  1 = moderate
  0 = severe

Note: Maximum total score is 10; patients scoring 9 or 10 are considered fit for discharge home.

cal, anesthetic, medical, or social. Combining all of these groups yields an overall incidence that ranges from 0.68 to 4.1% (6). Freestanding ambulatory units have a lower incidence of unanticipated hospital admission, whereas hospital-affiliated and university-based units tend to have a higher rate of unanticipated admission. The reason for this observed difference is not clear, but it may involve patient population and surgical case selection factors.

The Medical College of Virginia's Ambulatory Surgery Center had a 1.0% rate of unanticipated admission between 1981 and 1988 while performing 21,140 procedures (65). More than half of this 1.0% was due to surgical reasons, whereas 14% of those admitted were due to anesthetic reasons (see Table 20–5). The anesthetic reasons for admission are noted in Table 20–6 for this same time period (1981 through 1988).

The rate of unanticipated admission increases with advancing age and with increasing American Society of Anesthesiologists (ASA) physical status. The Phoenix Surgicenter reports an overall admission rate of 0.2%, which

Table 20–5. Reasons for Unanticipated Hospital Admissions for 21,140 Cases

REASONS	NO. OF PATIENTS ADMITTED
Surgical	127 (57.5)
Anesthesia	31 (14.0)
Medical	38 (17.2)
Social	25 (11.3)
Total admission number	211 (100)

Table 20–6. Anesthetic Reasons for Unanticipated Admission (Medical College of Virginia, 1981–1988)

REASONS	NO. OF PATIENTS (%)
Intractable vomiting	4 (13.0)
Aspiration	5 (16.1)
Delayed awakening	2 (6.4)
Hypertension	4 (13.0)
Arrhythmia	4 (13.0)
Syncope/hypotension	3 (9.7)
Drug reaction	2 (6.4)
Transfusion reaction	1 (3.2)
Congestive heart failure/pulmonary edema	1 (3.2)
Myocardial ischemia	1 (3.2)
Atypical pseudocholinesterase	1 (3.2)
Postoperative croup	1 (3.2)
Muscle stiffness	1 (3.2)
N_2O embolus	1 (3.2)

Total number of patients: 21,140; total number of admissions: 221; total number of admissions for anesthetic reasons: 31.

increases to 0.59% for patients older than 64 years of age. The same center has an admission rate of 1.4% for patients who are ASA physical status III (66).

MEETING NEW CHALLENGES

The volume of surgical procedures being performed on an ambulatory basis may exceed 70% of all surgical cases by the year 2000 as the scope and magnitude of procedures deemed appropriate for the ambulatory setting continues to increase. At the George Washington University Hospital, representative of a typical university hospital, the percentage of ambulatory patients increased from 41.1% to 50.9% of the total between 1985 and 1993, while the total surgical caseload remained essentially unchanged (Table 20–7). Of note is the changing use of the main operating rooms during the same time period. In 1985, the main operating suites handled 9.9% of the ambulatory patient population. This percentage increased to 38.3% by 1993 indicating a significant shift in operating room use. Finally, the length and complexity of cases being performed in the ambulatory unit has increased. Patients with more significant coexisting disease states will be shifted to the ambulatory setting and, as our population ages, the percentages of the surgical population constituting the geriatric group will increase as well. Finally, resources will be more tightly controlled as medicine moves into the era of cost containment and managed care. Therefore, the future challenge will be to continue to provide quality care as the volume and complexity of procedures and the acuity of patients increase while resources are limited. The care that patients receive in the PACU is crucial to the maintenance of high-quality care.

Table 20–7. George Washington University Hospital Surgical Case Distribution

	FY85	FY88	CY93
Total surgical caseload	10,969	10,656	11,220
Ambulatory caseload by location			
Main operating room	445	1,370	2,189
Ambulatory unit	3,447	2,808	2,244
Cystoscopy suite (outpatients)	617	800	1,278
Total ambulatory caseload	4,509	4,978	5,711
% of total surgical caseload	41.1	46.7	50.9

REFERENCES

1. Nicoll JM. The surgery of infancy. Br Med J 1909;2:753.
2. Waters RM. The "Down-Town" anesthesia clinic. Am J Surg 1919;33:71.
3. Cohen DO, Dillion JB. Anesthesia for out-patient surgery. JAMA 1966;196:1114.
4. Levy ML, Coakley CS. Survey of in and out surgery — first year. South Med J 1968;61:995.
5. Ford JL, Reed WA. The Surgicenter — an innovation in the delivery and cost of medical care. Ariz Med 1969;26:804.
6. Levy ML. Complications: prevention and quality assurance. Anesth Clin North Am 1987;5:113.
7. Korttila K, Ostman P, Faure E, et al. Randomized comparison of recovery after propofol nitrous oxide versus thiopentone-isflorane-nitrous oxide anaesthesia in patients undergoing ambulatory surgery. Acta Anaesthesiol Scand 1990;34:400–403.
8. Chouri AF, Bodner M, White PF. Recovery profile after desflurane-nitrous oxide versus isoflurane-nitrous oxide in outpatients. Anesthesiology 1991;74:419–424.
9. Andrews PLF, David CJ, Binham S, et al. The abdominal visceral innervation and the emetic reflex: pathways, pharmacology and plasticity. Can J Physiol Pharmacol 1990;68:325–345.
10. Borison HL. Area postrema: chemoreceptor circumventricular organ of the medulla oblongata. Prog Neurobiol 1989;32:351–390.
11. Watcha M, White P. Postoperative nausea and vomiting. Anesthesiology 1992;77:162–184.
12. Patasky AO, Kitz DS, Andrews RW, et al. Nausea and vomiting following ambulatory surgery: are all procedures created equal? [abstract]. Anesth Analg 1988;67(Suppl):S163.
13. Jaffe JH, Martin M. Opioid analgesics and antagonists. In: Gillman L, Cillman A, eds. The pharmaceutical basis of therapeutics. New York: Pergamon Press, 1990;497–504.
14. Enright AB, Parker JB. Double blind comparison of alfentanil N_2O with fentanyl N_2O for outpatient surgical procedures. Can J Anaesth 1988;35:462–467.
15. Sfez M, Le Mapihan Y, Gailard JL, et al. Analgesia for appendectomy: comparison of fentanyl and alfentanil. Anaesthesiol Scand 1990;34:30–34.
16. Bovill JG. Which potent opioid? Important criteria for selection. Drugs 1987;33:520–530.
17. White PF, Coe V, Shafer A, et al. Comparison of alfentanil with fentanyl for outpatient anesthesia. Anesthesiology 1986;64:99–106.
18. Phitayakorn P, Melnick BM, Vincinie AF 3rd. Comparison of sufentanil and fentanyl infusions for outpatient anaesthesia. Can J Anaesth 1987;34:242–245.
19. Flacke JW, Bloor BC, Kripke BJ, et al. Comparison of morphine, meperidine, fentanyl and sufentanil in balanced anesthesia: a double-blind study. Anesth Analg 1985;64:897–910.
20. Rising S, Dodgson MS, Steen PA. Isoflurane vs. fentanyl for outpatient laparoscopy. Acta Anaesthesiol Scand 1985;29:251–255.
21. Zuurmond WWA, van Leeuwen L. Alfentanil vs. isoflurane for outpatient arthroscopy. Acta Anaesthesiol Scand 1986;30:329–331.
22. Janhunen L, Tammisto T. Postoperative vomiting after different modes of general anaesthesia. Ann Chir Gynaecol 1972;61:152–159.
23. Haley S, Edelist G, Urbach G. Comparison of alfentanil, fentanyl and enflurane as supplements to general anaesthesia for outpatient gynecologic surgery. Can J Anaesth 1988;35:570–575.
24. Howie MB, Hoffer LJ, Krye J, et al. A comparison of enflurane with alfentanil anaesthesia for gynaecological surgery. Eur J Anaesthesiol 1989;6:281–294.
25. Sukhani R, Lurie J, Jabamoni R. Propofol for ambulatory gynecologic laparoscopy: does omission of nitrous oxide alter postoperative emetic sequelae and recovery? Anesth Analg 1994;78:831–835.
26. Hovorka J, Korttila K, Erkola O. Nitrous oxide does not increase nausea and vomiting after gynecological laparoscopy. Can J Anaesth 1989;36:145–148.
27. Lonie DS, Harper NJN. Nitrous oxide anaesthesia and vomiting. Anaesthesia 1086;41:703–707.
28. Muir JJ, Warner MA, Offord KJ, et al. Role of nitrous oxide and other factors in nausea and vomiting. A randomized and blinded prospective study. Anesthesiology 1987;66:513–518.
29. Ding Y, Fredman B, White P. Use of mivacurium during laparoscopic surgery: effect of reversal drugs on Postoperative recovery. Anesth Analg 1994;78:450–454.
30. Cohen MM, Cameron CB, Duncan PG. Pediatric anesthesia morbidity and mortality in the perioperative period. Anesth Analg 1990;70:160–167.
31. Patel RI, Hannallah RS. Anesthetic complications following pediatric ambulatory surgery: a 3-year study. Anesthesiology 1988;69:1009–1012.
32. Anderson R, Krohg K. Pain as a major cause of postoperative nausea. Can Anaesth Soc J 1976;23:366–369.
33. Palazzo MGA, Strunin L. Anaesthesia and emesis: I. etiology. Can Anaesth Soc J 1984;31:178–187.
34. White PF, Shafer A. Nausea and vomiting: causes and prophylaxis. Semin Anesth 1988;6:300–308.
35. Broadman L, Ceruzzi W, Patane P, et al. Metoclopramide reduces the incidence of vomiting following strabismus surgery in children. Anesthesiology 1990;72:245–248.
36. Melnick B, Sawyer R, Karambelkar D, et al. Delayed side effects of droperidol after ambulatory general anesthesia. Anesth Analg 1989;69:748–751.
37. Pandit SK, Kothary SP, Pandit UA, et al. Dose response study of droperidol and metoclopramide as antiemetics for outpatient anesthesia. Anesth Analg 1989;68:798–802.
38. Madej TH, Simpson KH. Comparison of the use of domperidone, droperidol and metoclopramide in the prevention of nausea and vomiting following major gynaecological surgery. Br J Anaesth 1986;58:884–887.
39. Cohen Se, Woods WA, Wyner J. Antiemetic efficacy of droperidol and metoclopramide. Anesthesiology 1984;60:67.
40. Doze VA, Shafer A, White PF. Nausea and vomiting after outpatient anesthesia: effectiveness of droperi-

dol alone and in combination with metoclopramide. Anesth Analg 1987;66:S41.

41. Scurderi P, Wetchler B, Sung Y, et al. Treatment of postoperative nausea and vomiting after outpatient surgery with the 5-HT3 antagonist ondansetron. Anesthesiology 1993;78:15–20.

42. McKenzie R, Kovac A, O'Connor T, et al. Comparison of ondansetron versus placebo to prevent postoperative nausea and vomiting in women undergoing ambulatory gynecologic surgery. Anesthesiology 1993;78:21–28.

43. Rosenberg D, Parnass S, Newman L. Ephedrine minimizes postoperative nausea and vomiting in outpatients [abstract]. Anesthesiology 1989;71:A322.

44. Bone ME, Dowson S, Smith G. A comparison of nalbuphine with fentanyl for postoperative pain relief following termination of pregnancy under day care anaesthesia. Anaesthesia 1988;43:194–197.

45. Wetchler BV, Alexander CD, Shariff MS, et al. A comparison of recovery in outpatients receiving fentanyl versus those receiving butorphanol. J Clin Anesth 1989;1:339–343.

46. Zelcer J, White PF, Chester S, et al. Intraoperative patient-controlled analgesia: an alternative to physician administration during outpatient monitored anesthesia care. Anesth Analg 1992;75:41–44.

47. Sevarino FB, Naulty JS, Sinatra R, et al. Transdermal fentanyl for postoperative pain management in patients recovering from abdominal gynecologic surgery. Anesthesiology 1992;77:463–466.

48. Caplan RA, Ready LB, Oden RV, et al. Transdermal fentanyl for postoperative pain management. A double-blind placebo study. JAMA 1989;261:1036–1039.

49. Striebel WH, Malewicz J, Hermanns K, et al. Intranasal meperidine titration for postoperative pain relief. Anesth Analg 1992;76:1047–1051.

50. Ashburn MA, Lind GH, Gillie MH, et al. Oral transmucosal fentanyl citrate (OTFC) for the treatment of postoperative pain. Anesth Analg 1993;76:377–381.

51. Ready L, Loper K, Nessly M, et al. Postoperative epidural morphine is safe on surgical wards. Anesthesiology 1991;75:452–456.

52. Joshi G, McCarroll S, McSwiney M, et al. Effects of intraarticular morphine on analgesic requirements after anterior cruciate ligament repair. Reg Anesth 1993;18:254–257.

53. Rosenblum M, Weller RS, Conard PL, et al. Ibuprofen provides longer lasting analgesia than fentanyl after laparoscopic surgery. Anesth Analg 1991;73:255–259.

54. O'Hara D, Fragen R, Kinzer M, et al. Ketorolac tromethamine as compared with morphine sulfate for treatment of postoperative pain. Clin Pharmacol Ther 1987;41:556–561.

55. Morley-Forster P, Newton P, Cook M. Ketorolac and Indomethacin are equally efficacious for relief of minor postoperative pain. Can J Anaesth 1993;40:1126–1130.

56. Higgins M, Givogre J, Marco A, et al. Recovery from outpatient laparoscopic tubal ligation is not improved by preoperative administration of ketorolac or ibuprofen. Anesth Analg 1992;79:274–280.

57. Ding Y, Fredman B, White P. Use of ketorolac and fentanyl during outpatient gynecologic surgery. Anesth Analg 1993;77:205–210.

58. Hannallah RS, Broadman LM, Belman AB, et al. Control of post-orchidopexy pain in pediatric outpatients: comparison of two regional techniques. Anesthesiology 1984;61:A429.

59. Narchi P, Benhamou D, Aubrun F, et al. Analgesia using mesosalpinx infiltration combined with intraperitoneal lidocaine for Yoon ring laparoscopy [abstract]. Anesthesiology 1992;77:A17.

60. Alexander CD, Wetchler BV, Thompson RE. Bupivacaine infiltration of the mesosalpinx in ambulatory surgical laparoscopic tubal sterilization. Can Anaesth J 1987;34:362.

61. Warner M, Shields S, Shute C. Major morbidity and mortality within one month of ambulatory surgery and anesthesia. JAMA 1993;270:1437–1441.

62. Korttila K. Recovery period and discharge. In: White P, ed. Outpatient anesthesia. New York: Churchill Livingstone, 1990;369–395.

63. Aldrete JA, Droulik D. A postoperative recovery score. Anesth Analg 1970;49:924.

64. Chung F. Are discharge criteria changing? J Clin Anesth 19;5(Suppl 1):645–685.

65. Kallar S, Jones G. Postoperative complications. In: White P, ed. Outpatient anesthesia. New York: Churchill Livingstone, 1990;397–415.

66. Dawson B, Reed WA. Anaesthesia for adult surgical outpatients. Can Anaesth Soc J 1980;27:409.

21

SURGICAL CONSIDERATIONS

O.W. Brown

Surgical complications that occur in the recovery room range from minor wound problems to life-threatening or limb-threatening occurrences. They must, therefore, be promptly identified if permanent morbidity or mortality is to be avoided. In addition, surgical complications that occur in the recovery room often require immediate reoperation, further emphasizing the need for prompt and accurate diagnosis.

WOUND COMPLICATIONS

Wound complications, which are usually quite easy to diagnose, consist of anything from a small hematoma at the incision site to life-threatening airway obstruction. For a patient who presents with a small wound hematoma, close observation is sufficient. However, the surgical team should be notified promptly if there is any increase in the size of the hematoma or if compression of a surrounding structure develops. Any hematoma that expands rapidly and/or results in hypotension, tachycardia, or overlying tissue ischemia requires prompt surgical exploration. Patients with significant hematomas after procedures such as thyroidectomy or carotid endarterectomy must be returned to the operating room immediately for prompt drainage if respiratory compromise and ensuing respiratory distress is to be avoided. For patients in whom the development of the hematoma is rapid, skin and subcutaneous sutures should be removed in the recovery room to allow

for immediate decompression and relief of the underlying respiratory compression.

After abdominal procedures, wound dehiscence and possible evisceration should be considered for any patient with profuse serosanguineous drainage from the abdominal incision. Although this complication occurs more commonly later in the postoperative period, it may occur at any time and must be promptly recognized and the patient must be returned to the operating room immediately.

Gastrointestinal Surgery

Most complications of surgery on the gastrointestinal tract do not occur until several days postoperatively. However, those that do occur are often life threatening and must be rapidly and accurately diagnosed.

The most common complication after instrumentation of the esophagus is esophageal perforation. Any patient who develops pain and fever after esophagoscopy is presumed to have an esophageal perforation until proven otherwise. Treatment consists of an immediate esophagram. Chest x-ray may also be helpful in making the diagnosis of esophageal perforation if air is identified in the soft tissues. However, a normal chest x-ray does not rule out an esophageal perforation. Although some controversy surrounds the treatment of esophageal perforations, most agree that the most 'conservative'' approach is surgery.

Bleeding complications after surgery on the gastrointestinal tract should be considered in any patient who develops hypotension and tachycardia in the recovery room. The bleeding may be present as bright red blood per rectum or as bleeding via the nasogastric tube. In patients who have undergone some type of gastric or bowel resection, the source of the bleeding may be at the anastomotic site. If the bleeding is not excessive, these patients may be observed initially. However, if such bleeding produces hypotension and tachycardia or if the patient is particularly debilitated, these patients necessarily require immediate surgical reexploration. For patients without external manifestations of bleeding, occult intra-abdominal bleeding should be considered. In the setting of hypovolemic shock, this also often requires immediate surgical attention.

Another early complication after surgery on the gastrointestinal tract is oliguria and anuria. Although this is most often the result of hypovolemia, mechanical obstruction of the ureters or transection of the ureters must be considered. For any patient in whom ureter obstruction is a possibility, cystoscopy and ureterography should be performed immediately. Any type of mechanical ureteral obstruction requires immediate exploration and repair.

Although uncommon in the recovery room setting, the complication of ischemia of an intestinal stoma may occur. It is important that any stoma be thoroughly examined at multiple time periods while the patient is in the recovery room to rule out the presence or development of stomal ischemia. If identified, it will most often require surgical reexploration with resection of the ischemic segment.

Patients undergoing upper abdominal procedures may develop a pneumothorax. This may occur during splenectomy or liver resection. Patients usually present with respiratory insufficiency and chest pain. Treatment consists of chest tube placement.

Breast Surgery

Recovery room complications after breast surgery include hematoma, pneumothorax, and nerve injury. Hematoma, as discussed previously, may jeopardize the viability of the overlying tissue. In addition, hematomas predispose a wound to infection. Therefore, any patient with a significantly sized hematoma should be returned to the operating room immediately for drainage.

Patients undergoing mastectomy, especially radical mastectomy, may develop a pneumothorax in the recovery room. This is most often secondary to the use of a small hemostat to control a perforating blood vessel. The patient may present with respiratory difficulty, chest pain, or in extreme cases, respiratory distress with cardiovascular collapse. Prompt chest tube placement is the treatment of choice.

Injuries to the intercostobrachial nerve, producing numbness over the upper medial portion of the arm, and to the long thoracic nerve, producing winging of the scapula, may also occur after surgery of the breast. These injuries should be diagnosed in the recovery room, but no surgical treatment is indicated.

Pulmonary Surgery

Bleeding following thoracotomy is most often identified by an increase in the amount of chest tube drainage. Patients with greater than 100cc/hr should be returned to the operating room for exploration. Another early complication following thoracotomy is torsion of a lobe following pulmonary resection. This can be identified on chest x-ray by an area of homogenous density in the operative hemithorax and can result in gangrene. Treatment is immediate reexploration. Patients can also develop mechanical obstruction secondary to retained blood in the airway following pulmonary resection. This may be avoided by the use of a double lumen (Carlen's) endotracheal tube during the thoracotomy.

Bronchopleural fistula may occur at 1 to 7 days postoperatively. These patients often present with an increase in the amount of air leak or hemoptysis. Chest x-ray may reveal a new air fluid level. If a bronchopleural fistula is suspected, bronchoscopy followed by immediate thoracotomy for closure is often necessary.

The recurrent laryngeal nerve may be injured during thoracotomy. This occurs more commonly on the left than on the right. Patients often display a hoarseness of the voice. If there has been a previous injury to the contralateral nerve, acute respiratory distress may ensue requiring emergency thoracotomy.

VASCULAR SURGICAL COMPLICATIONS

Unlike the major complications after most surgical procedures, which most often occur days to weeks after the initial procedure, complications following vascular reconstructions often manifest in the recovery room or during the very early postoperative period.

Aortic Surgery

Aortic reconstruction is associated with several early life-threatening and limb-threatening complications. As with other surgical procedures, patients may develop postoperative hemorrhage. This often presents as hypotension with associated tachycardia. Urine output is also often decreased. Abdominal distension may also be present. Any patient suspected of having intra-abdominal bleeding after aortic reconstruction should be returned to the operating room immediately. A direct correlation between the amount of blood transfused and the morbidity and mortality of aortic surgery has been established.

Poor urinary output after aortic reconstruction may be the result of many different factors. Surgical etiologies include mechanical obstruction or injury of the ureters or significant renal artery occlusive disease. If physiologic causes of oliguria and anuria can be excluded, measures such as cystoscopy or even surgical exploration must be undertaken to rule out this possibility. If not addressed in a timely fashion, permanent renal failure can occur.

Graft occlusion is uncommon after aortic reconstruction. It is easily diagnosed by the loss of the femoral pulse on the affected side.

The patient may also exhibit increasing ischemia of the lower extremity. However, for patients who have had longstanding lower extremity ischemia, the limb may not show any evidence of acute ischemia. Therefore, loss of pulse alone is sufficient to require immediate surgical reexploration.

Colon ischemia may occur in up to 4.3% of patients undergoing aortic reconstruction. Patients who have a bowel movement in the early postoperative period after aortic reconstruction, should be presumed to have some degree of colon ischemia until proven otherwise. These patients should undergo immediate colonoscopy and surgical exploration if indicated.

Embolization is another possible complication after aortic reconstruction. Patients often present with bluish discoloration of the feet and toes, giving rise to the entity known as "blue toe syndrome." In addition, embolization may occur in the area of the thigh or buttock, producing a similar type of skin pattern. If the patient has palpable pedal pulses, no acute surgical therapy is indicated.

Paraplegia is an uncommon complication after infrarenal aortic reconstruction, occurring in 0.2% of patients undergoing elective aortic aneurysm resection. It does, however, occur in 5 to 10% of patients undergoing resection of a descending thoracic aortic aneurysm. It is believed to develop as a result of interruption of the blood flow through the artery of Adamkiewicz, the origin of which had been found to occur between T8 and L4. The most appropriate course of medical treatment remains controversial. At present, no surgical treatment has proven beneficial.

Lower Extremity Revascularization

The most common major complication after upper or lower extremity revascularization is acute graft occlusion. It most often results in acute limb-threatening ischemia and requires prompt diagnosis and immediate return to the operating room if limb loss is to be prevented.

The diagnosis is often made because the patient develops the acute onset of excruciating pain. However, loss of sensation or motion in the extremity, as well as the loss of a pulse or Doppler signal are all important signs of acute graft occlusion requiring immediate reexploration.

Another complication after extremity revascularization, especially in the lower extremity, is the development of the reperfusion syndrome with an accompanying compartment syndrome. Diagnosis is made by the presence of increased pain, tense swelling, and loss of motor and sensory function in the affected extremity. Treatment consists of immediate return to the operating room for fasciotomy.

Carotid Endarterectomy

Stroke is the most easily recognized major complication after carotid endarterectomy. It occurs in 1 to 3% of all patients undergoing carotid endarterectomy. Patients in the recovery room who exhibit signs of hemispheric stroke, including unilateral extremity weakness or unilateral facial droop, should be returned to the operating room immediately for reexploration.

Wound hematomas are especially dangerous because of the possibility of compression of the trachea and the development of respiratory distress. Treatment consists of immediate removal of skin and subcutaneous sutures to provide acute decompression followed by return to the operating room for exploration.

Injury to the cranial nerves, although not usually requiring any type of formal treatment, may occur in up to 16% of patients undergoing carotid endarterectomy. Injury to the hypoglossal nerve is diagnosed by noting protrusion of the tongue and a deviation toward the side of the injury. Injury to the marginal mandibular branch of the facial nerve is evidenced by an inability to retract inferiorly the corner of the mouth on the affected side. This can be evaluated easily by asking the patient to show his teeth. This inability to retract the corner of the affected side is often incorrectly interpreted as a drooping of the contralateral corner of the mouth. Consequently, a diagnosis of postoperative stroke made be made incorrectly. It is essential for the physician in the recovery room to be able to differentiate these to clinical situations.

Renal Artery Surgery

Acute graft occlusion after renal artery reconstruction is suggested by the abrupt recurrence of severe hypertension in the recovery room. Hematuria is unusual. Depending on the clinical situation, oliguria also may be present. Immediate angiography is mandatory to confirm the diagnosis. Treatment consists of immediate reexploration.

Deep Vein Thrombosis and Pulmonary Embolism

Patients undergoing surgical procedures are at increased risk for deep vein thrombosis. Although it is unusual to make this diagnosis in the recovery room, it should be considered in any patient who presents with the acute onset of a swollen tender extremity. Similarly, pulmonary embolism should be considered in any patient who develops the acute onset of otherwise unexplained respiratory distress.

Cardiac Surgery

Excessive bleeding requiring reexploration occurs in 1 to 10% of patients undergoing cardiac surgery. Although several protocols exist for determining exactly when to reexplore a patient for bleeding, chest tube drainage of 200 to 300 mL per hour for several hours usually requires surgical reexploration. It is important to correct all hematologic causes of bleeding before undertaking direct surgical exploration.

Several peripheral nerve injuries may occur after cardiac surgery, including injury to the brachial plexus, the phrenic nerve, the recurrent laryngeal nerve, and the sympathetic chain. Most of these injuries are secondary to pressure and are temporary in nature. No specific surgical therapy is indicated.

Cardiac tamponade is a potentially life-threatening complication after cardiac surgery. These patients may present with excessive bleeding, a widening of the mediastinum on chest x-ray, elevated and equalized right and left heart filling pressures, hypotension, and a paradoxical pulse. After the diagnosis has been made, the patient should be returned to the operating room immediately for evacuation of clots and control of the bleeding. If the patient's clinical status does not allow time to return the patient to the operating room, the sternal incision should be opened at the bedside and the clots should be removed. The patient should then be taken to the operating room for exploration and control of bleeding.

Thyroid and Parathyroid Surgery

Bleeding after thyroid and parathyroid surgery is an uncommon but potentially life-threatening complication. It may result in respiratory distress secondary to compression of the underlying trachea. Prompt removal of sutures and relief of tracheal compression followed by surgical exploration is the treatment of choice.

The most common cause of postoperative respiratory distress after surgery in the neck is edema of the larynx. High doses of anti-inflammatory steroids have been suggested in these cases. However, when significant respiratory difficulty persists, tracheostomy is the treatment of choice.

Injury to the recurrent laryngeal may occur, especially in surgery of the thyroid. It can result in anything from mild hoarseness of the voice to severe respiratory distress, depending on the clinical situation and whether one or both of the recurrent nerves is injured. Treatment in the case of severe distress is tracheostomy.

Finally, metabolic abnormalities such as hypercalcemia and hypocalcemia and hyperthyroidism and hypothyroidism must be considered for all patients undergoing this type of surgery. Appropriate laboratory tests should be drawn as soon as the patient arrives in the recovery room.

Laparoscopic procedures have similar complications to open procedures. In addition, vascular injury, especially to the aorta and iliac vessels, must be considered after laparoscopy for a patient who presents with persistent hypotension, tachycardia, and increasing abdominal girth. This may be caused by the trocar or by the needle used to inflate the abdomen. Prompt recognition is imperative if life-threatening hemorrhage is to be avoided.

Surgical complications that occur in the recovery room are often potentially life-threatening or limb-threatening and require immediate diagnosis and treatment. In many cases, patients must be returned to the operating room immediately for appropriate therapy. Failure to diagnose these complications may result in the transfer of a potentially unstable patient to the surgical floor. It may also produce significant delays in treatment, which all too often will result in permanent morbidity or mortality. Any patient who presents with signs or symptoms that can not be explained readily on the basis of a physiologic problem must be considered to have a surgical problem and should undergo thorough surgical evaluation.

REFERENCES

1. Hertzer NR, et al. A prospective study of the incidence of injury to the cranial nerves during carotid endarterectomy. Surg Gynecol Obstet 1980;151:781.
2. Thompson JE. Complications of endarterectomy and their prevention. World J Surg 1979;3:155.
3. Moore W, ed. Vascular surgery; a comprehensive review. Philadelphia: WB Saunders, 1993.
4. Greenfield L, ed. Complications in surgery and trauma. Philadelphia: JB Lippincott Company, 1990.
5. Hagihara PF, et al. Incidence of ischemic colitis following abdominal aortic reconstruction. Surg Gynecol Obstet 1979;149:571–573.
6. Szilagyi DE, et al. Spinal cord damage in surgery of the abdominal aorta. Surgery 1978;83:38–56.
7. Budd DC, et al. Surgical morbidity after mastectomy operations. Am J Surg 1978;135:218–220.
8. Loop FD, Groves LK. Esophageal perforations. Ann Thorac Surg 1970;10:571.
9. Schuler JG. Intraoperative lobar torsion producing pulmonary infarction. J Thorac Cardiovasc Surg 1973;65:951.

10. Loop FD, et al. An 11-year evolution of coronary artery surgery (1967—1978). Ann Surg 1979;190:444.

11. Fairman RM, et al. Emergency thoracotomy in the surgical intensive care unit after open cardiac operation. Ann Thorac Surg 1987;44:169.

III
Administrative Considerations

22

ADMINISTRATIVE STRUCTURE

Geraldine Mitchell

INTRODUCTION

The focus of this chapter is on the administrative structure of a postanesthesia care unit. It contains components of universally accepted principles of organizational design and management theory that are common elements in all organizations. Although understanding essential elements of administrative structure provides the management staff with a basic framework for management style and structure, it does not really provide practitioners with principles that guarantee universal success. Instead, these principles are intended to identify a framework for the administrative manager to integrate into independent approaches for the successful development of the administrative structure of a postanesthesia care unit.

This decade has presented administrators with a rapidly changing healthcare environment. Key phases and concepts tied to financial reimbursement have emerged to challenge the survival of many healthcare organizations. In the competitive healthcare market, mission statements and strategic planning have taken on new meaning. To survive, health service organizations must now compete vigorously for their share of fixed or shrinking financial resources. It is imperative for administrative staff on all levels of management to understand the complex shifts in private and governmental payment policies and adjust the administrative structure of the organization, division, and individual working unit to meet these demands. The administrative staff of the post anesthesia care unit needs to identify their role in the institution's strategic plan and have a working understanding of basic administrative structure principles to insure the successful management of a post anesthesia care unit (PACU).

ORGANIZATION AND ADMINISTRATIVE DESIGN

Administrative structure and design have been studied and researched for the past sixty years. A general concept developed proposes that organizations are created for the purpose of achieving goals. These goals are interwoven in the mission, vision, and strategies of the organization. Whether the organization is a family owned country store, a computer industry mega giant, or a major metropolitan hospital, the question still remains as to how the activities of administration, work groups, and the individual should be organized and coordinated so that the desired outcomes are achieved. How should the activities of individuals assembling the components of a computer at IBM be coordinated to produce outputs that will minimize cost and encourage product development? Similarly, how should the activities of the surgeon, anesthesiologist, registered nurse, and other ancillary personnel be coordinated so that the patients' needs are served in a cost efficient manner?

Health care organizations have struggled with this question of administrative design especially when being compared with other industries. It has become the challenge of our times to convince administrators and medical professionals that health (n) care is an industry with a product that requires a high level of quality control. Regardless of the type of organization, whether the organization is the mega giant IBM, or the small non-profit community hospital, the basic concepts and components of administrative structure and design apply.

In both industry and the health care setting, organizational structure can be defined as the patterns of coordination and control, authority style, communication channels, and the system of work flow that produce the desired outcomes (1). Organizational structure provides the framework for function. Based on how an organization develops its patterns of control, authority style, and system of work flow will determine how the work units will function. This is a dynamic process influenced by changes in both the internal and the external environment. Competition for market share, changes in goods and services, technology, and organizational goals contribute to the liquity of organization structure. Organizations are continually redesigning to meet the demands of a changing economic industry. Management must recognize some of the basic administrative structure patterns that can be manipulated in order to achieve the goals of the organization. An understanding of the basic structural concepts of formalization, centralization, and job specialization and a knowledge of how these concepts influence the overall attitudes and behaviors within an organization will provide the administrative staff a diagram for the organization as a whole, the divisions within the organization, and the individual working unit structure.

Formalization is the degree to which policies, procedures, standards, and norms regulate the functions of the organization (2). It can be viewed as a continuum with formal at one end and informal at the other end. In a highly formal environment, typically there are expected outputs, defined procedures and policies, standardized practice, and less input by the employee to alter performance. Research shows that generally the unskilled jobs in industry have the highest degree of formalization and the more professional the level of the job the less formalization is likely. However, exceptions can be found in many professions. For example, in the medical field the registered nurse can change the pattern of care given to each patient, but the standardization of practice to meet some basic patient needs without exception requires extremely formalized policies and procedures. A post anesthesia care unit (PACU) tends to have a formalized structure combined with a high percentage of professional staff. This structure has evolved over time due to the formal rules, policies, and procedures imposed on the medical practice in a PACU by the hospital, professional organizations, and regulatory agencies in an effort to set standards of care that will provide a quality product.

The second component influencing administrative structural design is centralization. The concept of **centralization** can be defined as the degree or extent to which decision-making have been empowered to lower levels within the organization (1). A completely centralized organization places the decision making power in one person. The direct counter part of complete centralization is then the concept of complete decentralization or organizational democracy where every employee has a vote in decision making. Organizations usually fall somewhere on the continuum of the two extremes. An organization's degree of centralization is directly related to the dispersion of authority within the organization.

In order to evaluate an organization's degree of centralization, the following questions should be asked. Does lower management have decision making ability? At what level of importance are the decisions made by lower management? Does the decision that is made need approvals by higher levels? Answers to these questions measure the degree of centralization in administrative structure of a PACU. Despite the apparent simplicity of the centralization concept, it is difficult in practical application.

There are various sources that make application difficult. First, people in the same job description or level of responsibility can and usually do have different decision making authority throughout the organization.

Second, not all decisions are of equal importance in organizations. An example would be a PACU manager could delegate authority to an assistant for routine daily operating decisions, but retain decision making authority over staffing and scheduling. The last factor that affects centralization concept is the perception of decision making. Many supervisors' job descriptions may include the authority to make decisions but the individuals do not perceive that they have the authority; thus, objectively they have authority (decentralization), but subjectively they do not (centralization) (3).

The third concept that affects the administrative structure or design especially when examining the structure of a PACU is job specialization. **Job specialization** denotes the choices managers makes in assigning or designing the division of labor within an organization (4). Frederick W. Taylor, the "father of scientific management" first developed this concept in the 1940s. He developed what was termed horizontal specialization. This concept explains the employees' involvement in the creation of the total product or scope of the job. Today, the concept of job specialization is divided into **vertical** and **horizontal** specialization. **Horizontal** specialization applies to simple task oriented jobs very common in an assembly line environment where various workers assemble the product and no one person completes the project from start to finish.

Vertical specialization refers to the degree to which the employee has control over the performance of the job. Vertical independence depends on the number of rules, policies, procedures, and direct supervision that control the job. Professional jobs such as a physician, a registered nurse, or pharmacist possess components of both horizontal and vertical job specialization.

In the 1970s Henry Mentzberg, a leading researcher of organizational structure, developed the concept of a relationship structure between the components of formalization, centralization, specialization. He postulated that there must be consistent patterns of fits between these three components in order to maintain an effective organization or administrative structure (5). It is important to emphasize that these basic administrative concepts apply to all organizations (for-profit or nonprofit) and can be further divided within the internal administrative structure of a division, department, or unit of any organization. A division or department in a hospital may have low formalization, decentralization and varying degrees of job specialization, but an individual unit within that same division or department may have a totally different organizational structure. Generally the higher the job specialization, the greater the centralization and formalization.

This relationship holds because highly specialized jobs usually are regulated by policies and strict standards of performance that are not at the discretion of authority. The PACU is a unit that has a high degree of centralization, is more formalized than the divisional structure, and has a combination of horizontal and vertical job specialization. In a unit that has 85 percent or greater professional personnel (anesthesiologist and registered nurses) there is an extremely controlled environment; however these controls have been mandated overtime through the growth and development of various professional and regulatory agencies.

CONTROLLING FACTORS OF PACU

ASA, ASPAN, JCAHO

There are several organizations that contribute to the administrative structure of a postanesthesia care unit (PACU). The ASA (America Society of Anesthesiologists, AS-PAN (The American Society of Post Anesthesia Nurses), and JCAHO (The Joint Commission on Accreditation of Healthcare Organizations) influence the formalized structure of a PACU. These organizations define standards of practice for patient care which translate into formal rules, policies and procedures that validate the practices of the physician, nurse, and axillary personnel.

The ASA and ASPAN have jointly agreed on basic standards that directly affect the practices of the anesthesiologist and the registered nurse in the PACU. These standards apply to postanesthesia care practice in all geographic locations and specialized settings. The following PACU standards were jointly agreed upon and implemented in January, 1992 amended in 1994, and are currently the standards for PACU practice.

Standard I: All patients who have received general anesthesia, regional anesthesia, or monitored anesthesia care shall receive appropriate postanesthesia management.

1. A postanesthesia care unit (PACU) or an area which provides equivalent postanesthesia care shall be available to receive patients after surgery and anesthesia. All patients who receive anesthesia shall be admitted to the PACU except by specific order of the anesthesiologist responsible for the patient's care.
2. The medical aspects of care in the PACU shall be governed by policies and procedures which have been reviewed and approved by the Department of Anesthesiology.
3. The design, equipment and staffing of the PACU shall meet requirements of the facility's accrediting and licensing bodies.
4. The nursing standards of practice shall be consistent with those approved in 1986 by the American Society of Post Anesthesia Nurses (ASPAN).

Standard II: A patient transported to the PACU shall be accompanied by a member of the anesthesia care team who is knowledgeable about the patient's condition. The patient shall be continually evaluated and treated during transport with monitoring and support appropriate to the patient's condition.

Standard III: Upon arrival in the PACU, the patient shall be re-evaluated and a verbal report provided to the responsible PACU nurse by the member of the anesthesia care team who accompanies the patient.

1. The patient's status on arrival in the PACU shall be documented.
2. Information concerning the perioperative condition and the surgical/anesthetic course shall be transmitted to the PACU nurse.
3. The member of the Anesthesia Care Team shall remain in the PACU until the PACU nurse accepts responsibility for the nursing care of the patient.

Standard IV: The patient's condition shall be evaluated continually in the PACU.

1. The patient shall be observed and monitored by methods appropriate to the patient's medical condition. Particular attention should be given to monitoring oxygenation, ventilation and circulation. During recovery from all anesthetics, a quantitative method of assessing oxygenation such as pulse oximetry shall be employed in the initial phase of recovery. This is not intended for application during the recovery of the obstetrical patient in whom regional anesthesia was used for labor and vaginal delivery.
2. An accurate written report of the PACU period shall be maintained. Use of an appropriate PACU scoring system is encouraged for each patient on admission, at appropriate intervals prior to discharge, and at the time of discharge.
3. General medical supervision and coordination of patient care in the PACU should be the responsibility of an anesthesiologist.
4. There shall be a policy to assure the availability in the facility of a physician capable of managing complications and providing cardiopulmonary resuscitation for patients in the PACU.

Standard V: A physician is responsible for the discharge of the patient from the postanesthesia care unit.

1. When discharge criteria are used, they must be approved by the Department of Anesthesiology and the medical staff. They may vary depending upon whether the patient is discharged to a hospital room, to the ICU, to a short stay unit, or home.

2. In the absence of the physician responsible for the discharge, the PACU nurse shall determine that the patient meets the discharge criteria. The name of the physician accepting responsibility for discharge shall be noted on the record (6).

As stated, these are basic standards and may be exceeded based on the judgement of the anesthesiologist. The third organization to greatly influence the practices in postanesthesia care is the JCAHO.

The JCAHO is the premier accreditation body in the United States and strongly influences the practices of hospitals and physicians within the hospital seeking accreditation. The term *strongly influences* is truly an erroneous term. Although the participation in JCAHO review is considered voluntary, repercussions for not participating are far reaching. First, if the hospital accepts Medicare and Medicaid payment from the federal and local government for patient services, it is mandated by the federal government that the hospital must be accredited by JCAHO or payment is withheld. Second, if the hospital has a residency program, accreditation is usually required by the residency regulatory body. Third, in some states the Department of Public Health base their inspection and the frequency of inspection on whether the health care institution is accredited. So, the JCAHO accreditation program is considered voluntary but in reality, has been given informal authority to regulate practices in a health care setting.

The current JCAHO standards are formatted in what can be described as an interdisciplinary narrative. The PACU administrator needs to be aware of the integrated style of the standards and be able to locate within the JCAHO standards publication the areas that pertain to the PACU. The JCAHO has a scoring process based on the existence of a standard in the organization or department and how long the standard has been implemented. Scores range from one to five. A score of one indicates 91 to 100% of the medical records, policies, standards of care, and practices have been followed according to the JCAHO guidelines. A score of five, on the other hand, indicates that the standard was implemented less than 26% of the time or less than 12 months. The site visit and accreditation process from JCAHO is every three years. However, any scores of four or five in key areas will precipitate a visit annually and a conditional accreditation until all citations in key areas are corrected. If the hospital does not agree with the findings in the accreditation report, it does have the opportunity to appeal the decision to the accreditation board for reconsideration.

The site visit from JCAHO usually is composed of a three-person panel. A combination of a physician, a registered nurse, and an administrator make up the panel so that all areas of expertise are represented to evaluate the medical and non-medical practices of the institution.

Currently the JCAHO Manual has three distinct sections. The first is titled the Patient Focused Functions. Within this section there are five subgroups each group will be discussed based on its application to the PACU. The first subgroup, Patient Rights and Organizational Ethics (RI), addresses the recognition of the patient's rights both functional and ethical as it applies to his/her involvement in their care planning.

For the PACU administration such issues as informed consent, advance directives, privacy, security, resolutions of patient complaints are addressed in this subgroup.

The second subgroup, Assessment of Patients (PE), encompasses the criteria for the initial screening or assessment of each patient's physical, psychological, and social status to determine the need for care, type of care, and the need for any further assessment. It emphasizes the key periods of time a patient receiving anesthesia must be assessed by each discipline. In addition to the preanesthesia assessment, the patient must be assessed immediately before the induction of anesthesia and reevaluated on admission and discharge from the postanesthesia care unit by the anesthesiologist (7). Documentation of these evaluation periods will be discussed later in the chapter.

Also, identified is the responsibility of a registered nurse to assess the patients' need for nursing care in all settings in which nursing care is to be provided.

Subgroup number three of the Patient-Focused Functions is Care of Patients (TX). This section has very specific criteria regarding Anesthesia Care and Operative and Other Invasive Procedures. It reiterates some of the identical criteria as the PE section and emphasizes the reassessment of the patient postoperatively and medically approved discharge criteria from the PACU. The criteria for discharge can be individualized for each institution, but policies and documentation must support that the criteria has been implemented is an applicable standard for each patient. Figure 22–1 is an example of the amount of detail the JCAHO expects to find in the discharge criteria to receive a score of one. The patient's charts are reviewed during the JCAHO site visit in order to substantiate that the criteria was implemented and reviewed prior to the discharge from the PACU.

PF (Education) addresses the interdisciplinary approach to patient and family education after anesthesia. It requires that adequate instruction be given to the patient and family regarding the anesthetic agents used and the limiting physical activities associated with the types of anesthesia. Such instruction must be presented in ways understandable to the patient and/or family. It is usually the responsibility of the registered nurse to consolidate the instructions of the surgeon and the anesthesiologist and review the instructions with the outpatient and the responsible person accompanying the patient. It is also necessary to validate that the patient or responsible person verbalizes understanding of the PACU instructions. In the case of an inpatient, the registered nurse is responsible to give a detailed report to a RN on the receiving hospital unit of the patient's post anesthesia and post surgical condition.

CC (Continuum of Care) is the final component of section one of the JCAHO standards. It addresses the process by which pa-

tients have access to the appropriate level of care, health professionals, and settings based on the patients needs.

The Nursing Care section was eliminated from the JCAHO standards in 1995. Instead, nursing care is integrated through all the Patient-Focused Functions. Assessment and reassessment by a registered nurse remain key components of this section. JCAHO recognizes the limited length of stay in a PACU and looks for patient care standards/protocols that are key to patient outcomes. It stresses that nursing staff collaborate, as appropriate, with physicians and other disciplines in making decisions regarding each patient's care needs (7). It emphasizes the necessity to develop protocols to ensure that the same level of care is provided to each patient in a PACU.

Section two of the JCAHO standards entitled Organization Functions includes areas that affect all areas of the organizations functions including the PACU. It is the astute PACU administrator that can interrupt this standards in relationship to PACU functions. Improving Organization Performance (PI) is the redefinition of quality improvement and looks at the organization as a whole entity in its planning, measuring, assessing, and improving performance. Management of the Environment of Care (EC) includes all areas of safety, security, hazardous materials and waste, emergency preparedness, life safety, medical equipment and utility systems. It is the responsibility of the PACU administrator to integrate these standards in the functions of the PACU and to articulate to all members of the PACU staff their role in meeting these standards.

JCAHO is an agency that is continually upgrading and revising its protocols based on changes in patient's needs and medical practice. It is necessary for Administration to remain current on all annual revisions associated with the PACU.

Other key areas in section two are Leadership (LD), Management of Information (IM), and Surveillance, Preventions and Control of

PURPOSE: To establish guidelines for transfer of outpatients after anesthesia and surgery.

PROCEDURE: The following are guidelines for transfer of outpatients from phase I to phase II.

1.0 Patient must be alert and oriented.
2.0 Patient must have swallow, cough, and gag reflexes present.
3.0 Absence of respiratory distress.
4.0 Patient has minimal signs or symptoms of nausea, vomiting, and/or dizziness.
5.0 Patient has two measurements of stable vital signs per postanesthesia care unit (PACU) protocol after administration of intramuscular or intravenous pain medication.
6.0 Patient has oxygen saturation on room air greater than 90% unless otherwise approved by the anesthesiologist.
7.0 Patient is able to assume a 90° angle sitting position on the cart.
8.0 Patients who have spinal anesthesia must have return of motor function.

PROCEDURE: In addition to the guidelines for transfer of outpatients from phase I to Phase II, the following are guidelines for discharge of outpatients.

1.0 Patient must be able to ambulate (unless previous procedure, medical history, or surgery dictates otherwise).
2.0 Patient has satisfactory oxygen saturation level based on preoperative level.
3.0 Patient has satisfactory temperature on discharge based on preoperative level.
4.0 Ability to retain oral fluids is desirable but not an absolute requirement.
5.0 Patients who have pelvic or pelvic-related surgery or spinal anesthesia must be able to void unless otherwise approved by the anesthesiologist.
6.0 Patient has acceptable level of pain control.
7.0 Patient has responsible person as an escort home.
8.0 Patient and responsible person received written and verbal discharge instructions.
9.0 Final discharge decision made by the anesthesiologist.

Fig. 22–1. Guidelines for patient transfer.

Infections (IC), and each section impacts on the practices of a post anesthesia care unit.

One of the newest sections of JCAHO, Management of Human Resources (HR), addresses the competence of all personnel delivering any component of patient care. Measurement of competency for hospital accreditation and professional practice requires annual review and an educational tracking method. Licensing is no longer considered a measurement for clinical competency. The question remains as to how the administrator validates the competency of a professional who has been licensed to practice over five years, ten years, or twenty years.

The administrator for the medical staff and the hospital personnel needs to devise a method to validate clinical competency of the physician, registered nurse, and any axillary personnel participating in patient care. With current computer technology it is relatively easy to track the types of care given to patients by both physician and registered nurse in a PACU. It is also feasible to require annual review and testing of personnel to measure levels of competency. Figure 22–2 is one example of a skills checklist that can be utilized by the PACU clinical instructor or manager to evaluate a new nursing employee, or used as an annual needs assessment to formulate

POHA/PACU
CLINICAL COMPETENCY SELF ASSESSMENT

Name: _____   Year: _____

Unit Specific Basic	Competent Performing	Need a Review
Central IV Line:		
A. Assist with insertion	_____	_____
B. Site care	_____	_____
Catheter:		
A. Texas drainage	_____	_____
B. Indwelling catheter insertion	_____	_____
C. Straight catheter	_____	_____
D. Removal of indwelling catheter	_____	_____
E. Foley catheter care	_____	_____
Compresses:		
Moist heat	_____	_____
CVP measurement	_____	_____
Underwater seal (chest drainage)	_____	_____

Unit Specific Complex		
Delivery of blood products	_____	_____
IV Insertion	_____	_____
Suctioning endotrach and trach.	_____	_____
IVP Drugs in POHA/PACU	_____	_____
Use of oximeter	_____	_____
Drawing blood from arterial line	_____	_____
Autotransfusion	_____	_____
Administration of patient-controlled analgesia (PCA) therapy	_____	_____
A. PCA bolus	_____	_____
Oxygen setup: Mask, T-tube, ventimask	_____	_____
USN — Pre-op xylocaine tx.	_____	_____
Sequential pump	_____	_____
Hemodynamic monitor setup	_____	_____
EKG/hemo monitoring	_____	_____
Obtaining CO	_____	_____
Defibrillator	_____	_____
Escort transport monitor	_____	_____

What type of inservices would you like to see presented this year? Check off all of the following of interest to you.

_____ IV drug calculation
_____ Drugs in a code
_____ Conscious sedation
_____ Insulins (types and differences)
_____ Issues of abuse (suspected, recognize, Tx, etc.)
_____ PACU emergencies: all _____ Malignant hyperthermia _____ HTN
       _____ Respiratory _____ Cardiac _____ Shock
_____ Transculture nursing
_____ Charge/delegation
_____ Professional image
_____ Motivation
_____ Stress reduction
_____ Disaster response
_____ Surgical suite evacuation routine

What other topics would you like to see presented? Specify a specific surgery, disease, drug, anesthetic agent or type, management issue, etc.

_____
_____
_____

Signature: _____   Date: _____

Fig. 22–2. Clinical competency self assessment.

an individualized education plan to validate competency. JCAHO has further defined competency by specific age groups. Identifying the individual needs of the patient by age incorporates the physical as well as the psychosocial and emotional needs of each age group. Commonly many organizations have identified four primary age groups. The pediatric, adolescent, adult, and geriatric patient have specific needs for care and education that requires the health care provider to possess and display those skills associated with the recognition and understanding of age specific needs.

Again, these competencies can be validated in many creative methods. Self-learning modules, formal classroom instruction, and individually developed standards of care are just some methods currently practiced. It is up to each facility to devise its own validation process that can be consistently applied in the PACU to all personnel.

ASPAN in the standards publication for 1995 has addressed the JCAHO competency requirements for registered nurses and licensed practical nurses by outlining some critical elements of PACU competency. The following fourteen items are criteria recommended by ASPAN but not intended to be all inclusive:

1. Appropriate state license.
2. Completion of formal orientation program.
3. One year previous experience in a critical care setting.
4. Baccalaureate degree in Nursing for the RN.
5. Successful completion of an ACLS course or equivalent and certification.
6. CPR reviewed annually. Renewal every two years.
7. Displays characteristics essential to the profession:
   a. accountability
   b. autonomy
   c. authority
   d. leadership
8. Displays the ability to document pertinent patient data, nursing interventions and patient responses. Documentation is accurate, timely, concise, and legible.

9. Demonstrates the ability to perform rapid assessments, differentiating between short and long term needs.
10. Certification of RNs in perianesthesia nursing (CAPA and/or CPAN), as recognized by ASPAN, validates the defined body of knowledge for the perianesthesia nurse.
11. Displays the ability to educate self, teach patients/significant others, the community and other members of the heath care team.
12. Participates in nursing research in order to provide and promote the highest quality of patient care.
13. Protects the rights of the patient, the perianesthesia nurse and the facility by providing legal and ethical health care by ethical conduct and a clear understanding of legal guidelines.
14. Maintains competency by seeking educational opportunities in order to provide and promote the highest quality of patient care (8).

JCAHO further addresses competency in the Leadership section by address the need for competency based job descriptions and performance evaluations for all employees within the organization.

The final section in the JCAHO manual contains Governance (GO), Management (MA), Medical Staff (MS), and Nursing (NR). These sections address such issues as by-laws for the organization, medical staff appointment/reappointment and nursing licenses.

Obviously, there must be a mechanism in place to validate that the ASA and ASPAN standards are followed and the JCAHO requirements are met. This validation comes through the creation of policies and procedures as minimal care criteria, and the documentation process so that the standards of care are followed in the various post anesthesia care settings.

POLICIES AND PROCEDURES

Formal policies and procedures are a necessity of every PACU. Whether the PACU is in a free standing outpatient environment or inpatient acute care facility, the policies and procedures will not vary greatly in content. All policies should be written, approved, and signed by the Medical Director (usually an anesthesiologist) and the Administrative Director of the postanesthesia care unit. It must be stressed that policies and procedures answer the "who", "what", "why" and "how" patient care is delivered. Verbal practices have no validity to the JCAHO or in a court of law.

The terms **policy** and **procedure** are not interchangeable; and, therefore, one cannot take the place of the other. A policy is a statement that constitutes legitimate authorization for a designated agent to act in a particular way whenever a particular condition exists (9). Whereas a procedure contents the steps in a process by which a policy can be implemented or followed. Policies usually dictate "what" will be done and "why." Procedures explain the "how" and "who" of a policy. Policies can exist independent of a procedure and every policy does not necessitate the creation of procedure. However, every written procedure should have a written policy that supports the steps in the procedure. For policies to be successful, the following questions and conditions should be explored when developing and implementing a policy.

1. Does the user of the policy have the capability and resources to carry out the policy?
2. Will the actions by the user produce the expected goals of the policy?
3. Is the policy's purpose justified?

Figure 22–3 gives an example in which a policy and procedure has been combined into one document to address the reporting for a unplanned hospital or patient accident or incident. As indicated in the example, the policy document should include date of review and dates of any supersedes policies. This is especially important for cases in litigation. It is the policy that existed at the time of the incident or accident that will be considered during a law suit; not the policy in existence at date of trial. A **purpose** statement should be part of the policy. The purpose statement answers the questions "what" and "why" for the reader of the policy. The process of combining the policy and procedure into one document provides an ease of usage by the employee for implementation into practice. The policies and procedures can be combined in one volume or a separate manual for policies and a separate manual for procedures can be developed depending on the style the PACU chooses to use. The important factor is that every member of the PACU team (physician, nurse, axillary personnel) are familiar with the policies and procedures and that each employee has easy access to where the unit Policy and Procedure manual is stored. A content of a PACU policy manual should have, as a minimum requirement, the following items to comply with ASA, ASPAN and JCAHO standards.

1. A content review sheet that has an annual update and is signed and dated by both the medical director and administrative director.
2. An organizational chart identifying where the PACU appears in the organizational structure.
3. Table of content.
4. Listing of all hospital approved abbreviations.
5. Written scope of practice of all personnel. Scope of practice is an essential part of JCAHO review. It identifies the purpose of a post anesthesia care unit. It also itemizes the hours that the area is staffed and the type and mix of staffing on each shift if the PACU is a 24-hour operation. In addition, it identifies the patient population by age group and the patient-nurse ratio in compliance to ASA and ASPAN standards. Hospital infection control and safety practices that apply to the PACU must be stated or referenced in the scope of practice policy.
6. Hospital approved job descriptions for all personnel in the PACU.
7. Policies that address all aspects of care from admission to discharge of a PACU patient.
8. Education and competency policies related to professional and axillary personnel working in a PACU.

It is imperative that the PACU administrator and the management staff validate that policies are current and practice of the professional and axillary personnel reflects the con-

PACU POLICY/PROCEDURE MANUAL

SECTION: PACU
ISSUE OR
REVISION DATE: 9/91 SUBJECT: A&I REPORTING

PURPOSE: To provide a system for use by the Surgical Suite to identify, assess, and investigate significant accidents/incidents and to assist in the management of such occurrences that present a risk to Sinai Hospital, its employees, patients, or visitors.

POLICY:
1.0 An A&I report is completed for reportable occurrences immediately upon knowledge of an incident. Reportable incidents are as follows:

1) Accidents of patients, visitors, employees, volunteers, and physicians.
2) Non-routine patient care.
3) Damage, theft, or loss of articles.
4) Incidents on hospital grounds.
5) Any deviation from Informed Consent (see Informed Consent policy).

2.0 The Security Department must be notified immediately for incidents involving thefts, loss of articles, or incidents on hospital grounds.
3.0 The A&I report shall be initiated by the person who witnessed the incident or the person to whom the incident was reported.
4.0 The A&I form must be completed by the hospital employee.
5.0 All A&I reports are confidential and are maintained in a confidential manner.

PROCEDURE:
1.0 Completion and processing of the A&I report (print or type)
1.1 Sections I and II shall be completed by a witnessing person or the person.
1.2 The A&I will be sent by the employee witnessing or reporting the incident to the Nurse Manager/Supervisor responsible for the area in which the incident occurred.
1.3 Section III shall be completed, when applicable, by the physician performing the examination.
1.4 The A&I report is forwarded to the Director of Risk Management after it has been reviewed and signed by Nurse Manager/Supervisor and the Director of Nursing/Surgical Suite/Anesthesia.

Written By: **Approved By:**

Fig. 22–3. PACU policy/procedure manual.

tent of the policies. Validation of care given to each patient can be accomplished through documentation development and review.

DOCUMENTATION

In today's national health care environment, documentation has become a key component in the survival of health care institutions. There is an old saying in the medical and legal profession which sums up the level of importance of accurate documentation: "If it wasn't written, it wasn't done." Large medical malpractice monetary awards have been awarded because medical practice and standards of care could not be validated by what was written in the patient's record. In the postanesthesia care unit, the documentation component is critical to the efficiency of the unit. When developing documentation forms, the administrative staff must consider two major factors that influence the design of the documents. First, the charting must incorporate all the requirements in the ASA and ASPAN standards cited previously in this charter, the assessment and reassessment criteria from the JCAHO standards, and any legal recommendations that are reflective of the state's legal requirements in which the PACU is located.

Second, the document must be streamlined and designed in a style that will not impede the efficiency of the unit. Time is a crucial factor in the PACU. Long, cumbersome charting can slow down patient flow and increase the length of stay for the patient resulting in increased cost to the institution. Narrative type documentation should be kept to a minimum so that the PACU personnel and anesthesiologist can spend the majority of their time in patient care activities.

In many modern free-standing outpatient facilities, computer technology has facilitated the streamlining of the documentation process. All patient required forms can be computer generated and a check box system for assessment and reassessment can be utilized in the PACU. This method provides speed for the registered nurse in the documentation process, ease of billing for the data processing department, and hard copy storage of records is eliminated since records are stored on computer disc. However, most acute care facilities and ambulatory services connected with a major hospital still rely on the hard copy system for the PACU record and the complete patient chart. Documentation depends on the PACU environment. In an outpatient facility where the average length of stay in the PACU is 60 to 90 minutes, documentation can easily be accommodated by a single computerized sheet of paper or a small bedside computer. Figure 22–4 is an example of a computer generated form that includes the complete preoperative, intraoperative, and post anesthesia nursing documentation record. In the acute care setting, where length of stay could be

as long as 24 hours, documentation becomes more complex. It is not unusual for a PACU in an acute setting to have two types of documentation. Figure 22–5 and Figure 22–6 are an example of a documentation record typically used for a short stay outpatient or inpatient. It utilizes the check box system in order to streamline the process for the registered nurse while meeting all the standards of care requirements by ASA, ASPAN, and JCAHO. Note in Figure 22–6 that the discharge criteria and reassessment of the patient is documented by both the registered nurse and anesthesiologist to meet the JCAHO, ASA, ASPAN requirements. It is not unusual for the post anesthesia unit to be used as a critical care overflow unit when the intensive care units are full. The documentation for these patients cannot be accomplished through the short PACU form. Therefore, Figures 22–7, 22–8 and 22–9 indicate the changes in documentation for the patient who will remain in the post anesthesia care area for longer than 24 hours. In this model, the document is a fan folded, four part flow sheet that can contain critical patient data that can be tracked and trended for a 24 hour period.

STAFFING

Staffing like documentation is very individualized for the type of post anesthesia care unit and the classifications of the patients. The post anesthesia care unit has been recognized nationally as a critical care unit by the ASA and ASPAN.

Both organizations have acknowledge that professional nursing care in the immediate and second phase post anesthesia settings is essential for the delivery of quality care to the patient. ASPAN defines the professional registered nurse as one who possesses the analytical skills normally obtained through a baccalaureate degree in nursing. Because of the vulnerability of patients in a perioperative setting, professional nurses with specific education, experience, and knowledge about the immediate postoperative period are required in order

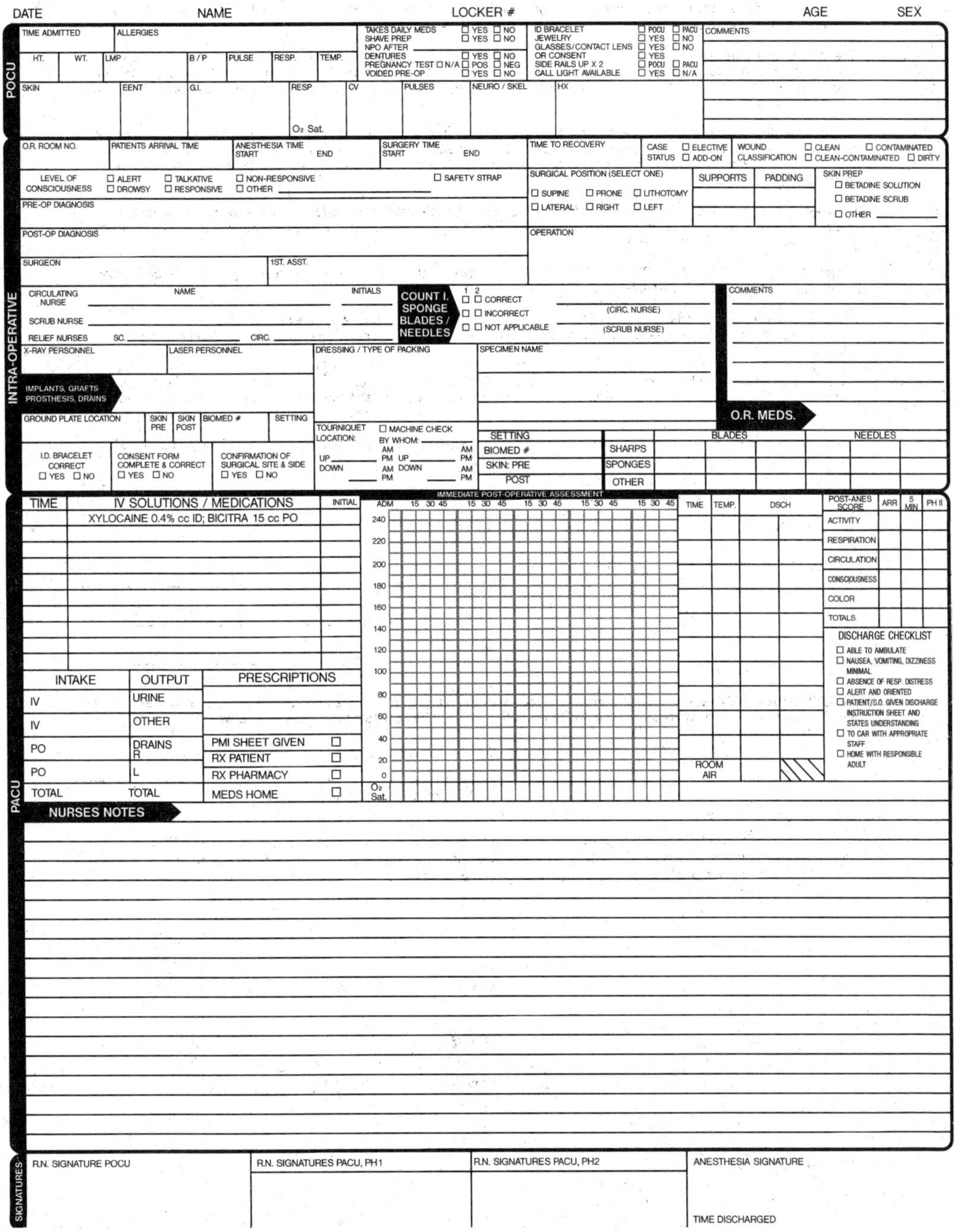

DATE   NAME   LOCKER #   AGE   SEX

POCU

| TIME ADMITTED | ALLERGIES | | | | | | TAKES DAILY MEDS ☐ YES ☐ NO | ID BRACELET ☐ POCU ☐ PACU | COMMENTS |
SHAVE PREP ☐ YES ☐ NO
NPO AFTER
DENTURES ☐ YES ☐ NO
PREGNANCY TEST ☐ N/A ☐ POS ☐ NEG
VOIDED PRE-OP ☐ YES ☐ NO

HT.   WT.   LMP   B/P   PULSE   RESP.   TEMP.

JEWELRY ☐ YES ☐ NO
GLASSES/CONTACT LENS ☐ YES ☐ NO
OR CONSENT ☐ YES
SIDE RAILS UP X 2 ☐ POCU ☐ PACU
CALL LIGHT AVAILABLE ☐ YES ☐ N/A

SKIN   EENT   G.I.   RESP   CV   PULSES   NEURO / SKEL   HX

O₂ Sat.

INTRA-OPERATIVE

O.R. ROOM NO.   PATIENTS ARRIVAL TIME   ANESTHESIA TIME START / END   SURGERY TIME START / END   TIME TO RECOVERY   CASE STATUS ☐ ELECTIVE ☐ ADD-ON   WOUND CLASSIFICATION ☐ CLEAN ☐ CLEAN-CONTAMINATED ☐ CONTAMINATED ☐ DIRTY

LEVEL OF CONSCIOUSNESS ☐ ALERT ☐ TALKATIVE ☐ NON-RESPONSIVE ☐ DROWSY ☐ RESPONSIVE ☐ OTHER   ☐ SAFETY STRAP

SURGICAL POSITION (SELECT ONE) ☐ SUPINE ☐ PRONE ☐ LITHOTOMY ☐ LATERAL ☐ RIGHT ☐ LEFT   SUPPORTS   PADDING   SKIN PREP ☐ BETADINE SOLUTION ☐ BETADINE SCRUB ☐ OTHER

PRE-OP DIAGNOSIS

POST-OP DIAGNOSIS   OPERATION

SURGEON   1ST. ASST.

CIRCULATING NURSE   NAME   INITIALS   COUNT I. SPONGE BLADES / NEEDLES   1 2 ☐ ☐ CORRECT ☐ ☐ INCORRECT ☐ ☐ NOT APPLICABLE   (CIRC. NURSE) (SCRUB NURSE)   COMMENTS

SCRUB NURSE

RELIEF NURSES   SC.   CIRC.

X-RAY PERSONNEL   LASER PERSONNEL   DRESSING / TYPE OF PACKING   SPECIMEN NAME

IMPLANTS, GRAFTS PROSTHESIS, DRAINS

O.R. MEDS.

GROUND PLATE LOCATION   SKIN PRE   SKIN POST   BIOMED #   SETTING   TOURNIQUET LOCATION: ☐ MACHINE CHECK   BY WHOM: BLADES   NEEDLES

UP _____ AM/PM   UP _____ AM/PM
DOWN _____ AM/PM   DOWN _____ AM/PM

SETTING   BIOMED #   SKIN: PRE   POST   SHARPS   SPONGES   OTHER

I.D. BRACELET CORRECT ☐ YES ☐ NO   CONSENT FORM COMPLETE & CORRECT ☐ YES ☐ NO   CONFIRMATION OF SURGICAL SITE & SIDE ☐ YES ☐ NO

PACU

| TIME | IV SOLUTIONS / MEDICATIONS | INITIAL | IMMEDIATE POST-OPERATIVE ASSESSMENT | | TIME | TEMP. | DSCH | POST-ANES SCORE | ARR | 5 MIN | PH II |

XYLOCAINE 0.4% cc ID; BICITRA 15 cc PO

ADM   15 30 45   15 30 45   15 30 45   15 30 45   15 30 45

240 220 200 180 160 140 120 100 80 60 40 20 0   O₂ Sat.

ROOM AIR

ACTIVITY
RESPIRATION
CIRCULATION
CONSCIOUSNESS
COLOR
TOTALS

DISCHARGE CHECKLIST
☐ ABLE TO AMBULATE
☐ NAUSEA, VOMITING, DIZZINESS MINIMAL
☐ ABSENCE OF RESP. DISTRESS
☐ ALERT AND ORIENTED
☐ PATIENT/S.O. GIVEN DISCHARGE INSTRUCTION SHEET AND STATES UNDERSTANDING
☐ TO CAR WITH APPROPRIATE STAFF
☐ HOME WITH RESPONSIBLE ADULT

INTAKE	OUTPUT	PRESCRIPTIONS
IV	URINE	
IV	OTHER	
PO	DRAINS R	PMI SHEET GIVEN ☐
		RX PATIENT ☐
PO	L	RX PHARMACY ☐
TOTAL	TOTAL	MEDS HOME ☐

NURSES NOTES

SIGNATURES

R.N. SIGNATURE POCU   R.N. SIGNATURES PACU, PH1   R.N. SIGNATURES PACU, PH2   ANESTHESIA SIGNATURE

TIME DISCHARGED

Figure 22–4. Computer generated charting record.

POST ANESTHESIA
NURSING ASSESSMENT RECORD

REPORT GIVEN:

SURGERY
TYPE OF ANESTHESIA: ☐ GENERAL   ☐ SPINAL   ☐ MAC
OTHER:

DATE	ADMISSION TIME	DISCHARGE TIME

PRE-OP:
☐ BP _____ SaO₂ _____
☐ PULSE _____ OR EBL _____

ADMISSION ASSESSMENT
L.O.C.
☐ ALERT   ☐ DROWSY
☐ ORIENTED ☐ CONFUSED
☐ RESPONSIVE TO VERBAL STIMULI
☐ RESPONSIVE TO TACTILE STIMULI
☐ UNRESPONSIVE

EMOTIONAL STATUS
☐ CALM ☐ CRYING ☐ COMBATIVE

RESPIRATORY
☐ LUNGS CTA
☐ CHEST EXPANSION SYMMETRICAL
☐ REGULAR   ☐ FULL
☐ O₂ THERAPY

CARDIOVASCULAR
☐ APICAL RATE REGULAR
☐ PALPABLE PULSES X 4 EXTREMITIES

GASTROINTESTINAL
☐ ABDOMEN SOFT NON-DISTENDED
☐ BOWEL SOUNDS PRESENT
☐ NGT _____ ☐ COLOR

GENITOURINARY
☐ BLADDER NON-PALPABLE
☐ FOLEY: _____

MUSCULAR/SKELETAL
☐ DERMATOME LEVEL _____
☐ MOVES EXTREMITIES X 4

SURGICAL SITE
☐ LOCATION: _____
☐ DRESSING D & I
☐ HEMOVAC _____
☐ JP _____
☐ ATS   ☐ LWS

IV THERAPY
☐ SITE _____
☐ PATENT
SEE PROGRESS NOTES ☐
PROTOCOLS/STANDARDS FOR
CARE IMPLEMENTED ☐

ADMITTING NURSE'S INITIALS: _____

Time / PAIN SCALE / Temp.

220, 200, 180, 160, 140, 120, 100, 80, 60, 40, 20, 0

O₂ THERAPY
SAO₂

POST-ANESTHETIC RECOVERY SCORE	AT ARRIVAL	ONE HOUR	AT DISCHARGE
Activity			
Respiration			
Circulation			
Consciousness			
Color			
Totals			

TIME	INIT.	MEDICATION - DOSE - ROUTE	TIME	INIT.	MEDICATION - DOSE - ROUTE

LAB TESTS					CXR, EKG, OTHER
TIME					

HG 408 (5/94)

Fig. 22–5. Postanesthesia nursing assessment record (page 1).

TIME	IV SOLUTIONS	INTAKE					OUTPUT					
		IV SOLUTIONS			BLD	ORAL	Hourly & Cumulative Total	Gastric	Drains	Chest Tubes	CBI Intake / Total	Urine Output	Hourly & Cumulative Total
	INTRAOPERATIVE TOTALS												

TOTAL INTAKE ☐   **TOTAL OUTPUT** ☐

REASSESSMENT FOR DISCHARGE
INPATIENTS + PHASE 1 OUTPATIENT
☐ A + 0 X 3
☐ SURGICAL DRESSING D + I
☐ IV SITE WITHOUT REDNESS OR SWELLING
☐ ABSENCE OF RESPIRATORY DISTRESS
☐ MINIMAL S/S N/V, DIZZINESS
☐ SEE PROGRESS NOTES
☐ REPORT GIVEN AND TRANSFERRED TO:
  ☐ PHASE 2   ☐ UNIT   ☐ ICU

TRANSFERRED WITH:
  ☐ 0$_2$ ☐ VENOUS PUMP   ☐ PCA
  ☐ OTHER: _____

PHASE 2 OUTPATIENT
☐ A + 0 X 3
☐ TOLERATED FLUIDS
☐ SURGICAL DRESSING D + I

HOME INSTRUCTIONS GIVEN:
☐ TO PATIENT
☐ TO RESPONSIBLE ADULT
☐ VERBALIZED UNDERSTANDING

☐ IV DC'd: ☐ NO REDNESS
  ☐ NO SWELLING   ☐ DENIES NUMBNESS
☐ DRESSED SELF
☐ DRESSED WITH ASSISTANCE
☐ AMBULATED - GAIT STEADY
☐ SEE PROGRESS NOTE
☐ DISCHARGED PER W/C WITH:
  ☐ RESPONSIBLE ADULT ☐ OTHER: _____
PATIENT OUTCOMES MET: PROTOCOLS/
STANDARDS FOR CARE RESOLVED ☐

DISCHARGE NURSE'S INITIALS: _____

PROGRESS NOTES

SIGNATURE	INITIALS	SIGNATURE	INITIALS
SIGNATURE	INITIALS	SIGNATURE	INITIALS

☐ **PATIENT REASSESSED AND MEETS DISCHARGE CRITERIA**   DATE: _____   TIME: _____

SIGNATURE _____

TRANSFER TO
☐ HOME ☐ FLOOR ☐ ICU

POST ANESTHESIA EVALUATION

NO KNOWN COMPLICATIONS OF ANESTHESIA
COMMENTS:

ANESTHESIA SURVEILLANCE TERMINATED   Date: _____ Time: _____ Sig. _____

Fig. 22–6.   Postanesthesia nursing assessment record (page 2).

POST ANESTHESIA
LONG TERM & CRITICAL CARE
NURSING ASSESSMENT RECORD

REPORT GIVEN:

SURGERY

TYPE OF ANESTHESIA: ☐ GENERAL ☐ SPINAL ☐ MAC

OTHER:

DATE | ADMISSION TIME | DATE | DISCHARGE TIME

TIME	BLOOD PRESSURE				HEART RATE				RESP.				PAP				MAP		PCWP	RAP	TEMP.	LOC	SaO_2	E.C.G.	LUNG SOUNDS
	00	15	30	45	00	15	30	45	00	15	30	45	00	15	30	45	00	30							
11 PM																									
12 AM																									
1 AM																									
2 AM																									
3 AM																									
4 AM																									
5 AM																									
6 AM																									
	B/P				HR				RESP.				PAP				MAP								
7 AM																									
8 AM																									
9 AM																									
10 AM																									
11 AM																									
12 PM																									
1 PM																									
2 PM																									
	B/P				HR				RESP.				PAP				MAP								
3 PM																									
4 PM																									
5 PM																									
6 PM																									
7 PM																									
8 PM																									
9 PM																									
10 PM																									

HL-1086 (10-94)

Fig. 22–7. Postanesthesia long-term and critical care nursing assessment record (page 1).

**POST ANESTHESIA
LONG TERM & CRITICAL CARE
NURSING ASSESSMENT RECORD**

Date _____ Time _____

NEUROMUSCULAR:	GASTROINTESTINAL:
	GENITOURINARY:
RESPIRATORY:	SURGICAL SITE:
CARDIOVASCULAR:	IV THERAPY:
	PROTOCOLS IMPLEMENTED:
	SIGNATURE:

Fig. 22–8. Postanesthesia long-term and critical care nursing assessment record (page 2).

**POST ANESTHESIA
NURSING ASSESSMENT RECORD
CONTINUATION FORM**

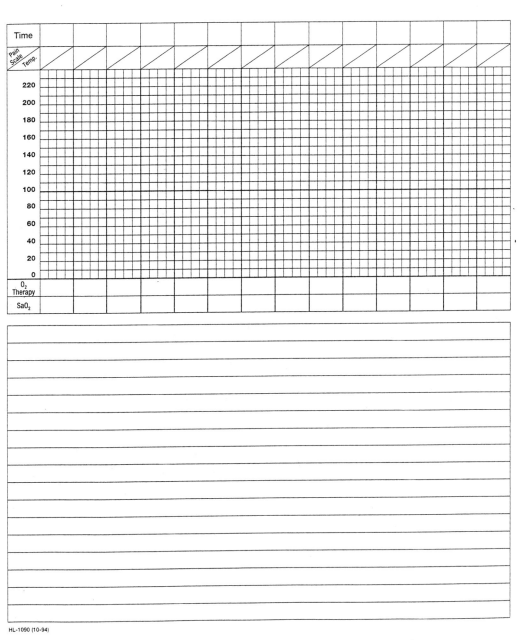

HL-1090 (10-94)

Fig. 22–9. Postanesthesia nursing assessment record continuation form.

to recognize and help manage anesthesia and surgery related complications. Auxillary or support personnel are utilized to enhance patient care and must function under the supervision of a professional registered nurse. Specific competencies for support staff should include but are not limited to the following dependent on the actual job description of the auxiliary personnel:

1. Basic life support
2. Basic airway care
3. Basic oral/nasal suctioning
4. Care of the patient with emesis
   a. positioning patient
   b. prevention of aspiration
5. Care of the patient with vasovagal reactions
   a. positioning of patient
   b. care of patient airway
   c. application of O_2 delivery system
6. Care of the patient with thermo-regulatory problems
   a. recognition and notification of hypothermia to RN
      (1) application of warm blankets
      (2) application of warming devices
      (3) monitoring of body temperature
      (4) discontinuance of warming devices
   b. recognition and notification of hyperthermia to RN
      (1) application of ice packs to "hot spots" (i.e., axilla and groin)
      (2) application of cooling devices
      (3) discontinuance of cooling devices
7. Care of the patient with intravenous fluids
   (a) recognition and notification of aberrant IV rate to RN
   (b) recognition and notification of alarming IV pump to RN
   (c) recognition and notification of infiltrated IV to RN
8. Care of the patient with seizure disorder
9. Care of the patient with drains, catheters
10. Care of the patient of cardiac/pulse oximetry/ pneumatic blood pressure monitors
    (a) application of electrodes/probes/BP cuffs
    (b) recognition of monitor alarms (EKG/ pulse oximetry/BP)
    (c) notification of monitor alarms to RN
    (d) discontinuance of monitoring equipment
11. Care of the patient on continual anti-embolism compression stocking
12. Care and safe transport of the PACU patient via stretcher/crib to:
    (a) bed
    (b) recliner chair (8)

An anesthesiologist must be readily available to manage, assist, and advise the registered nurse in the management of the patient in the post anesthesia phase. ASPAN has developed a patient classification system that is followed in the majority of PACU settings. It states that a professional registered nurse assesses the patient and develops a plan of care designed to meet the patient's preprocedual needs (8). This requirement is also interlaced through the JCAHO standards. Figure 22–10 lists the ASPAN staffing recommendations based on patient acuity and age.

It should also be noted that patient acuity and age are not the only factors that affect staffing. The physical layout of the PACU must be considered in order to maximize the nurse:patient ratio. One and one half or two beds should be available in the PACU for every operating room. It should be designed in such a manner that one registered nurse can readily oversee three to five patients without obstruction. Pillars and full dividing walls should be avoided in the construction of a post anesthesia care area. Poor design can only increase staffing requirements and, in the long term, personnel cost. A well designed PACU will facilitate the functional needs of the various user groups. (i.e., patients, family, physicians, nurses, axillary personnel). Other components of staffing that must be considered by the PACU administrator are the short term personnel scheduling and the daily staffing requirements.

Daily Requirements

The first step is to determine the daily nursing and auxiliary staffing requirements. The workload of the PACU is directly related to the operating room activity schedule. The daily registered nurse requirements for the

PATIENT CLASSIFICATION

PHASE I

CLASS 1:2   ONE NURSE TO TWO PATIENTS WHO ARE
    a. one unconscious, stable without artificial airway, and over the age of 9 years and one conscious, stable, and free of complications
    b. two conscious stable and free of complications
    c. two conscious stable, 11 years of age and under; with family or competent support staff present

CLASS 1:1   ONE NURSE TO ONE PATIENT
    a. at the time of admission, until the critical elements are met
    b. requiring mechanical life support and/or artificial airway
    c. any unconscious patient 9 years of age and under
    d. a second nurse must be available to assist as necessary

CLASS 2:1   TWO NURSES TO ONE PATIENT
    a. one critically ill, unstable, complicated patient

PHASE II

CLASS 1:3   ONE NURSE TO THREE PATIENTS
    a. older than 5 years of age within 1/2 hour of procedure/discharge from phase I
    b. 5 years of age and under within 1/2 hour of procedure/discharge from phase I with family present

CLASS 1:2   ONE NURSE TO TWO PATIENTS
    a. 5 years of age and under without family or support staff present
    b. initial admission of postprocedure

CLASS 1:1   ONE NURSE TO ONE PATIENT
    a. unstable patient of any age requiring transfer

    Staffing is based on patient acuity, census, and physical facility. Two licensed nurses, one of whom is an RN, are present whenever a patient is recovering in phase I. Two competent personnel, one of whom is an RN, are present whenever a patient is recovering in phase II. An RN must be present at all times in Phase II. When the patient census increases to greater than three, the RN staff-to-patient census increases to greater than three, the RN staff-to-patient ratio must be increased to maintain the minimum 1:3 ratio

Fig. 22–10.   Patient classification: phase I and phase II.

PACU will vary based on the following criteria for operating room usage. Does the health care center facilitate long or short procedures? Is the operating room an 8-hour, Monday-to-Friday operation, starting at 8 A.M., with the final surgery start time of 3:30 P.M.? Is the operating room open 24 hours a day, Monday to Friday only? Is it a trauma center? Are weekends staffed by an "on-call" system? Are there four, twelve, twenty or more operating rooms?

The answers to these questions will be used by the management group to individualize staffing to service the PACU patient population, volume and activity.

Figure 22–11 and Figure 22–12 demonstrate two very diverse staffing patterns for post anesthesia care units.

Figure 22–11 is an example of staffing for a free standing ambulatory setting with four operating suites open Monday to Friday. Surgery start time is 8 A.M and last scheduled surgery start is 3:30 P.M. The center has two postanesthesia beds for each operating room and has a 60% pediatric patient population. Note that, in the diagram, staffing starts at

DAILY STAFFING REQUIREMENTS
FOR AMBULATORY SETTING — PACU

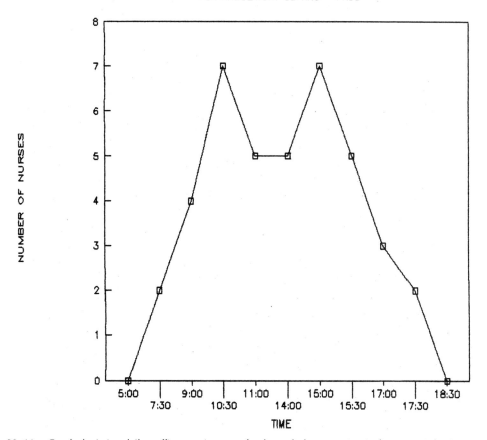

Fig. 22–11. Graph depicting daily staffing requirements for the ambulatory setting in the postanesthesia care unit.

a zero base and has staggered increasing staffing numbers peaking at 10:30 A.M. This staggered personnel model facilitates the required number of personnel needed when the PACU is fully utilized. The peak hours are at 10:30 A.M. and 2 P.M. to accommodate lunch and rest periods for the staff.

Figure 22–12, in contrast, depicts a PACU that is staffed Monday to Friday, 24 hours a day in an acute care facility. In this setting, work schedules are more flexible with the utilization of every half hour start times and staggered shifts based on eight, ten, or twelve hours. This example is based on ten to twelve operating room suites and 10,000 to 11,000

patients annually. The model includes a unit facilitator or charge assistant nurse manager who directs the flow of the patients in the PACU, coordinates the transfer of patients throughout the hospital, and generally problem solves in relationship to the daily schedule. It should be noted in the diagram that the base number never goes below two nursing personnel. This facilitates overnight patients for intensive care unit overflow and complies with the ASPAN staffing standards for coverage of urgent and emergency cases. Peak staffing is again at 10:30 A.M. and 2 P.M. to facilitate lunch and rest periods for personnel.

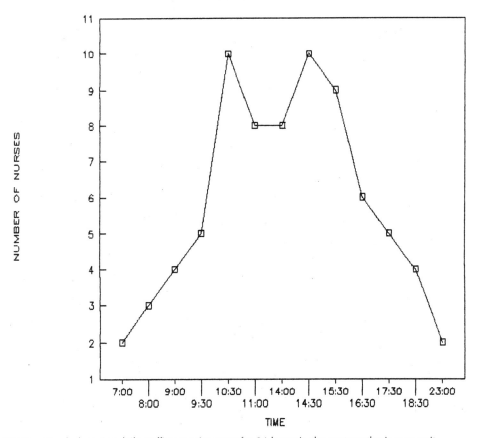

Fig. 22–12. Graph depicting daily staffing requirements for 24 hours in the postanesthesia care unit.

PERSONNEL SCHEDULING PROCESS

The next personnel issue for the administrative staff is the short term personnel scheduling process. This is not to be confused with the annual budget decisions that will be decided later in this chapter under budget requirements. Short term scheduling of staff is a two- to six-week schedule that commits staff to work based on the daily staffing requirements. Preparing this schedule can be a time consuming process since various factors dictate how the schedule should be completed. Minimum daily staffing requirements must be met in the final staff schedule. Other factors that affect the schedule are the availability of contingent staff to cover staff requests for days off and vacations, seasonal peak volume times, and staggered shift requirements. The staffing schedule usually includes the employee's name, shift start time, day, and date. Figure 22–13 is a sample of one type of PACU staffing schedule for a six-week period.

Staffing is a complex process in the PACU. It must meet the demands of unexpected urgencies or emergencies, the time of the day, rapid turnover of patient population, and varying daily volume in order to meet the standards of care to produce a quality product.

STAFFING SCHEDULE

TIME PERIOD: October 2–October 8
6-WEEK SCHEDULE

EMPLOYEE	DATES						
	S 2	M 3	T 4	W 5	TH 6	F 7	S 8
W. Stefl	C	/	/	/	/	/	C
B. Jones	X	/	/	/	X	/	X
A. Smith	C	C	/	/	/	/	/
T. Collins	X	/	/	/	/	/	X
D. Givens	X	/	/	/	/	/	X
K. Long	X	/	/	/	/	/	X
T. Sturdivant	X	/	/	/	/	/	X
W. Buford	X	/	/	/	/	/	X
J. Blain	X	/	/	/	/	/	X

"/" indicates days worked.
"X" indicates days off.
"C" indicates on-call coverage.

Fig. 22–13. Sample staffing schedule for a 6-week time period.

Usually staffing issues are the responsibility of the direct clinical manager of the PACU.

DELINEATION OF RESPONSIBILITY

When discussing the delineation of responsibility in a PACU, it is important to explore the broad concept of management. It is not a concept easily defined. Based on the product or group to be managed, the term lends itself to various definitions. Human resources management does not present with the same characteristics as product management. This diversity in role, therefore, leads to multiple descriptions of what is management. However, organizational design researchers now agree that management is indeed a separate legitimate field and requires special skills, education, and training (3). Historically, management in the health care industry has perpetuated the concept that talent doing manual, technical, or professional work guarantees the presence of talent if that person is promoted to a manager. This practice has led to the failure of many excellent practice specialists in their roles as manager. Laurence J. Peter was concerned about this dilemma when in 1969 he published *The Peter Principle*. Peter's commentary contains a great deal of truth. His "principle" states that every person in a hierarchy system tends to rise to his level of incompetence (10). Peter concluded that the outstanding worker at any level is likely to be promoted to the next level in the hierarchy.

This practice continues until the person reaches a level where performance is mediocre at best. At this point all promotions stop and the person is left, probably until retirement, one level above the level of good performance. This is not to imply that a practice specialist cannot be an effective manager. However, it must be recognized that a worker promoted to management must be mentored with supplementary education and training for optimal success.

The management team in health care has the responsibility of directing all the activities of employees toward the achievement of the institution's goals and objectives as defined in its mission, vision, and strategic plan. Management has some broad responsibilities connected to the health institution's strategic plan. First, management is responsible for moving patients through the health care system and assuring that the patients receive the best possible care at the lowest possible cost. Second, management is responsible to employees and must provide an environment that recognizes that each employee has reasonable needs for fair treatment, fair compensation, security, approval, and a sense of accomplishment. Third, management is responsible to the board of trustees in their capacity as managers of the institution's resources. Fourth, management's responsibility to the community it serves is to determine how best to meet current health care needs.

In looking at the management structure of the PACU, the organizational chart places the PACU in the administrative tree leading ultimately to the Chief Executive Officer (CEO). This ladder of authority can extend up through the Vice President of Nursing or the Chief Operations Officer (COO). This is strictly based on the organizational structure decisions of the CEO. There are no current regulatory criteria mandating either structural design. The JCAHO, however, has two requirements that directly affect the direct reporting requirements for clinical practice of the medical staff and nursing personnel. The medical practices in the PACU are the direct responsibility of the Anesthesia Chairman or an appointed anesthesiologist as the director of medical practice in the PACU. The Anesthesia Department has the responsibility to validate that hospital policies and procedures demonstrates consistent practice in all areas of the hospital where anesthetics are used. In addition, the clinical nursing practices must have related reporting mechanism to the Nursing Division; and, also, demonstrate consistent clinical practice in similar settings such as labor and delivery suites, catherization laboratories, and endoscopy suites. Therefore, if the PACU does not have a direct reporting relationship to the nursing department, it must facilitate this requirement for clinical practice through a liaison relationship through a registered nurse manager or a certified registered nurse anesthetist (CRNA). In a large health care system there is an administrative manager or director of surgical services who has a broad scope of responsibilities to coordinate the activities of all units in a functional department. A **functional** department can be defined as one made up of units and jobs that are similar in nature, or one in which the activities of the various units are interdependent and necessitate the coordination of one top manager or administration (3). The PACU can be considered a unit in the functional department of surgical services (i.e., Preoperative Holding Area, Operating Room, PACU, as well as surgical units and surgical intensive care units). This administrative director has the responsibility for the strategic planning of the complete perioperative process, annual budget planning, policy and procedure approval, and the overall coordination of the various axillary services. This position should be held by a person with advance skills in management and finance. The typical job description for an administrative director should include the requirement of a master's degree in business, health administration or related field. The next level of management in the PACU is the first-line supervisor. This role is usually a registered nurse, who usually functions as both clinician and supervisor. As a practice specialist the first-line supervisor does some of the actual work in the PACU. At various peak times in the PACU, it is the first-line supervisor who performs hands-on tasks to deliver patient care and ensure the efficiency of the PACU. On the other hand, as the management generalist the first-line supervisor is responsible for guiding and directing the work of others in the PACU. The first-line supervisor's management responsibility is more operational planning–oriented, in contrast to the director or administrator's responsibility for broader strategic planning. Therefore, this level of management coordinates the daily PACU volume as well as staffing and scheduling for the department.

In a small PACU it might also be the responsibility of the nurse manager to develop and monitor the budget. Usually, a large institution places that responsibility on the administrative level.

BUDGETS AND COST CONTAINMENT

There are many managers who have not received any formal training in finance or accounting and who tend to think there is only one correct way to perform financial analyses. In fact, every financial planning system is unique to the individual organization. Each organization designs its own budget procedure and the special documents and forms associated with this process. Budgeting is unique for each institution and will depend as much on the specific individuals working in the organization as it will on any formalized mechanical steps involved in the budget preparation and use. Therefore, this section on PACU budgets will focus more on budget concepts than on a specific step-by-step approach to the PACU fiscal planning.

The amount of participation that any individual administrator or PACU manager has in the budget process depends on the approach or philosophy of the organization's top management. In some institutions there is a great deal of management and employee participation in deciding a realistic minimum spending for the PACU. On the other hand, many PACU managers have to suffer with unrealistic budgets imposed upon them from above.

Teachers of finance and financial consultants stress the importance of participation in the budget process by individuals in all levels in the organization. The lower the organization goes to understand the specific circumstances and conditions of a PACU, the more likely it is to get an accurate understanding of the cost structure needed to operate the unit.

It is important for managers to understand that a **budget** is a process where plans are made and an effort is made to meet or exceed the objectives of the plan. In a health care system there are many types of budgets (i.e., Program Budget, Operation Budget, Capital Budget, Cash Budget, etc). For purposes related to the function of the PACU, the administrator is most concerned with two main budgets: the operating budget and the capital budget.

Operating Budget

The operating budget is probably the most familiar to PACU managers. It is the plan for the daily operating revenues and expenses and usually covers a time period of one year. The PACU is a revenue generating department and the monthly budget statement will include revenues generated from Medicare, Medicaid, Blue Cross, other private insurers, and self-pay patients. Although revenues are a part of all operating budgets, some managers are only shown the part of the operating budget known as expenses. The PACU administrator or manager generally has direct control and responsibility for the PACU expense budget. Most health care systems use a similar identification system for each functional unit. This financial structure is divided into **cost centers**. The expense part of the operating budget of a PACU will have a single cost center number. The financial reporting system—usually called the budget variance report (BVR)—for the cost center identifies the expenses incurred for the hospital's accounting cycle (usually one calendar month). The expense report will also show fiscal year-to-date cumulative totals. The expenses are separated into two major categories: salary and non-salary expenses.

The two categories are usually subdivided into line item accounts based on a more specifically described expense (i.e., overtime, RN salaries, medical supplies). Figure 22–14 is a sample of a cost center account showing expenses for a PACU. Note that the report shows both an actual gross revenue and a projected budgeted revenue. Also, the report shows a variance which reflects the budgeted amount of dollars minus actual dollars. In the variance column, the mathematical sign indicates actual performance against budget. Negative variance (minus sign) means the PACU spent more than what was budgeted. The positive variance (no sign) means the unit spend less than was budgeted. Some institutions use the signs in a reverse pattern with positive variance indicating unfavorable variance. Either method is acceptable as long as the institution is consistent. Some budget variance reports will include indirect operating expenses such as utilities, housekeeping expenses, and so forth. However, it is not unusual for these indirect expenses to appear on the facility's master budget. It is usually the PACU manager or administrator who reviews the monthly variance report and develops a written explanation of the positive and negative deviations from the budgeted plan. There are numerous justifications for deviations in the PACU report. Variables such as volume changes, patient acuity, late posting in the accounts payable department, and simply human error can greatly distort the monthly BVR. It is the PACU administrator's responsibility to justify increased or decreased spending, as well as to correct all input errors. Earlier in this chapter, staffing for the PACU was discussed in great detail regarding scheduling. Personal budget reports are also part of the budget variance report process.

Salary and Non-Salary Expenses

The personnel report describes the employees of the PACU in terms of positions and hours. Personnel is defined in the concept of **full-time equivalent** (F.T.E.). A full-time equivalent is a conversion of hours into one employee working eight hours a day, five days a week, fifty-two weeks a year. A person working eighty hours in a two week payroll period equates to 2,080 hours yearly or one full time equivalent (1 F.T.E.). Determining the reasonable amount of F.T.E.'s needed in a PACU is justified based on some type of indicator. It can be based on patient volume, patient hours, or some other predetermined productivity monitoring system set by the organization. These F.T.E.'s are converted to the annual dollar equivalent and reflected in the BVR as a salary experience by job classification. An F.T.E. factor should also be computed to reflect coverage for education and vacations. However, fringe benefits such as medical and dental coverage are not usually included in the cost center budget report.

The non-salary budget projects the direct expenses of the PACU cost center. Generally these expenses include all routine patient care items as well as items for maintaining the functioning of the PACU such as office supplies, repairs, and maintenance of equipment. Again, calculating non-salary expenses is similar to projecting the F.T.E.'s budget (salary expenses). The simplest method is to identify a cost per unit of activity (patient volume or patient hours) multiplied by the projected volume or activity, and include an inflation adjustment. This method provides the annual operational budget for the PACU and is reflected under budgeted dollar amounts in the monthly BVR. The PACU cost center budget is then added to the departmental budget, and the total departmental budgets make up the operational budget for the organization.

Capital Budgets

The second area in which the PACU manager, administrator, and medical director have considerable input is the capital budget requests for the PACU. Capital budgeting is the common name for the analysis of long term investments for the unit. These investments can range from projects as large as complete rebuilding of the PACU or as small as acquisitions like a PACU patient chair. Organizations usually have two criteria in evaluating capital equipment. First, the acquired asset has a useful life of greater than one year. Second, a minimum cost requirement is set by the organization. If the facility receives Medicare funding, then the capital expenditure is $500 or greater. However, some organizations may consider anything over $250 as capital equipment.

Funds are usually not available for an organization to acquire all the items it desires. The capital budget process requires choices to be made in the allocation of resources. The administrator of the PACU, in describing proposed capital expenses, needs to accurately provide justification for each purchase. This justification should include a description of the item, its cost, urgency of the purchase, the proposed purchase date, life of the item to be purchased, and salvage value of current equipment being replaced. The PACU management staff should rank all capital items before submitting them to the capital committee or organizational body that approves capital purchases.

Most capital items for the PACU do not generate additional revenue for the department. Instead, PACU capital is usually directed to enhance patient care. Therefore, it is difficult to formulate justification for capital equipment based on some of the conventional financial methods such as cash payback approach, discounted cash flow approach, or net present value. Justification approaches for capital equipment in a PACU rely on regulatory requirements, patient safety issues, or obsolescence of current equipment. Earlier in this chapter the responsibilities of management were discussed. As previously noted, the first responsibility of management is to move patients through the health care system and as-

sure that patients receive the best possible care at the lowest possible cost. Therefore, an administrative structure chapter would not be complete without addressing cost containment.

Cost Containment

Cost containment is not new in health care. In 1946 the federal government passed the Hill-Burton Act and tried to regulate health care cost by mandating consumer participation in health care planning and the CON process (Certificate of Need) (9). President Truman introduced National Health Care to Congress during his administration and his proposal was defeated in Congress. With the passing of the Medicare/Medicaid Act of 1965, the federal government tried to contain health care costs by requiring all recipients of Medicare funds to manage fiscal affairs through an annual budgeting process. Prior to this bill, hospitals paid little attention to the financial management process. One of the major reason for the failure of all these cost containment regulations was the concept of fee-for-service. Prior to 1965 all health care revenues were paid on a fee-for-service scale. This meant that the more the health care system did for the patient the more money that institution made. By 1980 revenues exceeding expenses were at an all time high in the health care industry. Then, in the 1980s the Reagan administration introduced Diagnosis Related Groups (DRG's) for Medicare payments. The DRG's introduced the concept of one fixed payment for certain types of diagnosis. Today, health care is an extremely changeable environment. Managed care is quickly engulfing the health care industry, and those health care systems that are slow to react and make plans to contain costs will not survive this transition. The days of plenty seem to be over and there is acknowledgement in healthcare that resources are not infinite and need to be carefully used and allocated.

In the very near future, PACU's will no longer generate revenues for the institution

	CURRENT MONTH					YEAR-TO-DATE				
	ACTUAL AMOUNT	BUDGET AMOUNT	VARIANCE AMOUNT	VARIANCE %	LAST YR AMOUNT	ACTUAL AMOUNT	BUDGET AMOUNT	VARIANCE AMOUNT	VARIANCE %	LAST YR AMOUNT
REVENUE										
DIRECT PAY ICU	769	0	769	.0	0	34	0	34	.0	0
DIRECT PAY IP OTH	1,534	3,319	1,785-	53.8-	7,482	23,010	36,393	13,383-	36.8-	22,398
DIRECT PAY E/R OP	0	0	0	.0	691	2,841	0	2,841	.0	1,227
DIRECT PAY OP OTH	13,999	34,081	20,082-	58.9-	5,459	117,396	353,472	236,076-	66.8-	127,276
BLUE CROSS ICU	769	0	769	.0	1,471	16,408	0	16,408	.0	5,915
BLUE CROSS IP OTH	40,287	32,344	7,943	24.6	43,493	450,243	354,661	95,582	27.0	464,098
BLUE CROSS E/R OP	329	0	329	.0	0	2,210	0	2,210	.0	896
BLUE CROSS OP OTH	86,517	72,287	14,230	19.7	62,536	865,585	749,721	115,864	15.5	811,607
COMMERCIAL ICU	0	0	0	.0	0	1,251	0	1,251	.0	805
COMMERCIAL IP OTH	6,738	16,404	9,666-	58.9-	11,245	128,647	179,879	51,232-	28.5-	155,177
COMMERCIAL E/R OP	0	0	0	.0	0	426	0	426	.0	0
COMMERCIAL OP OTH	16,993	72,359	55,366-	76.5-	28,343	280,088	750,469	470,381-	62.7-	314,025
IHP ICU	0	0	0	.0	0	1,632	0	1,632	.0	0
IHP INPATIENT OTH	4,531	0	4,531	.0	2,861	18,896	0	18,896	.0	11,126
IHP E/R OUTPAIENT	0	0	0	.0	1,578	532	0	532	.0	0
IHP OUTPAT OTHERS	5,880	0	5,880	.0	1,578	25,580	0	25,580	.0	10,887
MEDICARE A ICU	6,499	0	6,499	.0	0	38,974	0	38,974	.0	21,301
MEDICARE A IP OTH	84,498	102,379	17,881-	17.5-	90,090	962,810	1,122,623	159,813-	14.2-	852,873
MEDICARE A E/R OP	383	0	383	.0	0	383	0	383	.0	0
MEDICARE A OP OTH	106,037	101,303	4,734	4.7	85,585	993,761	1,050,658	56,897-	5.4-	841,053
MEDICAID ICU	0	0	0	.0	886-	7,567	0	7,567	.0	1,642
MEDICAID IP OTHRS	26,755	36,233	9,478-	26.2-	20,892	280,808	397,312	116,504-	29.3-	223,392
MEDICAID E/R OP	0	0	0	.0	0	6,465	0	6,465	.0	3,268
MEDICAID OP OTHRS	44,386	40,521	3,865	9.5	37,888	425,128	420,263	4,865	1.2	349,612
MCC INPATIENT OTH	329	0	329	.0	0	492	0	492	.0	0
MAN CARE ICU	0	0	0	.0	0	4,667	0	4,667	.0	492
MAN CARE IP OTHER	34,010	20,717	13,293	64.2	33,445	371,921	227,168	144,753	63.7	292,149
MAN CARE E/R OP	0	0	0	.0	0	957	0	957	.0	628
MAN CARE OP OTHER	91,848	41,245	50,603	122.7	70,872	980,831	427,768	553,063	129.3	697,046
TOTAL	573,091	573,192	101-	.0	504,623	6,009,543	6,070,387	60,844-	1.0-	5,208,893
REVENUE ADJ										
EXPENSES										
001 MGT/SUPERVISO	11,128	11,127	1-	.0	6,454	120,001	120,287	286	.2	71,881
003 REG NURSES	59,896	56,161	3,735-	6.7-	59,258	643,024	607,121	35,903-	5.9-	647,583
005 NUR ASSISTANT	5,706	5,219	487-	9.3-	3,236	55,481	56,419	938	1.7	40,345
007 RESIDENTS	1,735	0	1,735-	.0	1,638	4,575	0	4,575-	.0	1,481
010 OFFICE STAFF	937	1,963	1,026	52.3	0	17,417	21,222	3,805	17.9	12,120
019 HOLIDAY PREM P	0	0	0	.0	0	491	0	491-	.0	199
021 OVERTIME	3,216	223	2,993-	1,342.2-	903	16,159	2,419	13,740-	568.0-	16,532

518

9206283 RECOVERY ROOM   CLASS B/W VAR   REPORT 014-09   (WHOLE DOLLAR)   PER ENDING 05/31/95   ISSUED 06/10/95

	CURRENT MONTH					YEAR-TO-DATE				
	ACTUAL AMOUNT	BUDGET AMOUNT	VARIANCE AMOUNT	%	LAST YR AMOUNT	ACTUAL AMOUNT	BUDGET AMOUNT	VARIANCE AMOUNT	%	LAST YR AMOUNT
022 SHIFT PREMIUM	2,033	1,556	477-	30.7-	1,665	19,969	16,819	3,150-	18.7-	19,217
026 ON CALL	431	679	248	36.5	519	5,452	7,342	1,890	25.7	6,793
027 SALAR CHARGED	352-	0	352	.0	576-	5,019-	0	5,019	.0	145-
	84,729	76,928	7,801-	10.1-	74,579	877,551	831,629	45,922-	5.5-	816,006
020 FICA	7,211	5,696	1,515-	26.6-	5,707	70,068	61,576	8,492-	13.8-	62,613
041 OFF/ADMIN SUP	92	167	75	44.9	376	2,579	1,837	742	40.4-	2,033
042 MED/SURG SUPP	2,807	2,499	308-	12.3-	2,395	28,976	27,489	1,487-	5.4-	25,665
043 DRUG/PHARM	1,118	750	368-	49.1-	804	7,107	8,250	1,143	13.9	6,694
044 IV SOLUTIONS	1,990	1,666	324-	19.4-	2,003	25,186	18,326	6,860-	37.4-	21,286
049 ORTHOPED SUPP	61	0	61-	.0	0	304	0	304	.0	0
050 LAB SUPPLIES	0	0	0	.0	0	31	0	31-	.0	59
052 DIETARY FOOD	571	0	571-	.0	28	2,493	0	2,493-	.0	28
054 DIETARY PAPER	55	58	3	5.2	44	503	638	135	21.2	585
055 CLEANING PROD	12	0	12-	.0	20	72	0	72	.0	102
056 REP/MAINT SUP	0	0	0	.0	0	256	0	256	.0	0
058 LINEN REPLACE	74	0	74-	.0	19	541	0	541	.0	271
059 POST/FREIGHT	0	12	12	100.0	59	154	132	22-	16.7-	71
065 MINOR MED EQ	0	83	83	100.0	0	0	913	913	100.0	150
066 OTHR MINR EQ	0	0	0	.0	0	641	0	641-	.0	80
067 OTHR SUP/MATE	0	0	0	.0	0	136	0	136-	.0	0
094 REP/MAINT EQ	0	0	0	.0	0	512	0	512-	.0	0
102 SUBSCRIP/BOOK	65	8	57-	712.5-	0	109	88	21-	23.9-	0
104 TRAVEL/MEET	0	42	42	100.0	209	450	462	12	2.6	459
	14,054	10,981	3,073-	28.0-	11,665	140,120	119,711	20,409-	17.0-	120,096
TOTAL	98,783	87,909	10,874-	12.4-	86,243	1,017,671	951,340	66,331-	7.0-	936,102
EXCESS/(DEFICIT)	474,308	485,283	10,975-	2.3-	418,380	4,991,873	5,119,047	127,174-	2.5-	4,272,791

Fig. 22-14. Sample budget variance.

and, instead, need to concentrate on providing quick, quality service at a very low cost. Alternative staffing patterns must be explored to minimize personnel cost since it is the highest expense in the PACU operating budget. Educating the staff on the new concepts of managed care (i.e., HMO, PPO, PHO) is the first step to cost containment.

The PACU staff must facilitate cost containment measures by practicing economical care. The bedside care giver is in the best position to reduce medical supply cost. However, awareness and improvisation is no longer enough and every staff member of the PACU and the health care institution must conserve and preserve scarce resources for the viability of the organization.

Recently, the term, capitation, has entered the health care area. **Capitation** is a payment agreement between a health care provider (HMO, PPO, etc.) and a health care organization, usually a physician-hospital organization (PHO). A set monthly fee for each member who signs up to participate as a client or patient in a designated PHO is paid to the PHO by the health care provider. In exchange, the PHO agrees to provide all the medical care agreed upon by the health care provider. This is basically a paradigm shift in health care. It is now the health care organization that is at financial risk in the care of the patient, not the health care provider. Cost containment under this new payment agreement becomes paramount in the survival of the organization. The management responsibility to provide quality care at the **lowest** cost and the **quickest** service is the main focus of capitation. Capitation programs concentrate on preventive health care measures to reduce the risk of hospitalization, which equates to a larger profit margin for the PHO. It is too early to evaluate whether capitation will bring financial success to health care organizations; but it is clear that, in a capitation program, the PACU will no longer generate revenues for the organization. The PACU in this system becomes a cost center.

This new wave of reimbursement mandates that the administrative staff and all PACU personnel find creative ways to reduce both salary and non-salary expenses, reduce LOS for each patient, and maintain a quality product.

SUMMARY

With the flurry of change taking place within the health care marketplace during the 1990s, it is difficult to accurately forecast what will be the design of the successful hospital of the twenty-first century. This is the time when alert administrators need to take a business approach in the strategic planning for the post anesthesia care unit. As the PACU shifts from a revenue center to a cost center, management is faced with a time of revised expectations, overwhelming challenges, and an era of downsizing. Now, more than ever before in the history of health care, successful PACU managers need to have the skills necessary to preserve, conserve, and manage resources. They need the background knowledge of organizational design, the understanding of the jargon used by financial people, and the reorganization of a quality care product. Ambulatory centers have been the fastest growing health care service in the country, and the hospital of the future will need to reach out into homes and extend its influence into residential communities—following their patients after they have crossed its threshold for care. The administrative structure of the PACU must be flexibly designed to accommodate this transition, and its managers must possess the skills need to recognize the role of the PACU in the health care organization of the future.

REFERENCES

1. Bedeian AG, Zammuto RF. Organizations: theory and design. New York: Dryden Press, 1991;117.
2. Robbins SP. Essential of organizational behavior. 2nd ed. Englewood Cliffs, NJ: Prentice Hall, 1988;168.
3. Gibson JL, Ivancevich JM, Donnelly JH. Organizations: behavior, structure, processes. 8th ed. Bur Ridge, IL, Irwin, Inc., 1994;496-497.
4. Ford JD. Institutional versus questionnaire measures of organizational structure. Acad Manage J 1979;10:601–610.

5. Mintzburg H. The structure of organizations. Englewood Cliffs, NJ, Prentice Hall, 1979;188-199.
6. American Society of Anesthesiologists. Standards for post anesthesia care, effective date January 1, 1992. Park Ridge, IL: American Society of Anesthesiologists, 1994.
7. Joint Commission on Accreditation of Healthcare Organizations. The Joint Commission accreditation manual for hospitals. Vol. 1. Oakbrook Terrace, IL: Joint Commission on Accreditation of Healthcare Organizations, 1995.
8. American Society of Post Anesthesia Nurses. Standards of post anesthesia nursing practice. Richmond, VA: American Society of Post Anesthesia Nurses, 1995.
9. Reeves PN, Corle RC. Introduction to health planning. 4th ed. Arlington, VA, Resource Information Press, 1989;71.
10. Peter LJ. The Peter principle. New York: William Morrow & Company, 1969:26.

ADDITIONAL READINGS

Gordon, Judith R., *Human Resource Management.* Allyn and Bacon, Inc., Boston. 1986: Chapter 1.

Harvey, Donald F., Brown, Donald R. *An Experiential Approach to Organization Development.* Prentice Hall, Englewood Cliffs, N.J. 3rd Edition. 1988: Chapter 1.

Hersey, Paul, Blanchard, Kenneth H. *Management of Organizational Behavior.* Prentice Hall, Englewood Cliffs, N.J. 5th Edition. Chapter 5.

Momaril, Myrna. *Standard of Care: Legal Implications in the PACU,* Journal of Post Anesthesia Nursing. *8* (1); 1993: 13-20.

McConnell, Charles R. *The Effective Health CareSupervisor.* Aspen Publishers, Gaithersburg, Maryland, 2nd Edition, 1988: Chapter 4.

Pritchard, Virginia, Erkard, Janet M. *Standards of Nursing Care in the PACU,* Journal of Post Anesthesia Nursing. *5,* (3) 199: 163-167.

Tubbs, Stewart L. *A Systems Approach to Small Group Interaction.* Random House, N.Y., 3rd Edition. 1988: Chapter 4.

23

PHYSICAL DESIGN

John H. Eichhorn

As was demonstrated in Chapter 2, "Equipment and Monitoring Requirements," the needs of a postanesthesia care unit (PACU) vary widely among healthcare facilities. In the same way, the physical design of a PACU will incorporate many features specific to the institution, its character, its physical plant, its staff, the patient population, and particularly the number and type of surgical procedures performed. Basic construction guidelines and standards exist (1–3) and are primarily oriented toward building and safety codes that should be familiar to architects designing healthcare facilities. However, it is important that the physician staff, nursing staff, and facility administrative staff review this basic material so that they will know the terminology the architects use and where some of the things they are talking about originate.

The PACU exists to provide a centralized location for the care of patients leaving the operating room, who often in an altered state of consciousness and with potentially labile (or even unstable) vital signs. Its design must reflect this mission. It is a highly specialized facility that has many of the features of an intensive care unit but is still oriented to relatively brief periods of admission. Therefore, questions of traffic flow, supply storage and distribution, and housekeeping are more important than in a traditional intensive care unit (ICU). The design must provide immediate proximity to the necessary facilities and personnel, especially the concentrated expertise of the PACU nursing staff.

PACU LOCATION

Ideally, all PACUs would be immediately adjacent to the operating room (OR) with the entrance door directly off a main OR outer corridor. Clearly, this arrangement is not always possible because of the realities of the physical plants of various healthcare facilities. In almost all circumstances, the PACU should be on the same floor as the OR because of the dangers associated with an elevator ride (even of one floor in a dedicated elevator) for a patient just emerging from anesthesia. It should be as close to the OR as physically possible, if not immediately contiguous. The optimal design would make the maximum transport time for a stretcher pushed at normal speed from the OR or procedure room most distant from the PACU no more than 90 seconds.

The entrance and exit doors must be extra wide, even wider than the usual hospital room door. It is difficult to turn stretchers with intravenous poles and monitors into hallways through even the usual "wide" door. It is sometimes difficult to convince hospital architects of this fact. A staged demonstration with the architect pushing a stretcher similar to that which would exist in a "worst-case scenario" will quickly convince all involved. If at all possible, it is highly desirable to design the PACU with separate entrance and exit doors for patients. Ideally, the entrance door would be an automatic sliding or swing-open glass door directly from an OR corridor. The exit door (powered opening with a push-button control on the wall) would be at the opposite end of the unit and open out on to a major hospital patient-transport corridor readily accessible to the outpatient staging area and also to the elevators to the inpatient units. This "flow-through" concept helps maintain an orderly flow of stretcher traffic, avoiding in-out conflicts at a single entry-exit door. Also, this arrangement creates a minor but important psychological mindset for both patients and staff with the exit door as an unspoken goal symbolizing progress in the recovery/healing process.

HOW MANY BEDSPACES ARE NEEDED?

This discussion is limited to "phase I recovery" considerations, i.e., patients coming directly out of the OR. Phase II recovery is concerned with outpatients progressing toward discharge home and is best covered in material that specifically addresses ambulatory surgery (see Chapter 21).

As long ago as 1981 (4), it was recognized that the traditional concept of one recovery room bed for each OR served was out of date. A modern PACU might be adequate with a one-to-one ratio of beds to ORs in the very unusual circumstance of a very limited number of procedures being performed in an OR. Modern reality, however, dictates that with the relatively high turnover of patients, particularly outpatients or "short-stay" patients, a regular, general-purpose PACU with a good mix of a wide variety of patients should have bedspaces numbering approximately 1.5 times the number of ORs served. Truly high-volume ORs in outpatient surgery facilities will need bedspaces numbering up to two times the number of ORs.

FLOOR PLAN

The basic shape of the PACU may well be governed by the physical realities of the parent facility. The suggestion concerning separate patient entrance and exit doors and the consequent "flow-through" concept is outlined above. The ideal general shape is square, with patient bedspaces on three walls. The entrance and exit doors, the nurses' station, and the support and supply areas occupy the fourth wall and extend out into the floor space, making a gentle horseshoe-shaped arrangement. One benefit of this basic idea is that the distance from the nurses's station and control desk to each patient bedspace will be as short as possible.

It is reasonable to budget a total of approximately 200 square feet per bedspace and then add the central support space. This arrangement allows for reasonably sized bedspaces and generous aisles to avoid crowding, particularly when there is extra equipment at the foot of one bedspace. A 10-bed unit might need 200×10 plus an additional 800 or more square feet of support space for the central station, clean and dirty utility, medication area (or room), storage, and staff toilets — for a total of 2800 square feet. This does not include provision for rest area for the staff, call rooms, or associated locker room areas, if applicable.

In very large PACUs, it may be administratively desirable to divide a very large unit into subsections, each of which may have a specialized function. In all cases, lines of sight are critical in a PACU. Specific architectural drawings must be made for this purpose alone so that the ability to see the patient and the monitors on the headwall from the various places that staff are located can be verified in advance. Accordingly, solid corners (such as might be used to demarcate sections) within the unit are usually counterproductive to uninhibited lines of sight.

Emergency stations, such as the location of the crash cart and the location of the difficulty intubation/airway cart (often profitably put in small alcoves), must be specified early in the design process.

Likewise, supply stations must be specified early. An ideal arrangement would be for the main supply room to be on a border wall and accessible from a hospital corridor so that supply carts do not need to be wheeled through the patient care area. Smaller PACUs probably only need one supply room and substation rolling cart to supplement the supplies kept on shelves in each bedspace. Large units may have multiple strategically located supply rooms in a pattern to be thoroughly reviewed and approved by the nursing and support staffs who will be the main users of these key components of the PACU's design.

Lastly, it is important to have at least one patient isolation room. Ideally, this room would be accessible through a door from the PACU core and also via another door on the opposite side of the isolation room, which opens onto a hospital patient transport corridor. This arrangement allows transfer of the patient without traversing the main PACU area.

PACU TRAFFIC

The concept of "patient through-put" emphasized by separate entrance and exit doors at opposite ends of the PACU has been presented. It has the theoretical value of encouraging orderly patient progress. Practical considerations along the way include the need for aisles in the PACU that are unusually wide — wide enough for a regular bed with full suspension traction to make a full 180° turn. If possible, it would be desirable to have a separate door, or even two separate doors, for "pedestrian" traffic to facilitate movement by the staff and visitors. Concerning visitors, it is highly desirable to design the unit in such a manner that parents of pediatric patients and other visitors can enter the unit and access the requisite bedspace with as little exposure to other patients as possible.

BEDSPACES

All of the patient bedspaces should be identical in configuration, layout, equipment, and supply stock. This arrangement will minimize confusion in an emergency. Hard partitions between bedspaces are possible and probably would increase the sense of privacy for patients capable of appreciating this subtlety. Privacy curtains on long tracks that can completely enclose each bedspace are much more practical. There should be at least 100 square feet in the actual bedspace (creating the ability to work around all four sides of a regular hospital bed with 3-foot clearances). There should be at least 12 square feet of shelf storage space. This shelving often is attached to the headwall but may take the form of a rolling cart. If the latter is chosen, additional square feet of floor space must be allotted to accommodate the cart. These carts are advantageous because restocking can take place in the central station with no need to carry armloads of supplies to each bedspace. There must be a readily accessible writing surface. Some PACUs are equipped with the narrow rolling tables found in most hospital rooms for each bedspace. Ceiling-mounted tracks with hanging intravenous poles should extend up and down both sides of the bedspace. Lastly, there must be a pull-chain emergency call buzzer that alerts the PACU central station control desk to a call for help by staff or a patient who is sufficiently awake to use the buzzer.

GENERAL PACU FEATURES

There must be at least two fire exits and the design will be inspected to verify that they meet all applicable safety codes. There should be a nonslip tile floor of one uniform color (easier to see objects on the floor, less likely for staff to trip). The walls should be light, neutral colors. It is important that there be a large clock on each wall in an unobstructed location that is clearly visible from all places in the unit. The clocks should be electronically connected to be synchronized to the identical time (important in arrest or other emergency record keeping). There should be handwashing sinks throughout the unit, one for each six to eight bedspaces. The clean supply and utility room should have oversized storage space (no matter how carefully planned, it will be barely adequate in actual use) with a blanket warmer. The dirty supply and utility room should be on a border wall, preferably with its own door to an outside corridor so that contaminated items can be removed without passing by patients in bedspaces. This area needs three sinks: regular, instrument wash, and flushing. Whether there should be an autoclave depends on the institution's central supply system and infection control policies.

Staff support space is critical and often overlooked by architects who do not have to work in the spaces they create. Consideration must be given to adequate lavatories, secure personal belonging storage, accessibility of rest areas, etc. There must be dedicated space for physicians to write notes and dictate into the central recording system. Finally, some provision for integral office space, particularly for the head nurse, should be made. If there is a staff room or similar appropriate location, there should be a cabinet for reference books for the medical and nursing staffs.

LIGHTING

At least some entry of daylight is highly desirable if at all possible. General lighting should be the routine hospital "bright white" fluorescent tubes. Each bedspace must have three levels of lighting: a soft "night-light" setting, regular full fluorescent, and a ceiling mounted spotlight directly over the stretcher in each bedspace. There also must be at least one large roll-around procedure light that can become functionally a mobile OR light to be used for the performing of procedures.

ENVIRONMENTAL CONTROL

The average temperature should be 75°F. The relative humidity should be maintained between 40 and 60% at all times. There should be positive air pressure compared to adjacent patient-care areas (important for infection control, particularly relative to fresh surgical wounds). There must be a minimum of six air changes per hour, two of which are fresh outside air. Formal testing is required to demonstrate compliance with the OSHA standards for operating room environments on waste/trace gases.

ELECTRIC POWER

There must be *at least* six to eight standard hospital-grade electric outlets on the headwall of every bedspace. There should also be at least two of these (with red faceplates) on the emergency power system (10-second kick-in) and ventilators and other life-sustaining equipment should always be plugged into these outlets. If the associated OR uses plugs of different design (e.g., "Hubble" plugs), there should be one outlet on each headwall of this design to accommodate OR equipment without the need for plug adapters. There should be one 220-volt x-ray machine outlet for each two bedspaces.

MEDICAL GASES

There are extensive regulations that must be observed with regard to medical gases (5). There should be *at least* three oxygen outlets (one with a flowmeter installed at all times) on the headwall of each bedspace. There should be four or five suction outlets on each headwall, with at least one tracheal and one gastrointestinal suction regulator/bottle installed at all times. There should be one compressed air outlet on each bedspace headwall.

COMMUNICATIONS

In every PACU, there must be an adequate number of telephones. Although it is not wise to promote casual telephone use, it is remarkable how many people in a busy PACU must be on the telephone at the same time. Exact specification of desk phones at the central station and wall phones around the unit must be made once the traffic and use patterns have been thoroughly studied and planned. An internal paging system within the PACU should exist unless it is a small enough unit that normal speaking voices carry throughout. One of the most annoying features of a busy PACU is staff shouting back and forth to each other, most messages indicating the need to pick up the telephone.

A "panic button" arrangement that sounds an alarm in the OR and possibly also in the anesthesia department is absolutely mandatory. The need to summon help in an emergency cannot be thwarted by occupied telephones at a busy OR control desk. Finally, it is desirable to have an intercom system separate from the regular telephones that connects the PACU, each OR room, the OR desk, the preoperative holding area, anesthesia personnel (office and workroom), and other related locations. Again, architects seem skeptical of this suggestion until they visit a facility with this type of system in place and see its singular value in speeding effective communication in a busy PACU.

MONITORS

Outfitting a PACU with equipment, particularly all the classes of patient monitors mounted on the headwall in each bedspace, is covered extensively in Chapter 2, "Equipment and Monitoring Requirements."

CONCLUSION

The adage about an ounce of prevention being worth a pound of cure certainly applies to many of the patients who traverse a busy PACU, but it also applies specifically to the physical design of a PACU about to be built or renovated. All of the staff members involved need thoughtful representative spokespersons who can provide insight and input into the planning process. Combining this wisdom with the principles outlined above will result in an extremely well designed PACU that functions with maximal smoothness and efficiency.

REFERENCES

1. American Institute of Architects (AIA). Guidelines for construction of hospital and medical facilities. Washington, DC: American Institute of Architects, 1993.
2. National Fire Protection Association. NFPA 99 — standard for health care facilities. Quincy, MA: National Fire Protection Association, 1993.
3. National Fire Protection Association. NFPA 101 — life safety code. Quincy, MA: National Fire Protection Association, 1991.
4. Warfield CA, Warfield CG. The postanesthetic recovery room. In: Lisbon A, ed. Anesthetic considerations in setting up a new medical facility. Int Anesthesiol Clin 1981;19(2):63–75.
5. ECRI. Medical gas and vacuum systems. Health Devices 1994;23:1–53.

24

CONTINUOUS QUALITY IMPROVEMENT IN POSTANESTHESIA CARE

Eli M. Brown, Krishnaprasad Deepika

The quality of medical care in the postanesthesia period is an integral part of the total quality management (TQM) program of a healthcare organization. The current concept of TQM, or continuous quality improvement (CQI), is based on concepts advanced by W. Edwards Deming (1). The Deming philosophy represents a holistic approach for management. Deming views the organization as an integrated whole, provides a framework for consistent action, is driven by force of quality, and defines quality as a never-ending improvement of all processes. The never-ending improvement process should result in improved service, fewer errors, greater productivity, and reduced cost. In the modern era of managed competition, an effective CQI program places the healthcare organization at a competitive advantage (2). The five stages of the Deming philosophy are (3):

Stage I: Create a Positive Environment
Stage II: Identify Process Objectives
Stage III: Identify Measurement Characteristics
Stage IV: Manage Process Variation
Stage V: Improve the Process

STAGE I: CREATE A POSITIVE ENVIRONMENT

A CQI program cannot succeed unless definitive steps are taken by management to create a positive environment. The physician(s) in charge of the postanesthesia care unit (PACU) or intensive care unit (ICU) and the nursing supervisor(s) of the unit form the management team. It is the responsibility of this team to create a positive environment by using positive reinforcement, understanding the concerns of the staff and addressing their problems, seeking input from all levels of staff before making decisions, providing information and feedback in a timely manner, not overmanaging or undermanaging, and treating people with respect.

Adherence to the principles outlined above will help establish a positive, nonpunitive environment. The presence of a positive environment encourages all levels of personnel to participate actively in the CQI program. It is important to recognize that input from both professional and technical staff is essential to process improvement. The people in the "trenches" are in the best position to know what problems are encountered most frequently. Input from staff can be obtained through formal meetings, informal discussion, or written suggestions. If the staff feel that they are part of the decision-making process, they are more likely to support the decisions that are made.

Another way to obtain maximum cooperation of staff is to clearly define job responsibilities and allow people to make decisions within their scope of responsibility without "second guessing" those decisions. An effective manager will be available and accessible to offer advice without interfering in getting the job done.

STAGE II: IDENTIFY PROCESS OBJECTIVES

For a PACU or ICU to function effectively, there must be a process or system. The terms "process" and "system" are used interchangeably. A process (system) is defined by Kritchevsky and Simmons (4) as a sequence of actions by and interactions between functional units that bring about the manufacture of a product or the delivery of a service. In a PACU or ICU, the functional units include nursing staff, physicians, and other hospital staff members who act and interact to provide services to patients. The nature of the actions and interactions are usually defined in a written set of rules and regulations supplemented by actions implicitly defined by the norms of local culture.

Process objectives are derived from the expectations of the manager and the customer. In the case of a PACU, the manager's expectations would include, at a very minimum, adherence to the American Society of Anesthesiologists (ASA) Standards of Postanesthesia Care (see Fig. 2.1) and the Joint Commission on Accreditation of Healthcare Organizations (JCAHO) Standards (Fig. 24–1). In addition, there are explicit and implicit actions that the manager expects, such as appropriate assignment of personnel, communication among personnel, and adherence to safety standards.

The customers include the patient primarily but also may include the surgeon and anesthesiologist who cared for the patient. Their expectations include careful monitoring of the patient, carrying out physicians' orders, adequate pain relief, prevention and/or treatment of nausea and vomiting, early detection of complications, appropriate management of emergencies, and timely discharge of the patient under safe conditions.

STAGE III: IDENTIFY MEASUREMENT CHARACTERISTICS

This aspect of CQI is perhaps the most difficult because it involves the gathering of data that are both measurable and reliable. The development of measurement characteristics begins with a performance objective. The following are examples of performance objectives that relate to the PACU:

1. No delay in admission of patients to PACU. To be measured, this performance objective must be converted into a general performance characteristic, i.e., "time from completion of anesthesia until admission to PACU."
2. Appropriate transfer of patient from anesthesia staff to PACU staff. The general performance characteristic for this objective would be "the number of patients for whom there is no documentation of status on arrival in the PACU." It is implicit in this statement that the anesthesia staff person who accompanies the patient to the PACU will convey appropriate information concerning the preoperative condition and the surgical/anesthesia course to the PACU nurse who accepts the patient. Because this report usually is given verbally, it can only be measured through the subjective reporting of delinquencies.
3. Adequate monitoring of the patient. The general performance characteristic for this objective might be "the number or percentage of patients for which there is no documentation that oxygenation, ventilation, circulation, and temperature are being monitored at least every 15 minutes."
4. Timely discharge from the PACU. The general performance characteristic for this objective is length of stay in the PACU.

All of the above performance objectives relate to the process by which the PACU staff working as a team serves its customers. There are many variables that impact the ability of the PACU staff to serve their

Standards

TX.2.4.   *The patient's postprocedure status is assessed on admission to the postanesthesia recovery area and before discharge from the postanesthesia recovery area or the setting.*

TX.2.4.1   *The patient is discharged either by a qualified licensed independent practitioner or by the use of medical staff–approved criteria.*

TX.2.4.1.1   *When medical staff–approved criteria are used, compliance with the criteria is fully documented in the patient's medical record.*

Intent of TX.2.4 through TX.2.4.1.1

To ensure successful postanesthesia recovery, the level of care is based on the patient's status on admission to the postanesthesia recovery area. The ongoing and systematic collection and analysis of patient status information is used as a trigger for progression through the recovery period and ultimately as an indicator for discharge.

Organizations often quantify and stadardize criteria for discharge from the postanesthesia recovery area (for example, by the use of medical staff-approved criteria). To ensure a successful outcome when these criteria are used, it is important to provide evidence of compliance with the criteria in the patient's medical record.

Example of Implementation for TX.2.4 through TX.2.4.1.1

Findings from the assessment of the patient's physiological status and the outcomes of anesthesia and/ or operative or other invasive procedures are documented in the medical record in accordance with approved organizational policy. Such policy addresses either the use of medical staff-approved criteria or requires that the patient's status comply with those criteria before discharge from either the postanesthesia recovery area and/or from the setting or facility. A licensed independent practitioner makes the decision, or medical staff–approved discharge criteria are used.

Policies and procedures address the discharge of patients from the setting or facility and require accompaniment by a responsible adult.

Fig. 24–1.   Joint Commission standards for postanesthesia care. (Reproduced with permission from the Joint Committee on Accreditation of Healthcare Organizations.)

customers well. Structural factors that affect the quality of service include the ratio of PACU beds to the number of surgical procedures performed, the quantity and quality of personnel, the types and quality of monitoring equipment available, and the availability of equipment and personnel to transport patients upon discharge.

Other factors that impact the process are the physical condition of patients on entry to the PACU, the extensiveness of the surgical procedure performed, and the physical status of patients admitted to the healthcare facility. Therefore, all measurement characteristics exhibit variation. The goal is to reduce variation as much as possible.

STAGE IV: MANAGE PROCESS VARIATION

The types of variation that occur are either normal or abnormal. Normal variation is present in every process and is due to the common causes outlined above. These variations are predictable. Conversely, abnormal variation is an extraordinary occurrence in a process that is due to a special cause and therefore is unpredictable. Control of abnormal variation requires a problem-solving approach. This type of approach will be discussed later in this chapter.

Deming proposes a statistical methodology for detecting and managing process variation.

Although this approach has proven very effective in the business world, its applicability to medical practice is not as obvious. Still, some of the principles can be adapted very well to the evaluation of both process and outcome.

The management of process variation and identification of fail points must include both subjective and objective data. The subjective data are obtained from both external and internal customers. Whenever possible, the subjective data should be converted into some type of scoring system so that the information can be evaluated statistically for variations in the process. One example would be the patient's impression of care given in the PACU. A set of questions would need to be developed that might seek information concerning politeness and attentiveness of PACU personnel, comfort of the patient, treatment of common adverse effects such as nausea and vomiting, and any adverse experiences. A weighted score should be assigned to each item in accordance with its perceived importance. This approach would make it possible to establish a range of acceptable scores and to follow variations. When variations indicate a fail point, the matter should be investigated and corrected. A second example might relate to the PACU nurse as an internal customer. The nurse could rate anesthesia personnel and surgeons on a continuing basis with regard to adherence to establish policies and procedures. An overall rating could be given for adequacy of communication of pertinent information, clarity of orders given for care of the patient, appropriateness of mode of transfer of the patient from the OR to the PACU (were appropriate monitoring devices in place?), appropriateness of length of time that the anesthesia personnel remained with the patient after transfer, and presence of iatrogenic problems such as inadequate reversal of muscle relaxant.

Conversely, anesthesia personnel could rate PACU nurses with regard to such items as availability of nursing personnel to accept the patient on entry to PACU, adequacy of initial assessment of the patient and communication of that information to the responsible anesthesia person, appropriateness of carrying out of physicians' orders, and recognition of problems and appropriate management thereof.

There is considerable additional subjective information that can be gathered and converted into a numerical system that can be evaluated statistically. This information need not be threatening to personnel and it should not be used for punitive purposes. Indeed, the person who evaluates the statistical information gathered would not have knowledge of any specific individual's contribution to the accumulated data.

Objective data are somewhat easier to gather and evaluate. Examples of objective data include the overall PACU score for various time intervals, information concerning vital signs, oxygen saturation readings, accuracy and timeliness of charting, and incidence of adverse events. For all of these objective data, it is necessary to establish criteria and thresholds. Figure 24–2 is an example of a manual form that is in use at the University of Miami/Jackson Memorial Medical Center for this purpose. Today, the technology is available so that much of this information can be gathered by automation and collated so that it can be presented in statistical terms to those responsible for evaluating the data.

Evaluation of both the subjective and objective data should tell us whether or not our process (system) is in control. If the process exhibits an unfavorable trend as, for example, an increase in the number of patients whose temperature remains below 34°C for a prolonged period of time, we need to examine our methods for rewarming patients. The fail point might be insufficient or inadequate equipment for rewarming (structural) or inappropriate use of the equipment (process). Conversely, if we note a favorable trend as, for example, a significant decrease in the number of patients who develop significant hypertension in the

PARU/PATU QUALITY MANAGEMENT DATA COLLECTION SCREEN

ADMISSION DATE/TIME:_____(HUS)   READY FOR DISCHARGE:_____
ADM. RN SIGNATURE:_____   DISCHARGE DATE/TIME:_____
DC RN SIGNATURE:_____ `   TOTAL LENGTH OF STAY:_____

_____

TYPE OF PATIENT:
    ( ) PARU/PATU PATIENT WITH NO COMPLICATIONS/INTERVENTIONS
    ( ) ROUTINE ADULT PATIENT WITH COMPLICATIONS / INTERVENTIONS CHECKED BELOW
    ( ) PEDIATRIC PATIENT   ( ) NO COMPLICATIONS   ( ) COMPLICATIONS/CHECKED BELOW
    ( ) ICU/MONITORED PATIENT   ( ) PLANNED ICU/MON.   ( )UNPLANNED ICU/MONITORED
TYPE OF ANESTHESIA:
    ( )GENERAL   ( )SPINAL   ( )EPIDURAL   ( )BLOCK   ( )MAC   ( )OTHER
ASA CLASSIFICATION:
    ( ) 1   ( ) 2   ( ) 3   ( ) 4   ( ) 5   ( ) NOT DOCUMENTED
INVASIVE MONITORING:
    ( ) A-LINE   ( ) CVP/ INTROD.   ( )PA CATH   ( ) ICP ( ) OTHER   ( ) NONE
    DID PT. EXPERIENCE COMPLICATION OF INVASIVE MONITORING   ( ) YES ( ) NO
    IF YES, LIST COMPLICATION_____
ADMITTED FROM:
    ( ) OR   ( ) AMSU   ( ) RADIOLOGY   ( ) OTHER_____(_LIST)
DISCHARGED TO:
    ( ) PCC   ( ) AMSU   ( ) MONITORED ( ) ICU ( ) OTHER_____(LIST)

RESPIRATORY DYSFUNCTION:
    ( ) INTUBATED FROM OR
    ( ) REINTUBATED IN PARU/PATU
    ( ) VENTILATED
    ( ) CPAP
    ( ) SaO2< 90 > 1 MIN.
    ( ) BRONCHOSPASM
    ( ) PNEUMO/HEMOTHORAX
    ( ) ASPIRATION/PNEUMONIA
    ( ) PUL. EDEMA-CARDIOGENIC
    ( ) PUL. EDEMA-NON-CARDIOGENIC
    ( ) AIRWAY OBST.
    ( ) OTHER(LIST)_____
ALTERATION IN CARDIAC OUTPUT:
    ( ) HYPERTENSION DBP>100 FOR >2MIN/ RX. SYSTOLIC
    ( ) HYPOTENSION SBP<90 FOR >2MIN.
    ( ) TACHYCARDIA > 100 FOR > 5 MIN.
    ( ) BRADYCARDIA < 60 (SYMPTOMATIC)
    ( ) R/O M.I.
    ( ) SVO2 < 65
    ( ) R/O SEPSIS
    ( ) DYSRHYTHMIA (LIST)_____
    ( ) OTHER(LIST)_____

ALTERATION IN FL./ELECTROLYTE STATUS:
    ( ) U.O.< 0.5CC/KG/HR
    ( ) HYPOVOLEMIA/BOLUS
    ( ) HEMORRHAGE/ COAGULOPHATHY
    ( ) ELECTROLYTE INBALANCE
        ( )< H/H
        ( )< CALCIUM
        ( )< NA
        ( ) < / > BL. SUGAR
        ( ) < K
        ( ) OTHER(LIST)_____

ALTERATION IN BODY TEMP:
    ( ) TEMP. < 95 F-R
    ( ) TEMP. > 101F-R
ALTERATION IN NEURO /MOBILITY STATUS:
    ( ) MENTAL STATUS CHANGE
    ( ) DROWSY > 20 MIN.
    ( ) GLASCOW < 8
    ( ) SENSORY/MOTOR CHANGE
    ( ) SPINAL/EPIDURAL > 3 HRS.
    ( ) PULSE CHECKS
    ( ) OTHER(LIST)_____
ALTERATION IN COMFORT:
    ( ) NAUSEA
    ( ) VOMITING
    ( ) MEDICATED FOR PAIN
    ( ) SHIVERING
    ( ) OTHER(LIST)_____
ALTERATION IN SKIN INTEGRITY:
    ( ) REDNESS >30 MIN/STAGE 1
    ( ) BROKEN SKIN/STAGE 2
    ( ) ON BACKBOARD_____HRS.
    OTHER(LIST)_____
MISC.
    ( ) RN TO TRANSPORT_____MIN/HR
    ( ) ALLERGIC REACTION
    ( ) EQUIPMENT PROBLEM
    ( ) SUPPLY PROBLEM
DELAY IN DISCHARGE
    ( ) TRANSPORT DELAY_____MIN/HR
    ( ) NO BED ASSIGNMENT_____MIN/HR
    ( ) NO AVAILABLE PCC BED_____MIN/HR
    ( ) NO AVAILABLE UNIT BED_____MIN/HR
    ( )M.D. DELAY_____MIN/HR
    ( ) UNCLEAR SPINE_____MIN/HR
    ( ) OTHER _____

ADDITIONAL COMMENTS:_____

_____

Fig. 24–2.   Quality management data collection screening form.

PACU, we must try to identify the reason for the change and incorporate it into our process. The most obvious reason would be more effective and timely methods of postanesthesia pain control.

STAGE V: IMPROVE THE PROCESS

The management of process variation together with the identification and appropriate correction of fail points should result in a continuous improvement in the process of the PACU.

THE ROLE OF THE JOINT COMMISSION ON ACCREDITATION OF HEALTHCARE ORGANIZATION (JCAHO)

The JCAHO has recognized the changing milieu in CQI. The current Accreditation Manual for Hospitals shifts the primary focus from the performance of individuals to the performance of the Health Care Organization's (HCO) system or processes while continuing to recognize the importance of the individual competence of medical staff members and other staff. Current competence of medical staff is assessed by examining the criteria for granting clinical privileges, a discussion that is beyond the scope of this chapter. However, improving performance in postanesthesia management is very much a concern of JCAHO. The JCAHO defines performance in terms of what is done and how well it is done. These characteristics are called the "dimensions of performance." The definitions of dimensions of performance appears in Figure 24–3.

The JCAHO does not require that a healthcare organization adopt a specific CQI or TQM system. The JCAHO only requires that the healthcare organization incorporate several core concepts of CQI such as the key role that leaders (individually and collectively) play in enabling the systemic assessment and improvement of performance; the fact that most problems or opportunities for improvement derive from process weaknesses, not individual incompetence; the need for careful coordination of work and collaboration among departments and professional groups; the importance of seeking judgments from patients and others and using such judgments to identify areas for improvement; the importance of setting priorities for improvement; and the need for both systematically improving the performance of important functions and maintaining the stability of these functions (5).

EFFECT OF CQI ON OUTCOME

Those who are cynical concerning the cost effectiveness of CQI ask for scientific evidence that CQI has a significant effect on outcome. Some of the problems associated with looking at outcome data include paucity of data, presentation of adverse outcomes with no denominators and a lack of integration between process and outcome data (6). These problems can be overcome to a great extent by the use of currently available automation. It should be possible to gather data that indicate whether an adverse incident was initiated before admission to the PACU or occurred while the patient was in the PACU. It has been estimated that approximately one-third of adverse incidents related to anesthesia originate in the PACU, whereas the other two-thirds originate in the operating room (7).

The two items of outcome data that are of greatest concern to government agencies, managed care programs, and consumer groups are risk and cost. The bottom line is what proportion of our patients survive surgery and anesthesia and leave the hospital without permanent sequelae, and at what cost. Although many physicians recoil at consideration of cost in a CQI program, expenditure can provide important information concerning quality of care. A patient may be discharged without permanent sequelae, but because of a variety of adverse events, the patient may have needed an excessive period of care in an ICU requiring the use of expensive technology and laboratory testing. In such cases, cost can be an indication of a fail point in our system because of either structural or procedural deficiencies. The same might be true of a patient who requires more than usual care in a PACU.

Aside from these considerations, however, the fact is that the cost of medical care now exceeds 10% of the gross national product

I.   Doing the Right Thing

The **efficacy** of the procedure or treatment in relation to the patient's condition

The degree to which the care/intervention for the patient has been shown to accomplish the desired/projected outcome(s)

The **appropriateness** of a specific test, procedure, or service to meet the patient's needs

The degree to which the care/intervention provided is relevant to the patient's clinical needs, given the current state of knowledge

II.   Doing the Right Thing Well

The **availability** of a needed test, procedure, treatment, or service to the patient who needs it

The degree to which appropriate care/intervention is available to meet the patient's needs

The **timeliness** with which a needed test, procedure, treatment, or service is provided to the patient

The degree to which the care/intervention is provided to the patient at the most beneficial or necessary time

The **effectiveness** with which tests, procedures, treatments, and services are provided

The degree to which the care/intervention is provided in the correct manner, given the current state of knowledge, in order to achieve the desired/projected outcome for the patient

The **continuity** of the services provided to the patient with respect to other services, practitioners, and providers and over time

the degree to which the care/intervention for the patient is coordinated among practitioners, among organizations, and over time

The **safety** of the patient (and others) to whom the services are provided

The degree to which the risk of an intervention and the risk in the care environment are reduced for the patient and others, including the health care provider

The **efficiency** with which services are provided

The relationship between the outcomes (results of care) and the resources used to deliver patient care

The **respect and caring** with which services are provided

The degree to which the patient or a designee is involved in his/her own care decisions and to which those providing services do so with sensitivity and respect for the patient's needs, expectations, and individual differences

Fig. 24–3. Definitions of dimensions of performance. (Reproduced with permission of the JCAHO from the Accreditation Manual for Hospitals, 1994.)

(GNP), which has resulted in changes in medical care financing (8). Consequently, a TQM program must include consideration of costs.

In the PACU, the most obvious methods for controlling costs are to avoid iatrogenic errors such as improper selection or administration of drugs, close attention to the airway and oxygenation, and reduction in laboratory use. Many laboratory tests are generated out of habit or through the use of routine orders.

It has been demonstrated that in both PACUs and ICUs the ordering of laboratory tests only on specific indication will result in significant reduction in cost (8).

Perioperative risk related to anesthesia is usually perceived in terms of the presence or absence of adverse events. Indeed, the indicators of anesthesia quality outlined by the JCAHO in recent years focus on adverse events such as those outlined in Figures 24–4 and 24–5. Although following the trend of these indicators is extremely important to the individual HCO, the implication that these data can be used reliably to compare the performance among various institutions may not be true. There are a large number of variables that are difficult to control, such as the mix of patients involved, the scope of services provided, and the methods used to gather and report data. Although these comparisons are attractive to federal health agencies and consumer groups, they may actually contribute very little to CQI. Indeed, this approach may hinder CQI because it promotes competition among anesthesia departments to "put the best face" on the reporting of statistics and it fosters fear among individual anesthesiologists.

Patients developing central nervous system **(CNS) complications within 2 days postprocedure** of procedures involving anesthesia administration.

Patients developing a **peripheral neurological deficit** within 2 days postprocedure.

Acute **myocardial infarction** within 2 days postprocedure.

Cardiac arrest in 48 hours.

Intrahospital mortality in 48 hours.

Fig. 24–4. Joint commission indicators for anesthesia (1995): indicator measurement system.

Conversely, the study of both positive and negative aspects of anesthesia care in a specific institution can be very useful in promoting CQI if the data are used to develop protocols of care. Examples of positive aspects of anesthesia care that contribute to CQI are as follows:

1. Use of supplemental oxygen during transport. In 1991, at the University of Miami/Jackson Memorial Medical Center (JMH), it was noted that many patients were entering the PACU with a low SpO_2. Even though no direct correlation had been established between the low SpO_2 and adverse events, we deemed it desirable to study this issue. Accordingly, data were gathered on all patients entering the PACU. We found that 16.2% of these patients had an SpO_2 below 90, which persisted for at least 1 minute despite the application of oxygen. The quality management council recommended that all patients be transported with oxygen. In the years after this practice was instituted, the incidence fell dramatically (Fig. 24–6). Although it is apparent that some variation has continued in subsequent years, it is a "normal variation" of a process that is in control. Whether or not this practice changed outcome is really irrelevant, because we know instinctively that an SpO_2 below 90 is undesirable. Consequently, it is not always necessary to establish a cause-and-effect relationship between process and outcome before altering a practice protocol.
2. Use of warming devices in the operating room and PACU. One does not need to study the incidence of adverse outcomes to know that persistent hypothermia in the PACU is undesirable. The institution of use of warming devices (Baier Huggers) to decrease the loss of heat to the environment and warming of fluids has decreased the incidence of hypothermia in the PACU and has resulted in a decreased length of stay in the PACU at JMH (Fig. 24–7).
3. Acute pain control. The institution of improved methods of alleviating acute pain has had many beneficial effects, including a decreased incidence of hypertension, decreased length of stay in the PACU, and greatly improved patient satisfaction.

All of the above examples represent CQI, which resulted from a change in practice

AN-A	Fulminating pulmonary edema during procedure or within first postoperative day.
AN-B	**Aspiration pneumonitis** during procedures involving anesthesia or within 2 postoperative days.
AN-C	Postural headache with 4 days postprocedure involving spinal or epidural anesthesia.
AN-D	Dental Injury
AN-E	Ocular Injury
AN-F	Unplanned hospital admission within 2 days postprocedure after outpatient anesthesia.
AN-G	Unplanned admission of patients to an intensive care unit within 2 days postprocedure involving anesthesia administration and with an intensive care unit stay greater than 1 day.

Fig. 24–5. Indicators for internal healthcare organization use.

CQI - USE OF OXYGEN DURING TRANSPORT
O2 SATURATION ON ADMISSION TO PACU

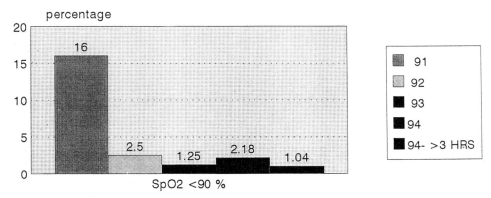

1991-PRIOR TO TRANSPORT WITH O2
1992-94 WITH O2 TRANSPORT
JACKSON MEMORIAL HOSPITAL,MIAMI

Fig. 24–6. Graph depicting continuous quality improvement: use of oxygen during transport.

C.Q.I.-EFFECT OF WARMING DEVICES ON HYPOTHERMIA
PACU-1991-1994

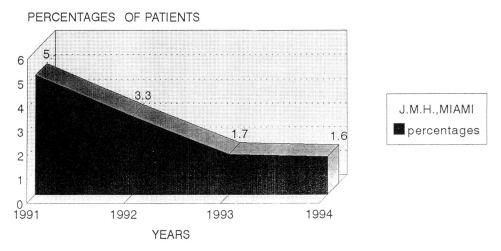

1991 Q.M.DATA INDICATED 5%HYPOTHERMIA IN PACU.
1992 WARMING DEVICES (BAIER HUGGER,HOT LINE FOR
FLUID WARMIG) WERE INSTITUTED.

Fig. 24–7. Graph depicting continuous quality improvement: effect of warming devices on hypothermia.

protocols due to improved technology, increased scientific information, or both. Conversely, despite all of our efforts, anesthesia-related-impact events continue to occur. An anesthesia-related-impact event is defined as an unanticipated, undesirable, possible anesthesia-related effect that requires intervention, is pertinent to recovery room care, and could have or actually did cause mortality or at least moderate morbidity (9).

Each impact event should be analyzed to determine whether the established protocols of care were followed. If the protocols of care, both explicit and implicit, were not followed, it might be the result of either a structural problem (inadequate equipment, inadequate personnel, etc.) or a process problem (lack of knowledge, unclear orders, or technical error such as wrong medication or improper use of equipment). If structural or process problems are identified, they usually can be readily corrected by purchase of new equipment, increasing or reassigning personnel, and conducting

a timely and effective in-training program. The recent introduction of anesthesia simulators provides an effective method for evaluating the performance of PACU personnel and preparing them to respond appropriately to adverse events.

Conversely, if it seems that the protocols of management were followed appropriately, then it behooves us to reevaluate our policies and procedures to determine whether they are adequate to meet our present requirements. Policies and procedures, as well as specific protocols of management, must be continually reexamined and updated in accordance with current concepts and practice.

PRACTICE PARAMETERS

Practice parameters include guidelines, standards, and other strategies of patient management. To further this concept, the American Medical Association (AMA) organized the Practice Parameter Partnership and Forum.

The partnership consists of representatives from the AMA and a variety of specialty societies. The ASA has representation on both the partnership and the forum. To date, the ASA House of Delegates has approved practice guidelines for three areas of practice: Pulmonary Artery Catheterization, Management of the Difficult Airway, and Management of Acute, Chronic, and Cancer Pain. A number of other areas are under consideration, including PACU discharge criteria (10).

To be effective and useful, practice parameters must be based on scientific principles, reflect current practice, have a positive cost-benefit ratio, and be sufficiently flexible so as to be applicable to a wide variety of practice situations. Parameters that contain these attributes can be adapted to rural as well as urban hospitals, community hospitals as well as academic institutions, and outpatient as well as inpatient facilities.

Practice parameters that relate to postanesthesia management in addition to discharge criteria from the PACU include management of the comatose patient, indications and interpretation of various monitoring techniques, application of various types of drug therapy, and ventilator management, among others.

It is not necessary for a healthcare organization to wait for the ASA or other organizations to develop these guidelines. They can and should be developed locally. Indeed, the development and testing of guidelines at the local level will help to provide the input necessary for the development of practice parameters related to postanesthesia management at the national level.

Whether or not the incorporation of practice parameters will improve patient outcome and reduce medical costs is yet to be deter-mined, but the concept is certainly in concert with Deming's philosophy of TQM.

SUMMARY

The quality of medical care in the postanesthesia period is an integral part of TQM. The concepts advanced by W. Edwards Deming are the basis for the CQI program described in this chapter. Deming's concepts include five stages of development that should ultimately result in a process that can be effectively managed and improved continuously over time. The JCAHO has recognized the wisdom of shifting the primary focus of CQI from the performance of individuals to the performance of the healthcare organization's process (system). The introduction of practice parameters will hopefully aid in the development of a process that will improve patient outcome and reduce the cost of medical care.

REFERENCES

1. Deming WE. Out of the crisis. Cambridge, MA: Massachusetts Institute of Technology, Center for Advanced Engineering Study, 1986.
2. Walton M. The Deming management method. New York: Putnam Publishing Group, 1986.
3. Hertz P. Quality improvement training manual. Miami, FL: Paul Hertz Group, 1989.
4. Kritchevsky S, Simmons B. Continuous quality improvement. JAMA 1991;266(13):1817–1822.
5. JCAHO. Accreditation manual for hospitals. Section 2 — Improving organizational improvement. Oakbrook Terrace, IL: Joint Commission on Accreditation of Healthcare Organizations, 1995;220.
6. Edsel D. Quality review bulletin. Vol. 17, No. 6. Oakbrook Terrace, IL: Joint Commission on Accreditation of Healthcare Organizations, 1991;182–192.
7. Narbone RF. Quality assurance in the postanesthesia care unit. In: Vender J, Speiss B, eds. Post anesthesia care. Philadelphia: WB Saunders, 1992;364.
8. Civetta J, Kirby R. Prediction and definition of outcome. Adv Anesth 1992;9:138.
9. Cullen DJ. Risk modification in the postanesthesia care unit. Int Anesthesiol Clin 1989;27(3):184–187.
10. Arens JF. A practice parameters overview. Anesthesiology 1993;78:229–230.

INDEX

Note: Page numbers followed by "f" indicate figures; page numbers followed by "t" indicate tables.

BUSINESS REPLY MAIL

FIRST CLASS   PERMIT NO. 724   BALTIMORE, MD

POSTAGE WILL BE PAID BY ADDRESSEE

Williams & Wilkins
P.O. Box 1496
Baltimore, Maryland 21298-9656